Marine Anti-Inflammatory and Antioxidant Agents 3.0

Marine Anti-Inflammatory and Antioxidant Agents 3.0

Editors

Donatella Degl'Innocenti
Marzia Vasarri

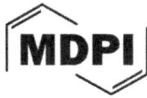

Basel • Beijing • Wuhan • Barcelona • Belgrade • Novi Sad • Cluj • Manchester

Editors

Donatella Degl'Innocenti
Department of Experimental
and Clinical
Biomedical Sciences
University of Florence
Florence
Italy

Marzia Vasarri
Department of Experimental
and Clinical
Biomedical Sciences
University of Florence
Florence
Italy

Editorial Office
MDPI AG
Grosspeteranlage 5
4052 Basel, Switzerland

This is a reprint of articles from the Special Issue published online in the open access journal *Marine Drugs* (ISSN 1660-3397) (available at: https://www.mdpi.com/journal/marinedrugs/special_issues/8695SJOR67).

For citation purposes, cite each article independently as indicated on the article page online and as indicated below:

Lastname, A.A.; Lastname, B.B. Article Title. *Journal Name* **Year**, *Volume Number*, Page Range.

ISBN 978-3-7258-2153-2 (Hbk)
ISBN 978-3-7258-2154-9 (PDF)
doi.org/10.3390/books978-3-7258-2154-9

© 2024 by the authors. Articles in this book are Open Access and distributed under the Creative Commons Attribution (CC BY) license. The book as a whole is distributed by MDPI under the terms and conditions of the Creative Commons Attribution-NonCommercial-NoDerivs (CC BY-NC-ND) license.

Contents

About the Editors vii

Preface ix

Marzia Vasarri and Donatella Degl'Innocenti
Marine Products and Their Anti-Inflammatory Potential: Latest Updates
Reprinted from: *Mar. Drugs* **2024**, *22*, 376, doi:10.3390/md22080376 1

Laura Micheli, Marzia Vasarri, Donatella Degl'Innocenti, Lorenzo Di Cesare Mannelli, Carla Ghelardini, Antiga Emiliano, et al.
Posidonia oceanica (L.) Delile Is a Promising Marine Source Able to Alleviate Imiquimod-Induced Psoriatic Skin Inflammation
Reprinted from: *Mar. Drugs* **2024**, *22*, 300, doi:10.3390/md22070300 5

Luisa Frusciante, Michela Geminiani, Alfonso Trezza, Tommaso Olmastroni, Pierfrancesco Mastroeni, Laura Salvini, et al.
Phytochemical Composition, Anti-Inflammatory Property, and Anti-Atopic Effect of *Chaetomorpha linum* Extract
Reprinted from: *Mar. Drugs* **2024**, *22*, 226, doi:10.3390/md22050226 21

Yena Park, Lei Cao, Suhyeon Baek, Seungjin Jeong, Hyun Jung Yun, Mi-Bo Kim and Sang Gil Lee
The Role of Sargahydroquinoic Acid and Sargachromenol in the Anti-Inflammatory Effect of *Sargassum yezoense*
Reprinted from: *Mar. Drugs* **2024**, *22*, 107, doi:10.3390/md22030107 47

N. M. Liyanage, Hyo-Geun Lee, D. P. Nagahawatta, H. H. A. C. K. Jayawardhana, Kyung-Mo Song, Yun-Sang Choi, et al.
Fucoidan from *Sargassum autumnale* Inhibits Potential Inflammatory Responses via NF-κB and MAPK Pathway Suppression in Lipopolysaccharide-Induced RAW 264.7 Macrophages
Reprinted from: *Mar. Drugs* **2023**, *21*, 374, doi:10.3390/md21070374 63

Serena Mirata, Valentina Asnaghi, Mariachiara Chiantore, Annalisa Salis, Mirko Benvenuti, Gianluca Damonte and Sonia Scarfì
Photoprotective and Anti-Aging Properties of the Apical Frond Extracts from the Mediterranean Seaweed *Ericaria amentacea*
Reprinted from: *Mar. Drugs* **2023**, *21*, 306, doi:10.3390/md21050306 77

Yi-Fen Chiang, Ko-Chieh Huang, Kai-Lee Wang, Yun-Ju Huang, Hsin-Yuan Chen, Mohamed Ali, et al.
Protective Effects of an Oligo-Fucoidan-Based Formula against Osteoarthritis Development via iNOS and COX-2 Suppression following Monosodium Iodoacetate Injection
Reprinted from: *Mar. Drugs* **2024**, *22*, 211, doi:10.3390/md22050211 106

Yawen Wang, Longjian Zhou, Minqi Chen, Yayue Liu, Yu Yang, Tiantian Lu, et al.
Mining Xanthine Oxidase Inhibitors from an Edible Seaweed *Pterocladiella capillacea* by Using In Vitro Bioassays, Affinity Ultrafiltration LC-MS/MS, Metabolomics Tools, and In Silico Prediction
Reprinted from: *Mar. Drugs* **2023**, *21*, 502, doi:10.3390/md21100502 120

Cecilie Græsholt, Tore Brembu, Charlotte Volpe, Zdenka Bartosova, Manuel Serif, Per Winge and Marianne Nymark
Zeaxanthin epoxidase 3 Knockout Mutants of the Model Diatom *Phaeodactylum tricornutum* Enable Commercial Production of the Bioactive Carotenoid Diatoxanthin
Reprinted from: *Mar. Drugs* **2024**, *22*, 185, doi:10.3390/md22040185 . . . . **138**

Mario D'Ambrosio, Elisabetta Bigagli, Lorenzo Cinci, Manuela Gencarelli, Sofia Chioccioli, Natascia Biondi, et al.
Tisochrysis lutea F&M-M36 Mitigates Risk Factors of Metabolic Syndrome and Promotes Visceral Fat Browning through β3-Adrenergic Receptor/UCP1 Signaling
Reprinted from: *Mar. Drugs* **2023**, *21*, 303, doi:10.3390/md21050303 . . . . **153**

Jan Seeger, Volker F. Wendisch and Nadja A. Henke
Extraction and Purification of Highly Active Astaxanthin from *Corynebacterium glutamicum* Fermentation Broth
Reprinted from: *Mar. Drugs* **2023**, *21*, 530, doi:10.3390/md21100530 . . . . **168**

Fatma H. Al-Awadhi, Emily F. Simon, Na Liu, Ranjala Ratnayake, Valerie J. Paul and Hendrik Luesch
Discovery and Anti-Inflammatory Activity of a Cyanobacterial Fatty Acid Targeting the Keap1/Nrf2 Pathway
Reprinted from: *Mar. Drugs* **2023**, *21*, 553, doi:10.3390/md21110553 . . . . **182**

Md Khursheed, Hardik Ghelani, Reem K. Jan and Thomas E. Adrian
Anti-Inflammatory Effects of Bioactive Compounds from Seaweeds, Bryozoans, Jellyfish, Shellfish and Peanut Worms
Reprinted from: *Mar. Drugs* **2023**, *21*, 524, doi:10.3390/md21100524 . . . . **202**

Ngoc Bao An Nguyen, Mohamed El-Shazly, Po-Jen Chen, Bo-Rong Peng, Lo-Yun Chen, Tsong-Long Hwang and Kuei-Hung Lai
Unlocking the Potential of Octocoral-Derived Secondary Metabolites against Neutrophilic Inflammatory Response
Reprinted from: *Mar. Drugs* **2023**, *21*, 456, doi:10.3390/md21080456 . . . . **227**

About the Editors

Donatella Degl'Innocenti

Prof. Donatella Degl'Innocenti is a distinguished Associate Professor of Biochemistry at the Department of Experimental and Clinical Biomedical Sciences "Mario Serio" at the University of Florence, Italy, where she has served since 2001. She holds a Ph.D. in Biochemistry and has established herself as a prominent figure in the field, building a robust network of national and international scientific collaborations throughout her career.

As an active researcher, Prof. Degl'Innocenti leads a dedicated laboratory within her department, which is known for its significant contributions to biochemical research. Her independent research experience is underscored by numerous publications as a senior author in high-impact, peer-reviewed international journals. Her work has made substantial contributions to the understanding of biochemical processes, particularly in the context of natural and marine compounds and their health implications.

Prof. Degl'Innocenti's recent research has concentrated on the health-promoting properties of natural and marine-derived compounds. Notably, she has explored the amyloid aggregation process, investigating potential inhibitory mechanisms of natural compounds and extracts from Mediterranean red seaweed.

Additionally, her studies on the biological properties of extracts from the Posidonia oceanica (L.) Delile marine plant have shed light on their role in modulating pathophysiological cellular processes, including inflammation, oxidative stress, cancer cell migration, and protein glycation. Beyond her research, Prof. Degl'Innocenti is a valued member of the Scientific Committee of the Interuniversity Center of Marine Biology and Applied Ecology (CIBM) in Livorno, Italy. Her expertise in biochemistry and marine biology continues to drive advancements in understanding the intricate relationships between marine natural products and human health.

Marzia Vasarri

Dr. Marzia Vasarri is a Postdoctoral Fellow at the Department of Experimental and Clinical Biomedical Sciences "Mario Serio" at the University of Florence, Italy. She earned her bachelor's degree in biotechnology in 2014 and her master's degree in medical and Pharmaceutical Biotechnology in 2016, both of which equipped her with strong technical and scientific expertise in biochemistry and molecular biology.

Dr. Vasarri's research is centered on the bioactive properties of natural products, with a particular emphasis on marine-derived substances. A significant portion of her work has been dedicated to studying the marine plant *Posidonia oceanica* (L.) Delile. Her investigations have explored the plant's effects on various pathophysiological cellular processes, including inflammation, oxidative stress, cancer cell migration, protein glycation processes, lipid accumulation in hepatic cells, and its potential to induce autophagy.

She has also contributed to research on the biological properties of natural products delivered within nanoformulations, enhancing the efficacy and bioavailability of encapsulated compounds and phytocomplexes to fully harness their therapeutic potential.

Preface

Chronic diseases linked to oxidative stress and inflammation are becoming increasingly prevalent, posing significant challenges to global health. Oxidative stress occurs when the balance between oxidants and antioxidants is disrupted, leading to the excessive production of reactive oxygen and nitrogen species (ROS/RNS). This imbalance damages cellular structures, nucleic acids, and proteins, with long-lasting effects. Inflammation, triggered by elevated ROS/RNS or pro-inflammatory agents, further exacerbates this damage through pathways such as NF-κB, releasing cytokines and chemokines. The complex interaction between oxidative stress and inflammation has sparked growing interest regarding the development of novel therapeutic strategies to regulate these processes.

One promising area of research is the use of natural products with inherent antioxidant and anti-inflammatory properties. In recent decades, marine ecosystems have emerged as valuable sources of bioactive compounds with significant therapeutic potential. The structural diversity of marine-derived molecules offers a rich platform for developing new, safer alternatives to conventional treatments for managing oxidative stress and inflammation.

The purpose of this reprint is to offer a comprehensive overview of recent research on marine-derived bioactive compounds and their role in regulating oxidative stress and inflammation. It includes in vitro and in vivo experimental studies that explore the mechanisms of action and molecular interactions among these compounds, along with review articles that synthesize current knowledge on marine bioactives and their potential applications in supporting human health.

The motivation behind this Special Issue stems from the urgent need to identify novel, safe, and effective therapeutic agents to address the growing burden of chronic diseases. As conventional therapies often come with significant side effects, there is a pressing need for natural alternatives that can modulate inflammation and oxidative stress without adverse outcomes. The marine environment offers a largely untapped reservoir of compounds with immense therapeutic potential, and this Special Issue seeks to highlight their relevance in the modern therapeutic landscape.

This reprint is intended for a broad audience, including researchers, clinicians, and healthcare professionals interested in the fields of oxidative stress, inflammation, and natural product pharmacology. It will also serve as a valuable resource for graduate students and academics seeking to deepen their understanding of the therapeutic potential of marine bioactives.

We hope that this reprint will inspire further research into the fascinating world of marine-derived compounds and their role in addressing global health challenges.

Donatella Degl'Innocenti and Marzia Vasarri
Editors

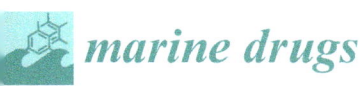

Editorial

Marine Products and Their Anti-Inflammatory Potential: Latest Updates

Marzia Vasarri and Donatella Degl'Innocenti *

Department of Experimental and Clinical Biomedical Sciences, University of Florence, Viale Morgagni 50, 50134 Florence, Italy; marzia.vasarri@unifi.it
* Correspondence: donatella.deglinnocenti@unifi.it

The depths of the sea are a rich source of biologically active compounds with therapeutic potential for various human diseases, including inflammatory conditions. The growing need for new and effective health products continuously drives scientific research to discover new marine natural compounds and their biological properties. This fascinating field of study has led to the success of this Special Issue "Marine Anti-inflammatory and Antioxidant Agents 3.0" of the journal *Marine Drugs*, which gathered 13 innovative and original scientific publications. These publications highlight the value of marine natural resources in developing new anti-inflammatory treatments and functional products, aligning with the principles of sustainability and circular bioeconomy, thereby contributing to environmental conservation.

This editorial aims to review recent scientific advances in marine natural products with anti-inflammatory potential, as published in this Special Issue "Marine Anti-inflammatory and Antioxidant Agents 3.0". It highlights the roles and mechanisms of these products in various applications, including health care for treating inflammation-related disorders, industry for producing functional foods, and environmental conservation within the context of the circular economy. Specifically, this editorial compiles scientific studies on a marine plant, green algae, four brown algae, red algae, two microalgae, and two bacterial strains. Additionally, two reviews are included in this Issue.

Micheli et al. focused their study on the well-known anti-inflammatory properties of the marine plant *Posidonia oceanica* (L.) Delile, demonstrating its potential anti-psoriatic application. Administering an oral hydroalcoholic extract of *P. oceanica* leaves (POE) to C57BL/6 mice with Imiquimod (IMQ)-induced psoriatic dermatitis showed that POE treatment significantly reduced PASI scores, skin thickness, and temperature. Histological improvements and decreased levels of inflammatory cytokines and lipocalin-2 further supported POE's potential as a natural anti-inflammatory agent for psoriasis, suggesting its possible integration into complementary medicine (Micheli, L.; Vasarri, M.; Deg'Innocenti, D.; Di Cesare Mannelli, L.; Ghelardini, C.; Antiga, E.; Verdelli, A.; Caproni, M.; Barletta, E. *Posidonia oceanica* (L.) Delile Is a Promising Marine Source Able to Alleviate Imiquimod-Induced Psoriatic Skin Inflammation. *Mar. Drugs* 2024, 22, 300. https://doi.org/10.3390/md22070300 [1]).

The study conducted by Frusciante et al. represents the forefront in research supporting the circular economy and environmental sustainability. The anti-inflammatory property of an extract obtained from the invasive green macroalga *Chaetomorpha linum*, present in the Orbetello Lagoon, was examined. This alga, typically harvested mechanically and treated as plant waste, revealed unexpected potential. The *C. linum* extract demonstrated potent inhibitory activity on the production of ROS, NO, and PGE2 in cell-based tests, as well as reduced expression of iNOS and COX-2. These results indicate that the extract is promising as a therapeutic candidate for chronic inflammatory conditions like atopic dermatitis. The research underscores the potential value of utilizing underexploited marine biomass for extracting bioactive compounds, offering new opportunities for medical and environmental

Citation: Vasarri, M.; Degl'Innocenti, D. Marine Products and Their Anti-Inflammatory Potential: Latest Updates. *Mar. Drugs* 2024, 22, 376. https://doi.org/10.3390/md22080376

Received: 10 August 2024
Accepted: 20 August 2024
Published: 21 August 2024

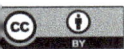

Copyright: © 2024 by the authors. Licensee MDPI, Basel, Switzerland. This article is an open access article distributed under the terms and conditions of the Creative Commons Attribution (CC BY) license (https://creativecommons.org/licenses/by/4.0/).

innovation (Frusciante, L.; Geminiani, M.; Trezza, A.; Olmastroni, T.; Mastroeni, P.; Salvini, L.; Lamponi, S.; Bernini, A.; Grasso, D.; Dreassi, E.; et al. Phytochemical Composition, Anti-Inflammatory Property, and Anti-Atopic Effect of *Chaetomorpha linum* Extract. *Mar. Drugs* 2024, 22, 226. https://doi.org/10.3390/md22050226 [1]).

For the first time, Park et al. demonstrated the anti-inflammatory properties of an extract from the brown alga *Sargassum yezoense*, a prevalent species along Korea's eastern coast, and its fractions. The ethanolic extract significantly reduced inflammation in lipopolysaccharide (LPS)-stimulated RAW 264.7 macrophages and suppressed M1 polarization in bone marrow-derived murine macrophages. Five fractions were obtained through liquid–liquid extraction, with the chloroform fraction (SYCF) showing the highest phenolic content and antioxidant capacity. SYCF, rich in sargahydroquinoic acid (SHQA) and sargachromenol (SCM), exhibited robust anti-inflammatory effects, inhibiting NO production and cytokine expression in macrophages and suppressing NF-κB and MAPK signaling pathways. This indicates SYCF's potential as a functional food ingredient or therapeutic agent for inflammation-related disorders (Park, Y.; Cao, L.; Baek, S.; Jeong, S.; Yun, H.J.; Kim, M.-B.; Lee, S.G. The Role of Sargahydroquinoic Acid and Sargachromenol in the Anti-Inflammatory Effect of *Sargassum yezoense*. *Mar. Drugs* 2024, 22, 107. https://doi.org/10.3390/md22030107 [1]).

Liyanage et al. also used the RAW 264.7 macrophage cell model stimulated with LPS to study the anti-inflammatory properties of fucoidan from the brown alga *Sargassum autumnale*. Among various fucoidan fractions, SAF3 showed the most significant protective effect, inhibiting NO and PGE2 production by downregulating iNOS and COX-2 expression. Additionally, SAF3 reduced the pro-inflammatory cytokines IL-1β, TNF-α, and IL-6, suppressing NF-κB and MAPK signaling pathways in a dose-dependent manner. These results suggest SAF3's potential as a functional food ingredient or treatment for inflammatory disorders (Liyanage, N.M.; Lee, H.-G.; Nagahawatta, D.P.; Jayawardhana, H.H.A.C.K.; Song, K.-M.; Choi, Y.-S.; Jeon, Y.-J.; Kang, M.-C. Fucoidan from *Sargassum autumnale* Inhibits Potential Inflammatory Responses via NF-κB and MAPK Pathway Suppression in Lipopolysaccharide-Induced RAW 264.7 Macrophages. *Mar. Drugs* 2023, 21, 374 https://doi.org/10.3390/md21070374 [1]).

Belonging to the brown algae family, *Ericaria amentacea* was studied by Mirata et al. who analyzed the anti-aging and photoprotective properties of two ethanolic extracts obtained from different parts, namely apices and thalli. Comparing the apices and thalli extracts in HaCaT keratinocyte and L929 fibroblast cell models exposed to UV rays, it was observed that the apices hydroalcoholic extracts showed the highest potential, blocking UV-induced damage and oxidative stress. This study highlighted the importance of *E amentacea* apices derivatives as ideal components for counteracting sunburn symptoms and for anti-aging cosmetic lotions (Mirata, S.; Asnaghi, V.; Chiantore, M.; Salis, A.; Benvenuti, M.; Damonte, G.; Scarfi, S. Photoprotective and Anti-Aging Properties of the Apical Frond Extracts from the Mediterranean Seaweed *Ericaria amentacea*. *Mar. Drugs* 2023, 21, 306. https://doi.org/10.3390/md21050306 [1]).

A formula based on oligo-fucoidan (FF) has shown protective effects against osteoarthritis, reducing inflammation and cartilage damage. The key ingredient, oligo-fucoidan (over 30% of the formula), is derived from the brown algae *Laminaria japonica*. In a study by Chiang and colleagues using a monosodium iodoacetate (MIA) model of osteoarthritis (OA), the formula modulated p38 signaling and reduced COX-2 and iNOS levels. These findings suggest its potential for managing osteoarthritis by improving joint function, reducing inflammation, and protecting cartilage. However, further clinical validation is needed. A better understanding of fucoidan's therapeutic properties could lead to personalized treatments for osteoarthritis tailored to individual patient needs (Chiang, Y.-F.; Huang, K.-C.; Wang, K.-L.; Huang, Y.-J.; Chen, H.-Y.; Ali, M.; Shieh, T.-M.; Hsia, S.-M. Protective Effects of an Oligo-Fucoidan-Based Formula against Osteoarthritis Development via iNOS and COX-2 Suppression following Monosodium Iodoacetate Injection. *Mar. Drugs* 2024, 22, 211. https://doi.org/10.3390/md22050211 [1]).

The edible red alga *Pterocladiella capillacea* is known for its anti-inflammatory properties. Wang et al. demonstrated the xanthine oxidase inhibitory and anti-inflammatory activities of various fractions of *P. capillacea* extract for potential anti-gout applications. These findings support the value of further investigation into *P. capillacea* as part of the development of anti-gout drugs or related functional foods (Wang, Y.; Zhou, L.; Chen, M.; Liu, Y.; Yang, Y.; Lu, T.; Ban, F.; Hu, X.; Qian, Z.; Hong, P.; et al. Mining Xanthine Oxidase Inhibitors from an Edible Seaweed *Pterocladiella capillacea* by Using In Vitro Bioassays, Affinity Ultrafiltration LC-MS/MS, Metabolomics Tools, and In Silico Prediction. *Mar. Drugs* **2023**, *21*, 502. https://doi.org/10.3390/md21100502 [1]).

Research led by Græsholt and colleagues revealed intriguing findings regarding the genetic engineering of the microalga *Phaeodactylum tricornutum* to enhance the production of diatoxanthin, a carotenoid known for its antioxidant and anti-inflammatory benefits. By employing CRISPR/Cas9 gene editing to deactivate the ZEP2 and ZEP3 genes, the study demonstrated that zep3 mutant strains maintained more stable diatoxanthin levels in low-light environments, offering a promising approach for commercial production (Græsholt, C.; Brembu, T.; Volpe, C.; Bartosova, Z.; Serif, M.; Winge, P.; Nymark, M. *Zeaxanthin epoxidase 3* Knockout Mutants of the Model Diatom *Phaeodactylum tricornutum* Enable Commercial Production of the Bioactive Carotenoid Diatoxanthin. *Mar. Drugs* **2024**, *22*, 185. https://doi.org/10.3390/md22040185 [1]).

The marine microalga *Tisochrysis lutea* was also studied for its effects on pre-metabolic syndrome in rats. D'Ambrosio et al. demonstrated that *T. lutea* could reduce triglycerides, glucose levels, and improve adiponectin levels without causing the adverse effects seen with other treatments. The multifaceted impact of *T. lutea* on energy metabolism and inflammation suggests its potential for mitigating metabolic syndrome risks (D'Ambrosio, M.; Bigagli, E.; Cinci, L.; Gencarelli, M.; Chioccioli, S.; Biondi, N.; Rodolfi, L.; Niccolai, A.; Zambelli, F.; Laurino, A.; et al. *Tisochrysis lutea* F&M-M36 Mitigates Risk Factors of Metabolic Syndrome and Promotes Visceral Fat Browning through β3-Adrenergic Receptor/UCP1 Signaling. *Mar. Drugs* **2023**, *21*, 303. https://doi.org/10.3390/md21050303 [1]).

The Gram-positive bacterium *Corynebacterium glutamicum* was the focus of Seeger et al.'s study, who developed an innovative method for ethanol extraction of astaxanthin, a potent antioxidant carotenoid, from genetically modified *C. glutamicum*. Optimal extraction conditions were identified with high recovery and purity of astaxanthin, and the natural astaxanthin showed high antioxidant activity, comparable to or exceeding synthetic variants. This highlights astaxanthin's potential in cosmetics and nutraceuticals (Seeger, J.; Wendisch, V.F.; Henke, N.A. Extraction and Purification of Highly Active Astaxanthin from *Corynebacterium glutamicum* Fermentation Broth. *Mar. Drugs* **2023**, *21*, 530. https://doi.org/10.3390/md21100530 [1]).

Al-Awadhi et al. identified 7(E)-9-keto-hexadec-7-enoic acid and related analogs from a marine cyanobacterial mat. This compound activated the Keap1/Nrf2 pathway, showing significant anti-inflammatory potential. It reduced nitric oxide levels and modulated inflammatory pathways, suggesting its potential as a dietary intervention for managing inflammation and related diseases (Al-Awadhi, F.H.; Simon, E.F.; Liu, N.; Ratnayake, R.; Paul, V.J.; Luesch, H. Discovery and Anti-Inflammatory Activity of a Cyanobacterial Fatty Acid Targeting the Keap1/Nrf2 Pathway. *Mar. Drugs* **2023**, *21*, 553. https://doi.org/10.3390/md21110553 [1]).

This Special Issue was enhanced by two reviews that offered the latest insights into the anti-inflammatory properties of natural marine products. Khursheed and colleagues present an overview of research on anti-inflammatory compounds derived from marine sources, highlighting their potential as new therapeutic drugs (Khursheed, M.; Ghelani, H.; Jan, R.K.; Adrian, T.E. Anti-Inflammatory Effects of Bioactive Compounds from Seaweeds, Bryozoans, Jellyfish, Shellfish and Peanut Worms. *Mar. Drugs* **2023**, *21*, 524. https://doi.org/10.3390/md21100524 [1]). Meanwhile, Nguyen and co-authors compiled studies on the anti-inflammatory properties of octocorals, summarizing findings from 46 studies conducted between 1995 and April 2023. This review provides a thorough overview of the anti-inflammatory potential of octocorals and aims to inspire further research to develop these compounds into therapeutic agents (Nguyen, N.B.A.; El-Shazly, M.; Chen, P.-J.; Peng, B.-R.; Chen, L.-Y.; Hwang, T.-L.; Lai, K.-H. Unlocking the Potential of Octocoral-Derived Secondary Metabolites against Neutrophilic Inflammatory Response. *Mar. Drugs* **2023**, *21*, 456. https://doi.org/10.3390/md21080456 [1]).

In summary, this Special Issue "Marine Anti-inflammatory and Antioxidant Agents 3.0" emphasized the vast potential of the marine environment as a source of bioactive compounds with promising anti-inflammatory properties. Ranging from plant extracts to carotenoids, fucoidans, and cyanobacterial metabolites, these substances offer new avenues for treating inflammatory diseases and contribute to sustainable therapeutic solutions. The reviewed studies highlight significant advances in understanding the mechanisms of these marine compounds and their potential applications in healthcare, functional foods, and environmental sustainability. Looking forward, continued exploration and research into marine natural products are crucial to fully unlocking their therapeutic potential.

Conflicts of Interest: The authors declare no conflict of interest.

Reference

1. Special Issue website "Marine Anti-inflammatory and Antioxidant Agents 3.0". Available online: https://www.mdpi.com/journal/marinedrugs/special_issues/8695SJOR67 (accessed on 20 August 2024).

Disclaimer/Publisher's Note: The statements, opinions and data contained in all publications are solely those of the individual author(s) and contributor(s) and not of MDPI and/or the editor(s). MDPI and/or the editor(s) disclaim responsibility for any injury to people or property resulting from any ideas, methods, instructions or products referred to in the content.

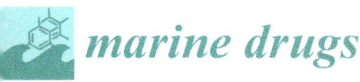

Article

Posidonia oceanica (L.) Delile Is a Promising Marine Source Able to Alleviate Imiquimod-Induced Psoriatic Skin Inflammation

Laura Micheli [1,†], Marzia Vasarri [2,†], Donatella Degl'Innocenti [2,3], Lorenzo Di Cesare Mannelli [1], Carla Ghelardini [1], Antiga Emiliano [4], Alice Verdelli [5], Marzia Caproni [4] and Emanuela Barletta [6,*]

1. Department of Neuroscience, Psychology, Drug Research and Child Health (NEUROFARBA), Pharmacology and Toxicology Section, University of Florence, 50139 Firenze, Italy; laura.micheli@unifi.it (L.M.); lorenzo.mannelli@unifi.it (L.D.C.M.); carla.ghelardini@unifi.it (C.G.)
2. Department of Experimental and Clinical Biomedical Sciences "Mario Serio", Biochemistry Section, University of Florence, 50134 Firenze, Italy; marzia.vasarri@unifi.it (M.V.); donatella.deglinnocenti@unifi.it (D.D.)
3. CIBM, Applied Ecology and Marine Biology Interuniversity Centre "G. Bacci", 57128 Livorno, Italy
4. Department of Health Sciences, Dermatology Section, University of Florence, 50125 Firenze, Italy; emiliano.antiga@unifi.it (A.E.); marzia.caproni@unifi.it (M.C.)
5. Central Tuscany Local Health Authority, Department of Multidimensional Medicine, Immuno-Rheumatology and Infectious Diseases Area, Dermatology SOC, Dermatological Rare Diseases SOS, 50125 Firenze, Italy; alice.verdelli@hotmail.it
6. Department of Experimental and Clinical Biomedical Sciences "Mario Serio", Experimental Pathology and Oncology Section, University of Florence, 50134 Firenze, Italy
* Correspondence: emanuela.barletta@unifi.it
† These authors contributed equally to this work.

Abstract: Psoriasis is a chronic immune-mediated inflammatory cutaneous disease characterized by elevated levels of inflammatory cytokines and adipokine Lipocalin-2 (LCN-2). Recently, natural plant-based products have been studied as new antipsoriatic compounds. We investigate the ability of a leaf extract of the marine plant *Posidonia oceanica* (POE) to inhibit psoriatic dermatitis in C57BL/6 mice treated with Imiquimod (IMQ). One group of mice was topically treated with IMQ (IMQ mice) for 5 days, and a second group received POE orally before each topical IMQ treatment (IMQ-POE mice). Psoriasis Area Severity Index (PASI) score, thickness, and temperature of the skin area treated with IMQ were measured in both groups. Upon sacrifice, the organs were weighed, and skin biopsies and blood samples were collected. Plasma and lesional skin protein expression of IL-17, IL-23, IFN-γ, IL-2, and TNF-α and plasma LCN-2 concentration were evaluated by ELISA. PASI score, thickness, and temperature of lesional skin were reduced in IMQ-POE mice, as were histological features of psoriatic dermatitis and expression of inflammatory cytokines and LCN-2 levels. This preliminary study aims to propose *P. oceanica* as a promising naturopathic anti-inflammatory treatment that could be introduced in Complementary Medicine for psoriasis.

Keywords: *Posidonia oceanica*; Imiquimod; inflammation; psoriasis; IL-17; IL-23; TNF-α; Lipocalin-2

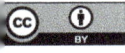

1. Introduction

Psoriasis is an immune-mediated chronic inflammatory disease of the skin with an estimated worldwide prevalence of about 2–3% which results from interactions between genetic predisposition and environmental stimuli. Besides the dermatological manifestations, it can also affect other organs. Therefore, psoriasis can be considered a systemic inflammatory disease rather than merely a cutaneous disease. Psoriasis severity is assessed and graded by the Psoriasis Area and Severity Index (PASI) [1], which evaluates the percentage of the affected body area and measures the intensity of redness (erythema), infiltration (thickness), and desquamation (scaliness). Histologically, skin lesions are characterized by an inflammatory infiltration of the dermis and epidermis consisting of macrophages, lymphocytes, neutrophils, and dendritic cells, and by an increase in keratinocyte proliferation, acanthosis (thickening of the stratum spinosum), and parakeratosis (cell nuclei within stratum corneum) [2].

A pivotal role in the pathogenesis of the psoriatic disease is played by cytokines such as tumor necrosis factor alpha (TNF-α), interleukin-23 (IL-23, composed of the IL-12B p40 subunits shared with IL-12, and the IL-23A p19 subunit), and the interleukin-17 family (IL-17A through IL-17F), secreted by activated keratinocytes, by dendritic Langerhans cells, and by Th17 and Th22 subpopulations of T helper lymphocytes [3–5]. Moreover, IL-17 can act with TNF-α to induce amplification of the initial inflammatory trigger by activating the NF-κB pathway [6,7]. Furthermore, TNF-α and the IL-23/IL-17 axis are among the main targets of biological therapies that use monoclonal antibodies against these cytokines [8,9]. In the last few years, several studies have also revealed that adipokine Lipocalin-2 (LCN-2) is highly expressed in psoriatic patients and in psoriasis mouse models [10]. LCN-2, also known as neutrophil gelatinase-associated lipocalin (NGAL), is a 25 kDa protein covalently bound to the matrix metalloproteinase 9. LCN-2 participates in several biological functions, such as immune response, cell growth, iron transport, and synthesis of inflammatory mediators. LCN-2 plays many roles in the pathogenesis of psoriasis both in the differentiation and proliferation of keratinocytes and in the recruitment of inflammatory cells such as lymphocytes and neutrophils via the IL-23/IL-17 axis [11]; thus, LCN-2 might be considered a marker of psoriasis [12].

In recent years, a mouse psoriasis-like model has been developed by topical application to the skin surface of the imidazoquinoline compound Imiquimod (IMQ) [13–15], a well-known ligand of Toll-like receptors 7 and 8 [16]. The IMQ-induced mouse model of psoriasis displays skin lesions closely related to human cutaneous psoriasis, clinically characterized by erythema, skin thickening, and scaling. Typical histological alterations such as acanthosis and parakeratosis, and inflammatory infiltrates of lymphocytes, macrophages, neutrophils, and dendritic cells are also reproduced. In addition, in this model, IMQ-treated skin displays a higher expression of IL-17 and IL-23 than untreated skin, indicating the involvement of the IL-23/IL-17 axis. Therefore, the IMQ-induced mouse model of psoriasis is widely used to study the pathogenesis of psoriatic skin lesions as well as the development of new therapies [13,15]. The therapeutical management of psoriasis provides different approaches depending on disease severity. Mild psoriasis is treated with topical therapies and phototherapy, while moderate and severe psoriasis are treated with systemic therapy, including biological agents against specific cytokines. [17,18]. Although biologics are usually considered safer than conventional immunosuppressive treatments, not all psoriatic patients are good candidates for biological therapies. For example, patients with malignant neoplasms and with active infections or systemic diseases cannot be treated with biologics since biological agents can induce side effects such as infections and malignancies [19–21].

In recent years, several natural products from plants have been considered as new potential anti-psoriatic agents with the aim of finding a complementary/alternative drug characterized by the absence of long-term toxicity, leading to better patient compliance than conventional therapies [22,23].

Although plants have historically been one of the main sources of pharmacological substances, in recent years, more attention has been paid to the marine world as an exceptional reservoir of new bioactive molecules that are safe and effective for human health, including anti-inflammatory agents [24].

Posidonia oceanica L. Delile is a Mediterranean angiosperm traditionally used as a medicinal plant for the treatment of various human diseases [25]. The healing properties of *P. oceanica* have been described in ancient Egypt, where it was said to be used for sore throats and skin problems [26]. Recently, phytotherapy has focused attention on *P. oceanica* for its bioactive properties and, in addition to its ecological importance, as a potential source of new drugs [25]. New findings on the bioactive properties of *P. oceanica* make this plant a promising source of natural therapeutic products for human health [25]. Studies conducted on in vitro cell models and in vivo animal models pave the way for research into new alternative and complementary therapeutic strategies based on *P. oceanica* against a wide range of pathological conditions.

Our laboratory has revealed that the hydroalcoholic extract obtained from *P. oceanica* leaves (POE) has no toxicity both in vitro and in vivo and, among other activities, has anti-inflammatory properties [27,28]. Indeed, in the murine macrophage RAW264.7 cell line stimulated with lipopolysaccharide, POE has inhibited intracellular ROS levels and the activity of the proinflammatory enzymes iNOS and COX-2, as well as the NF-κB signalling pathway [27]. Furthermore, in CD1 mice, oral administration of POE has inhibited carrageenan-induced inflammation by reducing pain and paw edema, by suppressing tissue myeloperoxidase activity and reducing the tissue concentration of the proinflammatory cytokines IL-1β and TNF-α [28], suggesting that oral administration of POE may exert anti-inflammatory effects both locally and systemically.

Given the demonstrated anti-inflammatory properties of POE, this preliminary study aims to verify the ability of POE to prevent the main inflammatory aspects of psoriatic-like lesions in the IMQ-induced mouse model, thus providing a new potential source of natural compounds to be used in alternative medicine of psoriasis.

2. Results

2.1. Body and Internal Organ Weight

To verify the systemic effects of topical IMQ treatment, the body weight in control mice and in experimental mice was recorded daily during the 5-day period. As shown in 1a, topical application of IMQ induced a body weight loss of less than 18% of the initial body weight in both IMQ and IMQ-POE mice; body weight in control mice was unaffected by topical application of vehicle cream and oral administration with POE vehicle during all five days. In addition, at the end of the experimental period (day 5), the organ's relative weight was evaluated. As shown in Figure 1b, the relative weight of the liver and kidney in both IMQ and IMQ-POE mice did not differ from the relative weight of the liver and kidney of control mice. However, during the topical application of IMQ, both groups of experimental mice displayed a statistically significant increase ($p < 0.05$) in the relative weight of the spleen compared to the control group (IMQ mice, 1.1 ± 0.1; IMQ-POE mice 0.7 ± 0.02; control mice 0.3 ± 0.02). However, IMQ-POE mice displayed a lesser increase in spleen weight than IMQ mice (0.7 ± 0.02 versus 1.1 ± 0.1, $p < 0.05$). These results suggest that topical IMQ treatment with or without oral administration of POE has no toxic effect since there was no change in the organ weight-to-body weight ratio of the liver and kidney compared to the control group. In addition, although topical application of IMQ induces splenomegaly according to previous findings [14,29–31], a recent study has revealed that the spleen is not directly involved in the development of psoriatic lesions in IMQ-treated mice [31].

2.2. Clinical Evaluation of Skin Inflammation

To clinically assess the severity of skin inflammation during topical application of IMQ and to verify whether oral administration of POE could improve inflammatory status, PASI score, thickness, and temperature of the treated skin area were evaluated. PASI score was equal to 0 in control mice during all five days (Figure 2d). When compared to control mice, after 24 h from the first application of IMQ (day 2), erythema had already appeared in IMQ mice (Figure 2a), while desquamation and induration were evident after 48 h (day 3, Figure 2b,c) with a PASI score > 3 (PASI = 3.1 ± 0.5, day 3, Figure 2d). At the end of the experimental period, the PASI score was 9.5 in IMQ mice (PASI = 9.5 ± 0.3, day 5, Figure 2d). During oral administration of POE, signs of skin inflammation related to IMQ topical application were less severe; erythema appeared after 48 h in comparison to control mice (day 3, Figure 2a), with a PASI score lower than the PASI score observed in IMQ mice (PASI = 1.1 ± 0.3 versus PASI = 3.1 ± 0.5, $p < 0.05$, day 3, Figure 2d), while desquamation and induration appeared after 72 h in comparison to control mice (day 4, Figure 2b,c), with a PASI score still lower than the PASI score observed in IMQ mice (PASI = 3.8 ± 0.6

versus PASI = 7.1 ± 0.6, $p < 0.05$, day 4, Figure 2d). At the end of the experimental period, the PASI score in IMQ-POE mice was still lower than the PASI observed in IMQ mice (PASI = 6.3 ± 0.8 versus PASI = 9.5 ± 0.3, $p < 0.05$, day 5, Figure 2d). Figure 2e shows clinical pictures of psoriatic lesions developed during each day in IMQ mice and the attenuation of lesional severity during oral administration of POE. Application of vehicle cream in control mice never induces any skin alteration.

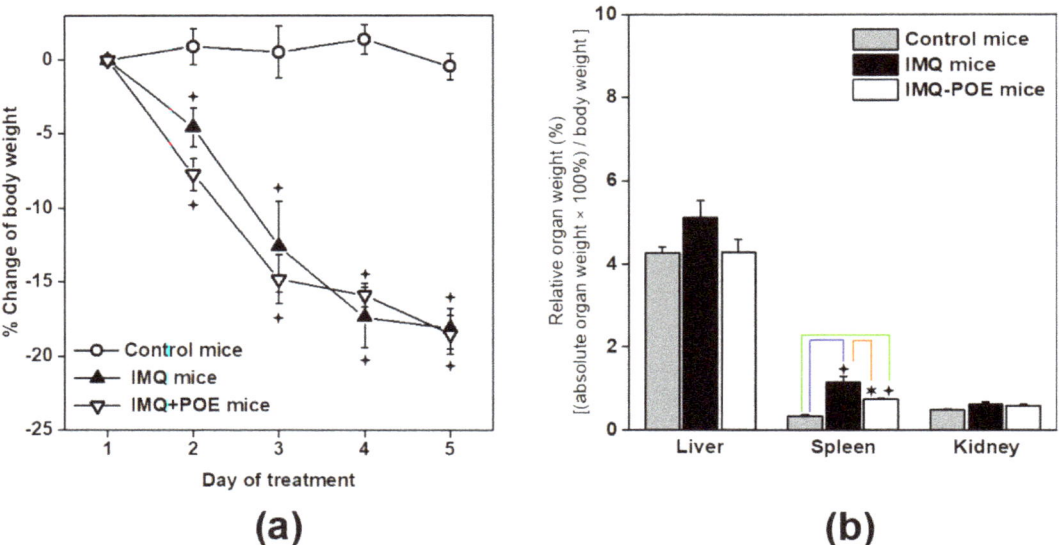

Figure 1. Body weight and organ weight changes. (**a**) Changes in body weight are expressed as a percentage of the initial value (day 1) in control mice (white circle), IMQ mice (black triangle), and IMQ-POE mice (white triangle). Values are mean ± SEM ($n = 6$/group) measured at different time points. (**b**) Changes in liver, spleen, and kidney weights are expressed as organ-relative weight at the end of the experimental period (day 5) in control mice (grey bar), IMQ mice (black bar), and IMQ-POE mice (white bar). The bar graph represents the mean ± SEM ($n = 6$/group). extFourStar $p < 0.05$ IMQ mice or IMQ-POE mice vs. control mice by one-way ANOVA with Bonferroni post hoc test; extSixStar $p < 0.05$ IMQ-POE mice vs. IMQ mice by one-way ANOVA with Bonferroni post hoc test; if it is not indicated, the differences are statistically non-significant.

Since the thickness of the inflamed skin area is related to the intensity of oedema, changes in the double-fold thickness of the treated skin area were recorded during the 5 days of treatment. In control mice, the thickness of skin treated with vehicle cream did not change over the 5 days, while the thickness of Imiquimod-treated skin was increased in both IMQ and IMQ-POE mice (Figure 3). However, in IMQ mice, the thickness of the treated skin area was higher than in IMQ-POE mice after 48 h from topical application of IMQ (Figure 3, day 3, 0.9 ± 0.06 mm versus 0.7 ± 0.03 mm, $p < 0.05$) and it remained at higher levels until the end of treatment. These results are consistent with a lower intensity of skin inflammation during POE treatment.

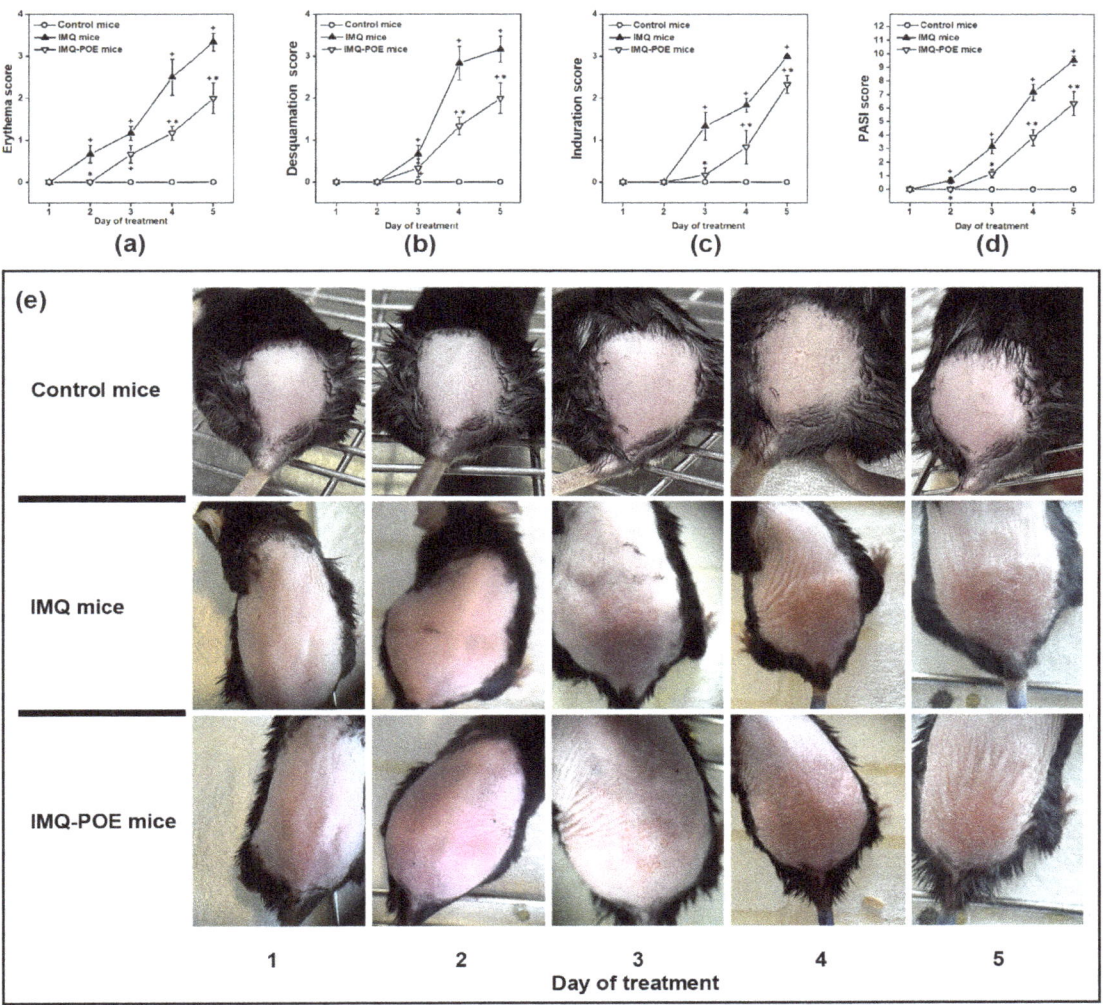

Figure 2. Evaluation of psoriatic skin inflammation. (**a**) Erythema score, range 0–4. (**b**) Desquamation score, range 0–4. (**c**) Induration score, range 0–4. (**d**) PASI cumulative index (sum of the three a, b, and c scores), range from 0 to 12. The line graph represents the mean of each score ± SEM ($n = 6$/group) measured at different time points in control mice (white circle), IMQ mice (black triangle), and IMQ-POE mice (white triangle). **** $p < 0.05$ IMQ mice or IMQ-POE mice vs. control mice by one-way ANOVA with Bonferroni post hoc test; ****** $p < 0.05$ IMQ-POE mice vs. IMQ mice by one-way ANOVA with Bonferroni post hoc test; if it is not indicated, the differences are statistically non-significant. (**e**) Representative pictures of the dorsal treated skin area of control mice, IMQ mice, and IMQ-POE mice during each day of the treatment period.

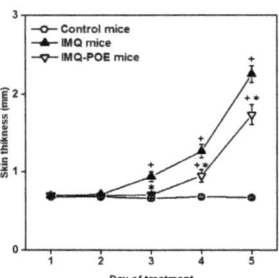

Figure 3. Measurement of dorsal skin thickness. Double-fold dorsal skin thickness was measured in the dorsal treated area by an engineer's micrometer in control mice (white circle), IMQ mice (black triangle), or IMQ-POE mice (white triangle). Values are reported in millimeters and expressed as mean ± SEM (n = 6/group). extFourStar $p < 0.05$ IMQ mice or IMQ-POE mice vs. control mice by one-way ANOVA with Bonferroni post hoc test; extSixStar $p < 0.05$ IMQ-POE mice vs. IMQ mice by one-way ANOVA with Bonferroni post hoc test; if iAt is not indicated, the differences are statistically non-significant.

Finally, the temperature of the treated skin area was measured, since temperature increase is one of the four cardinal signs of inflammation. While skin temperature in control mice did not change over the 5 days, after 24 h from IMQ topical application (day 2), both groups of IMQ and IMQ-POE mice displayed an increase in skin temperature; however in the treated skin area, the temperature in IMQ mice was higher than in IMQ-POE mice (Figure 4, 33.1 ± 0.3 °C versus 32.0 ± 0.04 °C, $p < 0.05$) and it remained higher in IMQ mice than in IMQ-POE mice for the subsequent days. These results confirm that POE oral administration improves inflammatory status induced by topical application of IMQ.

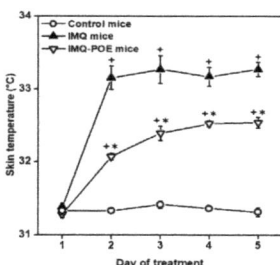

Figure 4. Changes in dorsal skin temperature. Skin temperature was measured in the dorsal treated area of control mice (white circle), IMQ mice (black triangle), or IMQ-POE mice (white triangle) by an infrared camera during the 5 days of treatment. Values are reported in °C and expressed as mean ± SEM (n = 6/group). extFourStar $p < 0.05$ IMQ mice or IMQ-POE mice vs. control mice by one-way ANOVA with Bonferroni post hoc test; extSixStar $p < 0.05$ IMQ-POE mice vs. IMQ mice by one-way ANOVA with Bonferroni post hoc test; if it is not indicated, the differences are statistically non-significant.

2.3. Histological Examination and Immunodetection of Macrophages and Lymphocytes

To check whether the characteristic features of psoriasis were also present at the microscopic level, at the end of the five days of treatment, we performed a histological examination by hematoxylin and eosin staining of the dorsal skin area treated with vehicle cream (control mice), or with IMQ (IMQ mice), or with IMQ and oral administration of POE (IMQ-POE mice). In comparison to control mice (Figure 5a), IMQ topical application induced in both IMQ and IMQ-POE mice the characteristic psoriatic changes of the stratified squamous epithelium [32] represented by (a) acanthosis (Figure 5b,c, black arrowheads), i.e., epidermal hyperplasia with an increased thickness of stratum spinosum;

(b) hyperkeratosis and parakeratosis (Figure 5b,c, double black arrowheads), i.e., thickening of the stratum corneum and retention of nuclei in the stratum corneum; (c) agranulosis (Figure 5b,c, white arrowheads), i.e., reduction in the stratum granulosum. However, when epidermal hyperplasia was evaluated by measurement of epidermal thickness, excluding stratum corneum and rete pegs, during oral administration of POE, there was a statistically significant reduction ($p < 0.05$) in epidermal hyperplasia in IMQ-POE mice compared to that observed in IMQ mice (Figure 5d, 59.4 ± 1.5 μm versus 90.1 ± 2.7 μm, $p < 0.05$), although oral administration of POE was not able to completely revert normal epidermal thickness observed in control mice (Figure 5d, 23.9 ± 0.7 μm). In addition, during oral administration of POE, the height of dermal papillae was reduced in IMQ-POE mice compared to IMQ mice (Figure 5e, 86.0 ± 2.8 μm versus 120.0 ± 1.9 μm, $p < 0.05$), although it remains greater than control mice (Figure 5e, 25.1 ± 0.6 μm). Furthermore, while the signs of skin inflammation were evident in IMQ mice, they were largely absent in specimens of lesional skin of IMQ-POE mice. Indeed, the lesional skin of IMQ mice showed dilatation and congestion of the dermal capillaries (Figure 5b, black arrows), and the presence of Munro's microabscesses, i.e., aggregates of pyknotic neutrophils in the stratum corneum (Figure 5b, double white arrowheads), which are one of the hallmarks of early psoriasis [32]. The improvement of psoriatic inflammatory characteristics induced by oral administration of POE was also confirmed by ELISA detection of the CD86 marker of inflammatory macrophages and CD3 marker of lymphocytes in the skin specimens. As shown in Figure 5e, while in control mice, CD86 and CD3 markers were almost undetectable, in IMQ mice, the levels of both CD86 and CD3 markers were expressed at a higher level than in IMQ-POE mice (CD86, 0.9 ± 0.01 pg/mg versus 0.7 ± 0.008 pg/mg, $p < 0.05$; CD3 2.2 ± 0.07 pg/mg versus 1.8 ± 0.02 pg/mg, $p < 0.05$).

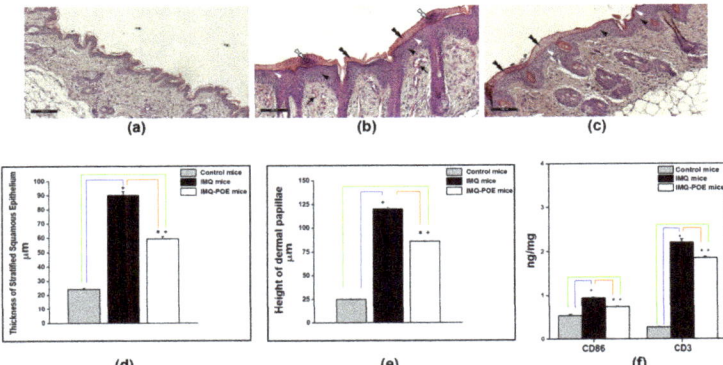

Figure 5. Histological examination. Representative pictures of hematoxylin and eosin-stained skin sections obtained from the dorsal skin area treated with (**a**) vehicle cream (control mice); (**b**) Imiquimod (IMQ mice); (**c**) Imiquimod and oral administration of POE (IMQ-POE mice). Scale bar, 100 μm. Black arrowheads indicate epidermal hyperplasia; double black arrowheads indicate hyperkeratosis and parakeratosis; white arrowheads indicate agranulosis; black arrows indicate dilatation and congestion of the dermal capillaries; double white arrowheads indicate Munro's micro abscesses. Microscopic evaluation of the thickness of stratified squamous epithelium (**d**) and the height of dermal papillae (**e**), in skin sections of control mice (grey bar), skin sections of IMQ mice (black bar), and skin sections of IMQ-POE mice (white bar); values are reported in micrometres and expressed as mean ± SEM. (**f**) The levels of CD86 marker of inflammatory macrophages and CD3 marker of T lymphocytes were detected by ELISA in the treated dorsal skin area; values are reported in ng/mg of tissue and expressed as mean ± SEM. **** $p < 0.05$ IMQ mice or IMQ-POE mice vs. control mice by one-way ANOVA with Bonferroni post hoc test; ****** $p < 0.05$ IMQ-POE mice vs. IMQ mice by one-way ANOVA with Bonferroni post hoc test.

2.4. Evaluation of Cytokines and LCN-2 Expression

To verify the effect of oral administration of POE on the expression of IL-23 and TNF-α, of the Th17-associated IL-17A and IL-17F cytokines, of Th1-associated IFN-γ and IL-2 cytokines, the protein expression of cytokines was evaluated by ELISA in the treated dorsal skin area and in plasma at the end of the experimental period (day 5).

As shown in Figure 6a, protein expression of IL-23 and TNF-α, of the Th17-associated cytokines IL-17A and IL-17F, and of the Th1-associated IFN-γ was higher in the dorsal treated skin area of IMQ and IMQ-POE mice than in control mice, while only the Th1-associated IL-2 was almost unexpressed in skin samples. However, all these cytokines were lower in IMQ-POE mice than in IMQ mice (IL-23, 5.5 ± 0.06 pg/mg versus 8.4 ± 0.08 pg/mg, $p < 0.05$; TNF-α, 9.5 ± 0.08 pg/mg versus 14.9 ± 0.2 pg/mg, $p < 0.05$; IL-17A, 4.6 ± 0.04 pg/mg versus 6.4 ± 0.2 pg/mg, $p < 0.05$; IL-17F, 17.1 ± 0.04 pg/mg versus 23.1 ± 0.2 pg/mg, $p < 0.05$; IFN-γ, 17.5 ± 0.17 pg/mg versus 22.8 ± 0.2 pg/mg, $p < 0.05$).

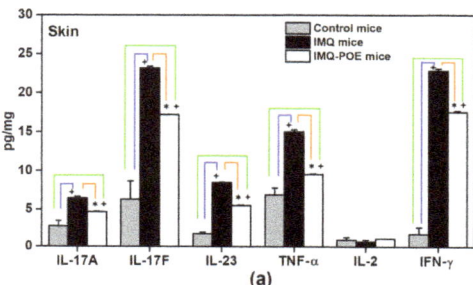

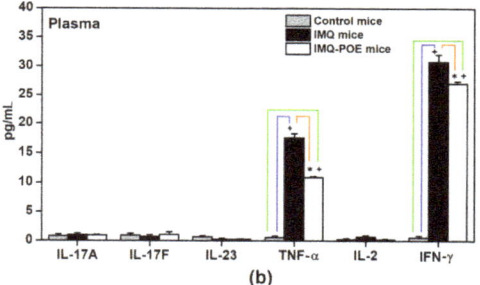

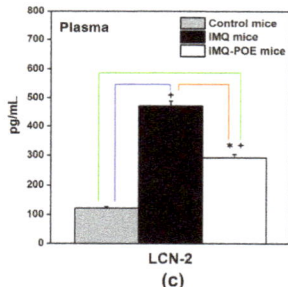

Figure 6. Protein expression of cytokines and LCN-2. The levels of cytokines and LCN-2 were measured by ELISA in control mice (grey bar), IMQ mice (black bar), and IMQ-POE mice (white bar). (**a**) The levels of IL-17A, IL-17F, IL-23, TNF-α, IL-2, and IFN-γ in the treated dorsal skin area are reported in pg/mg of tissue; (**b**) the level of IL-17A, IL-17F, IL-23, TNF-α, IL-2, and IFN-γ and (**c**) of LCN-2 in plasma is reported in pg/mL. Values are expressed as mean ± SEM ($n = 6$/group). extFourStar $p < 0.05$ IMQ mice or IMQ-POE mice vs. control mice by one-way ANOVA with Bonferroni post hoc test; extSixStar $p < 0.05$ IMQ-POE mice vs. IMQ mice by one-way ANOVA with Bonferroni post hoc test.

In plasma (Figure 6b), the expression of IL-23, IL-17A, IL-17F, and IL-2 was almost undetectable in all three groups of mice, and only TNF-α and IFN-γ were more highly expressed in IMQ mice and in IMQ-POE mice than in control mice. However, in IMQ mice, TNF-α and IFN-γ were expressed at a higher level than in IMQ-POE mice (TNF-α 17.5 ± 0.6 pg/mL versus 10.8 ± 0.2 pg/mL, $p < 0.05$; IFN-γ, 30.7 ± 1.2 pg/mL versus 27 ± 0.3 pg/mL, $p < 0.05$).

Detection of LCN-2 expression in plasma samples by ELISA at the end of the experimental period revealed that LCN-2 protein expression was higher in IMQ mice and in IMQ-POE mice compared to control mice. Moreover, in IMQ mice, LCN-2 concentration was about twice that in IMQ-POE mice (Figure 6c, 472.1 ± 15.6 pg/mL versus 291.6 ± 11.1 pg/mL, $p < 0.05$). These results further support the role of POE as a mitigator of proinflammatory effects associated with psoriatic lesions.

3. Discussion

Psoriasis is an immune-mediated chronic inflammatory dermatological and systemic disease influenced by genetic predisposition and environmental stimuli. The main histological characteristic is a dysregulated proliferation and differentiation of keratinocytes and infiltration of inflammatory cells such as T lymphocytes, neutrophils, and macrophages. Interactions between keratinocytes and immune cells play a pivotal role in the pathogenesis of psoriatic lesions. Keratinocytes activated by environmental and microbial stimuli secrete cytokines and antimicrobial peptides that activate dendritic cells, which in turn activate subsets of Th lymphocytes that release several cytokines such as IL-23, IL-17A, and IL-17F and TNF-α, which can promote proliferation and altered differentiation of keratinocytes, creating a loop of maintenance and amplification of inflammation [33,34]. Therefore, for the treatment of psoriasis, especially for the more serious forms, in recent decades, there has been a great development of biological drugs based on the use of antibodies against cytokines, particularly against TNF-α, IL-17A, IL-17F, and IL-23, which are not only involved in skin lesions, but they can also have systemic effects [18,35–37]. However, the use of biological drugs can be limited by several factors, such as the risk of immunogenicity [20,38,39], long-term administration, which can affect patient compliance, and the expensive cost. Thus, researchers' attention has recently been focused on the anti-inflammatory and immune response modulation activities of various natural products with the aim of helping traditional therapies improve patient's safety and adherence to treatment [40–42].

Modern science has recognized the millennia-long use of plants by humans to fight disease. *Posidonia oceanica* is a marine plant used since the time of ancient Egypt to treat various human ailments and for skin care. Our research group has studied the bioactive properties of a hydroalcoholic extract of *P. oceanica* leaves (POE) for years. Although the phytochemical extracts are highly heterogeneous, due to the presence of a mixture of different bioactive components, it has been observed that biological responses may not be due to a single bioactive compound, but to the mix of several bioactive compounds [43–46]. Furthermore, recent studies have revealed that proanthocyanidins, derived from grapes, apples, and other vegetables, are composed of a group of natural polyphenols that can alleviate psoriatic inflammation [47,48], supporting the role of synergism between bioactive compounds. The analysis of POE by UPLC allowed us to reveal that POE is made up of 88% polyphenols and is predominantly represented by (+) catechins and to a lesser extent by gallic acid, ferulic acid, epicatechin, and chlorogenic acid [49]. Nevertheless, we have revealed that neither single compounds nor even catechin alone can explain the biological effects of the entire *Posidonia oceanica* extract. [49]. Both in vitro and in vivo scientific studies of the leaf extract of this marine plant have shown that the phytocomplex can be exploited in various human health applications due to its nontoxicity [24]. Among other bioactivities, the anti-inflammatory role of POE has been described both in vitro and in vivo [27,28]. Because inflammation plays an important role in psoriasis, in this preliminary study, we have investigated the beneficial role of POE in the pathogenesis of psoriatic-like lesions in an IMQ-induced mouse model of psoriasis. We have chosen the oral administration route of POE, both due to the absence of its toxicity in vivo [28] and because psoriasis is now considered a systemic disease.

In this study, we have provided evidence that oral administration of POE can inhibit psoriasiform dermatitis induced in mice by IMQ treatment, an approved animal model for the in vivo experimental study of psoriasis [14,15].

First, PASI score, skin thickness, and lesional skin temperature, a cardinal sign of inflammation, were reduced in mice treated by oral administration of POE, indicating that POE can effectively reduce the classical clinical aspects of psoriatic skin lesions. Moreover, POE was able to inhibit the hallmark histological aspects of psoriasiform dermatitis, such as thickness of stratified squamous epithelium, hyperkeratosis, parakeratosis, agranulosis, dilatation, and congestion of the dermal capillaries and development of Munro's micro abscesses [32], and to reduce infiltration of inflammatory macrophages and T lymphocytes, as revealed by reduction in expression of CD86 and CD3 markers. These inhibitory effects are consistent with previous results from our laboratory which revealed that POE can reduce signs and symptoms of inflammation such as inflammatory pain and oedema in CD1 mice [28]. Furthermore, oral administration of POE in IMQ-treated mice was able to reduce the clinical and histopathological signs of psoriasis without additional systemic adverse effects, as demonstrated by the absence of significant changes in the relative organ weights of the liver and kidney compared to the control mice.

Second, POE was also able to inhibit, in lesional skin of IMQ mice, protein expression of the major inflammatory cytokines implicated in the pathogenesis of psoriasis, such as the Th1 hallmark cytokine TNF-α and IFN-γ and the Th17 product IL-17A and IL-17F, and the cytokine IL-23 secreted by dendritic cells, which activates Th1 and Th17 cells to produce IL-17, IFN-γ, and TNF-α. In addition, POE was able to reduce plasma levels of inflammatory cytokines TNF-α and IFN-γ, whose high serum levels correlate with disease severity in psoriatic patients [50]. These results agree with our previous study that revealed the inhibitory effect of POE on the protein expression of cytokines TNF-α and IL-1 in another murine inflammatory model [28]. Several biological effects of TNF are mediated by NF-κB activation [51], including cellular proliferation, differentiation, and apoptosis, so that NF-κB is considered an essential nuclear transcription factor in the pathogenesis of psoriasis [52]. Recently, our laboratory has shown that POE is able to inhibit NF-κB activation by preventing phosphorylation and nuclear translocation of the p65 subunit of NF-κB through inhibition of IκBα degradation [27].

In this regard, it might be interesting to extend our study on the role of POE in the immune-mediated pathogenesis of psoriasis not only by inhibiting upstream signaling agents, such as TNF expression, but also by inhibiting downstream signaling agents of the canonical NF-κB pathway. Therefore, we plan to verify in a future study the role of POE in an in vitro model of psoriasis using both the hyperproliferative model of LPS/IL-22-stimulated HaCaT cells and the inflammatory model of HaCaT cells stimulated with LPS/TNF-α [53,54].

Finally, in our psoriasis mouse model, we have revealed that plasma levels of LCN-2 were lowered during oral administration of POE. LCN-2 has recently been proposed as a potential target for psoriasis treatment, since it is involved in keratinocyte differentiation and pathogenesis of psoriasis by stimulating neutrophil function, Th17 activation, and secretion of IL-23 by dendritic cells [11]. Psoriatic patients display a higher risk of developing nonmelanoma skin cancer than healthy subjects, especially those patients with moderate to severe psoriasis [55]. Recently, it has been revealed that plasma levels of LCN-2 were significantly higher in psoriatic patients with nonmelanoma skin cancer than in patients with skin tumours without psoriasis [56]. Therefore, POE might also be involved in reducing the risk of developing skin cancers in psoriatic patients by inhibiting LCN-2 expression.

In conclusion, our preliminary study proposes POE as a promising natural source of bioactive compounds that might improve traditional pharmacological treatment of psoriasis.

4. Materials and Methods

4.1. Chemicals and Reagents

All chemicals and reagents were purchased from Sigma-Aldrich (Merck KGaA, Darmstadt, Germany) unless otherwise stated.

4.2. Animals and Ethical Statement

C57BL/6 mice were purchased from Envigo (Varese, Italy). Experiments were conducted with female C57BL/6 mice 10 weeks old, weighing 25–35 g at the beginning of the experimental procedure. Animals were housed in conventional cages in the CeSAL animal facility (Centro Stabulazione Animali da Laboratorio, University of Florence) under controlled environmental conditions (room temperature at 22 °C and 12 h light/12 h dark cycle) and provided with commercial solid food and tap water available ad libitum. All animal manipulations were carried out according to Directive 2010/63/EU of the European Parliament and of the European Union Council (22 September 2010) on the protection of animals used for scientific purposes. The ethical policy of the University of Florence complies with the Guide for the Care and Use of Laboratory Animals of the US National Institutes of Health (NIH Publication No. 85-23, revised 1996; University of Florence assurance number: A5278-01). All the experimental procedures carried out in this study were approved by the Italian Ministry of Health (No. 333/2020-PR) and by the Animal Subjects Review Board of the University of Florence. Experiments involving animals were performed according to the ARRIVE guidelines [57,58]. All efforts were made to minimize animal suffering and to reduce the number of animals used.

4.3. Preparation of Posidonia oceanica Leaf Extract (POE)

P. oceanica leaves were collected and extracted as previously described [49]. Briefly, 1 g of *P. oceanica* dried leaves after mincing was suspended in 10 mL EtOH/H2O (70:30 v/v) at 37 °C under stirring overnight and then stirred at 65 °C for an additional 3 h. After repeated centrifugations, the hydroalcoholic phase was mixed in a 1:1 ratio with n-hexane (v/v) under shaking. Then, the recovered hydroalcoholic fraction was dispensed in 1 mL aliquots and dried. The dry extract will be called POE. Specifically, in this study, the hydroalcoholic extract from 4 g of *P. oceanica* dried and minced leaves gave a yield of 0.2 g of POE. In order to analyze the biochemical composition of POE, 9.4 mg of dry extract was solubilized in 0.5 mL of EtOH/H2O (70:30 v/v) and POE was then assessed for total polyphenol content (Folin–Ciocâlteu method), and for its antioxidant (FRAP assay) and free-radical scavenging (DPPH assay) activities, as previously described [59]. The total polyphenol content in POE was 0.5 ± 0.06 mg/mL of gallic acid equivalents, and the antioxidant and radical-scavenging activities were 0.13 ± 0.07 mg/mL and 1.1 ± 0.2 mg/mL of ascorbic acid equivalents, respectively.

4.4. Imiquimod-Induced Psoriasis and POE Treatment

The animals were divided into 2 groups: (a) the control mice ($n = 6$) and (b) the experimental mice ($n = 12$). All the mice were housed individually, with 1 animal per cage to prevent licking each other. Psoriasis-like lesions were induced in the experimental mice according to the protocol employed in previous studies [14,15,60]. Briefly, a dose of 62.5 mg of commercially available Imiquimod 5% cream (Imunocare; Difa Cooper S.p.A., Milan, Italy), corresponding to 3.125 mg of Imiquimod, was topically applied daily on a 2 cm^2 shaved dorsal skin area for 5 consecutive days. This dose of IMQ was already demonstrated in various publications [14,15,60] to induce reproducible psoriatic-like skin inflammation in this mouse model. To analyze the effect of POE during treatment with IMQ, the experimental mice were divided into two subgroups: (a) the group of so-called IMQ mice ($n = 6$) treated topically with IMQ, which were orally administered by gastric gavage with vehicle solution (1% carboxymethyl cellulose sodium salt, CMC) at a volume of 10 mL/kg of the animal weight 1 h before each topical treatment with IMQ, and (b) the group of so-called IMQ-POE mice ($n = 6$), to which, 1 h before each topical treatment with IMQ, POE resuspended in the vehicle solution was orally administered by gastric gavage at a dose of 100 mg/kg of the animal body weight. The oral POE dosage at 100 mg/kg was chosen based on the anti-inflammatory effects of POE observed in mice in our previous study [28]. The control group was treated similarly by topical application of the vehicle cream (isostearic acid, benzyl alcohol, cetyl alcohol, stearyl alcohol, soft white paraffin, polysorbate 60, sorbitan stearate, glycerol, methyl hydroxybenzoate (E218), propyl hydroxybenzoate (E216), xanthan gum, purified water), and by oral administration with vehicle solution 1 h before each topical treatment with vehicle cream. The body weight of each group of mice was recorded every day starting on the day of application of each cream (day 1) until the end of the experimental period (day 5). To facilitate comprehension of the experimental design, we have provided a schematic workflow in Scheme 1.

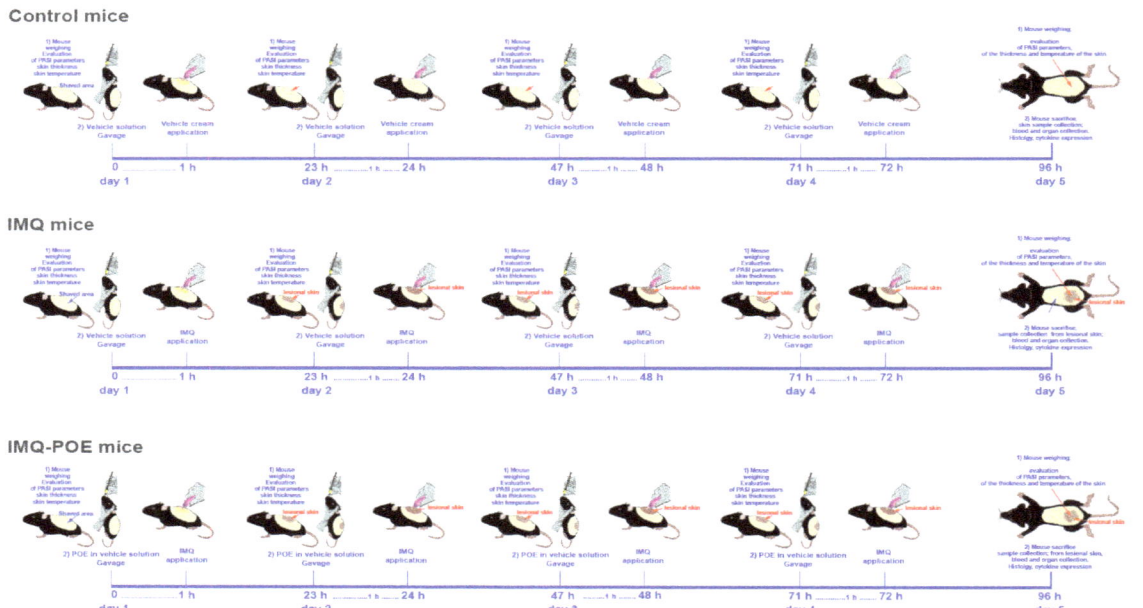

Scheme 1. Illustration of the experimental design.

4.5. Assessment of Inflammation Severity

In order to compare the severity of psoriatic-like lesions between control mice, IMQ mice, and IMQ-POE mice, a modified PASI score was assessed every day starting on day 1 until the end of the experiment (day 5). This evaluation was performed before the above daily treatments in all three groups of mice. Except for the extension of the area affected by psoriatic-like lesions, since the extension of the experimental treated area was the same and it was not related to spontaneously occurring psoriasis, a scale from 0 to 4 was used to evaluate erythema, desquamation, and infiltration, where 0 = none, 1 = mild, 2 = moderate, 3 = severe, and 4 = very severe. The cumulative index (sum of the three scores) was then evaluated as a measure of the overall inflammation severity comparable to the PASI score (maximum score = 12). In addition, we measured the double-fold dorsal skin thickness of the treated area using an electronic digital caliper, resolution: 0.01mm (150 mm Stainless Steel Electronic Digital Calliper, Juning, Shenzhen, Guangdong 518000, China). Finally, the temperature of the dorsal treated skin area was measured daily by an infrared camera (Pti120, Fluke s.r.l., Milan, Italy) during the 5 days of treatment in all three groups of mice. Images were analyzed by Fluke Connect Desktop Software (version 4.3).

4.6. Organ and Blood Collection and Tissue Histological Examination

At the end of the 5th day of treatment, mice were anesthetised with isoflurane (2%), and the blood was collected from the vena cava in the presence of 2% EDTA as anticoagulant and centrifuged (2500 RCF for 10 min at room temperature) to obtain the plasma fraction;

mice were then sacrificed by decapitation. The spleen, liver, and kidneys were immediately removed and weighed. The organ relative weight was calculated by the ratio of each animal's organ weight to body weight and expressed as the percentage of body weight. In addition, biopsies were taken from vehicle cream-treated skin areas in control mice and from Imiquimod-treated skin areas in IMQ and IMQ-POE mice by surgical excision from each mouse. Briefly, skin specimens were fixed in 10% phosphate-buffered formalin, dehydrated, cleared, and then embedded in paraffin. Skin sections (5 μm) were cut, mounted on glass slides, deparaffinized, and stained with hematoxylin and eosin. The mounted specimens were then observed under a bright-field light microscope (BX40 upright microscope, Olympus, Tokyo, Japan) equipped with a digital microscope camera (C B5, Optika, Bergamo, Italy). Epidermal thickness, excluding stratum corneum and rete pegs, and the height of dermal papillae, measured by the distance between the top of dermal papillae and the level showing no dermal papillae, were determined in 20 randomly chosen microscopic fields in each section from each mouse specimen using Aperio ImageScope software version 12.4.6 (Leica Biosystems, Nußloch, Germany).

4.7. Quantitation of Cytokines and LCN-2 Protein Expression

Levels of TNF-α, and IL-23, and of Th17-associated cytokines IL-17A and IL-17F, and of Th1-associated cytokines IFN-γ and IL-2 were measured by enzyme-linked immunosorbent assay (ELISA) in skin tissue samples and in plasma.

Proteins were extracted from skin sections at the end of the experimental period according to the method described by Kawashima et al. [61]. Briefly, twenty serial sections from each paraffin-embedded specimen were placed in 1.5 mL vials and deparaffinized by incubation for 10 min at room temperature in xylene and centrifuged for 3 min at $16,000 \times g$. The pellet was resuspended in xylene for an additional 10 min incubation and centrifuged again. The pellet was then hydrated in a series of graded ethanol, air-dried, and resuspended in 50 μL of lysis buffer (400 mM Tris–HCl pH 8.0, 150 mM NaCl, 1 mM EGTA, 1 mM EDTA, 1% Triton X-100, 0.5% sodium deoxycholate, 50 mM NaF, 1 mM PMSF, 1 mM AEBSF, 800 nM Aprotinin, 50 μM Bestatin, 15 μM E64, 20 μM Leupeptin, 10 μM Pepstatin A), homogenized using a micro pestle (Carl Roth GmbH + Co. KG), and incubated at 90 °C for 60 min. The debris was removed by centrifugation, and the total protein concentration in tissue lysates was determined by Lowry's method [62] using bovine serum albumin as a reference.

The expression of TNF-α, IL-23, IL-17A, IL-17F, IFN-γ, and IL-2 in tissue supernatant and in plasma was measured using commercial ELISA assay kits (TNF alpha Mouse Uncoated ELISA Kit, IL-12/IL-23 total p40 Uncoated ELISA kit, IL-17A homodimer Mouse Uncoated ELISA kit, IL-17F homodimer Mouse Uncoated ELISA kit, IFN-γ Mouse Uncoated ELISA kit, IL-2 Mouse Uncoated ELISA kit; Invitrogen Thermo Fisher Scientific, Inc., Waltham, MA, USA) following the standard protocol provided by the assay kit manufacturer. Concentrations were expressed as picogram of cytokine per milligram of extracted protein from tissue samples or as picogram of cytokine per milliliter of plasma.

Lipocalin-2 concentration was examined in plasma at the end of the experimental period by a commercial ELISA kit (Mouse NGAL ELISA Kit, Bioporto Diagnostics A/S, Hellerup, Denmark) according to manufacturer instructions. Concentrations were expressed as picogram of LCN-2 per milliliter of plasma.

4.8. Immunodetection of T-Lymphocytes and Macrophages in Skin Sections

Macrophage and lymphocyte T infiltration in vehicle cream-treated skin areas of control mice and in Imiquimod-treated skin areas of IMQ and IMQ-POE mice was evaluated by detecting the CD86 marker for inflammatory macrophages and the CD3 marker for T cells. Briefly, the expression of CD86 and CD3 was measured in tissue supernatant isolated from the paraffin-embedded specimen, as described above using commercial ELISA assay kits (CD86 ELISA Kit, CD3 ELISA Kit; Antibodies-online, GmbH, Aachen, Germany) according to manufacturer instructions. Concentrations were expressed as nanogram per milligram of extracted protein.

4.9. Statistical Analysis

Results were expressed as the mean ± SEM and were analyzed statistically using JASP software (JASP Team 2024 Version 0.18.3). The statistical difference between groups was analyzed using one-way ANOVA with a Bonferroni correction (Bonferroni post hoc test); statistical significance was defined as $p < 0.05$.

Author Contributions: Conceptualization, B.E.; methodology, B.E., D.D. and M.L.; validation, D.D.; formal analysis, V.M.; investigation, M.L. and V.M.; resources, G.C. and D.C.M.L.; writing—original draft preparation, B.E.; writing—review and editing, B.E., D.D., E.A., C.M. and V.A.; supervision, B.E.; project administration, B.E.; funding acquisition, B.E. and D.D. All authors have read and agreed to the published version of the manuscript.

Funding: This research was funded by University of Florence (Fondi di Ateneo 2021 and 2022 to E.B and D.D.).

Institutional Review Board Statement: The ethical policy of the University of Florence complies with the Guide for the Care and Use of Laboratory Animals of the US National Institutes of Health (NIH Publication No. 85–23, revised 1996; University of Florence assurance number: A5278-01) All the experimental procedures carried out in this study were approved by the Italian Ministry of Health (No. 333/2020-PR) and by the Animal Subjects Review Board of the University of Florence Experiments involving animals were performed according to the ARRIVE guidelines.

Data Availability Statement: The data presented in this study are available on request from the corresponding author.

Acknowledgments: We thank the "Optical Microscopy, Histochemistry and Immunohistochemistry" Service, Imaging Platform, at the Department of Experimental and Clinical Medicine, University of Florence, for histology slide preparation. We give our special thanks for providing us with *Posidonia oceanica* leaves to the Applied Ecology and Marine Biology Interuniversity Center "G. Bacci" (CIBM), Livorno, Italy.

Conflicts of Interest: The authors declare no conflicts of interest.

References

1. Fredriksson, T.; Pettersson, U. Severe psoriasis–oral therapy with a new retinoid. *Dermatologica* **1978**, *157*, 238–244. [CrossRef] [PubMed]
2. Rendon, A.; Schäkel, K. Psoriasis Pathogenesis and Treatment. *Int. J. Mol. Sci.* **2019**, *20*, 1475. [CrossRef] [PubMed]
3. Dascălu, R.C.; Bărbulescu, A.L.; Stoica, L.E.; Dinescu, Ș.C.; Biță, C.E.; Popoviciu, H.V.; Ionescu, R.A.; Vreju, F.A. Review: A Contemporary, Multifaced Insight into Psoriasis Pathogenesis. *J. Pers. Med.* **2024**, *14*, 535. [CrossRef] [PubMed]
4. Nong, Y.; Han, G.; Hawkes, J.E. Expanding the Psoriasis Framework: Immunopathogenesis and Treatment Updates. *Cutis* **2024**, *113*, 82–91. [CrossRef]
5. de Alcantara, C.C.; Reiche, E.M.V.; Simão, A.N.C. Cytokines in psoriasis. *Adv. Clin. Chem.* **2021**, *100*, 171–204. [PubMed]
6. Huangfu, L.; Li, R.; Huang, Y.; Wang, S. The IL-17 family in diseases: From bench to bedside. *Signal Transduct. Target. Ther.* **2023**, *8*, 402–423. [CrossRef]
7. Gu, C.; Wu, L.; Li, X. IL-17 family: Cytokines, receptors and signaling. *Cytokine* **2013**, *64*, 477–485. [CrossRef] [PubMed]
8. Strychalski, M.L.; Brown, H.S.; Bishop, S.C. Cytokine Modulators in Plaque Psoriasis—A Review of Current and Prospective Biologic Therapeutic Approaches. *JAAD Int.* **2022**, *27*, 82–91. [CrossRef]
9. Erichsen, C.Y.; Jensen, P.; Kofoed, K. Biologic therapies targeting the interleukin (IL)-23/IL-17 immune axis for the treatment of moderate-to-severe plaque psoriasis: A systematic review and meta-analysis. *J. Eur. Acad. Dermatol. Venereol.* **2020**, *34*, 30–38. [CrossRef]
10. Ren, K.; Xia, Y. Lipocalin 2 Participates in the Epidermal Differentiation and Inflammatory Processes of Psoriasis. *J. Inflamm. Res.* **2022**, *15*, 2157–2166. [CrossRef]
11. Xiao, X.; Yeoh, B.S.; Vijay-Kumar, M. Lipocalin 2: An Emerging Player in Iron Homeostasis and Inflammation. *Annu. Rev. Nutr.* **2017**, *37*, 103–130. [CrossRef] [PubMed]
12. Pourani, M.R.; Abdollahimajd, F.; Zargari, O.; Shahidi Dadras, M. Soluble biomarkers for diagnosis, monitoring, and therapeutic response assessment in psoriasis. *J. Dermatol. Treat.* **2022**, *33*, 1967–1974. [CrossRef] [PubMed]

13. Asbóth, D.; Bánfi, B.; Kocsis, D.; Erdő, F. Rodent models of dermatological disorders. *Ital. J. Dermatol. Venerol.* **2024**, *159*, 303–317. [CrossRef] [PubMed]
14. Jabeen, M.; Boisgard, A.S.; Danoy, A.; El Kholti, N.; Salvi, J.P.; Boulieu, R.; Fromy, B.; Verrier, B.; Lamrayah, M. Advanced Characterization of Imiquimod-Induced Psoriasis-Like Mouse Model. *Pharmaceutics* **2020**, *12*, 789. [CrossRef] [PubMed]
15. Chuang, S.Y.; Lin, C.H.; Sung, C.T.; Fang, J.Y. Murine models of psoriasis and their usefulness for drug discovery. *Expert. Opin. Drug Discov.* **2018**, *13*, 551–562. [CrossRef] [PubMed]
16. Meyer, T.; Stockfleth, E. Clinical investigations of Toll-like receptor agonists. *Expert Opin. Investig. Drugs* **2008**, *17*, 1051–1065. [CrossRef]
17. Wride, A.M.; Chen, G.F.; Spaulding, S.L.; Tkachenko, E.; Cohen, J.M. Biologics for Psoriasis. *Dermatol. Clin.* **2024**, *42*, 339–355. [CrossRef] [PubMed]
18. Armstrong, A.W.; Read, C. Pathophysiology, Clinical Presentation, and Treatment of Psoriasis: A Review. *JAMA* **2020**, *323*, 1945–1960. [CrossRef] [PubMed]
19. Sitek, A.N.; Li, J.T.; Pongdee, T. Risks and safety of biologics: A practical guide for allergists. *World Allergy Organ J.* **2023**, *16*, 100737–100749. [CrossRef] [PubMed]
20. Kamata, M.; Tada, Y. Efficacy and Safety of Biologics for Psoriasis and Psoriatic Arthritis and Their Impact on Comorbidities: A Literature Review. *Int. J. Mol. Sci.* **2020**, *21*, 1690. [CrossRef]
21. Kamata, M.; Tada, Y. Safety of biologics in psoriasis. *J. Dermatol.* **2018**, *45*, 279–286. [CrossRef] [PubMed]
22. Dinu, M.; Tatu, A.L.; Cocoș, D.I.; Nwabudike, L.C.; Chirilov, A.M.; Stefan, C.S.; Earar, K.; Dumitriu Buzia, O. Natural Sources of Therapeutic Agents Used in Skin Conditions. *Life* **2024**, *14*, 492. [CrossRef] [PubMed]
23. Nowak-Perlak, M.; Szpadel, K.; Jabłońska, I.; Pizon, M.; Woźniak, M. Promising Strategies in Plant-Derived Treatments of Psoriasis-Update of In Vitro, In Vivo, and Clinical Trials Studies. *Molecules* **2022**, *27*, 591. [CrossRef] [PubMed]
24. Vasarri, M.; Degl'Innocenti, D. Antioxidant and Anti-Inflammatory Agents from the Sea: A Molecular Treasure for New Potential Drugs. *Mar. Drugs* **2022**, *20*, 132. [CrossRef] [PubMed]
25. Vasarri, M.; De Biasi, A.M.; Barletta, E.; Pretti, C.; Degl'Innocenti, D. An Overview of New Insights into the Benefits of the Seagrass *Posidonia oceanica* for Human Health. *Mar. Drugs* **2021**, *19*, 476. [CrossRef] [PubMed]
26. Batanouny, K.H.; Aboutabl, E.; Shabana, M.; Soliman, F. Akādīmīyat al-Baḥth al- extturncommaIlmī wa-al-Tiknūlūjiyā. In *Wild Medicinal Plants in Egpyt [i.e. Egypt]: An Inventory to Support Conservation and Sustainable Use*; Academy of Scientific Research and Technology: Cairo, Egypt; International Union for Conservation: Gland, Switzerland, 1999; pp. 1–255.
27. Vasarri, M.; Leri, M.; Barletta, E.; Ramazzotti, M.; Marzocchini, R.; Degl'Innocenti, D. Anti-inflammatory properties of the marine plant *Posidonia oceanica* (L.) Delile. *J. Ethnopharmacol.* **2020**, *247*, 112252. [CrossRef] [PubMed]
28. Micheli, L.; Vasarri, M.; Barletta, E.; Lucarini, E.; Ghelardini, C.; Degl'Innocenti, D.; Di Cesare Mannelli, L. Efficacy of *Posidonia oceanica* Extract against Inflammatory Pain: In Vivo Studies in Mice. *Mar. Drugs* **2021**, *19*, 48. [CrossRef] [PubMed]
29. Badanthadka, M.; D'Souza, L.; Salwa, F. Strain specific response of mice to IMQ-induced psoriasis. *J. Basic Clin. Physiol. Pharmacol.* **2021**, *32*, 959–968. [CrossRef] [PubMed]
30. Horváth, S.; Kemény, Á.; Pintér, E.; Gyulai, R. A Localized Aldara (5% Imiquimod)-Induced Psoriasiform Dermatitis Model in Mice Using Finn Chambers. *Curr. Protoc. Pharmacol.* **2020**, *90*, e78. [CrossRef]
31. Shinno-Hashimoto, H.; Eguchi, A.; Sakamoto, A.; Wan, X.; Hashimoto, Y.; Fujita, Y.; Mori, C.; Hatano, M.; Matsue, H.; Hashimoto, K. Effects of splenectomy on skin inflammation and psoriasis-like phenotype of imiquimod-treated mice. *Sci. Rep.* **2022**, *12*, 14738. [CrossRef]
32. Balan, R.; Grigoraș, A.; Popovici, D.; Amălinei, C. The histopathological landscape of the major psoriasiform dermatoses. *Arch. Clin. Cases* **2021**, *6*, 59–68. [CrossRef]
33. Zhu, Q.; Zhao, L.; Ding, H.; Song, J.; Zhang, Q.; Yu, S.; Wang, Y.; Wang, H. Interleukins and Psoriasis. *J. Cutan. Med. Surg.* **2024**, *28*, NP19–NP35. [CrossRef]
34. Wu, M.; Dai, C.; Zeng, F. Cellular Mechanisms of Psoriasis Pathogenesis: A Systemic Review. *Clin. Cosmet. Investig. Dermatol.* **2023**, *16*, 2503–2515. [CrossRef] [PubMed]
35. Alzahrani, S.A.; Alzamil, F.M.; Aljuhni, A.M.; Al Thaqfan, N.A.; Alqahtani, N.Y.; Alwarwari, S.A.; Alkharashi, A.A.; Alzabadin, R.A.; Alzehairi, R.A.; Alhajlah, A.A.A. Systematic Review Evaluating the Effectiveness of Several Biological Therapies for the Treatment of Skin Psoriasis. *Cureus* **2023**, *15*, e50588. [CrossRef]
36. Reid, C.; Griffiths, C.E.M. Psoriasis and Treatment: Past, Present and Future Aspects. *Acta Derm. Venereol.* **2020**, *100*, adv00032. [CrossRef] [PubMed]
37. Ben Abdallah, H.; Johansen, C.; Iversen, L. Key Signaling Pathways in Psoriasis: Recent Insights from Antipsoriatic Therapeutics. *Psoriasis* **2021**, *11*, 83–97. [CrossRef]
38. Behrangi, E.; Moodi, F.; Jafarzadeh, A.; Goodarzi, A. Paradoxical and bimodal immune-mediated dermatological side effects of TNF-α inhibitors: A comprehensive review. *Ski. Res. Technol.* **2024**, *30*, e13718. [CrossRef]
39. Valenzuela, F.; Flores, R. Immunogenicity to biological drugs in psoriasis and psoriatic arthritis. *Clinics* **2021**, *76*, e3015. [CrossRef]
40. Semele, R.; Grewal, S.; Jeengar, M.K.; Singh, T.G.; Swami, R. From Traditional Medicine to Advanced Therapeutics: The Renaissance of Phyto-nano Interventions in Psoriasis. *Recent Adv. Inflamm. Allergy Drug Discov.* **2024**, *18*, 27–42. [CrossRef] [PubMed]

41. Moudgil, K.D.; Venkatesha, S.H. The Anti-Inflammatory and Immunomodulatory Activities of Natural Products to Control Autoimmune Inflammation. *Int. J. Mol. Sci.* **2022**, *24*, 95. [CrossRef]
42. Wang, Y.; Tian, Z.; Huang, S.; Dang, N. *Tripterygium wilfordii* Hook. F. and Its Extracts for Psoriasis: Efficacy and Mechanism. *Drug Des. Dev. Ther.* **2023**, *17*, 3767–3781. [CrossRef] [PubMed]
43. Ebrahimi, B.; Baroutian, S.; Li, J.; Zhang, B.; Ying, T.; Lu, J. Combination of marine bioactive compounds and extracts for the prevention and treatment of chronic diseases. *Front. Nutr.* **2023**, *9*, 1047026. [CrossRef] [PubMed]
44. Vaou, N.; Stavropoulou, E.; Voidarou, C.C.; Tsakris, Z.; Rozos, G.; Tsigalou, C.; Bezirtzoglou, E. Interactions between Medical Plant-Derived Bioactive Compounds: Focus on Antimicrobial Combination Effects. *Antibiotics* **2022**, *11*, 1014. [CrossRef] [PubMed]
45. Nasim, N.; Sandeep, I.S.; Mohanty, S. Plant-derived natural products for drug discovery: Current approaches and prospects. *Nucleus* **2022**, *65*, 399–411. [CrossRef] [PubMed]
46. Yang, Y.; Zhang, Z.; Li, S.; Ye, X.; Li, X.; He, K. Synergy effects of herb extracts: Pharmacokinetics and pharmacodynamic basis. *Fitoterapia* **2014**, *92*, 133–147. [CrossRef] [PubMed]
47. Zhou, L.; Luo, N.; Zhong, X.; Xu, T.; Hao, P. The immunoregulatory effects of natural products on psoriasis via its action on Th17 cells versus regulatory T cells balance. *Int. Immunopharmacol.* **2022**, *110*, 109032. [CrossRef]
48. Yang, Y.; Zhao, Y.; Lai, R.; Xian, L.; Lei, Q.; Xu, J.; Guo, M.; Xian, D.; Zhong, J. An Emerging Role of *Proanthocyanidins* on Psoriasis: Evidence from a Psoriasis-Like Mouse Model. *Oxidative Med. Cell. Longev.* **2022**, *2022*, 5800586. [CrossRef]
49. Barletta, E.; Ramazzotti, M.; Fratianni, F.; Pessani, D.; Degl'Innocenti, D. Hydrophilic extract from *Posidonia oceanica* inhibits activity and expression of gelatinases and prevents HT1080 human fibrosarcoma cell line invasion. *Cell Adhes. Migr.* **2015**, *9*, 422–431. [CrossRef]
50. Wang, Q.; Yan, D.; Zheng, S.; Li, M.; Li, J.; Fu, X.; Fu, D.; Hu, H.; Song, X.; Tian, Z. Cytokine Profiles and the Relationship of Disease Severity in Patients with Psoriasis. *Indian J. Dermatol.* **2022**, *67*, 204–211.
51. Preedy, M.K.; White, M.R.H.; Tergaonkar, V. Cellular heterogeneity in TNF/TNFR1 signalling: Live cell imaging of cell fate decisions in single cells. *Cell Death Dis.* **2024**, *15*, 202–213. [CrossRef]
52. Tomar, Y.; Gorantla, S.; Singhvi, G. Insight into the pivotal role of signaling pathways in psoriasis pathogenesis, potential therapeutic molecules and drug delivery approaches. *Drug Discov. Today* **2023**, *28*, 103465–103475. [CrossRef] [PubMed]
53. Ubago-Rodríguez, A.; Quiñones-Vico, M.I.; Sánchez-Díaz, M.; Sanabria-de la Torre, R.; Sierra-Sánchez, Á.; Montero-Vílchez, T.; Fernández-González, A.; Arias-Santiago, S. Challenges in Psoriasis Research: A Systematic Review of Preclinical Models. *Dermatology* **2024**. [CrossRef]
54. Bocheńska, K.; Smolińska, E.; Moskot, M.; Jakóbkiewicz-Banecka, J.; Gabig-Cimińska, M. Models in the Research Process of Psoriasis. *Int. J. Mol. Sci.* **2017**, *18*, 2514. [CrossRef] [PubMed]
55. Wang, X.; Liu, Q.; Wu, L.; Nie, Z.; Mei, Z. Risk of non-melanoma skin cancer in patients with psoriasis: An updated evidence from systematic review with meta-analysis. *J. Cancer* **2020**, *11*, 1047–1055. [CrossRef]
56. Verdelli, A.; Caproni, M.; Coi, A.; Corrà, A.; Degl'Innocenti, D.; Vasarri, M.; Quintarelli, L.; Volpi, V.; Cipollini, E.M.; Barletta, E. Neutrophil Gelatinase-Associated Lipocalin as Potential Predictive Biomarker of Melanoma and Non-Melanoma Skin Cancers in Psoriatic Patients: A Pilot Study. *Int. J. Mol. Sci.* **2022**, *23*, 12291. [CrossRef] [PubMed]
57. Kilkenny, C.; Browne, W.; Cuthill, I.C.; Emerson, M.; Altman, D.G.; NC3Rs Reporting Guidelines Working Group. Animal research: Reporting in vivo experiments: The ARRIVE guidelines. *Br. J. Pharmacol.* **2010**, *160*, 1577–1579. [CrossRef]
58. McGrath, J.C.; Lilley, E. Implementing guidelines on reporting research using animals (ARRIVE etc.): New requirements for publication in BJP. *Br. J. Pharmacol.* **2015**, *172*, 3189–3193. [CrossRef]
59. Leri, M.; Ramazzotti, M.; Vasarri, M.; Peri, S.; Barletta, E.; Pretti, C.; Degl'Innocenti, D. Bioactive Compounds from *Posidonia oceanica* (L.) Delile Impair Malignant Cell Migration through Autophagy Modulation. *Mar. Drugs* **2018**, *16*, 137. [CrossRef]
60. van der Fits, L.; Mourits, S.; Voerman, J.S.; Kant, M.; Boon, L.; Laman, J.D.; Cornelissen, F.; Mus, A.M.; Florencia, E.; Prens, E.P.; et al. Imiquimod-induced psoriasis-like skin inflammation in mice is mediated via the IL-23/IL-17 axis. *J. Immunol.* **2009**, *182*, 5836–5845. [CrossRef]
61. Kawashima, Y.; Kodera, Y.; Singh, A.; Matsumoto, M.; Matsumoto, H. Efficient extraction of proteins from formalin-fixed paraffin-embedded tissues requires higher concentration of tris(hydroxymethyl)aminomethane. *Clin. Proteom.* **2014**, *11*, 4. [CrossRef]
62. Lowry, O.H.; Rosebrough, N.J.; Farr, A.L.; Randall, R.J. Protein measurement with the Folin phenol reagent. *J. Biol. Chem.* **1951**, *193*, 265–275. [CrossRef] [PubMed]

Disclaimer/Publisher's Note: The statements, opinions and data contained in all publications are solely those of the individual author(s) and contributor(s) and not of MDPI and/or the editor(s). MDPI and/or the editor(s) disclaim responsibility for any injury to people or property resulting from any ideas, methods, instructions or products referred to in the content.

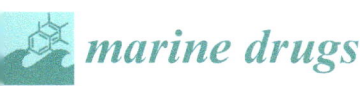

Article

Phytochemical Composition, Anti-Inflammatory Property, and Anti-Atopic Effect of *Chaetomorpha linum* Extract

Luisa Frusciante [1], Michela Geminiani [1,2,*], Alfonso Trezza [1], Tommaso Olmastroni [1], Pierfrancesco Mastroeni [1], Laura Salvini [3], Stefania Lamponi [1,2], Andrea Bernini [1], Daniela Grasso [1], Elena Dreassi [1], Ottavia Spiga [1,2,4] and Annalisa Santucci [1,2,4]

1. Dipartimento di Biotecnologie Chimica e Farmacia, Università di Siena, Via Aldo Moro, 53100 Siena, Italy; luisa.frusciante@unisi.it (L.F.); alfonso.trezza2@unisi.it (A.T.); tommaso.olmastroni@student.unisi.it (T.O.); p.mastroeni@student.unisi.it (P.M.); stefania.lamponi@unisi.it (S.L.); andrea.bernini@unisi.it (A.B.); daniela.grasso@student.unisi.it (D.G.); elena.dreassi@unisi.it (E.D.); ottavia.spiga@unisi.it (O.S.); annalisa.santucci@unisi.it (A.S.)
2. SienabioACTIVE, Università di Siena, Via Aldo Moro, 53100 Siena, Italy
3. Fondazione Toscana Life Sciences, Strada del Petriccio e Belriguardo, 53100 Siena, Italy; l.salvini@toscanalifesciences.org
4. Advanced Robotics and Enabling Digital TEchnologies & Systems 4.0 (ARTES 4.0), Viale Rinaldo Piaggio, 34, 56025 Pontedera, Italy
* Correspondence: geminiani2@unisi.it; Tel.: +39-0577-232534

Abstract: Utilizing plant-based resources, particularly their by-products, aligns with sustainability principles and circular bioeconomy, contributing to environmental preservation. The therapeutic potential of plant extracts is garnering increasing interest, and this study aimed to demonstrate promising outcomes from an extract obtained from an underutilized plant waste. *Chaetomorpha linum*, an invasive macroalga found in the Orbetello Lagoon, thrives in eutrophic conditions, forming persistent mats covering approximately 400 hectares since 2005. The biomass of *C. linum* undergoes mechanical harvesting and is treated as waste, requiring significant human efforts and economic resources—A critical concern for municipalities. Despite posing challenges to local ecosystems, the study identified *C. linum* as a natural source of bioactive metabolites. Phytochemical characterization revealed lipids, amino acids, and other compounds with potential anti-inflammatory activity in *C. linum* extract. In vitro assays with LPS-stimulated RAW 264.7 and TNF-α/IFN-γ-stimulated HaCaT cells showed the extract inhibited reactive oxygen species (ROS), nitric oxide (NO), and prostaglandin E2 (PGE2) productions, and reduced inducible nitric oxide synthase (iNOS) and cyclooxygenase-2 (COX-2) expressions via NF-κB nuclear translocation, in RAW 264.7 cells. It also reduced chemokines (TARC/CCL17, RANTES/CCL5, MCP-1/CCL2, and IL-8) and the cytokine IL-1β production in HaCaT cells, suggesting potential as a therapeutic candidate for chronic diseases like atopic dermatitis. Finally, in silico studies indicated palmitic acid as a significant contributor to the observed effect. This research not only uncovered the untapped potential of *C. linum* but also laid the foundation for its integration into the circular bioeconomy, promoting sustainable practices, and innovative applications across various industries.

Keywords: *Chaetomorpha linum*; macroalgae; UPLC-MS/MS; inflammation; RAW 264.7; HaCaT; atopic dermatitis; molecular modeling

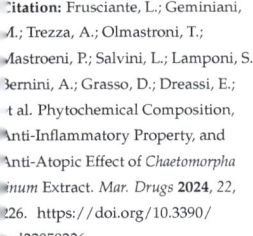

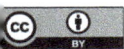

1. Introduction

Marine macroalgae, commonly called seaweeds, and their extracts have become increasingly important in developing nutraceutical products. This is attributed to their substantial content of bioactive compounds, which has captured considerable attention within the pharmaceutical industry as a valuable source of raw materials. Indeed, the high level of biodiversity of marine macroalgae makes them a considerable reservoir for active compounds, given their ability to produce a diverse range of secondary metabolites characterized by a broad spectrum of biological activities [1–4].

Currently, plant metabolites make up a significant portion of the pharmaceutical industry's revenue, and using plant materials as a source of bioactive compounds is of great economic importance [5,6]. Natural bioactive compounds derived from marine organisms, particularly invasive algal species, have garnered increased attention in scientific research due to their abundance and wide availability. Seaweeds are the ocean's living resources. Despite their widespread use in the food and feed industries, they are untapped as nutraceutical and medicinal products despite their significant antioxidative qualities. However, macroalgae are increasingly viewed as a source of secondary metabolites with great potential for developing new drugs. Many previous studies demonstrated the remarkable benefits of macroalgae on human health and protection against chronic diseases due to their content of proteins, lipids, fatty acids, polysaccharides, and antioxidant compounds [2,7–9]. Moreover, removing their biomass from invaded environments offers an exceptionally promising potential resource.

This study aimed to investigate the phytochemical composition and biological properties of an extract obtained from the invasive macroalga *Chaetomorpha linum* in LPS-stimulated RAW 264.7 murine macrophages and TNF-α/IFN-γ-stimulated HaCaT human keratinocytes. In silico studies were performed to obtain 3D structures of the entire RAW 264.7 and HaCaT anti-inflammatory target complement, and docking simulations provided findings about potential target/compound interactions. *C. linum* (Müller) Kützing (Basyonim: *Conferva linum* O.F. Müll.) is a macroalgae species in the Chlorophyceae family. It commonly manifests in opportunistic vegetative blooms, thriving in eutrophic environments, especially in ample orthophosphate availability [10]. *C. linum* mats exhibit remarkable resilience and tenacity, presenting significant challenges for their removal. Flourishing since 2005 in the Orbetello Lagoon of Tuscany, Italy, these mats form dense, self-sustaining coverings over approximately 400 hectares. With biomass levels ranging between 2 and 24 kg m^{-2} and the region experiencing mild winters, the mats' surfaces undergo nearly continuous growth. Their persistence poses challenges for local ecosystems, impacting water quality and the local fishing industry [10,11]. Furthermore, these biomasses are mechanically harvested and treated as waste, requiring significant human efforts and considerable financial resources, which are crucial for local governments. In the Orbetello Lagoon, from 2002 to 2006, an average of 27,098.02 tons (6774 tons per year) of macroalgae were harvested, incurring expenses of about 600,000 Euros per year [12]. However, macroalgae represents a potential resource.

Various potential uses have been explored for algae from the Orbetello Lagoon over the past decade. Among these, biodiesel production stands out as an intriguing alternative to fossil fuels, offering a sustainable energy supply that reduces greenhouse gas emissions and promotes efficiency [13]. The biomass of macrophytes has been utilized in the past for the production of bio-oil, yielding promising results in terms of extraction efficiency [12]; nonetheless, similar approaches applied to macroalgae from the Orbetello Lagoon have proven less efficient [14].

Therefore, this study aimed to contribute to the development of the "circular bioeconomy" mission by exploring possible biotechnological applications for *C. linum* harvested from the Orbetello Lagoon, particularly in the pharmaceutical and cosmeceutical sectors. Inflammatory responses and oxidative stress have recently emerged as significant factors in the pathogenesis and progression of various chronic, non-communicable diseases [15]. Among them, allergic diseases, including allergic rhinitis, food allergy, allergic asthma, atopic dermatitis, and eczema, are systemic conditions whose escalating incidence rates have become a growing concern [16], highlighting the need for comprehensive understanding and effective management strategies [17–19]. Common treatments for atopic dermatitis, such as corticosteroids, calcineurin inhibitors, and antihistamines, often result in significant side effects when used over long periods [20–23]. This emphasizes the potential of natural plant-derived remedies, which offer effective treatment with minimal adverse effects. Such botanical alternatives present a safer option for managing skin inflammation, with the potential to reduce or eliminate the occurrence of side effects [24]. In recent years, there has been a steady increase in the prevalence of allergic diseases [25–27]. Evidence suggests that cutaneous inflammatory conditions typically progress to more systemic inflammatory diseases such as allergic rhinitis and asthma, a phenomenon referred to as the "atopic march" [28–30]. Furthermore, the growing field of "cosmeceuticals", a recently coined term to describe products that blend cosmetic and pharmaceutical properties, refers to products capable of enhancing or altering skin functions and appearance, thereby providing skin benefits [31]. This expanding sector is renowned for its innovative approach, constantly searching for active molecules with improved properties to counteract undesired effects, primarily by integrating natural resources into cosmetic formulations. Natural resources present numerous advantages, including environmental friendliness, reduced toxicity, non-carcinogenic properties, accessibility, minimal side effects, and economic benefits [32,33]. With a specific focus on its anti-inflammatory properties, the objective was to repurpose and add value to *C. linum's* strategic and valuable biomass.

2. Results

2.1. Chemical Composition of C. linum Extract

The extraction process plays a key role in the recovery of biomolecules from natural matrices, as it affects their quality and quantity. There are several methodologies applicable for the extraction of bioactive compounds, and their choice is based on the chemical and physical characteristics of the molecules of interest as well as the starting raw material. Heat-reflux extraction of 10 g of oven-dried pulverized *C. linum* algae collected from the Orbetello lagoon with an ethanol–water (70:30 v/v) mixture produced 1.247 g of freeze-dried *C. linum* ethanolic (CLE) dry extract, resulting in a percentage yield of 12.47% (w/w). In order to assess the effectiveness of ethanol–water extraction, the crude extracts were subjected to NMR testing, where the molecular classes and relative fractions were closely examined. Proton NMR spectrum revealed the presence of both saturated and unsaturated fatty acids through a set of broad peaks that had a higher intensity (Figure S1) when compared to the peaks of polar species. Although peaks indicating amino acids, sugar, and aromatics were also detected, their presence was much lesser. These results suggested that the CLE dry extract was significantly enriched in fatty acid contents as compared to polar metabolites. Based on this evidence, further characterization of the mixture by proper separation methods was initiated.

2.1.1. UPLC-MS/MS Analysis

CLE extract was profiled by UPLC-MS/MS. A total of 19 metabolites were identified using Compound Discoverer 3.3 software integrated using the ChemSpider database and the mzCloud for data processing and compared with the literature data [34,35]. Overall, most of the metabolites detected in CLE were lipids, with compounds identified as free fatty acids (MUFA 18:1ω-9 Oleic acid, PUFA 18:4ω-3 stearidonic acid) and fatty acids derivatives. Matched metabolites were listed in Table 1, along with their retention time, molecular formulae, observed and theoretical m/z, and error (ppm). For all matched compounds, the error was lower than 5 ppm. Among them, one was a palmitic acid monoacylglycerol (MAG)-derivative (Palmitin), three were identified as hydroxy-derivatives of saturated fatty acids (Hydroxymyristic acid, Hydroxylauric acid, and Dihydroxypalmitic acid), two PUFA 18:3n-3 Alpha-linoleic acid-derived oxylipins (9(10)-EpODE, Hydroxylinoleic acid), a fatty acid amide (Lauramide), and a fatty aldehyde (8-Pentadecenal). The other matched metabolites were identified as amino acids (Valine, Norleucine, and Thymine), terpenes (Carnosic acid, Rosmanol, and Methyl dehydroabietate), and flavonoids (Kaempferol, Apigenin, and 3′-O-Methylequol).

Table 1. Matched metabolites in *Chaetomorpha linum* ethanolic extract.

Chemical Class	Name	Retention Time (min)	Formula	Calculated MW	m/z	Reference Ion	Mass Error (ppm)
Lipids	Palmitin	41.679	$C_{19}H_{38}O_4$	330.2777	331.2849	$[M+H]^+$	1.99
	Oleic acid	50.271	$C_{18}H_{34}O_2$	282.2555	281.2482	$[M-H]^-$	−1.54
	Stearidonic acid	24.921	$C_{18}H_{28}O_2$	276.2094	277.2167	$[M+H]^+$	1.81
	Hydroxymyristic acid	40.396	$C_{14}H_{28}O_3$	244.2033	243.196	$[M-H]^-$	−2.14
	Hydroxylauric acid	35.009	$C_{12}H_{24}O_3$	216.172	215.1647	$[M-H]^-$	−2.61
	Dihydroxypalmitic acid	37.957	$C_{16}H_{34}O_4$	290.2461	291.2534	$[M+H]^+$	1.38
	9(10)-EpODE	38.428	$C_{18}H_{30}O_3$	294.2204	295.2276	$[M+H]^+$	2.9
	Hydroxylinoleic acid	40.866	$C_{18}H_{32}O_3$	296.236	297.2432	$[M+H]^+$	2.8
	Lauramide	35.481	$C_{12}H_{25}NO$	199.1942	200.2014	$[M+H]^+$	2.71
	8-Pentadecenal	41.627	$C_{15}H_{28}O$	224.2136	223.2063	$[M-H]^-$	−2.03
Amino acids	Valine	2.043	$C_5H_{11}NO_2$	117.0793	118.0866	$[M+H]^+$	2.5
	Norleucine	1.877	$C_6H_{13}NO_2$	131.0948	132.1021	$[M+H]^+$	1.18
	Thymine	8.042	$C_5H_6N_2O_2$	126.0433	127.0505	$[M+H]^+$	2.52
Terpenoids	Carnosic acid	31.801	$C_{20}H_{28}O_4$	332.1984	333.2056	$[M+H]^+$	−1.23
	Rosmanol	28.817	$C_{20}H_{26}O_5$	346.1783	347.1856	$[M+H]^+$	0.89
	Methyl dehydroabietate	40.729	$C_{21}H_{30}O_2$	314.2241	315.2313	$[M+H]^+$	−1.7
Flavonoids	Kaempferol	12.302	$C_{15}H_{10}O_6$	286.0479	285.0407	$[M-H]^-$	0.66
	Apigenin	32.899	$C_{15}H_{10}O_5$	270.0532	269.0459	$[M-H]^-$	1.42
	3′-O-Methylequol	23.484	$C_{16}H_{16}O_4$	272.1052	271.0979	$[M-H]^-$	1.06

Note: MW —molecular weight; EpODE—epoxyoctadecadienoic acid.

2.1.2. GC-FID Analysis

CLE fatty acid pattern was further evaluated by GC-FID. The chromatographic profile and fatty acid methyl esters identified in CLE were reported in Figure 1 and Table 2, respectively.

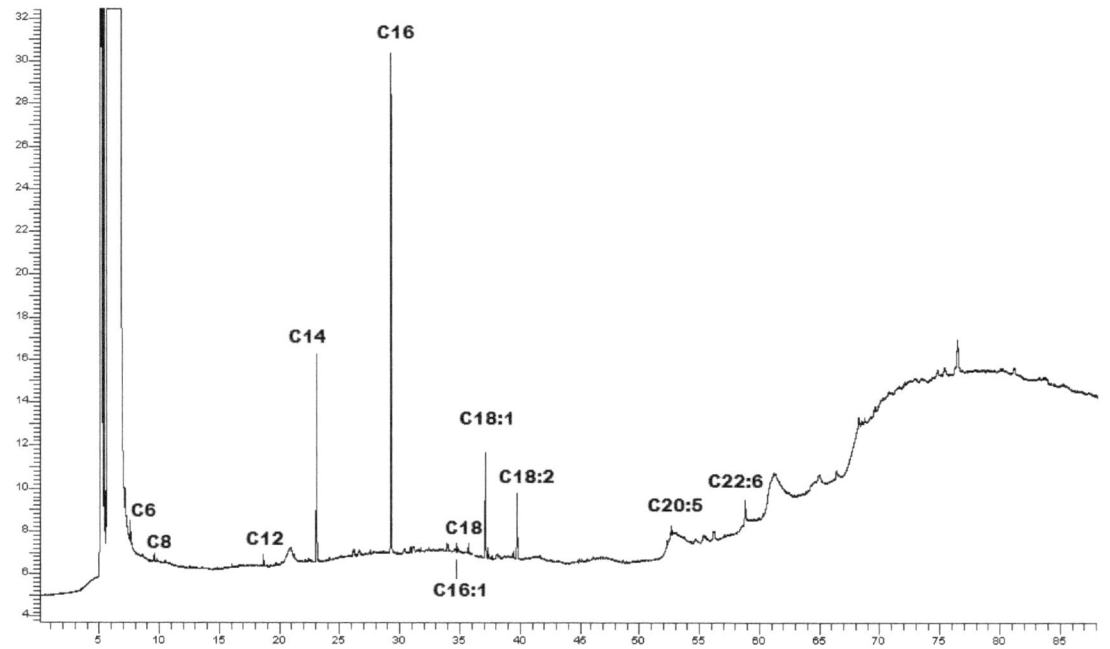

Figure 1. Chromatographic profile of CLE.

Table 2. Fatty acid methyl esters identified in CLE.

Fatty Acid	RT (min)	Area % *
Caproic acid C6:0	7.21	1.66 ± 0.19
Caprylic acid C8:0	9.53	0.33 ± 0.06
Lauric acid C12:0	18.68	1.06 ± 0.08
Tridecanoic acid C13:0	20.16	1.38 ± 0.09
Myristic C14:0	23.09	20.46 ± 2.12
Palmitic acid C16:0	29.27	52.18 ± 1.87
Palmitoleic acid C16:1	31.09	1.14 ± 0.15
Stearic acid C18:0	35.51	1.00 ± 0.07
Oleic acid C18:1	37.12	11.70 ± 1.24
Linoleic acid C18:2	39.74	7.35 ± 1.42
Eicosapentanoic acid C20:5	52.62	0.24 ± 0.05
Docosahexaenoic acid C22:6	58.81	2.65 ± 0.18

* % values were expressed in mean ± sd (n = 3).

The analysis revealed that the predominant fatty acid in CLE was palmitic acid (16:0) (52.18%), followed by myristic acid (14:0) (20.46%), and oleic acid (18:1ω9) (11.70%).

2.2. The Effect of CLE on Cell Viability of RAW 264.7 and HaCaT Cells

First, to exclude any cytotoxic effect of CLE, the viability of RAW 264.7 and HaCaT cells was measured with MTT and CCK-8 assay, respectively. The findings indicated that CLE was not cytotoxic at concentrations up to 100 µg/mL; a minor reduction in viability was observed at a concentration of 100 µg/mL after 24 h of treatment (Figure 2).

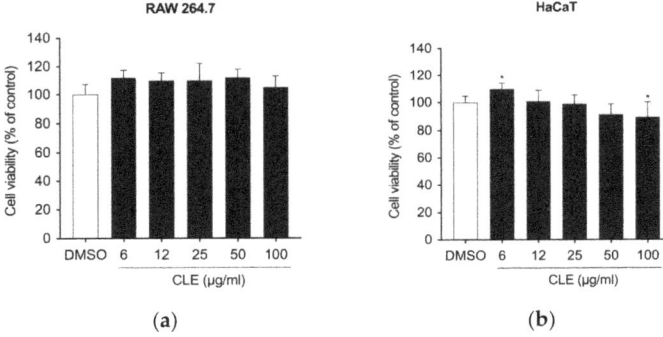

Figure 2. The effects of CLE on the viability of (**a**) RAW 264.7 and (**b**) HaCaT cells. After culturing the cells with CLE (0, 6, 12, 25, 50, and 100 µg/mL), cell viability was measured with the MTT and CCK-8 assays, respectively, after 24 h. All data showed mean ± SD values of three independent experiments. Statistically significant differences were denoted by * $p \leq 0.0207$ (vs. DMSO). p-values were calculated using one-way ANOVA with Dunnett's post hoc test.

2.3. The Effects of CLE on Inflammatory Mediators in LPS-Stimulated RAW 264.7 Cells

Reactive oxygen species (ROS) serve as signaling molecules crucial in the development of inflammatory disorders [36]. Therefore, we investigated the impact of pretreating RAW 264.7 cells stimulated with LPS with CLE on intracellular ROS production. Dexamethasone (DEX) at a concentration of 5 µg/mL was chosen as a reference for assessing anti-inflammatory efficacy. The cells were pre-treated with DEX and with varying concentrations of CLE (25, 50, and 100 µg/mL) before being stimulated with LPS. Treatment with DEX resulted in a statistically significant reduction in ROS production level in stimulated RAW 264.7 cells (Figure 3a), a decrease that was also evident following treatment with all tested concentrations of CLE. Notably, CLE demonstrated a significantly superior effect compared to 5 µg/mL DEX at all concentrations.

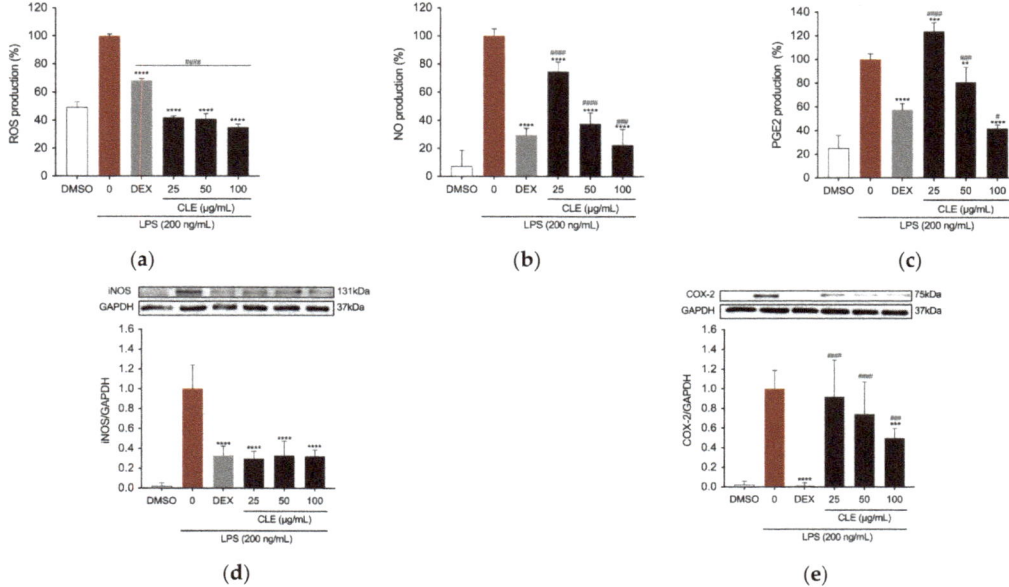

Figure 3. The effects of CLE on LPS-induced ROS, NO, and PGE2 production, and iNOS and COX-2 protein expression levels in RAW264.7 cells: (**a**) Intracellular ROS level was quantified after pretreatment with different concentrations of CLE followed by LPS stimulation (200 ng/mL) for 5 h. Data were presented as bar graphs for ROS level measured from relative fluorescence intensity normalized to cell count with Crystal Violet assay. Culture supernatants of RAW 264.7 cells pretreated with DEX or CLE for 4 h and then stimulated with 200 ng/mL LPS for 24 h were analyzed for (**b**) NO and (**c**) PGE2 production. iNOS (**d**) and COX-2 (**e**) expression levels were determined by Western blotting. All data showed mean ± SD values of three independent experiments. Statistically significant differences were denoted by ** $p = 0.0039$, *** $p = 0.0005$, and **** $p < 0.0001$ (vs. LPS). # $p = 0.0231$, ### $p \leq 0.0009$, and #### $p < 0.0001$ (vs. DEX as positive control). p-values were calculated using one-way ANOVA with Tukey's post hoc test.

A key response of RAW 264.7 cells to inflammatory stimuli was the secretion of proinflammatory cytokines and mediators, with nitric oxide (NO) being particularly notable. To assess CLE's anti-inflammatory properties, we measured NO levels in the culture supernatants of both untreated and CLE-treated LPS-stimulated RAW 264.7 cells with Griess assay. Positive control was achieved by treating the cells as described previously. Cells treated with LPS exhibited elevated levels of NO. Conversely, in the presence of CLE, there was a concentration-dependent reduction in NO production (Figure 3b). Specifically, CLE at concentrations of 25 and 50 µg/mL significantly reduced NO levels in LPS-stimulated RAW cells. Furthermore, treatment with 100 µg/mL CLE resulted in a decrease in NO level significantly greater than the positive control. Interestingly, CLE at concentrations of 50 and 100 µg/mL also inhibited PGE2 level in the supernatant of RAW 264.7 cells, with the highest concentration tested exhibiting an effect superior to the positive control (Figure 3c).

To further investigate the anti-inflammatory mechanism of CLE, the protein expression of iNOS and COX-2, precursor enzymes of NO and PGE2, respectively, was assessed using Western blotting. As reported in Figure 3d,e, the expression of iNOS and COX-2 was upregulated in the LPS-treated group. However, this increase was inhibited by CLE.

2.4. The Effect of CLE on NF-κB Activation in LPS-Stimulated RAW 264.7 Cells

The study examined whether CLE could hamper the activation of the NF-κB pathway, as the regulation of inflammatory mediators in LPS-stimulated macrophages involves NF-κB activated transcriptional processes [37]. Western blotting for NF-κB was conducted to verify whether CLE can suppress the nuclear translocation of NF-κB. Exposure to LPS alone increased the amount of NF-κB in the nucleus (Figure 4a). However, CLE at 100 μg/mL significantly inhibited increased levels of nuclear NF-κB p65 compared to the LPS group, with an effect comparable to that of DEX positive control ($p = 0.801$). The analysis of NF-κB localization by immunofluorescence staining and colocalization analysis confirmed that in untreated RAW 264.7 cells, the p65 protein was localized outside the nucleus. LPS stimulation induced the translocation of p65 from outside to inside the nucleus. However, DEX and CLE retained NF-κB in the cytoplasm of cells (Figure 4b).

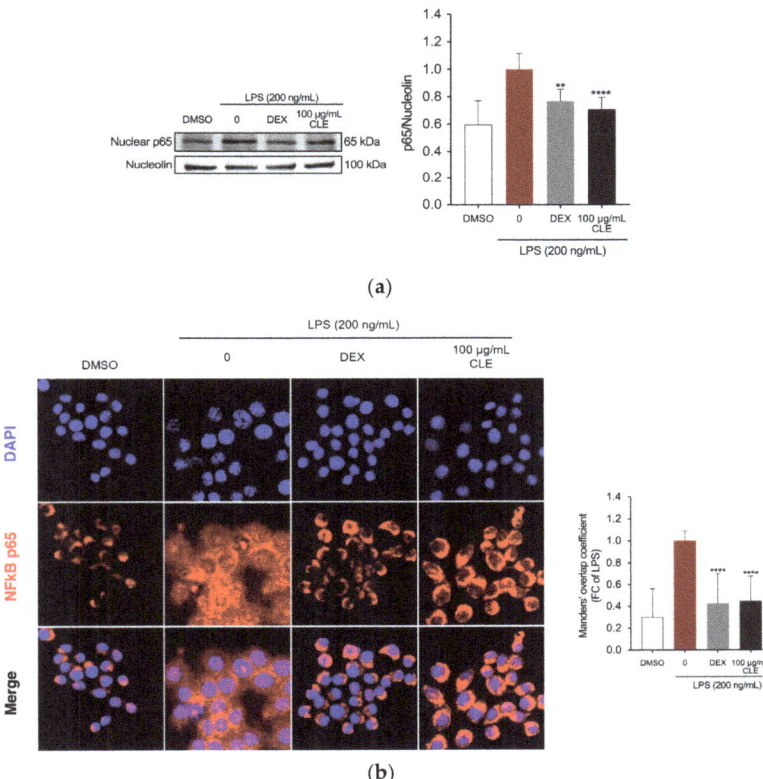

Figure 4. The effects of CLE on suppressing the upstream signaling for NF-κB activation in LPS-induced RAW264.7 cells. Cells were pre-treated with DEX or CLE for 4 h and then incubated with LPS (200 ng/mL) for 1 h. (**a**) NF-κB in LPS-stimulated RAW264.7 cells using Western blotting. Quantification of relative band intensities from three independent experimental results determined by densitometry. Data were presented as mean ± SD of three independent experiments. ** $p = 0.016$, **** $p < 0.0001$ (vs. LPS). (**b**) Localization of NF-κB visualized by a fluorescent microscope after staining for NF-κB (red). The nuclei of cells were stained with DAPI (blue). The bar graph shows the quantification (using Manders' coefficient) of NF-κB p65 co-localization with DAPI. **** $p < 0.0001$ (vs. LPS). Micrographs were captured with 40× magnification.

2.5. CLE Reduced Inflammation in TNF-α/IFN-γ Insulted HaCaT Cells

To investigate the therapeutic potential of CLE against skin inflammatory disorders, we assessed its protective effect on inflammatory responses in HaCaT human keratinocytes. Considering the results obtained from the CCK-8 assay, which indicated a slight decrease in cell viability of HaCaT cells following treatment with CLE at a concentration of 100 µg/mL, we proceeded with our investigations only using concentrations of 25 and 50 µg/mL. The cells were pretreated with concentrations of CLE for 4 h, followed by treatment with TNF-α/IFN-γ at 10 ng/mL for 24 h. Treatment with CLE at concentrations of 25 and 50 µg/mL significantly decreased the production of TARC/CCL17, RANTES/CCL5, and IL-8 in the supernatant of TNF-α/IFN-γ-induced HaCaT cells (Figure 5a–c). Additionally, the concentration of 50 µg/mL was capable of reducing the levels of the chemokine MCP-1/CCL2 and the cytokine IL-1β (Figure 5d,e).

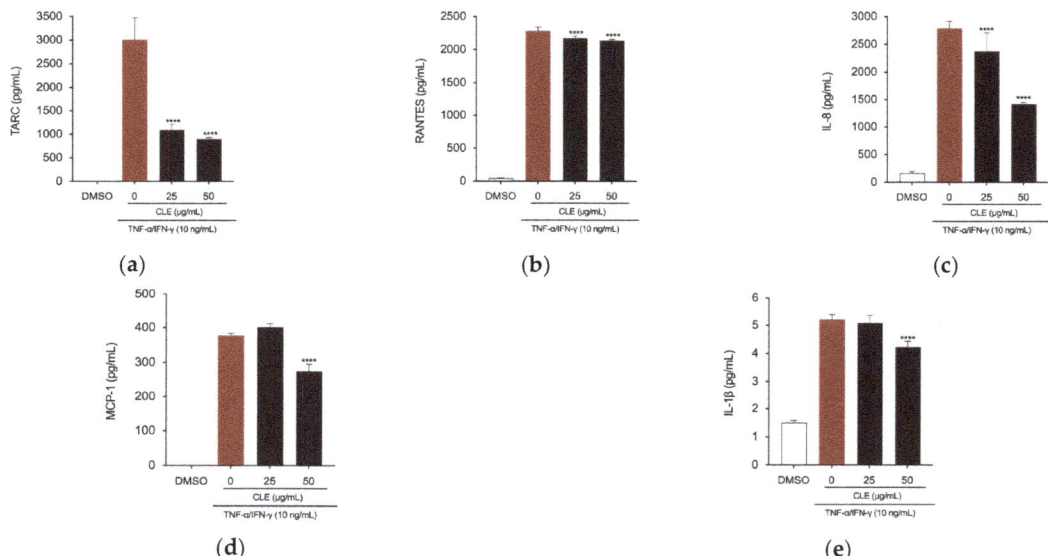

Figure 5. The effects of CLE on TNF-α/INF-γ-induced production of pro-inflammatory chemokines (upper) and cytokines (lower) in HaCaT cells. After pre-treating the cells with DEX or CLE for 4 h, cells were stimulated with 10 ng/mL TNF-α/INF-γ for 24 h. Levels of (**a**) TARC/CCL17, (**b**) RANTES/CCL5, (**c**) IL-8, (**d**) MCP-1/CCL2, and (**e**) IL-1β were measured using ELISA kits. Data showed mean ± SD values of three independent experiments. **** $p < 0.0001$ (vs. 10 ng/mL TNF-α/INF-γ). p-values were calculated using one-way ANOVA with Dunnett's post hoc test.

2.6. Mutagenicity Assay: Ames Test

Six distinct CLE concentrations were evaluated by the Ames test on TA98 and TA100 bacteria, both with and without S9 metabolic activation, in the Salmonella mutagenicity assay. The findings regarding the mutagenic impact of the specimens, as reported in Figure 6a,b, showed that CLE was non-genotoxic to TA98 and TA100 at all concentrations examined, both in the presence and absence of S9 fraction. Indeed, the number of revertants was smaller and significantly different from the positive control at the maximum concentration (1000 µg/mL) ($p \leq 0.01$). In every instance, the background level and positive control levels fell within the typical range observed in our lab.

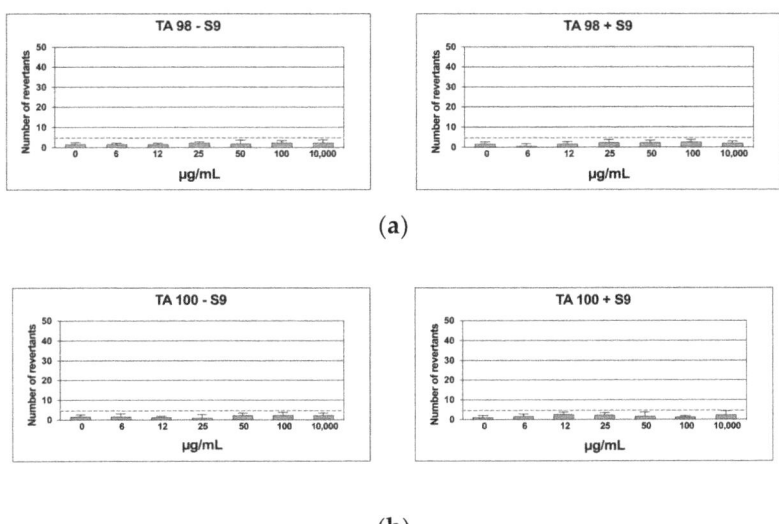

Figure 6. The number of revertants in TA98 (**a**) and TA100 (**b**) *S. typhimurium* strain exposed to different concentrations of CLE with S9 fraction and without S9 fraction. The results were reported as the mean of revertants $\pm$ SD; $n = 6$; $p \leq 0.01$.

2.7. In Silico Results

Target/Compound Virtual Screening

To identify potential targets involved in the interaction with CLE compounds, a ligand-based virtual screening was performed against the entire RAW264.7 and HaCaT cells anti-inflammatory target complement identified from the "target section" in the DrugBank database. Our study identified 53 targets indirectly or directly involved with the cell's anti-inflammatory condition for both cell lines. Each primary structure was downloaded from the UniProt database. To verify the availability of target 3D structures, a multiple sequence alignment (MSA) was performed using BLASTp against the "Protein Data Bank" database. Based on the MSA results, we obtained and downloaded a total of 35 protein 3D structures (Table S1).

Each structure was optimized through molecular modeling to resolve potential structural gaps and steric clashes; subsequently, virtual screening was performed among all targets and compounds extracted from our natural source. To standardize our analyses and enhance the reliability of our in silico results, we adopted two different strategies to select the best three complexes: (i) binding free energy (docking score) and (ii) evolution approach considering the interaction network consensus binding residues, as suggested in previous work [38]. As a result of the virtual screening, we selected the first three complexes with the highest binding free energy: the catalytic domain of human phosphodiesterase 3b (PDB code: 1SO2), the crystal structure of PDE4A10 (PDB code: 2QYK), and the crystal structure of PDE4C2 (PDB code: 2QYM). In detail, 1SO2/PA, 2QYK/PA, and 2QYM/PA complexes showed binding energies of -6.9 kcal/mol, -6.7 kcal/mol, and -6.5 kcal/mol, respectively. Interaction network analyses revealed that palmitic acid formed a wide polar and hydrophobic interaction network within the target binding pocket (Figure 7).

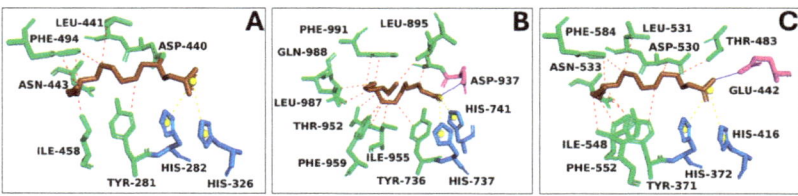

Figure 7. The overview of target/palmitic acid complexes. Three-dimensional structures of (**A**) PDE4C2 (PDB code: 2QYM), (**B**) PDE3B (PDB code: 1SO2), and (**C**) PDE4A10 (PDB code: 2QYK), in complex with palmitic acid represented in brown sticks. The binding residues involved in hydrophobic interactions, hydrogen bonds, and salt bridges were represented as green, pink, and blue sticks, respectively. Hydrophobic interactions were reported as red dotted lines, hydrogen bonds as a continuous blue line, and salt bridges as yellow dotted lines, with the charge center represented as a yellow sphere.

3. Discussion

The importance of developing new anti-inflammatory agents from natural sources is widely acknowledged today and represents a critical imperative to pursue. Seaweeds in this regard, have been suggested as promising anti-inflammatory candidates due to their composition of lipids, phenolic compounds, carotenoids, phytosterols, alkaloids and polysaccharides. In this study, we evaluated the anti-inflammatory activity and phytochemical composition of a hydroalcoholic extract obtained from the green macroalga *C. linum*, an invasive species in the Orbetello Lagoon (Tuscany, Italy), to determine the potential reuse of this "waste" that would otherwise require costly biomass treatment and management.

Plants can produce a variety of secondary (specialized) metabolites with significant biological activity due to their need to adapt to environmental changes. This is especially true for algae, which must ensure survival in one of the harshest and everchanging environments. As a result, even within the same species or depending on meteorological conditions and harvesting period, the production of metabolites varies significantly [3]. Because of this characteristic, analyzing the chemical composition of algae is particularly challenging. Yet, it makes them ideal contenders for screening candidate compounds with bioactive potential. While data concerning the anti-inflammatory activity of *C. linum* species remains limited, and comprehensive investigations into the phytochemical composition of *C. linum* from the Orbetello Lagoon are lacking; previous studies examined samples from various regions of the Mediterranean Sea for their lipid content. These studies reported different lipidic profiles for *C. linum* from different origins [7,8,35,39–41], thereby positioning it as an attractive candidate for further exploration of its potential anti-inflammatory properties.

Recent studies on *Chlorophyta* of genus Ulva, widely utilized as a model for investigating complex metabolic networks due to their rapid growth rate and ability to thrive under diverse environmental conditions, have shed light on changes in metabolic pathways involved in lipid biosynthesis. These pathways are utilized by algae to adapt to conditions of nutritional stress, particularly from nitrates and phosphates [42,43].

The phytochemical composition of CLE was evaluated using UPLC-MS/MS. The most prevalent class of secondary metabolites found in CLE was lipids. GC-FID analysis further indicated that the predominant fatty acid in CLE was palmitic acid (16:0) (52.18%), followed by myristic acid (14:0) (20.46%), and oleic acid (18:1ω9) (11.70%). In a study by Biandolino et al., *C. linum* collected from Mar Piccolo of Taranto was reported to contain both saturated and unsaturated fatty acids, with unsaturated fatty acids representing the predominant part. Among them, C18 PUFAs were the dominant unsaturated fatty acids. Palmitic acid (16:0) was the dominant saturated species, with a high proportion of myristic acid (14:0), whereas MUFAs were primarily represented by 18:1ω9 and 18:1ω7 [41]. Another study on *C. linum* from the Sea of Japan reported a percentage of MUFAs primarily represented by 18:1ω9 and 18:1ω7, but the highest proportion of saturated fatty acids was in that case of myristic acid (14:0) [44]. Extracts from *C. linum* growing wild in Corsican Pond, on the other hand, report saturated fatty acids as the main compounds from a pentane *C. linum* extract, whereas the components of the sterol's family were the major compounds from an ethyl acetate extract [35]. Differences may be attributed to the extraction method used for the analysis, but ecological conditions, the life cycle of the algae, and seasonal variations are also of extreme importance. The nutritional composition of several *Clorophyta* species from fishpond aquaculture systems, including *C. linum*, was also studied, along with their anti-inflammatory activities and the effects that their bioaccessibility could have on this property. It was found that in *C. linum*, the total PUFA content was low, and a high level of saturated fatty acids balanced this low PUFA content. However, of all the tested species, *C. linum* was the one with the highest ω3/ω6 ratio [7]. Among the unsaturated fatty acids, the most abundant ω3 PUFA was α-linolenic acid (18:3ω3) along with MUFA 18:1, while myristic (14:0) and palmitic (16:0) were the dominant saturated species. Moreover, in the same study, *C. linum* demonstrated the highest inhibitory activity on COX-2. The anti-inflammatory activity of *C. linum* and its bioaccessible fraction was measured as a percentage of COX-2 inhibition [7]. At 100 µg/mL, the extract displayed inhibitory properties in accordance with other works using the same COX-2 inhibition methodology [45]. It should be noted that following in vitro digestion studies, they found low bioaccessibility of the compounds under investigation for their anti-inflammatory activity, recommending that the seaweed be used as an extract and not as food so that the destruction of cell walls would make bioactive compounds more bioaccessible [7]. Seaweed-derived lipids have been extensively studied for their anti-inflammatory, antioxidant, antimicrobic, antitumoral, and cardioprotective properties [46]. The anti-inflammatory effect of lipid extracts from both microalgae and macroalgae is well-recognized, with *Ochrophyta* and *Rhodophyta* being the most investigated phyla among the macroalgae [47–50]. Nevertheless, the *Chlorophyta* phylum has, to date, received little attention on this side [51,52]. Investigations were primarily conducted in vitro using murine macrophage RAW 264.7 and human THP-1 monocytic cell lines, with COX-2 activity and NO level being the most often assessed parameters. Very few examples of in vivo tests are reported. Unsaturated fatty acids, and especially ω-3 PUFAs, are thought to be primarily responsible for the anti-inflammatory activity of seaweeds [48,53]. Notoriously, macroalgae, despite having a relatively modest (0.5% to 8.0% of DW) lipid content, are the main primary producers of both ω-3 and ω-6 PUFAs [2]. Lipid crude extracts, lipid fractions, or isolated complex lipids are typically produced using a methanol/chloroform (2:1) mixture [2], but other organic solvents have demonstrated good efficiency in extracting lipids from algal samples. For this study, we evaluated the practicability of analyzing the composition of *C. linum* using less aggressive and easier-to-handle solvents, opting for a mixture of ethanol and water (70:30 v/v), since the literature data report lipid-enriched extracts with similar solvents [39,54,55]. Despite having higher extraction efficiency, other organic solvents such as hexane, chloroform, and methanol have the drawback of being very toxic. The European Parliament and Council Directive 2009/32/EC of 23 April 2009 for the approximation of the laws of the Member States concerning the extraction solvents used in the preparation of food products and their "ingredients" establishes that ethanol and acetone can be used without concentration limits. Acetone and ethanol are part of the solvents defined as GRAS (Generally Recognized as Safe) since toxicological studies show no long-term adverse effects on human health. Acetone is considered a GRAS by the FDA on par with ethanol, but only ethanol can be used without any concentration limits [56,57].

Potential anti-inflammatory properties of *C. linum* ethanolic extract were assessed in LPS-stimulated RAW 264.7 macrophage cells and TNF-α/IFN-γ-stimulated HaCaT keratinocyte cells. According to the findings of the current investigation, CLE had no cytotoxic effects and did not dramatically influence the viability of macrophages or keratinocytes at any of the tested concentrations. Additionally, it was not found to be mutagenic. During the inflammatory process, the major functions of macrophages are antigen presentation, phagocytosis, and immunomodulation through the production of various cytokines and growth factors [21]. It is well known that iNOS and COX-2 play an important role in inflammation. Additionally, ROS acts as a crucial signaling molecules in the development of inflammatory disorders [36]. NO and PGE2, downstream signaling factors of iNOS and COX-2, and several other pro-inflammatory cytokines and chemokines, are involved in the regulation of immune and inflammatory responses, causing symptoms such as pain, fever, and edema [58]. NO, which is regulated by iNOS, is a potent reactive factor in inflammatory responses found in stimulated macrophages and in the sites of inflammation [59]. COX-2 catalyzes the conversion of arachidonic acid to prostaglandins, including PGE2, and COX-2 activity can contribute to inflammatory pain. All these molecular players, in concert, may induce the recruitment of further inflammatory cells, resulting in triggering acute generalized inflammatory responses characteristic of septic shock and multi-organ failure [60]. For this reason, therapeutic interventions that target macrophages and their products could open new avenues for anti-inflammatory treatments. Therefore, we evaluated the anti-inflammatory effects of CLE by measuring the levels of these inflammation-related factors in RAW 264.7 cells. Pre-treatment with CLE significantly reduced protein expression of LPS-induced increased levels of iNOS and COX-2 and the release of ROS, NO, and PGE2 in RAW 264.7 cells in a dose-dependent manner. Targeted inhibition of COX-2 is a promising approach to inhibit inflammation, with phytonutrients and phytochemicals holding the potential to act in this regulation.

NF-κB plays an important role in the control of gene-encoding pro-inflammatory cytokines, as well as inducible enzymes, including iNOS and COX-2 [37]. It comprises five members, c-Rel, p65/RelA, RelB, p50/NF-κB1, and p52/NF-κB2, which form various homo- or heterodimers to control target gene transcription [37]. While inactive, NF-κB remains in the cytoplasm bound to an inhibitor of κB (IκB) proteins. Cellular activation triggers IKK activation, leading to IκB phosphorylation and its dissociation from p65 NF-κB, thereby activating NF-κB. The activated NF-κB complex moves to the nucleus where it binds to NF-κB-binding sites in gene promoters, regulating their expression [61]. Increased activation of the NFκB signaling pathway triggers the production of downstream inflammation-related factors. Since we found that CLE modulates NF-κB downstream pro-inflammatory markers, we further elucidated if CLE could interfere with the activation of NF-κB signaling by examining its effect on inhibiting LPS-induced translocation of NF-κB into the nucleus. Our results showed that LPS treatment caused a significant decrease in NF-κB in the nucleus, but this effect could be reversed by pre-treatment with CLE, indicating that signal transduction pathways mediated by NFκB may be effectively blocked by CLE in activated macrophages.

Keratinocytes, a prominent group of epidermal cells crucial in the development of inflammatory skin lesions [62], and macrophages engage in crosstalk to serve as the primary defense against infections and regulate the skin's homeostatic and inflammatory responses. Beyond their physical barrier function, keratinocytes actively contribute to the pathophysiology of various skin diseases by working with macrophages to regulate inflammatory responses [63,64]. Keratinocytes release mediators that stimulate blood-borne monocytes to differentiate into M1 macrophages, which release pro-inflammatory cytokines that activate keratinocytes. The role of macrophages in the inflammatory process and the use of RAW 264.7 cells as a suitable in vitro model to study inflammation have been well established. Our extract effectively reduced LPS-induced ROS generation in RAW 264.7 macrophages. Oxidative stress is a central player in inflammatory conditions, as evidenced by recent research linking it to the pathogenesis of atopic dermatitis (AD) in humans [65]. Stressed keratinocytes release various chemokines like IL-8, which recruit neutrophils. ROS activation triggers NF-κB, modulating genes such as TNF-α, interleukins, and iNOS [66]. Skin inflammation induced by oxidative stress involves the release of inflammatory mediators like COX-2 and TNF-α, regulated by signaling pathways including NF-κB, MAPK, and JAK/STAT [67]. Our finding that CLE inhibited ROS generation, as well as the production of NO and PGE2 in the supernatant of stimulated RAW 264.7 cells and their progenitor enzymes, presented promising avenues for treating inflammatory skin conditions, including AD.

TNF-α and IFN-γ are pro-inflammatory mediators secreted by macrophages that can stimulate keratinocytes, activating various cell signaling mechanisms and increasing the expression of pro-inflammatory mediators in keratinocytes [68,69]. HaCaT keratinocyte cells stimulated with TNF-α/IFN-γ are a commonly used in vitro model for studying inflammatory skin diseases [70]. TNF-α and IFN-γ can work synergistically to induce the expression of inflammatory cytokines (IL-6 and IL-1β) and chemokines (TARC/CCL17, MCP-1/CCL2, IL-8, and RANTES/CCL5) in HaCaT keratinocytes [71]. Cytokines are well-known for mediating inflammatory cell migration, keratinocyte proliferation, and further cytokine production by keratinocytes. Prominent players in these processes include IL-1β and IL-6, while key inflammatory chemokines such as RANTES/CCL5 and TARC/CCL17 orchestrate the recruitment of leukocytes to inflammation sites. Moreover, MCP-1/CCL2 and IL-8 are closely linked to the onset and severity of chronic skin inflammation, with TARC/CCL17 levels showing a positive correlation with atopic dermatitis severity in affected individuals [71]. RANTES/CCL5 predominantly acts as a chemotactic agent, activating T-cells [61]. The NF-κB family, consisting of transcription factors activated by various stimuli, including LPS, TNF-α, and IFN-γ, plays a critical role in the expression of multiple proinflammatory genes [61]. These genes regulate the production of proinflammatory cytokines like IL-6 and IL-1β, as well as chemokines such as TARC/CCL17, RANTES/CCL5, and MPC-1/CCL2 in HaCaT cells [62].

In addition to reducing the production of inflammatory mediators in LPS-stimulated RAW 264.7 macrophage cells, potentially by inhibiting NF-κB nuclear translocation, CLE also dose-dependently decreased the levels of chemokines (TARC/CCL17, RANTES/CCL5, MCP-1/CCL2, and IL-8) and the cytokine IL-1β in TNF-α/IFN-γ-induced HaCaT cells. Considering these findings, the discovery that the ethanolic extract from *C. linum* biomass can significantly suppress key inflammatory factors in both macrophage and keratinocyte cells presents numerous possibilities for treating various serious inflammatory conditions, including skin diseases. Two studies demonstrated that allergic diseases follow a specific sequence, beginning with atopic dermatitis and food allergies in infancy and progressing gradually to allergic asthma and rhinitis in childhood [29,30]. However, the mechanisms underlying the so-called atopic march remain incompletely understood, given the complexity and heterogeneity of atopic diseases, which result from a combination of genetic, environmental, and epigenetic factors [29].

The UPLC-MS/MS analysis revealed that fatty acids and their oxygenated derivatives were the predominant class of lipids in CLE, alongside polar lipids. Among the fatty acids identified, MUFA ω-9 oleic acid (OA) and PUFA ω-3 stearidonic acid (SDA) were the only ones found in their free form. Studies describing the anti-inflammatory activity of dietary OA and SDA were found in the literature. OA demonstrated anti-inflammatory effects on LPS-stimulated THP-1 macrophages by blocking the NF-κB pathway and downstream production of pro-inflammatory cytokines, also promoting the production of the anti-inflammatory cytokine IL-10 [72]. In a study by Sung et al., it emerged that SDA also exerted anti-inflammatory effects via the inactivation of the NF-κB signaling pathway, suppressing iNOS-mediated NO production [73].

Oxygenated fatty acid derivatives were found in CLE, which included PUFA oxylipin derivatives and hydroxylated derivatives of saturated fatty acids. Oxylipins are interesting metabolites derived from PUFAs and are nowadays recognized as being involved in the defense mechanisms of macroalgae [74]. Indeed, since an acquired immune system is missing in macroalgae, they heavily rely on their secondary metabolites to mediate interactions with other organisms and the environment, and it was suggested that seaweed oxylipins, like mammals' leukotrienes and prostaglandins, have a role in their systemic defense mechanisms [42]. As members of *Chlorophyta* are typically rich in C18 PUFA [75], they mainly oxidize C18 substrates [42]. Accordingly, oxylipin derivatives found in CLE were the LA 18:2ω-6 derived hydroxy-linoleic (13-HODE) acid and the ALA C18:3ω-3 derivative 9(10)-EpODE, also known as 9(10)-epoxy-12Z,15Z-octadecadienoic acid. To the best of our knowledge, this is the first evidence of the presence of 9(10)-EpODE in *C. linum*, while a previous report of HODE fatty acid derivatives in this species was found in the literature [76]. Of note, the antinociceptive role of ω-3 epoxy-fatty acids, including 9(10)-EpODE, has been reported in a study on monoepoxides from eicosapentaenoic and docosahexaenoic acids from different sources [77]. As for the second-mentioned oxylipin found in CLE, Kumari et al. reported that in a study comparing the lipidic composition of several different species of macroalgae, *Chlorophyta* contained the highest amounts of hydroxy-oxylipins. Among them, *C. linum* presented a predominance of octadecanoids (C18-oxls) derived from C18 PUFAs (namely, linoleic acid [LA; C18:2ω6] and α-linolenic acid [ALA; C18:3ω3]), including hydroxy fatty acid 13-HODE [76], in accordance with what we found in CLE. This could prove to be very interesting since the esterified form of hydroxylated fatty acids is a recently discovered class of biologically active lipids whose role in inflammation and diabetes in mammals has been indicated to be very attractive [78]. Indeed, an LA ester of 13-HODE found in both mammals and plants has been reported to have anti-inflammatory activity in an LPS-induced cytokine secretion assay [79].

Polar lipid Palmitin, a palmitic acid (16:0) derivative, was also identified in CLE. In general, seaweed-derived fatty acids are mainly found as polar lipids, such as glycolipids (GL), which include monoacyl-, diacyl-, and triacylglycerol (MAG, DAG, and TAG) subclasses, and phospholipids (PL), but also betaine lipids. MAG is formed from TAG and DAG by hydrolysis, which also generates free fatty acids [75]. Although Stabili et al. previously reported the presence of glycerol moieties of monoacyl, diacyl, and triacylglycerol in *C. linum* from Mar Piccolo [39], to our knowledge, this is the first report of the identification of Palmitin in this species. Palmitin has recently been identified in the ethanolic extract of *Spirulina platensis*, a well-recognized superfood with extensively documented beneficial properties, as one of the metabolites responsible for the inhibition of NO production via the downregulation of iNOS, TNF-α, and IL-6 in LPS-induced BV2 microglia [80]. Moreover, it was detected in a methanolic extract of red seaweed *Kappaphycus malesianus*, which prevented the release of cytokines and other pro-inflammatory mediators by inhibiting the NF-κB pathway during microglia-mediated neuroinflammation [81].

In silico studies also revealed the potential anti-inflammatory role of palmitic acid in CLE. Despite its known pro-inflammatory nature, the findings of this investigation suggested that it can act as an agonist with biological targets within the receptor complement system considered here. Notably, palmitic acid's anti-inflammatory properties may result from its interaction with the phosphodiesterase enzyme family [82,83]. Previous research has shown the inhibition of various phosphodiesterase isoforms by free fatty acids [84], indicating that fatty acids could mitigate inflammatory processes mediated by this enzyme family, thus supporting the computational findings. Through docking simulations, palmitic acid demonstrated a high binding free energy score, forming robust polar interactions with the binding residues of known inhibitors of the target, sharing the same binding pocket [85,86].

The second most abundant class of secondary metabolites found in CLE was amino acids. Extensive data report a high content of proteins in *C. linum* [7,87,88]. Of note, the main nutritional value of green seaweeds is in their protein and carbohydrate content, and the composition of essential amino acids (EAA) especially determines the nutritional quality of such proteins [4]. Indeed, green seaweed proteins are known to contain an amount of EAA close to casein and legume proteins, recognized as the principal sources of EAA. One important EAA is Valine, which was among the identified amino acids in CLE as well as in *C. linum* from Mar Piccolo of Taranto, as previously reported by Stabili et al. [39]. Besides their nutritional value, seaweed proteins and peptides have also demonstrated remarkable antioxidant, antimicrobial, antitumoral, anti-hypertensive, anti-diabetic, and anti-inflammatory properties [89–95]. Among the proteins found in seaweed, lectins are more broadly characterized for their anti-inflammatory activity, but numerous studies have reported the ability of other seaweed-derived proteins and peptides to interfere with inflammatory pathways. These studies, mainly conducted in vitro, included inhibition of NF-κB in macrophagic models, resulting in a decrease in the production of COX-2, iNOS, and TNF-α [96–100].

The other two classes of compounds found in CLE through UPLC-MS/MS analysis were flavonoids and terpenoids. While flavonoids are renowned for their anti-inflammatory properties [101–106], terpenoids, particularly carnosic acid, also exhibit anti-inflammatory potential [107–109].

Based on in vitro studies and metabolic profiling, we were confident that CLE exerts anti-inflammatory properties. All these findings strongly suggest that CLE may regulate the release of inflammatory markers by blocking the NF-κB inflammatory pathway. However, additional research is required to elucidate specific inhibitory mechanisms and cellular targets of the found active metabolites to further understand how each interacts with the other, acting as parts of a complex anti-inflammatory matrix.

4. Materials and Methods

4.1. Materials

Dulbecco's Modified Eagle's Medium (DMEM), trypsin solution, and all the solvents used for cell culture were purchased from Merck (Darmstadt, Germany). Mouse immortalized fibroblasts (NIH3T3) and RAW 264.7 cells were from the American Type Culture Collection (Manassas, VA, USA). Ames test kit was supplied by Xenometrix (Allschwil, Switzerland).

4.2. The Collection of Chaetomorpha linum and the Preparation of Algae Extract (CLE)

The algae *C. linum* (Müller) Kützing was collected from the Orbetello Lagoon (Tuscany, Italy) in May 2021 (Table 3). The samples were harvested and then rinsed with water to remove salt and debris. After being thoroughly cleaned, the material was oven-dried at 55 °C until it reached a constant weight. It was then ground into a fine powder, and the pulverized algae were extracted with an ethanol–water (70:30 v/v) mixture using a sample/solvent ratio equal to 1:10 (g/mL) at 80 °C for 3 h. The supernatant was then separated from residual biomass, filtered, and subjected to rotary evaporation to remove organic solvent. Finally, the aqueous residue was freeze-dried to produce the dry extract. The extraction was carried out in duplicate. Following extraction, 100 mg of dry extract was dissolved in 1 mL of 100% DMSO to obtain a 100 mg/mL CLE stock solution. This solution was then aliquoted and stored in the refrigerator at −32 °C for subsequent analyses.

Table 3. *Chaetomorpha linum* specimens collected from the Orbetello Lagoon (Tuscany, Italy).

Collection Date	Voucher Number	Type	Species Name	Location	GPS Point
16 May 2021	CL01	Green	*Chaetomorpha linum*	Orbetello	42°26′15.1″ N 11°11′38.7″ E
18 May 2021	CL02	Green	*Chaetomorpha linum*	Orbetello	42°26′15.1″ N 11°11′38.7″ E
25 May 2021	CL03	Green	*Chaetomorpha linum*	Orbetello	42°26′15.1″ N 11°11′38.7″ E

4.3. NMR Spectroscopy

Samples for NMR spectroscopy were prepared by dissolving 1 mg/mL of CLE dry extract in DMSO-d6 (Cambridge Isotope Lab, Cambridge, MA, USA). Spectra were acquired on a Bruker Avance III 600 spectrometer operating at 14.1 T using a spectral with 8000 Hz and digitized over 32k points by accumulating 32 transients with a recycle delay of 5 s. The residual signal from DMSO was used as a chemical shift reference. Spectra were processed and analyzed using Chenomx 10 (Chenomx Inc., Edmonton, AB, Canada).

4.4. UPLC-MS/MS

To investigate the non-volatile profile of CLE, an Ultimate 3000 UPLC system (Thermo Fisher Scientific, Waltham, MA, USA) was used and was controlled using Thermo Xcalibur software (Thermo Fisher Scientific, Waltham, MA, USA). The dry *Chaetomorpha linum* extract was dissolved in the ethanol–water (70:30 v/v) mixture and injected into the UPLC-Q-Exactive plus system. The samples were separated using a column Acquity UPLC BEH C18 (2.1 mm × 15 cm, 1.7 μm, Waters, Waltham, MA, USA). Mobile phases consisted of solvent A (0.1% formic acid in water) and solvent B (0.1% formic acid in acetonitrile). The gradient started with 2% of B, which was maintained constant for 1 min. Then, the organic phase was increased up to 100% in 50 min. Phase B was maintained at 100% for another 2 min and then returned to the initial condition. The flow rate was maintained at 0.2 mL/min, and the injection volume of the sample was 10 μL. Additionally, the column temperature was kept at 35 °C. A Q-Exactive Plus™ quadrupole Orbitrap mass spectrometer (Thermo Fisher Scientific, Waltham, MA, USA) was used to perform mass spectrometry analyses in the negative and positive ion modes, with a scan mass range set at m/z 200–2000. HR-MS spectra were recorded in the positive and negative ion modes using the following parameters: spray voltage 3.5 kV (positive) and 3.0 kV (negative), sheath gas 20 (arbitrary units), auxiliary gas 5.0 (arbitrary units), capillary temperature 320 °C, and resolution 35,000. MS/MS spectra were obtained by a Higher Energy Collision Dissociation (HCD) of 30 (arbitrary units). The accuracy error threshold was fixed at 5 ppm. The final annotated metabolome dataset was generated by Compound Discoverer 3.3 (Thermo Fisher Scientific, Waltham, MA, USA). The Compound Discoverer 3.0 software is fully integrated with the ChemSpider database and the mzCloud for automated and expedited data processing. The retention time tolerance (RT) was set to 0.2 min, with mass tolerance equal to 5 ppm, and other parameters were selected as the default values for peak extraction and peak alignment.

4.5. GC-FID

The fatty acids profile of CLE was assessed using GC-FID with a Perkin Elmer Clarus 500 gas chromatograph equipped with a flame ionization detector (FID) and a split/splitless inlet. Detector and inlet temperatures were set at 230 °C and 280 °C, respectively. Helium served as the carrier gas at a flow rate of 1 mL/min. The split ratio was 1:10, and the injection volume was 1 μL. A SPTM-2380 fused silica capillary column (60 m × 0.25 mm I.D., Supelco, Bellefonte, PA, USA) was used. The oven temperature was programmed from 70 to 120 °C at 10°/min, increased to 243 °C at 2 °C/min, followed by another increase to 260 °C at a rate of 15 °C/min and held at 260 °C for 20 min. Data acquisition was performed using Perkin Elmer TotalChrom Navigator 6.3.1 software. The CLE was prepared for GC-FID analysis by converting triglycerides to fatty acid methyl esters (FAME) with 14% BF3 methanolic solution from Sigma-Aldrich S.r.l. (Milan, Italy). To the sample (3 mg), 1 mL of BF3 solution was added and kept for 30 min at 95 °C. After cooling, the sample was extracted with 1 mL of n-exane and centrifuged for 5 min (3400 × g). The n-exane phase was used for GC analysis after dilution with n-exane (1:10 v/v). Analyses were conducted in triplicate. Compound identification was performed by comparing chromatographic peaks with those of a 37-component FAME Mix from Sigma-Aldrich S.r.l. (Milan, Italy) analyzed in the same chromatographic conditions.

4.6. In Vitro Anti-Inflammatory Activity

4.6.1. Cell Cultures

RAW 264.7 and HaCaT cells were obtained from ATCC (ATCC, Manassas, VA, USA) and cultured in DMEM containing 10% v/v FBS, 100 mg/mL penicillin, and 100 mg/mL streptomycin. Cultures were maintained at 37 °C in a humidified atmosphere of 5% CO_2. Comparative analysis was performed with cell populations at the same generation.

4.6.2. RAW 264.7 and HaCaT Cells Viability

RAW 264.7 cells were seeded at a density of 1×10^4 cells/well in 96-well plates and cultured until sub-confluence (80–85% confluence). Cells were treated with different concentrations (6, 12, 25, 50, and 100 μg/mL) of CLE prepared in DMSO (Sigma-Aldrich) and diluted in medium, and the final DMSO concentration was kept below 0.1% v/v throughout the experiment. The control was treated with DMSO at a concentration of 0.1% v/v, corresponding to the highest concentration of the compound. After 24 h of treatment, cells were washed with sterile PBS, and MTT was added to a final concentration of 1 mg/mL. After a 2 h incubation, cells were lysed with 150 μL of DMSO. The absorbance was measured at 550 nm using an EnVision system (PerkinElmer, Waltham, MA, USA), and the percentage of cell viability was calculated relative to the control. The percentage of cell viability was calculated relative to the control. The viability of HaCaT cells was measured using the Cell Counting Kit-8 (CCK-8) (Sigma-Aldrich, Burlington, MA, USA) according to the manufacturer's instructions. The viability of cells, treated as before, was measured at 450 nm using a microplate reader (CLARIOstar, BMG Labtech, Ortenberg, Germany). The percentage of viable cells was determined relative to the vehicle control.

4.6.3. Cell Stimulation

RAW 264.7 and HaCaT cells were treated with CLE for 4 h prior to 24 h stimulation with Lipopolysaccharide (LPS) (obtained from Escherichia coli O111:B4, Sigma-Aldrich) or TNFα/IFN-γ (Sigma-Aldrich), respectively. Dexamethasone (DEX) (Sigma-Aldrich), commonly used to treat inflammation, was used as a positive control at a concentration of 5 μg/mL.

4.6.4. The Quantification of Intracellular ROS Generation

The generation of ROS in RAW 264.7 cells was determined in 96-well plates with 2′,7′-dichlorodihydrofluorescein diacetate (DCFH$_2$-DA, Sigma-Aldrich), which was intracellularly deacetylated and oxidized to highly fluorescent 2′,7′-dichlorofluorescein (DCF) [110]. After pre-treatment with different concentrations of CLE, cells were stimulated with LPS (200 ng/mL) for 5 h. DCFH$_2$-DA (10 μM) dissolved in HBSS was applied to the cells and incubated at 37 °C. The plate was scanned using an EnVision system (PerkinElmer) with an excitation wavelength of 485 nm and an emission wavelength of 535 nm. Afterward, the number of cells in each well was determined by Crystal Violet assay [111]. The results were normalized to the relative cell count for each well and expressed as the relative ROS production % (RFI) with respect to the LPS group.

4.6.5. The Determination of NO Production

The production of nitric oxide (NO) in the supernatant of RAW 264.7 cells was determined in 6-well plates (1×10^6 cells/well) cultured until sub-confluence (80–85%). After treatment with CLE at different concentrations (25, 50, and 100 μg/mL) for 4 h, the cells were stimulated with LPS (200 ng/mL) for 24 h. Following stimulation, 100 μL of conditioned medium from each well was transferred to a new 96-well plate and mixed with an equal volume of Griess reagent composed of 1% sulfanilamide and 0.1% N-(1-naphthyl) ethylenediamine dihydrochloride in 5% phosphoric acid. After incubation at room temperature for 10 min, the absorbance was measured at 540 nm using an EnVision system (PerkinElmer). Nitrite concentration was assessed by a sodium nitrite standard curve.

4.6.6. Immunofluorescence Study

RAW 264.7 cells were pre-treated with CLE at 100 μg/mL for 4 h and stimulated with LPS for 1 h. The cells were fixed with 4% paraformaldehyde dissolved in PBS for 15 min and then permeabilized with 0.5% TritonX-100 in PBS for 5 min. After blocking, cells were incubated overnight at 4 °C with anti-NF-κB p65 (clone 1G10.2) mouse monoclonal antibody (Sigma-Aldrich). Cells were then incubated at room temperature for 1 h with Alexa 594-conjugated goat anti-Mouse IgG (Life Technologies, Carlsbad, CA, USA). Finally, the samples were mounted with a fluoroshield mounting medium with

DAPI (Abcam, Cambridge, UK). Images were captured by fluorescence microscopy (Zeiss AxioLabA1, Oberkochen, Germany). The quantitative co-localization analysis of NF-κB p65 and DAPI signals was performed using ImageJ and the JACoP plug-in to determine Manders' coefficient [112], which represents the percentage of NF-κB p65 pixels that overlap DAPI pixels.

4.6.7. Protein Extraction

Whole-cell lysates were obtained with RIPA buffer, added with phosphate and protease inhibitors, and then disrupted by sonication for 15 min in an ice bath. Protein concentration was assessed using the BCA protein assay. Nuclear fractionations were obtained using the NE-PER™ Cytoplasmic and Nuclear Protein Extraction Kit (Thermo Fisher Scientific Rockford, IL, USA) according to the manufacturer's protocol.

4.6.8. Western Blotting

Twenty micrograms of protein was resolved by 8% SDS–PAGE and transferred onto a nitrocellulose membrane. The membrane was blocked in PBS 10% w/v nonfat dry milk at RT with gentle shaking for 2 h. The membrane was incubated with anti-iNOS (rabbit polyclonal IgG, 1:10,000 Sigma-Aldrich), anti-COX-2 (rabbit polyclonal IgG, 1:2000 Cell Signaling), anti-NF-κB p65 (clone 1G10.2, 1:500) mouse monoclonal antibody (Sigma-Aldrich), and anti-GAPDH HRP-conjugated (1:50,000) primary antibodies, at 4 °C. The blots were washed three times and incubated with anti-rabbit HRP-conjugated secondary antibody (Sigma-Aldrich) 1:80,000 or anti-mouse HRP-conjugated secondary antibody (Sigma-Aldrich) 1:50,000 for 1 h, RT. After washing three times, immunoreactive bands were detected using ECL (LuminataCrescendo, Merck Millipore, Burlington, MA, USA) and images acquired by LAS4000 (GE Healthcare, Chicago, IL, USA). The optical densities of immunoreactive bands were analyzed by ImageQuantTL software (GE Healthcare, Chicago, IL, USA, V 7.0) using GAPDH as a loading normalizing factor.

4.6.9. Enzyme-Linked Immunosorbent (ELISA) Assay

RAW 264.7 and HaCaT cells (5×10^6 cells/mL) were seeded in 6-well plates and cultured for 24 h. After treatment with CLE at different concentrations (25, 50, and 100 µg/mL) for 4 h, the cells were stimulated with LPS (200 ng/mL) or TNF-α/IFN-γ (10 ng/mL) for 24 h. DEX (5 µg/mL) was used as a positive control. Then, the culture supernatants were collected. The concentration of PGE2 in the supernatants of RAW 264.7 cells was detected using a PGE2 ELISA kit (Cat# E-EL-0034, Elabscience, Houston, TX, USA) according to the manufacturer's instructions. HaCaT cells' supernatants were analyzed using ELISA kits for TARC (EHCCL17, Invitrogen, Waltham, MA, USA), RANTES (EHRNTS, Invitrogen), Human IL-8 (BMS204-3, Invitrogen), Human Il-1β (RAB0273, Sigma Aldrich), and MCP-1 (BMS281, Invitrogen) according to the manufacturer's instructions.

4.7. Mutagenicity Assay: Ames Test

The TA100 and TA98 strains of Salmonella typhimurium were utilized for mutagenicity assay in the absence and presence of metabolic activation, i.e., with and without S9 liver fraction. The tester strains used were selected because they are sensitive, detect a large proportion of known bacterial mutagens, and are most commonly used routinely within the pharmaceutical industry [113]. The following specific positive controls were used, respectively, with and without S9 fraction: 2-Nitrofluorene (2-NF) 2 µg/mL + 4-Nitroquinoline N-oxide (4-NQO) 0.1 µg/mL, and 2-aminoanthracene (2-AA) 5 µg/mL. The final concentration of S9 in the culture was 4.5%.

Approximately 10^7 bacteria were exposed to 6 concentrations (0.025, 0.050, 0.10, 0.50, 1.0, and 10.0 mg/mL) of the CLE extract, as well as to positive and negative controls, for 90 min in a medium containing sufficient histidine to support approximately two cell divisions. After 90 min, the exposure cultures were diluted in a pH indicator medium lacking histidine and aliquoted into 48 wells of a 384-well plate. Within two days, cells that had undergone the reversion to His grew into colonies. Metabolism by the bacterial colonies reduced the pH of the medium, changing the color of that well. This color change can be detected visually. The number of wells containing revertant colonies was counted for each dose and compared to a zero dose control. Each dose was tested in six replicates. The material was regarded mutagenic if the number of histidine revertant colonies was twice or more than the spontaneous revertant colonies.

4.8. Statistical Analysis

Experiments were performed in triplicate. Statistical analyses were performed using GraphPad Prism 9.0 software (GraphPad Software, San Diego, CA, USA). Data were presented as mean ± SD and were compared using one-way ANOVA with appropriate post hoc test. A p-value of 0.05 or less was considered significant.

4.9. In Silico Studies

Structural Optimization and Resources

The anti-inflammatory target complement was retrieved from DrugBank [114] using the "target section" with the keyword "inflammatory". To select the RAW 264.7 and HaCaT anti-inflammatory target complement, we analyzed the RAW 264.7 transcriptome using the Harmonizome 3.0 database [115] and extracted all targets present in the anti-inflammatory target complement list of DrugBank. Their 3D structures and FASTA sequences were retrieved from the RCSB Protein Data Bank [116] and UniProt database [117], respectively. The 3D structures were obtained by performing multiple sequence alignments with BLASTp v.2.15.0 (National Center For Biotechnology Information, MD, USA) and choosing PDB as the search database; all parameters were used as default [118]. All targets considered in this study are reported in Table S1.

To avoid errors during the docking simulations, potential missing side chains and steric clashes in the 3D structures reported in PDB files were added/resolved with molecular/homology modeling using MODELLER v.9.3 implemented in PyMOD3.0 (PyMOL2.5 plugin, Schrödinger, Inc., New York, NY, USA) [119]. The 3D structures were then analyzed and validated using PROCHECK v.3.5.4 (European Bioinformatics Institute, Cambridge, UK) [120]. Prior to conducting the docking simulations, high-energy intramolecular interactions were minimized using GROMACS 2019.3 (Stockholm University and KTH-Royal Institute of Technology, and KTH-Royal Institute of Technology, Stockholm, Sweden) [121] with the charmm36 force field. CHARMM-GUI v.3.8 (Lehigh University, Bethlehem, Palestine) [122] was used to assign all parameters to the biological targets and ligands.

In detail, prior to conducting further simulations, the starting conformation sequence was aligned against its primary structure, allowing for the addition of potential missing side chains to the structure. Furthermore, loop modeling implemented in MODELLER v.9.3 (Departments of Biopharmaceutical Sciences and Pharmaceutical Chemistry, and California Institute for Quantitative Biomedical Research, Mission Bay Byers Hall, University of California San Francisco, San Francisco, CA, USA) was employed to optimize the best starting orientation of each loop within the structure. Lastly, each structure was analyzed using the PROCHECK tool, where a Ramachandran plot (which analyzes the backbone of ϕ and ψ angles and Chi1–Chi2 plots for side chains) confirmed the validity of the starting conformation. Then, we minimized the energy of each structure by performing energy minimization using GROMACS 2019.3 with the charmm36 force field. This step was taken to prevent the possibility of the structures from sterically hindering potential clashes and/or to optimize the energy values. The resulting structures were then immersed in a cubic box filled with TIP3P water molecules, and the system was neutralized with the addition of counter ions. Simulations were run by applying periodic boundary conditions. Energy minimization was performed with 5000 steps using the steepest descent as the algorithm, which converged to a minimum energy with forces less than 10 kJ/mol/nm.

To enhance the reliability of our simulations, we conducted docking simulations based on in vitro evidence. Therefore, we selectively chose targets for which their experimental 3D structures were in complex with an active compound. In cases where multiple 3D structures of the same target were combined with different ligands in different binding regions, such as allosteric pockets, we created a box capable of enclosing such binding regions. Consequently, a box was created for each target, and we set the grid box at the center of mass of the ligand in the experimental 3D structure of the target, using AutoDock/VinaXB v.1.1.2. (Center for Computational Structural Biology (CCSB), La Jolla, CA, USA) and MGLTOOLS v.1.5.7 (The Scripps Research Institute, La Jolla, CA, USA) [123] scripts. To provide a more consistent result for our docking simulation, we changed the default exhaustiveness from 8 to 32 and only selected binding poses with a root mean square deviation (RMSD) 2 Å lower than that of the best-docked pose. All parameters were used as default.

Three-dimensional structures of compounds were retrieved and downloaded in sdf format from the PubChem database [124]. Then, a virtual screening was carried out using the extracted compounds on the targets. OpenBabel v.3.1.0 (University of Cambridge, Cambridge, UK) [125] was used to convert protein and ligand files and to assign gasteiger partial charges, as proposed in previous works [126,127]. The interaction network was explored with the PLIP tool (Biotechnology Center TU Dresden (BIOTEC), Dresden, Germany) [128].

5. Conclusions

We identified *C. linum* as a natural source of various bioactive metabolites, making this invasive species from the Orbetello lagoon an attractive subject for further investigation. The CLE extract not only decreased the production of inflammatory mediators in LPS-stimulated RAW 264.7 macrophage cells, potentially through the inhibition of NF-κB nuclear translocation, but it also exhibited an anti-atopic effect by reducing the production of inflammatory chemokines and cytokines in TNF-α/IFN-γ-induced HaCaT cells. These findings suggested that the ethanolic extract from *C. linum* biomass held significant promise as a therapeutic agent for inflammation. By effectively suppressing key inflammatory factors in both macrophage and keratinocyte cells, this research may offer a basis for the identification and development of novel therapeutic anti-inflammatory candidates with fewer adverse effects.

Supplementary Materials: The following supporting information can be downloaded at: https://www.mdpi.com/article/10.3390/md22050226/s1, Figure S1: 1D-1H spectrum of CLE dry extract dissolved in DMSO-d6. Peck's characteristics of saturated and unsaturated fatty acids were labeled with proton originating the resonance underlined. Fatty acid peak intensities over other species were apparent. Table S1: Inflammatory targets.

Author Contributions: Conceptualization, A.S., M.G. and L.F.; methodology, L.F., M.G., S.L., A.B. and L.S.; validation, L.F., M.G. and A.S.; investigation, L.F., T.O., P.M., S.L., L.S., E.D., D.G. and M.G.; formal analysis, A.T.; resources, A.S.; data curation, L.F.; writing—original draft preparation, L.F.; writing—review and editing, L.F., A.S. and M.G.; visualization, L.F., M.G. and A.T.; supervision, A.S.; project administration, A.S. and O.S. All authors have read and agreed to the published version of the manuscript.

Funding: This research received no external funding.

Institutional Review Board Statement: Not applicable.

Data Availability Statement: The original contributions presented in the study are included in the article/Supplementary Material, further inquiries can be directed to the corresponding author.

Acknowledgments: The authors thank: PRIN: PROGETTI DI RICERCA DI RILEVANTE INTERESSE NAZIONALE—Bando 2022 Prot. 2022LW54KC; PRIN: PROGETTI DI RICERCA DI RILEVANTE INTERESSE NAZIONALE—Bando 2022 PNRR Prot. P2022RYR5W; F-Cur funds to M.G.; UE—FSE REACT-EU, PON Ricerca e Innovazione 2014–2020; Progetto ERICA ARTES 4.0, E87G23000100001 Agenzia Coesione Territoriale; Progetto "Bioeconomia circolare di Posidonia oceanica spiaggiata" Prot. NS0000021. Progetto OMNIALGAE—Ministero dell'Ambiente e della Tutela del Territorio e del Mare (MATTM).

Conflicts of Interest: The authors declare no conflicts of interest.

References

1. Deepika, C.; Ravishankar, G.A.; Rao, A.R. Potential Products from Macroalgae: An Overview. In *Sustainable Global Resources of Seaweeds Volume 1*; Springer International Publishing: Berlin, Germany, 2022; pp. 17–44.
2. Jaworowska, A.; Murtaza, A. Seaweed Derived Lipids Are a Potential Anti-Inflammatory Agent: A Review. *Int. J. Environ. Res. Public. Health* **2023**, *20*, 730. [CrossRef] [PubMed]
3. El-Beltagi, H.S.; Mohamed, A.A.; Mohamed, H.I.; Ramadan, K.M.A.; Barqawi, A.A.; Mansour, A.T. Phytochemical and Potential Properties of Seaweeds and Their Recent Applications: A Review. *Mar. Drugs* **2022**, *20*, 342. [CrossRef] [PubMed]
4. Echave, J.; Otero, P.; Garcia-Oliveira, P.; Munekata, P.E.S.; Pateiro, M.; Lorenzo, J.M.; Simal-Gandara, J.; Prieto, M.A. Seaweed-Derived Proteins and Peptides: Promising Marine Bioactives. *Antioxidants* **2022**, *11*, 176. [CrossRef] [PubMed]
5. Savchenko, T.; Degtyaryov, E.; Radzyukevich, Y.; Buryak, V. Therapeutic Potential of Plant Oxylipins. *Int. J. Mol. Sci.* **2022**, *23*, 14627. [CrossRef] [PubMed]
6. Market Analysis and Insights: Global Biomedical Materials Market. Available online: https://www.marketgrowthreports.com/global-biomedical-materials-market-21051012 (accessed on 28 March 2024).
7. Ripol, A.; Cardoso, C.; Afonso, C.; Varela, J.; Quental-Ferreira, H.; Pousão-Ferreira, P.; Bandarra, N.M. Composition, Anti-Inflammatory Activity, and Bioaccessibility of Green Seaweeds from Fish Pond Aquaculture. *Nat. Prod. Commun.* **2018**, *13*, 1934578X1801300. [CrossRef]
8. Cardoso, C.; Ripol, A.; Afonso, C.; Freire, M.; Varela, J.; Quental-Ferreira, H.; Pousão-Ferreira, P.; Bandarra, N. Fatty Acid Profiles of the Main Lipid Classes of Green Seaweeds from Fish Pond Aquaculture. *Food Sci. Nutr.* **2017**, *5*, 1186–1194. [CrossRef]
9. Amaro, H.M.; Pagels, F.; Tavares, T.G.; Costa, I.; Sousa-Pinto, I.; Guedes, A.C. Antioxidant and Anti-Inflammatory Potential of Seaweed Extracts as Functional Ingredients. *Hydrobiology* **2022**, *1*, 469–482. [CrossRef]
10. Lenzi, M. Artificial Top Layer Sediment Resuspension To Counteract Chaetomorpha Linum (Muller) Kutz Blooms In A Eutrophic Lagoon. Three Years Full-Scale Experience. *J. Aquac. Mar. Biol.* **2017**, *5*, 00114. [CrossRef]
11. Sorce, C.; Persiano Leporatti, M.; Lenzi, M. Growth and Physiological Features of Chaetomorpha Linum (Müller) Kütz. in High Density Mats. *Mar. Pollut. Bull.* **2018**, *129*, 772–781. [CrossRef]
12. Bastianoni, S.; Coppola, F.; Tiezzi, E.; Colacevich, A.; Borghini, F.; Focardi, S. Biofuel Potential Production from the Orbetello Lagoon Macroalgae: A Comparison with Sunflower Feedstock. *Biomass Bioenergy* **2008**, *32*, 619–628. [CrossRef]
13. Galletti, A.M.R.; Antonetti, C.; Licursi, D.; Mussi, L.; Balestri, E.; Lardicci, C. Levulinic Acid Production from the Green Macroalgae Chaetomorpha Linum and Valonia Aegagropila Harvested in the Orbetello Lagoon. *Chem. Eng. Trans.* **2019**, *74*, 103–108. [CrossRef]
14. Renzi, M.; Giovani, A.; Focardi, S.E. Biofuel Production from the Orbetello Lagoon Macrophytes: Efficiency of Lipid Extraction Using Accelerate Solvent Extraction Technique. *J. Environ. Prot.* **2013**, *4*, 1224–1229. [CrossRef]
15. Piovani, D.; Nikolopoulos, G.K.; Bonovas, S. Non-Communicable Diseases: The Invisible Epidemic. *J. Clin. Med.* **2022**, *11*, 5939. [CrossRef] [PubMed]
16. Wang, J.; Zhou, Y.; Zhang, H.; Hu, L.; Liu, J.; Wang, L.; Wang, T.; Zhang, H.; Cong, L.; Wang, Q. Pathogenesis of Allergic Diseases and Implications for Therapeutic Interventions. *Signal Transduct. Target. Ther.* **2023**, *8*, 138. [CrossRef]
17. Bertino, L.; Guarneri, F.; Cannavò, S.P.; Casciaro, M.; Pioggia, G.; Gangemi, S. Oxidative Stress and Atopic Dermatitis. *Antioxidants* **2020**, *9*, 196. [CrossRef]
18. Cadau, S.; Gault, M.; Berthelemy, N.; Hsu, C.-Y.; Danoux, L.; Pelletier, N.; Goudounèche, D.; Pons, C.; Leprince, C.; André-Frei, V.; et al. An Inflamed and Infected Reconstructed Human Epidermis to Study Atopic Dermatitis and Skin Care Ingredients. *Int. J. Mol. Sci.* **2022**, *23*, 12880. [CrossRef]
19. Ji, H.; Li, X.-K. Oxidative Stress in Atopic Dermatitis. *Oxid. Med. Cell Longev.* **2016**, *2016*, 2721469. [CrossRef] [PubMed]
20. Naesens, M.; Kuypers, D.R.J.; Sarwal, M. Calcineurin Inhibitor Nephrotoxicity. *Clin. J. Am. Soc. Nephrol.* **2009**, *4*, 481–508. [CrossRef]
21. Bechstein, W.O. Neurotoxicity of Calcineurin Inhibitors: Impact and Clinical Management. *Transpl. Int.* **2000**, *13*, 313–326. [CrossRef]
22. Li, L.; Liu, R.; Peng, C.; Chen, X.; Li, J. Pharmacogenomics for the Efficacy and Side Effects of Antihistamines. *Exp. Dermatol.* **2022**, *31*, 993–1004. [CrossRef]
23. Buchman, A.L. Side Effects of Corticosteroid Therapy. *J. Clin. Gastroenterol.* **2001**, *33*, 289–294. [CrossRef] [PubMed]
24. Hwang, D.H.; Koh, P.O.; Kang, C.; Kim, E. Rosa Davurica Pall. Improves DNCB-Induced Atopic Dermatitis in Mice and Regulated TNF-Alpa/IFN-Gamma-Induced Skin Inflammatory Responses in HaCaT Cells. *Phytomedicine* **2021**, *91*, 153708. [CrossRef]
25. Nur Husna, S.M.; Tan, H.-T.T.; Md Shukri, N.; Mohd Ashari, N.S.; Wong, K.K. Allergic Rhinitis: A Clinical and Pathophysiological Overview. *Front. Med.* **2022**, *9*, 874114. [CrossRef]
26. Dierick, B.J.H.; van der Molen, T.; Flokstra-de Blok, B.M.J.; Muraro, A.; Postma, M.J.; Kocks, J.W.H.; van Boven, J.F.M. Burden and Socioeconomics of Asthma, Allergic Rhinitis, Atopic Dermatitis and Food Allergy. *Expert. Rev. Pharmacoecon. Outcomes Res.* **2020**, *20*, 437–453. [CrossRef] [PubMed]
27. Zhang, Y.; Lan, F.; Zhang, L. Advances and Highlights in Allergic Rhinitis. *Allergy* **2021**, *76*, 3383–3389. [CrossRef] [PubMed]

28. Gil, T.-Y.; Kang, S.-C.; Jin, B.-R.; An, H.-J. Euphorbia Hirta Leaf Ethanol Extract Suppresses TNF-α/IFN-γ-Induced Inflammatory Response via Down-Regulating JNK or STAT1/3 Pathways in Human Keratinocytes. *Life* **2022**, *12*, 589. [CrossRef]
29. Maiello, N.; Comberiati, P.; Giannetti, A.; Ricci, G.; Carello, R.; Galli, E. New Directions in Understanding Atopic March Starting from Atopic Dermatitis. *Children* **2022**, *9*, 450. [CrossRef]
30. Yang, L.; Fu, J.; Zhou, Y. Research Progress in Atopic March. *Front. Immunol.* **2020**, *11*, 559823. [CrossRef]
31. Martin, K.I.; Glaser, D.A. Cosmeceuticals: The New Medicine of Beauty. *Mo. Med.* **2011**, *108*, 60.
32. Siahaan, E.A.; Agusman; Pangestuti, R.; Shin, K.H.; Kim, S.K. Potential Cosmetic Active Ingredients Derived from Marine By-Products. *Mar. Drugs* **2022**, *20*, 734. [CrossRef]
33. Lee, J.; Hyun, C.G. Natural Products for Cosmetic Applications. *Molecules* **2023**, *28*, 534. [CrossRef] [PubMed]
34. Ghallab, D.S.; Shawky, E.; Ibrahim, R.S.; Mohyeldin, M.M. Comprehensive Metabolomics Unveil the Discriminatory Metabolites of Some Mediterranean Sea Marine Algae in Relation to Their Cytotoxic Activities. *Sci. Rep.* **2022**, *12*, 8094. [CrossRef] [PubMed]
35. Sutour, S.; XU, T.; Casabianca, H.; Paoli, M.; de Rocca-Serra, D.; Garrido, M.; Pasqualini, V.; Aiello, A.; Castola, V.; Bighelli, A. Chemical Composition of Extracts from Chaetomorpha Linum (Miller) Kütz. A Potential Use in the Cosmetic Industry. *Int. J Phytocosmetics Nat. Ingred.* **2015**, *2*, 5. [CrossRef]
36. Forrester, S.J.; Kikuchi, D.S.; Hernandes, M.S.; Xu, Q.; Griendling, K.K. Reactive Oxygen Species in Metabolic and Inflammatory Signaling. *Circ. Res.* **2018**, *122*, 877–902. [CrossRef] [PubMed]
37. Sharif, O.; Bolshakov, V.N.; Raines, S.; Newham, P.; Perkins, N.D. Transcriptional Profiling of the LPS Induced NF-kB Response in Macrophages. *BMC Immunol.* **2007**, *8*, 1. [CrossRef]
38. Trezza, A.; Geminiani, M.; Cutrera, G.; Dreassi, E.; Frusciante, L.; Lamponi, S.; Spiga, O.; Santucci, A. A Drug Discovery Approach to a Reveal Novel Antioxidant Natural Source: The Case of Chestnut Burr Biomass. *Int. J. Mol. Sci.* **2024**, *25*, 2517. [CrossRef] [PubMed]
39. Stabili, L.; Acquaviva, M.I.; Angilé, F.; Cavallo, R.A.; Cecere, E.; Del Coco, L.; Fanizzi, F.P.; Gerardi, C.; Narracci, M.; Petrocelli, A. Screening of Chaetomorpha Linum Lipidic Extract as a New Potential Source of Bioactive Compounds. *Mar. Drugs* **2019**, *17*, 313. [CrossRef] [PubMed]
40. Stabili, L.; Cecere, E.; Licciano, M.; Petrocelli, A.; Sicuro, B.; Giangrande, A. Integrated Multitrophic Aquaculture By-Products with Added Value: The Polychaete Sabella Spallanzanii and the Seaweed Chaetomorpha Linum as Potential Dietary Ingredients. *Mar. Drugs* **2019**, *17*, 677. [CrossRef]
41. Biandolino, F.; Prato, E. A Preliminary Investigation of the Lipids and Fatty Acids Composition of *Gammarus Aequicauda* (*Crustacea: Amphipoda*) and Its Main Food Source. *J. Mar. Biol. Assoc. United Kingd.* **2006**, *86*, 345–348. [CrossRef]
42. Barbosa, M.; Valentão, P.; Andrade, P.B. Biologically Active Oxylipins from Enzymatic and Nonenzymatic Routes in Macroalgae. *Mar. Drugs* **2016**, *14*, 23. [CrossRef]
43. Kumari, P.; Kumar, M.; Reddy, C.R.K.; Jha, B. Nitrate and Phosphate Regimes Induced Lipidomic and Biochemical Changes in the Intertidal Macroalga Ulva Lactuca (*Ulvophyceae, Chlorophyta*). *Plant Cell Physiol.* **2014**, *55*, 52–63. [CrossRef] [PubMed]
44. Khotimchenko, S.V.; Vaskovsky, V.E.; Titlyanova, T.V. Fatty Acids of Marine Algae from the Pacific Coast of North California. *Bor. Mar.* **2002**, *45*, 17–22. [CrossRef]
45. George, A.; Chinnappan, S.; Chintamaneni, M.; Kotak, C.V.; Choudhary, Y.; Kueper, T.; Radhakrishnan, A.K. Anti-Inflammatory Effects of Polygonum Minus (Huds) Extract (Lineminus™) in in-Vitro Enzyme Assays and Carrageenan Induced Paw Edema. *BMC Complement. Altern. Med.* **2014**, *14*, 355. [CrossRef] [PubMed]
46. Terme, N.; Chénais, B.; Fournière, M.; Bourgougnon, N.; Bedoux, G. Algal Derived Functional Lipids and Their Role in Promoting Health. In *Recent Advances in Micro and Macroalgal Processing*; Wiley: Hoboken, NJ, USA, 2021; pp. 370–417.
47. Kim, H.; Shin, H.Y.; Jeong, E.J.; Lee, H.D.; Hwang, K.C.; Yu, K.W.; Lee, S.; Lee, S. Antioxidant and Anti-Inflammatory Activities of Sargassum Macrocarpum Extracts. *Antioxidants* **2022**, *11*, 2483. [CrossRef] [PubMed]
48. da Costa, E.; Melo, T.; Reis, M.; Domingues, P.; Calado, R.; Abreu, M.H.; Domingues, M.R. Polar Lipids Composition, Antioxidant and Anti-Inflammatory Activities of the Atlantic Red Seaweed Grateloupia Turuturu. *Mar. Drugs* **2021**, *19*, 414. [CrossRef] [PubMed]
49. Leitner, P.D.; Jakschitz, T.; Gstir, R.; Stuppner, S.; Perkams, S.; Kruus, M.; Trockenbacher, A.; Griesbeck, C.; Bonn, G.K.; Huber, L.A.; et al. Anti-Inflammatory Extract from Soil Algae Chromochloris Zofingiensis Targeting TNFR/NF-kB Signaling at Different Levels. *Cells* **2022**, *11*, 1407. [CrossRef] [PubMed]
50. Lopes, G.; Daletos, G.; Proksch, P.; Andrade, P.B.; Valentão, P. Anti-Inflammatory Potential of Monogalactosyl Diacylglycerols and a Monoacylglycerol from the Edible Brown Seaweed Fucus Spiralis Linnaeus. *Mar. Drugs* **2014**, *12*, 1406–1418. [CrossRef] [PubMed]
51. Lopes, D.; Melo, T.; Rey, F.; Meneses, J.; Monteiro, F.L.; Helguero, L.A.; Abreu, M.H.; Lillebø, A.I.; Calado, R.; Domingues, M.R. Valuing Bioactive Lipids from Green, Red and Brown Macroalgae from Aquaculture, to Foster Functionality and Biotechnological Applications. *Molecules* **2020**, *25*, 3883. [CrossRef] [PubMed]
52. McCauley, J.I.; Meyer, B.J.; Winberg, P.C.; Ranson, M.; Skropeta, D. Selecting Australian Marine Macroalgae Based on the Fatty Acid Composition and Anti-Inflammatory Activity. *J. Appl. Phycol.* **2015**, *27*, 2111–2121. [CrossRef]
53. Lopes, D.; Melo, T.; Rey, F.; Costa, E.; Moreira, A.S.P.; Abreu, M.H.; Domingues, P.; Lillebø, A.I.; Calado, R.; Rosário Domingues, M. Insights of Species-Specific Polar Lipidome Signatures of Seaweeds Fostering Their Valorization in the Blue Bioeconomy. *Algal Res.* **2021**, *55*, 102242. [CrossRef]

54. Arguelles-Peña, K.; Olguín-Rojas, A.; Acosta-Osorio, A.A.; Carrera, C.; Barbero, G.F.; Ángel García-Alvarado, M.; Del Carmen Rodríguez-Jimenes, G.; Olguín-Rojas, K.; Acosta-Osorio, J.A.; Carrera, A.A.; et al. An Evaluation of the Equilibrium Properties in Hexane and Ethanol Extractive Systems for Moringa Oleifera Seeds and Fatty Acid Profiles of the Extracts. *Separations* **2021**, *8*, 217. [CrossRef]
55. Grima, E.M.; Medina, A.R.; Giménez, A.G.; Sánchez Pérez, J.A.; Camacho, F.G.; García Sánchez, J.L. Comparison between Extraction of Lipids and Fatty Acids from Microalgal Biomass. *J. Am. Oil Chem. Soc.* **1994**, *71*, 955–959. [CrossRef]
56. Food and Drug Administration Substances Generally Recognized as Safe (Final Rule) RIA; 2016. Available online: https://www.fda.gov/about-fda/economic-impact-analyses-fda-regulations/summary-substances-generally-recognized-safe-final-rule (accessed on 28 March 2024).
57. Molino, A.; Rimauro, J.; Casella, P.; Cerbone, A.; Larocca, V.; Chianese, S.; Karatza, D.; Mehariya, S.; Ferraro, A.; Hristoforou, E.; et al. Extraction of Astaxanthin from Microalga Haematococcus Pluvialis in Red Phase by Using Generally Recognized as Safe Solvents and Accelerated Extraction. *J. Biotechnol.* **2018**, *283*, 51–61. [CrossRef] [PubMed]
58. Seibert, K.; Zhang, Y.; Leahy, K.; Hauser, S.; Masferrer, J.; Perkins, W.; Lee, L.; Isakson, P. Pharmacological and Biochemical Demonstration of the Role of Cyclooxygenase 2 in Inflammation and Pain. *Proc. Natl. Acad. Sci. USA* **1994**, *91*, 12013–12017. [CrossRef] [PubMed]
59. Zamora, R.; Vodovotz, Y.; Billiar, T.R. Inducible Nitric Oxide Synthase and Inflammatory Diseases. *Mol. Med.* **2000**, *6*, 347–373. [CrossRef] [PubMed]
60. Cianchi, F.; Perna, F.; Masini, E. INOS/COX-2 Pathway Interaction: A Good Molecular Target for Cancer Treatment. *Curr. Enzym. Inhib.* **2005**, *1*, 97–105. [CrossRef]
61. Yeo, H.; Lee, Y.H.; Koh, D.; Lim, Y.; Shin, S.Y. Chrysin Inhibits NF-κB-Dependent CCL5 Transcription by Targeting IκB Kinase in the Atopic Dermatitis-Like Inflammatory Microenvironment. *Int. J. Mol. Sci.* **2020**, *21*, 7348. [CrossRef] [PubMed]
62. Kim, M.-J.; Hwang, B.S.; Hwang, Y.; Jeong, Y.T.; Jeong, D.W.; Oh, Y.T. Anti-Inflammatory and Antiatopic Effects of Rorippa Cantoniensis (Lour.) Ohwi in RAW 264.7 and HaCaT Cells. *Molecules* **2023**, *28*, 5463. [CrossRef] [PubMed]
63. Bhattacharjee, O.; Ayyangar, U.; Kurbet, A.S.; Lakshmanan, V.; Palakodeti, D.; Ginhoux, F.; Raghavan, S. Epithelial-Macrophage Crosstalk Initiates Sterile Inflammation in Embryonic Skin. *Front. Immunol.* **2021**, *12*, 718005. [CrossRef] [PubMed]
64. Villarreal-Ponce, A.; Tiruneh, M.W.; Lee, J.; Guerrero-Juarez, C.F.; Kuhn, J.; David, J.A.; Dammeyer, K.; Mc Kell, R.; Kwong, J.; Rabbani, P.S.; et al. Keratinocyte-Macrophage Crosstalk by the Nrf2/Ccl2/EGF Signaling Axis Orchestrates Tissue Repair. *Cell Rep.* **2020**, *33*, 108417. [CrossRef]
65. Khan, A.Q.; Agha, M.V.; Sheikhan, K.S.A.M.; Younis, S.M.; Al Tamimi, M.; Alam, M.; Ahmad, A.; Uddin, S.; Buddenkotte, J.; Steinhoff, M. Targeting Deregulated Oxidative Stress in Skin Inflammatory Diseases: An Update on Clinical Importance. *Biomed. Pharmacother.* **2022**, *154*, 113601. [CrossRef] [PubMed]
66. Liu, H.-M.; Cheng, M.-Y.; Xun, M.-H.; Zhao, Z.-W.; Zhang, Y.; Tang, W.; Cheng, J.; Ni, J.; Wang, W. Possible Mechanisms of Oxidative Stress-Induced Skin Cellular Senescence, Inflammation, and Cancer and the Therapeutic Potential of Plant Polyphenols. *Int. J. Mol. Sci.* **2023**, *24*, 3755. [CrossRef] [PubMed]
67. Allen, R.G.; Tresini, M. Oxidative Stress and Gene Regulation. *Free Radic. Biol. Med.* **2000**, *28*, 463–499. [CrossRef] [PubMed]
68. Frank, S.; Kolb, N.; Werner, E.R.; Pfeilschifter, J. Coordinated Induction of Inducible Nitric Oxide Synthase and GTP-Cyclohydrolase I Is Dependent on Inflammatory Cytokines and Interferon-γ in HaCaT Keratinocytes: Implications for the Model of Cutaneous Wound Repair. *J. Investig. Dermatol.* **1998**, *111*, 1065–1071. [CrossRef] [PubMed]
69. Takuathung, M.N.; Potikanond, S.; Sookkhee, S.; Mungkornasawakul, P.; Jearanaikulvanich, T.; Chinda, K.; Wikan, N.; Nimlamool, W. Anti-Psoriatic and Anti-Inflammatory Effects of Kaempferia Parviflora in Keratinocytes and Macrophage Cells. *Biomed. Pharmacother.* **2021**, *143*, 112229. [CrossRef] [PubMed]
70. Viard-Leveugle, I.; Gaide, O.; Jankovic, D.; Feldmeyer, L.; Kerl, K.; Pickard, C.; Roques, S.; Friedmann, P.S.; Contassot, E.; French, L.E. TNF-α and IFN-γ Are Potential Inducers of Fas-Mediated Keratinocyte Apoptosis through Activation of Inducible Nitric Oxide Synthase in Toxic Epidermal Necrolysis. *J. Investig. Dermatol.* **2013**, *133*, 489–498. [CrossRef] [PubMed]
71. Shiu, P.H.T.; Li, J.; Zheng, C.; Rangsinth, P.; Li, R.; Cheung, Q.T.L.; Lau, A.H.Y.; Chan, J.C.K.; Kwan, Y.W.; Cheung, T.M.Y.; et al. Amauroderma Rugosum Extract Suppresses Inflammatory Responses in Tumor Necrosis Factor Alpha/Interferon Gamma-Induced HaCaT Keratinocytes. *Molecules* **2022**, *27*, 6533. [CrossRef] [PubMed]
72. Santamarina, A.B.; Pisani, L.P.; Baker, E.J.; Marat, A.D.; Valenzuela, C.A.; Miles, E.A.; Calder, P.C. Anti-Inflammatory Effects of Oleic Acid and the Anthocyanin Keracyanin Alone and in Combination: Effects on Monocyte and Macrophage Responses and the NF-κB Pathway. *Food Funct.* **2021**, *12*, 7909–7922. [CrossRef] [PubMed]
73. Sung, J.; Jeon, H.; Kim, I.-H.; Jeong, H.S.; Lee, J. Anti-Inflammatory Effects of Stearidonic Acid Mediated by Suppression of NF-κB and MAP-Kinase Pathways in Macrophages. *Lipids* **2017**, *52*, 781–787. [CrossRef]
74. Dyall, S.C.; Balas, L.; Bazan, N.G.; Brenna, J.T.; Chiang, N.; da Costa Souza, F.; Dalli, J.; Durand, T.; Galano, J.M.; Lein, P.J.; et al. Polyunsaturated Fatty Acids and Fatty Acid-Derived Lipid Mediators: Recent Advances in the Understanding of Their Biosynthesis, Structures, and Functions. *Prog. Lipid Res.* **2022**, *86*, 101165. [CrossRef]
75. Santos, F.; Monteiro, J.P.; Duarte, D.; Melo, T.; Lopes, D.; da Costa, E.; Domingues, M.R. Unraveling the Lipidome and Antioxidant Activity of Native Bifurcaria Bifurcata and Invasive Sargassum Muticum Seaweeds: A Lipid Perspective on How Systemic Intrusion May Present an Opportunity. *Antioxidants* **2020**, *9*, 642. [CrossRef] [PubMed]

76. Kumari, P.; Reddy, R.; Jha, B. Quantification of Selected Endogenous Hydroxy-Oxylipins from Tropical Marine Macroalgae. *Mar. Biotechnol.* **2014**, *16*, 74–87. [CrossRef] [PubMed]
77. Morisseau, C.; Inceoglu, B.; Schmelzer, K.; Tsai, H.-J.; Jinks, S.L.; Hegedus, C.M.; Hammock, B.D. Naturally Occurring Monoepoxides of Eicosapentaenoic Acid and Docosahexaenoic Acid Are Bioactive Antihyperalgesic Lipids. *J. Lipid Res.* **2010**, *51*, 3481–3490. [CrossRef] [PubMed]
78. Yore, M.M.; Syed, I.; Moraes-Vieira, P.M.; Zhang, T.; Herman, M.A.; Homan, E.A.; Patel, R.T.; Lee, J.; Chen, S.; Peroni, O.D.; et al. Discovery of a Class of Endogenous Mammalian Lipids with Anti-Diabetic and Anti-Inflammatory Effects. *Cell* **2014**, *159*, 318–332. [CrossRef] [PubMed]
79. Kolar, M.J.; Konduri, S.; Chang, T.; Wang, H.; McNerlin, C.; Ohlsson, L.; Härröd, M.; Siegel, D.; Saghatelian, A. Linoleic Acid Esters of Hydroxy Linoleic Acids Are Anti-Inflammatory Lipids Found in Plants and Mammals. *J. Biol. Chem.* **2019**, *294*, 10698–10707. [CrossRef] [PubMed]
80. Ngu, E.-L.; Tan, C.-Y.; Lai, N.J.-Y.; Wong, K.-H.; Lim, S.-H.; Ming, L.C.; Tan, K.-O.; Phang, S.-M.; Yow, Y.-Y. Spirulina Platensis Suppressed INOS and Proinflammatory Cytokines in Lipopolysaccharide-Induced BV2 Microglia. *Metabolites* **2022**, *12*, 1147. [CrossRef] [PubMed]
81. Lai, N.J.-Y.; Ngu, E.-L.; Pang, J.-R.; Wong, K.-H.; Ardianto, C.; Ming, L.C.; Lim, S.-H.; Walvekar, S.G.; Anwar, A.; Yow, Y.-Y. Carrageenophyte Kappaphycus Malesianus Inhibits Microglia-Mediated Neuroinflammation via Suppression of AKT/NF-KB and ERK Signaling Pathways. *Mar. Drugs* **2022**, *20*, 534. [CrossRef] [PubMed]
82. Li, H.; Zuo, J.; Tang, W. Phosphodiesterase-4 Inhibitors for the Treatment of Inflammatory Diseases. *Front. Pharmacol.* **2018**, *9*, 409585. [CrossRef]
83. O'Brien, J.J.; O'Callaghan, J.P.; Miller, D.B.; Chalgeri, S.; Wennogle, L.P.; Davis, R.E.; Snyder, G.L.; Hendrick, J.P. Inhibition of Calcium-Calmodulin-Dependent Phosphodiesterase (PDE1) Suppresses Inflammatory Responses. *Mol. Cell. Neurosci.* **2020**, *102*, 103449. [CrossRef]
84. Dubois, M.; Picq, M.; Némoz, G.; Lagarde, M.; Prigent, A.-F. Inhibition of the Different Phosphodiesterase Isoforms of Rat Heart Cytosol by Free Fatty Acids. *J. Cardiovasc. Pharmacol.* **1993**, *21*, 522–529. [CrossRef]
85. Scapin, G.; Patel, S.B.; Chung, C.; Varnerin, J.P.; Edmondson, S.D.; Mastracchio, A.; Parmee, E.R.; Singh, S.B.; Becker, J.W. Van der Ploeg, L.H.T.; et al. Crystal Structure of Human Phosphodiesterase 3B: Atomic Basis for Substrate and Inhibitor Specificity. *Biochemistry* **2004**, *43*, 6091–6100. [CrossRef] [PubMed]
86. Wang, H.; Peng, M.-S.; Chen, Y.; Geng, J.; Robinson, H.; Houslay, M.D.; Cai, J.; Ke, H. Structures of the Four Subfamilies of Phosphodiesterase-4 Provide Insight into the Selectivity of Their Inhibitors. *Biochem. J.* **2007**, *408*, 193–201. [CrossRef] [PubMed]
87. O' Connor, J.; Meaney, S.; Williams, G.A.; Hayes, M. Extraction of Protein from Four Different Seaweeds Using Three Different Physical Pre-Treatment Strategies. *Molecules* **2020**, *25*, 2005. [CrossRef] [PubMed]
88. Gentscheva, G.; Milkova-Tomova, I.; Pehlivanov, I.; Gugleva, V.; Nikolova, K.; Petkova, N.; Andonova, V.; Buhalova, D.; Pisanova, E. Chemical Characterization of Selected Algae and Cyanobacteria from Bulgaria as Sources of Compounds with Antioxidant Activity. *Appl. Sci.* **2022**, *12*, 9935. [CrossRef]
89. Beaulieu, L.; Bondu, S.; Doiron, K.; Rioux, L.-E.; Turgeon, S.L. Characterization of Antibacterial Activity from Protein Hydrolysates of the Macroalga Saccharina Longicruris and Identification of Peptides Implied in Bioactivity. *J. Funct. Foods* **2015**, *17*, 685–697. [CrossRef]
90. Cian, R.E.; Martínez-Augustin, O.; Drago, S.R. Bioactive Properties of Peptides Obtained by Enzymatic Hydrolysis from Protein Byproducts of Porphyra Columbina. *Food Res. Int.* **2012**, *49*, 364–372. [CrossRef]
91. SAITO, M. Antihypertensive Effect of Nori-Peptides Derived from Red Alga Porphyra Yezoensis in Hypertensive Patients. *Am. J. Hypertens.* **2002**, *15*, A210. [CrossRef]
92. Admassu, H.; Gasmalla, M.A.A.; Yang, R.; Zhao, W. Identification of Bioactive Peptides with α-Amylase Inhibitory Potential from Enzymatic Protein Hydrolysates of Red Seaweed (*Porphyra* Spp). *J. Agric. Food Chem.* **2018**, *66*, 4872–4882. [CrossRef] [PubMed]
93. Cao, D.; Lv, X.; Xu, X.; Yu, H.; Sun, X.; Xu, N. Purification and Identification of a Novel ACE Inhibitory Peptide from Marine Alga Gracilariopsis Lemaneiformis Protein Hydrolysate. *Eur. Food Res. Technol.* **2017**, *243*, 1829–1837. [CrossRef]
94. Li, P.; Ying, J.; Chang, Q.; Zhu, W.; Yang, G.; Xu, T.; Yi, H.; Pan, R.; Zhang, E.; Zeng, X.; et al. Effects of Phycoerythrin from Gracilaria Lemaneiformis in Proliferation and Apoptosis of SW480 Cells. *Oncol. Rep.* **2016**, *36*, 3536–3544. [CrossRef]
95. Hung, L.D.; Hirayama, M.; Ly, B.M.; Hori, K. Biological Activity, CDNA Cloning and Primary Structure of Lectin KSA-2 from the Cultivated Red Alga Kappaphycus Striatum (Schmitz) Doty Ex Silva. *Phytochem. Lett.* **2015**, *14*, 99–105. [CrossRef]
96. Nam, T.-J. A Glycoprotein from Porphyra Yezoensis Produces Anti-Inflammatory Effects in Liposaccharide-Stimulated Macrophages via the TLR4 Signaling Pathway. *Int. J. Mol. Med.* **2011**, *28*, 809–815. [CrossRef] [PubMed]
97. de Queiroz, I.N.L.; Quinderé, A.L.G.; Rodrigues, J.A.G.; de Sousa Oliveira Vanderlei, E.; Ribeiro, N.A.; da Conceição Rivanor, R.L.; Ribeiro, K.A.; Coura, C.O.; Pereira, K.M.A.; Chaves, H.V.; et al. Dual Effects of a Lectin from the Green Seaweed Caulerpa Cupressoides Var. Lycopodium on Inflammatory Mediators in Classical Models of Inflammation. *Inflamm. Res.* **2015**, *64*, 971–982. [CrossRef] [PubMed]
98. Abu Bakar, N.; Anyanji, V.U.; Mustapha, N.M.; Lim, S.-L.; Mohamed, S. Seaweed (Eucheuma Cottonii) Reduced Inflammation, Mucin Synthesis, Eosinophil Infiltration and MMP-9 Expressions in Asthma-Induced Rats Compared to Loratadine. *J. Funct. Foods* **2015**, *19*, 710–722. [CrossRef]

99. Lee, H.-A.; Kim, I.-H.; Nam, T.-J. Bioactive Peptide from Pyropia Yezoensis and Its Anti-Inflammatory Activities. *Int. J. Mol. Med.* **2015**, *36*, 1701–1706. [CrossRef] [PubMed]
100. Mesquita, J.X.; de Brito, T.V.; Fontenelle, T.P.C.; Damasceno, R.O.S.; de Souza, M.H.L.P.; de Souza Lopes, J.L.; Beltramini, L.M.; dos Reis Barbosa, A.L.; Freitas, A.L.P. Lectin from Red Algae Amansia Multifida Lamouroux: Extraction, Characterization and Anti-Inflammatory Activity. *Int. J. Biol. Macromol.* **2021**, *170*, 532–539. [CrossRef] [PubMed]
101. Lim, H.; Heo, M.Y.; Kim, H.P. Flavonoids: Broad Spectrum Agents on Chronic Inflammation. *Biomol. Ther.* **2019**, *27*, 241–253. [CrossRef] [PubMed]
102. Vernarelli, J.A.; Lambert, J.D. Flavonoid Intake Is Inversely Associated with Obesity and C-Reactive Protein, a Marker for Inflammation, in US Adults. *Nutr. Diabetes* **2017**, *7*, e276. [CrossRef] [PubMed]
103. Alam, W.; Khan, H.; Shah, M.A.; Cauli, O.; Saso, L. Kaempferol as a Dietary Anti-Inflammatory Agent: Current Therapeutic Standing. *Molecules* **2020**, *25*, 4073. [CrossRef]
104. Yoon, J.H.; Kim, M.-Y.; Cho, J.Y. Apigenin: A Therapeutic Agent for Treatment of Skin Inflammatory Diseases and Cancer. *Int. J. Mol. Sci.* **2023**, *24*, 1498. [CrossRef]
105. Ginwala, R.; Bhavsar, R.; Chigbu, D.I.; Jain, P.; Khan, Z.K. Potential Role of Flavonoids in Treating Chronic Inflammatory Diseases with a Special Focus on the Anti-Inflammatory Activity of Apigenin. *Antioxidants* **2019**, *8*, 35. [CrossRef]
106. Li, K.; Hu, W.; Yang, Y.; Wen, H.; Li, W.; Wang, B. Anti-Inflammation of Hydrogenated Isoflavones in LPS-Stimulated RAW264.7 Cells via Inhibition of NF-κB and MAPK Signaling Pathways. *Mol. Immunol.* **2023**, *153*, 126–134. [CrossRef]
107. Michalak, I.; Tiwari, R.; Dhawan, M.; Alagawany, M.; Farag, M.R.; Sharun, K.; Bin Emran, T.; Dhama, K. Antioxidant Effects of Seaweeds and Their Active Compounds on Animal Health and Production—A Review. *Vet. Q.* **2022**, *42*, 48–67. [CrossRef] [PubMed]
108. Habtemariam, S. Anti-Inflammatory Therapeutic Mechanisms of Natural Products: Insight from Rosemary Diterpenes, Carnosic Acid and Carnosol. *Biomedicines* **2023**, *11*, 545. [CrossRef]
109. Yeo, I.J.; Park, J.H.; Jang, J.S.; Lee, D.Y.; Park, J.E.; Choi, Y.E.; Joo, J.H.; Song, J.K.; Jeon, H.O.; Hong, J.T. Inhibitory Effect of Carnosol on UVB-Induced Inflammation via Inhibition of STAT3. *Arch. Pharm. Res.* **2019**, *42*, 274–283. [CrossRef] [PubMed]
110. Ng, N.; Ooi, L. A Simple Microplate Assay for Reactive Oxygen Species Generation and Rapid Cellular Protein Normalization. *Bio-protocol* **2021**, *11*, e3877. [CrossRef]
111. Feoktistova, M.; Geserick, P.; Leverkus, M. Crystal Violet Assay for Determining Viability of Cultured Cells. *Cold Spring Harb. Protoc.* **2016**, *2016*, pdb.prot087379. [CrossRef]
112. Geminiani, M.; Gambassi, S.; Millucci, L.; Lupetti, P.; Collodel, G.; Mazzi, L.; Frediani, B.; Braconi, D.; Marzocchi, B.; Laschi, M.; et al. Cytoskeleton Aberrations in Alkaptonuric Chondrocytes. *J. Cell Physiol.* **2017**, *232*, 1728–1738. [CrossRef]
113. Mortelmans, K.; Zeiger, E. The Ames Salmonella/Microsome Mutagenicity Assay. *Mutat. Res./Fundam. Mol. Mech. Mutagen.* **2000**, *455*, 29–60. [CrossRef] [PubMed]
114. Wishart, D.S.; Feunang, Y.D.; Guo, A.C.; Lo, E.J.; Marcu, A.; Grant, J.R.; Sajed, T.; Johnson, D.; Li, C.; Sayeeda, Z.; et al. DrugBank 5.0: A Major Update to the DrugBank Database for 2018. *Nucleic Acids Res.* **2018**, *46*, D1074–D1082. [CrossRef]
115. Rouillard, A.D.; Gundersen, G.W.; Fernandez, N.F.; Wang, Z.; Monteiro, C.D.; McDermott, M.G.; Ma'ayan, A. The Harmonizome: A Collection of Processed Datasets Gathered to Serve and Mine Knowledge about Genes and Proteins. *Database* **2016**, *2016*, baw100. [CrossRef] [PubMed]
116. Berman, H.M.; Westbrook, J.; Feng, Z.; Gilliland, G.; Bhat, T.N.; Weissig, H.; Shindyalov, I.N.; Bourne, P.E. The Protein Data Bank. *Nucleic Acids Res.* **2000**, *28*, 235–242. [CrossRef] [PubMed]
117. Bateman, A.; Martin, M.J.; O'Donovan, C.; Magrane, M.; Alpi, E.; Antunes, R.; Bely, B.; Bingley, M.; Bonilla, C.; Britto, R.; et al. UniProt: The Universal Protein Knowledgebase. *Nucleic Acids Res.* **2017**, *45*, D158–D169. [CrossRef] [PubMed]
118. Johnson, M.; Zaretskaya, I.; Raytselis, Y.; Merezhuk, Y.; McGinnis, S.; Madden, T.L. NCBI BLAST: A Better Web Interface. *Nucleic Acids Res.* **2008**, *36*, W5–W9. [CrossRef] [PubMed]
119. Janson, G.; Paiardini, A. PyMod 3: A Complete Suite for Structural Bioinformatics in PyMOL. *Bioinformatics* **2021**, *37*, 1471–1472. [CrossRef] [PubMed]
120. Laskowski, R.A.; MacArthur, M.W.; Moss, D.S.; Thornton, J.M. PROCHECK: A Program to Check the Stereochemical Quality of Protein Structures. *J. Appl. Crystallogr.* **1993**, *26*, 283–291. [CrossRef]
121. Berendsen, H.J.C.; van der Spoel, D.; van Drunen, R. GROMACS: A Message-Passing Parallel Molecular Dynamics Implementation. *Comput. Phys. Commun.* **1995**, *91*, 43–56. [CrossRef]
122. Jo, S.; Kim, T.; Iyer, V.G.; Im, W. CHARMM-GUI: A Web-based Graphical User Interface for CHARMM. *J. Comput. Chem.* **2008**, *29*, 1859–1865. [CrossRef] [PubMed]
123. Koebel, M.R.; Schmadeke, G.; Posner, R.G.; Sirimulla, S. AutoDock VinaXB: Implementation of XBSF, New Empirical Halogen Bond Scoring Function, into AutoDock Vina. *J. Cheminform.* **2016**, *8*, 27. [CrossRef]
124. Kim, S.; Chen, J.; Cheng, T.; Gindulyte, A.; He, J.; He, S.; Li, Q.; Shoemaker, B.A.; Thiessen, P.A.; Yu, B.; et al. PubChem 2019 Update: Improved Access to Chemical Data. *Nucleic Acids Res.* **2019**, *47*, D1102–D1109. [CrossRef]
125. O'Boyle, N.M.; Banck, M.; James, C.A.; Morley, C.; Vandermeersch, T.; Hutchison, G.R. Open Babel: An Open Chemical Toolbox. *J. Cheminformatics* **2011**, *3*, 33. [CrossRef] [PubMed]

126. Fusi, F.; Trezza, A.; Spiga, O.; Sgaragli, G.; Bova, S. Ca v 1.2 Channel Current Block by the PKA Inhibitor H-89 in Rat Tail Artery Myocytes via a PKA-Independent Mechanism: Electrophysiological, Functional, and Molecular Docking Studies. *Biochem. Pharmacol.* **2017**, *140*, 53–63. [CrossRef] [PubMed]
127. Fusi, F.; Durante, M.; Spiga, O.; Trezza, A.; Frosini, M.; Floriddia, E.; Teodori, E.; Dei, S.; Saponara, S. In Vitro and in Silico Analysis of the Vascular Effects of Asymmetrical N,N-Bis(Alkanol)Amine Aryl Esters, Novel Multidrug Resistance-Reverting Agents. *Naunyn Schmiedebergs Arch. Pharmacol.* **2016**, *389*, 1033–1043. [CrossRef]
128. Adasme, M.F.; Linnemann, K.L.; Bolz, S.N.; Kaiser, F.; Salentin, S.; Haupt, V.J.; Schroeder, M. PLIP 2021: Expanding the Scope of the Protein–Ligand Interaction Profiler to DNA and RNA. *Nucleic Acids Res.* **2021**, *49*, W530–W534. [CrossRef]

Disclaimer/Publisher's Note: The statements, opinions and data contained in all publications are solely those of the individual author(s) and contributor(s) and not of MDPI and/or the editor(s). MDPI and/or the editor(s) disclaim responsibility for any injury to people or property resulting from any ideas, methods, instructions or products referred to in the content.

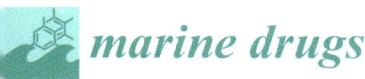

Article

The Role of Sargahydroquinoic Acid and Sargachromenol in the Anti-Inflammatory Effect of *Sargassum yezoense*

Yena Park [1,†], Lei Cao [2,†], Suhyeon Baek [1], Seungjin Jeong [1], Hyun Jung Yun [3], Mi-Bo Kim [4,*] and Sang Gil Lee [1,4,*]

1. Department of Smart Green Technology Engineering, Pukyong National University, Busan 48513, Republic of Korea; qkrdpsk1141@gmail.com (Y.P.); bmh46750@gmail.com (S.B.); wtw3737@gmail.com (S.J.)
2. Department of Food Science and Biotechnology, Gachon University, Seongnam 13120, Republic of Korea; caolei@gachon.ac.kr
3. Food Safety and Processing Research Division, National Institute of Fisheries Science, Busan 46083, Republic of Korea; yhj0412@korea.kr
4. Department of Food Science and Nutrition, College of Fisheries Science, Pukyong National University, Busan 48513, Republic of Korea
* Correspondence: mibokim1120@gmail.com (M.-B.K.); sglee1125@pknu.ac.kr (S.G.L.); Tel.: +82-051-629-5842 (M.-B.K.); +82-051-629-5851 (S.G.L.)
† These authors contributed equally to this work.

Abstract: The anti-inflammatory effect of the ethanol extract of *Sargassum yezoense* and its fractions were investigated in this study. The ethanol extract exhibited a strong anti-inflammatory effect on lipopolysaccharide-stimulated RAW 264.7 macrophages and effectively suppressed the M1 polarization of murine bone-marrow-derived macrophages stimulated by lipopolysaccharides and IFN-γ (interferon-gamma). Through a liquid–liquid extraction process, five fractions (n-hexane, chloroform, ethyl acetate, butanol, and aqueous) were acquired. Among these fractions, the chloroform fraction (SYCF) was found to contain the highest concentration of phenolic compounds, along with two primary meroterpenoids, sargahydroquinoic acid (SHQA) and sargachromenol (SCM), and exhibit significant antioxidant capacity. It also demonstrated a robust anti-inflammatory effect. A direct comparison was conducted to assess the relative contribution of SHQA and SCM to the anti-inflammatory properties of SYCF. The concentrations of SHQA and SCM tested were determined based on their relative abundance in SYCF. SHQA contributed to a significant portion of the anti-inflammatory property of SYCF, while SCM played a limited role. These findings not only highlight the potential of the chloroform–ethanol fractionation approach for concentrating meroterpenoids in *S. yezoense* but also demonstrate that SHQA and other bioactive compounds work additively or synergistically to produce the potent anti-inflammatory effect of SYCF.

Keywords: *Sargassum yezoense*; anti-inflammation; liquid–liquid partition; sargahydroquinoic acid; sargachromenol

Citation: Park, Y.; Cao, L.; Baek, S.; Jeong, S.; Yun, H.J.; Kim, M.-B.; Lee, S.G. The Role of Sargahydroquinoic Acid and Sargachromenol in the Anti-Inflammatory Effect of *Sargassum yezoense*. *Mar. Drugs* **2024**, *22*, 107. https://doi.org/10.3390/md22030107

Academic Editors: Donatella Degl'Innocenti and Marzia Vasarri

Received: 22 January 2024
Revised: 21 February 2024
Accepted: 24 February 2024
Published: 26 February 2024

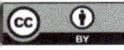

Copyright: © 2024 by the authors. Licensee MDPI, Basel, Switzerland. This article is an open access article distributed under the terms and conditions of the Creative Commons Attribution (CC BY) license (https://creativecommons.org/licenses/by/4.0/).

1. Introduction

Sargassum species, belonging to the phylum of brown algae, predominantly inhabit tropical and subtropical marine environments. These species form marine ecosystems that support a diverse array of marine life through the provision of food and habitat. Notably, specific *Sargassum* species, such as *Sargassum fusiforme* and *Sargassum horneri*, have been traditionally utilized for culinary and medicinal purposes in Asian countries, including Korea, China, and Japan [1,2]. Pharmacological investigations have also revealed that *Sargassum* species exhibit diverse therapeutic properties, such as anticancer, anti-inflammatory, antibacterial, and antiviral activities. These effects are largely attributed to the presence of bioactive metabolites, including polyphenols, carotenoids, polysaccharides, and meroterpenoids [2,3].

Sargassum yezoense (Yamada), a prevalent species along the eastern coast of Korea, is recognized for its abundance and wide distribution [4]. The methanol extract of this species has demonstrated significant potential in regulating adipogeneisis [5]. Despite this, research focusing on the bioactive components of *S. yezoense*, particularly meroterpenoids, remains relatively scarce compared to other extensively studied *Sargassum* species.

Meroterpenoids are natural secondary metabolites, with their structure partially derived from terpenoid pathways. Notable examples include coenzyme Q10 and α-tocopherol (vitamin E) [6]. Synthesized by diverse organisms, including algae, meroterpenoids exhibit structural diversity based on their origin and biosynthesis. This diversity underpins their broad spectrum of biological activities, encompassing anti-cholinesterase, anti-diabetic, antioxidative, anti-inflammatory, and antineoplastic properties, alongside renal, cardioprotective, and neuroprotective effects [7]. *Sargassum* species are also rich sources of meroterpenoid compounds, including sargahydroquinoic acid (SHQA), sargachromenol (SCM), and sargaquinoic acid (SQA) [8]. Importantly, meroterpenoids from *Sargassum* species have demonstrated inhibitory effects on the expression of nitric oxide, tumor necrosis factor (TNF), and other inflammatory mediators [9–11].

In both the food and pharmaceutical industries, various separation techniques are utilized to isolate and purify natural products from complex extracts. These include adsorption column chromatography, gel filtration chromatography, membrane filtration, and liquid–liquid extraction (LLE) [12]. LLE, in particular, is a commonly employed method for separating compounds or complexes, based on differential solubility in immiscible solvents. It finds extensive application in the food industry for purposes, such as flavor analysis, separation of food colorings, and detection of antibiotics in food products [13–15]. Employed as a fractionation method for crude extracts, LLE enables the recovery of secondary metabolite-enriched fractions using solvents of varying polarities [6]. For instance, LLE using solvents like n-hexane and ethyl acetate has been effective in isolating meroterpenoid compounds from ethanol extracts of *S. serratifolium* and marine-drived fungus *Aspergillus vesicolor* [8,16].

The present study aims to evaluate the anti-inflammatory effects and bioactive components of ethanol extracts and various fractions of *S. yezoense*, with a particular focus on the reliable roles of two key meroterpenoids, SHQA and SCM.

2. Results

2.1. Anti-Inflammatory Effect of Ethanol Extract of S. yezoense

The ethanol extract of *S. yezoense* (SYEE) did not show any toxicity towards RAW 264.7 cells up to 25 μg/mL (Figure 1a). Moreover, SYEE exhibited significant inhibition in lipopolysaccharide (LPS)-induced elevation of mRNA levels of pro-inflammatory factors, including *Tnf*, interleukin-1 beta (*Il1b*), cyclooxygenase-2 (*Cox2*), nitric oxide synthase 2 (*Nos2*), and NADPH oxidase 2 (*Nox2*) (Figure 1b). The inhibitory effect was also observed on the protein expression levels of NOS2 and COX2 (Figure 1c). Specifically, when treated at a concentration of 5 μg/mL, SYEE effectively mitigated the induction of COX2 and NOS2, reducing their expression to levels comparable to those in non-exposed samples. In accordance with the mRNA expression of *Tnf*, the secretion of TNF was significantly suppressed when exposed to SYEE at concentrations of 5.0 and 10 μg/mL (Figure 1d).

Furthermore, a combined treatment of LPS and interferon-gamma (IFN-γ) was adopted to induce the M1 polarization of bone-marrow-derived macrophages (BMDMs). This treatment significantly upregulated the mRNA expression levels of M1 markers, such as *Il1b*, *Nos2*, and a surface marker cluster of differentiation 86 (*Cd86*) [17,18]. SYEE effectively inhibited their induction (Figure 2). SYEE also markedly ameliorated the mRNA levels of another pro-inflammatory factor, *Cox2*. SYEE also showed intracellular antixodaint capacity by supressing the induction of *Nox1* and *Nox2*.

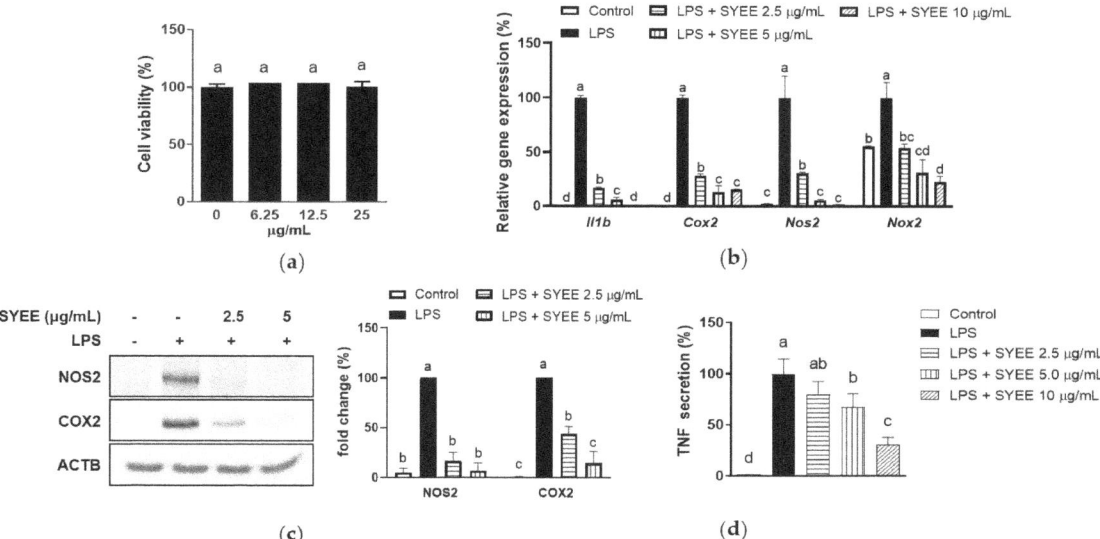

Figure 1. Effect of SYEE on LPS-stimulated RAW 264.7 macrophages. (**a**) Effect of SYEE on cell viability of RAW 264.7 macrophages were measured. (**b**) Levels of mRNA expression of *Tnf*, *Il6*, *Cox2*, *Nos2*, and *Nox2* were presented as fold changes relative to the LPS-stimulated samples; (**c**) Level of protein expression of COX2 and NOS2 were presented as fold changes relative to the LPS-stimulated samples. β-Actin (ACTB) was used as the internal control. (**d**) Level of secreted TNF was presented as fold changes relative to the LPS-stimulated samples. The data are expressed as mean ± standard deviation (n = 3). Columns without a common letter differ from each other significantly (p < 0.05).

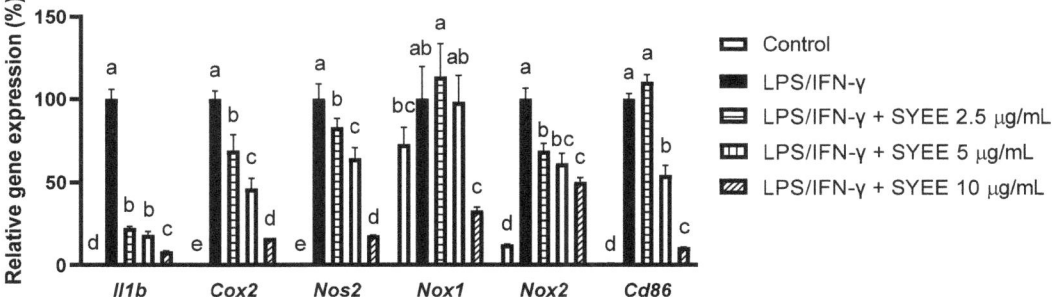

Figure 2. Effect of SYEE on LPS- and IFN-γ-stimulated mouse BMDMs. Level of mRNA expression of *Il1b*, *Cox2*, *Nos2*, *Nox1*, *Nox2*, and *Cd86* were presented as fold changes relative to the LPS-stimulated samples. The data are expressed as mean ± standard deviation (n = 3). Columns without a common letter differ from each other significantly (p < 0.05).

To examine the effect of SYEE treatment on the cell cycle, the cells were sorted based on their cell cycle stages (Figure 3a,b). LPS treatment increased the percentage of cells in the G0/G1 phase and decreased the cells at the S and G2/M stages. SYEE significantly recovered this LPS-led cell cycle disruption.

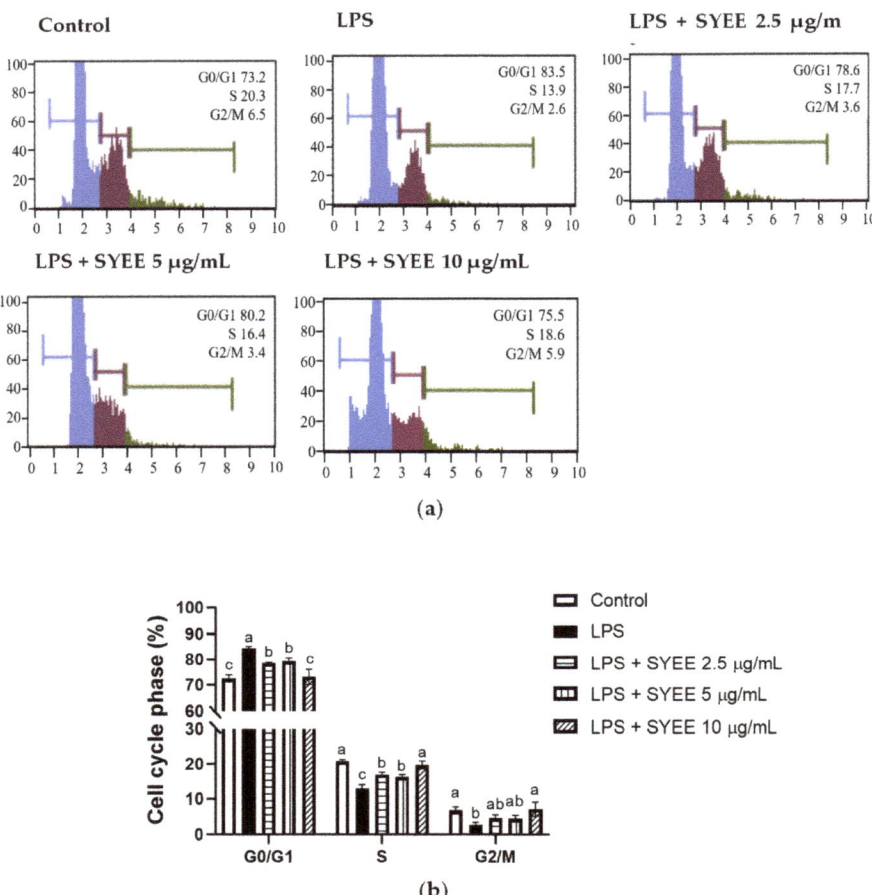

Figure 3. Effect of SYEE on cell cycle arrest analysis. The cell cycle distribution was determined by flow cytometric analysis of the DNA content of RAW 264.7 cells following staining with Muse™ Cell Cycle Reagent. After indicated treatment, the number of cells in the G0/G1, S, and G2/M stages was determined. (**a**) Fluorescence-activated cell sorting analysis; (**b**) the percentage of cells in different cell cycle phases. The data are expressed as mean ± standard deviation (n = 3). Columns not sharing a common letter are significantly different from each other ($p < 0.05$).

2.2. Phenolic Content and Antioxidant Capcaties of SYEE and its Fractions

The SYEE was partitioned into a hexane fraction (SYHF), chloroform fraction (SYCF), ethyl acetate fraction (SYEtF), butanol fraction (SYBF), and aqueous fraction (SYWF) by LLE. Among the five fractions, SYWF had the highest overall yield at 54%, followed by SYHF 20%, SYCF 14%, SYEtF 2%, and SYBF 2%. Their total phenolic content (TPC) and total antioxidant capacities were analyzed (Table 1).

Among the fractions, SYCF emerged with the highest phenolic content (80.46 mg phloroglucinol equivalent/g) and demonstrated superior antioxidant capacity (158.28 mg vitamin C equivalent/g for DPPH assay, 182.48 mg vitamin C equivalent/g for ABTS assay, and 0.47 mmol FeSO4 equivalent/g for FRAP assay). SYEtF possessed the second-highest phenolic content and antioxidant capacity. While SYBF showed a comparable TPC and FRAP capacity with SYEE, its DPPH and ABTS activities were slightly lower. In addition, SYWF exhibited the lowest antioxidant capacity and TPC among all fractions.

Table 1. The phenolic content and antioxidant activities SYEE and different fractions.

	Yield (%)	TPC (mg PGE/g)	DPPH (mg VCE/g)	ABTS (mg VCE/g)	FRAP (mmol FSE/g)
SYEE	3.4	25.20 ± 6.17 [d]	42.17 ± 1.27 [c]	97.65 ± 0.87 [b]	0.18 ± 0.02 [d]
SYHF	20	43.01 ± 3.69 [c]	58.83 ± 1.73 [b]	98.32 ± 3.33 [b]	0.28 ± 0.04 [c]
SYCF	14	80.46 ± 4.05 [a]	158.28 ± 2.10 [a]	182.48 ± 15.22 [a]	0.47 ± 0.02 [a]
SYEtF	2	58.36 ± 1.84 [b]	65.22 ± 7.64 [b]	108.32 ± 6.45 [b]	0.40 ± 0.02 [b]
SYBF	2	32.75 ± 6.54 [cd]	23.56 ± 3.63 [d]	59.15 ± 1.73 [c]	0.24 ± 0.01 [cd]
SYWF	54	8.45 ± 2.45 [e]	14.39 ± 4.17 [d]	27.65 ± 1.80 [d]	0.02 ± 0.00 [e]

TPC, total phenolic content; DPPH, 2,2-diphenyl-1-picrylhydrazyl radical scavenging capacity; ABTS, 2,2′-azino-bis (3-ethylbenzthiazoline-6-sulfonic acid radical scavenging capacity; FRAP, ferric-reducing antioxidant power. PGE, phloroglucinol equivalent; VCE, vitamin C equivalent; FSE, FeSO$_4$ equivalent. The data are expressed as mean ± standard deviation (n = 3). Numbers that do not share a common letter are significantly different ($p < 0.05$).

2.3. Anti-Inflammatory Activities of Fractions of SYEE

Given the enhanced phenolic content and robust antioxidant capacity observed in the three fractions (SYHF, SYCF, and SYEtF), we proceeded to investigate their anti-inflammatory effect on LPS-stimulated macrophages. The cytotoxicity of these three fractions on RAW 264.7 cells were tested (Figure 4a–c). SYEtF exhibited no toxicity at concentrations up to 25 µg/mL, while SYHF and SYCF showed no toxicity at concentrations up to 12.5 µg/mL.

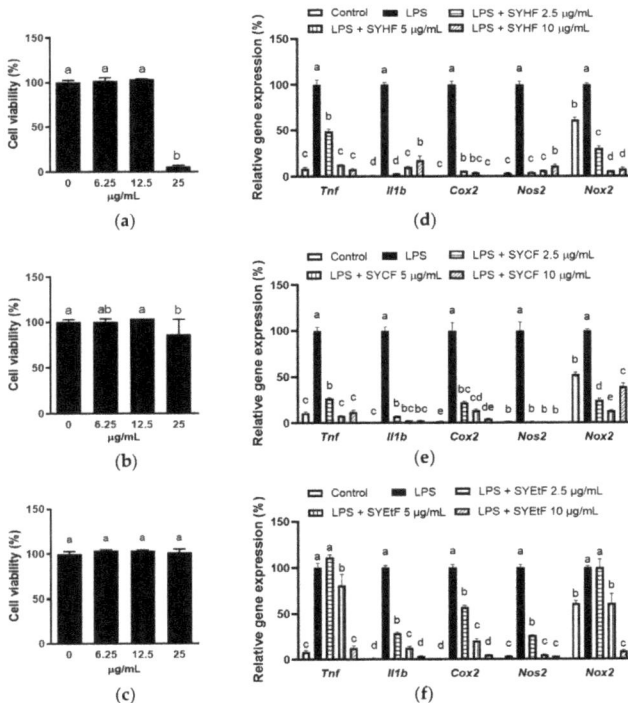

Figure 4. Effect of SYHF, SYCF, and SYEtF on LPS-stimulated RAW 264.7 macrophages. The effect of (**a**) SYHF, (**b**) SYCF, and (**c**) SYEtF on cell viablity of RAW 264.7 macrophages. The effect of (**d**) SYHF, (**e**) SYCF, and (**f**) SYEtF on mRNA expression of *Tnf*, *Il6*, *Cox2*, *Nos2*, and *Nox2*. The data are expressed as mean ± standard deviation (n = 3). Columns without a common letter differ from each other significantly ($p < 0.05$).

As shown in Figure 4d,e, both SYHF and SYCF exhibited a significant reduction in the mRNA expression of pro-inflammatory factors, beginning at the lowest concentration tested (2.5 μg/mL). Specifically, at 2.5 μg/mL, SYCF suppressed the levels of *Tnf*, *Il1b*, *Cox2*, *Nos2*, and *Nox2* to 26.79%, 7.15%, 21.88 %, 1.5%, and 24.23%, respectively, compared to LPS-stimulated samples. Concurrently, SYHF achieved reductions of 48.65%, 2.99%, 5.72%, 4.38%, and 29.70% for the same pro-inflammatory factors.

On the contrary, SYEtF, at a concentration of 2.5 μg/mL, did not exhibit significant inhibition in the elevation of *Tnf* and *Nox2* (Figure 4f). This suggests a comparatively weaker anti-inflammatory effect of SYEtF when compared to the robust effects observed in SYHF and SYCF.

Although both SYHF and SYCF inhibited the mRNA expression of *Tnf* at 2.5 μg/mL, these concentrations of SYCF did not inhibit the secretion of TNF (Figure 5a–c). Compared to SYCF, SYHF showed a more pronounced inhibition on the secretion of TNF. With regard to SYEtF, contrary to the *Tnf* mRNA expression level, the TNF secretion level remained unaffected across all three tested concentrations.

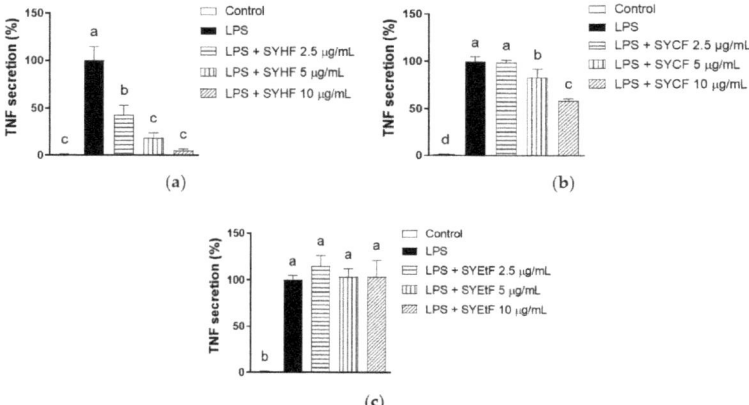

Figure 5. Effect of (**a**) SYHF, (**b**) SYCF and (**c**) SYEtF on TNF secretion of LPS-simulated RAW 264.7 macrophages. The data are expressed as mean ± standard deviation (n = 3). Columns without a common letter differ from each other significantly ($p < 0.05$).

2.4. Quantification of SHQA and SCM

The quantification of two key meroterpenoids in *Sargassum* species, SHQA and SCM, was carried out in both SYEE and its hexane, chloroform, and ethyl acetate fractions through HPLC (Supplementary Figure S1). The spectra of SHQA and SCM were also presented.

In SYEE, SYHF, SYCF, and SYEtF, SHQA was found to constitute 5.89%, 6.49%, 15.01%, and 2.89% of the total composition, respectively (Table 2). The abundance of SCM was relatively lower compared to SHQA, ranging approximately between 0.53% and 1.96% of the total yield. SYCF exhibited the highest content of both SHQA and SCM, surpassing the levels observed in the ethanol extract and the other two fractions. This observation suggests that the ethanol–chloroform partition may serve as an efficient method for concentrating SHQA and SCM from *S. yezoense*.

Table 2. Quantification of SHQA and SCM in the ethanol extract and three fractions of *S. yezoense*.

	SHQA (mg/g)	SCM (mg/g)
SYEE	58.9	5.3
SYHF	64.9	11.6
SYCF	150.1	19.6
SYEtF	28.9	5.5

2.5. Contribution of SHQA and SCM to Anti-Inflammatory Effect of SYCF

Previously, the anti-inflammatory effect of SHQA and SCM was studied individually [9,10,19]. To better understand its contribution to the anti-inflammatory properties of SYCF, a direct comparison between SYCF, SHQA, and SCM was conducted, based on their relative abundance in SYCF.

As shown in Figure 6a,b, both SYCF (at a concentration of 2.5 µg/mL) and its corresponding SHQA (at a concentration of 0.375 µg/mL or 0.89 µM) effectively suppressed the induction of *Tnf*, *Il1b*, *Il6*, *Nos2*, *Cox2*, and *Nox2*. On the other hand, SCM (at a concentration of 0.05 µg/mL or 0.12 µM) demonstrated a suppressive effect only on the the expression of *Tnf* and *Nox2*. Noteworthily, SCM at 0.12 µM significantly increased the mRNA expression of *Nos2*. Compared to SHQA, SYCF suppressed the level of *Tnf*, *Il1b*, *Nos2* and *Cox2* to a stronger extent.

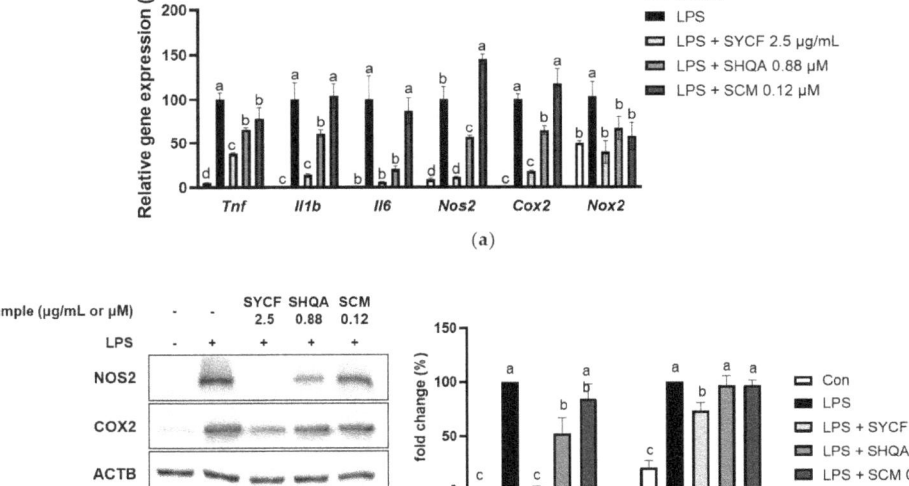

Figure 6. Contribution of SHQA and SCM on inhibition of LPS-induced inflammation. (**a**) The effect of SYCF, and corresponding concentration of SHQA and SCM on mRNA expression of *Tnf*, *Il1b*, *Il6*, *Nos2*, *Cox2*, and *Nox2*. (**b**) The effect of SYCF, and corresponding concentration of SHQA and SCM on protein expression of NOS2 and COX2. The data are expressed as mean ± standard deviation (n = 3). Columns without a common letter differ from each other significantly (p < 0.05).

Based on the protein expression level of NOS2 and COX2, SYCF completely inhibited the LPS-induced NOS2 expression, whereas SHQA reduced NOS2 expression to approximately 30%, and SCM did not show a significant impact. In addition, SYCF also reduced COX2 expression, while SHQA and SCM had no effect on it. This suggests that SHQA, along with other bioactive compounds, may work additively or synergistically to produce the potent anti-inflammatory effect of SYCF. SCM, which is present in low abundance, may have a limited contribution to these effects.

The nuclear factor-κB (NF-κB) pathway is critical in regulating inflammatory responses. The nuclear translocation of NF-κB was assessed via immunofluorescence (Figure 7a,b). A significant inhibition of the nuclear translocation of NF-κB by both SYCF and SHQA was observed, with SYCF showing a more potent supression than SHQA.

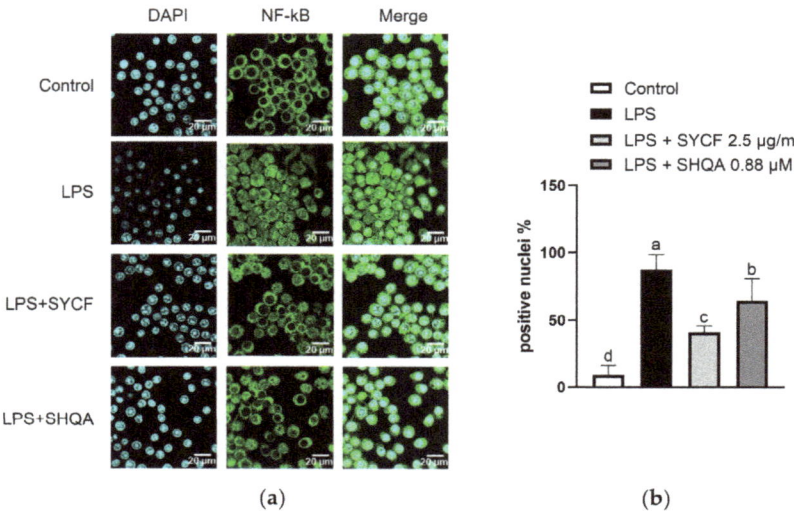

Figure 7. Effect of SYCF and SHQA on nuclear translocation of NF-κB. (**a**) NF-κB immunolocalization in RAW 264.7 cells treated with LPS, analyzing using NF-kB antibody (green). Nuclei were DAPI stained (blue). (**b**) Percentage of NF-κB-positive nuclei observed and counted. Data represent as mean ± standard deviation ($n = 4$ field of observation). Columns without a common letter differ from each other significantly ($p < 0.05$). Scale bar indicates 20 µm.

3. Discussion

Previous studies showed that the meroterpenoids SHQA and SCM, isolated from *S. macrocarpa* and *S. siliquastrum*, exert anti-inflammatory effects in LPS-induced macrophages [10,11]. However, few studies have examined the contribution of meroterpenoids to the antioxidant and anti-inflammatory effects of *Sargassum* species based on their real abundancy. In this study, the anti-inflammatory property of an ethanol extract of *S. yezoense* and its fractions were investigated. Also, our study determined the tested concentration of SHQA and SCM based on their real abundance in SYCF; therefore, a direct comparison between SYCF, SHQA, and SCM could provide more insights into their respective contributions to the overall anti-inflammatory effect of *S. yezoense*.

LPS, a component of Gram-negative bacterial cell walls, is a potent macrophage activator that induces inflammatory responses and cell cycle arrest in macrophages [20]. LPS activates macrophages to produce pro-inflammatory cytokines, such as TNF, IL-1β, IL-6, and secondary mediators, like nitric oxide by the enzyme NOS2 and prostaglandins by COX2, which are critical regulators of immunity [21,22]. However, their uncontrolled expression can cause chronic inflammatory conditions. Therefore, it is necessary to improve the chronic inflammatory condition by regulating the inflammatory response. The protective effect of SYEE against the LPS-induced inflammatory response in RAW 264.7 macrophages was demonstrated by its inhibition on the mRNA expression of *Il1b*, *Il6*, and *Nos2*, as well as its inhibition on the protein expression of COX2 and NOS2.

Macrophages are characterized by possessing high plasticity and an ability to undergo differentiation in response to specific stimuli. Particularly, the combination of IFN-γ and the toll-like receptor 4 agonist LPS synergistically induces M1 polarization in macrophages [23,24]. M1 polarization is pivotal in the inflammatory response, characterized by a high expression of pro-inflammatory cytokines, such as *Il1b*, *Il6*, and surface markers, such as *Cd86* [18]. It is worth noting that primary macrophages directly isolated and cultivated from BMDMs exhibit distinct phagocytic activity, cytokine production, and the regulation of oxidative burst, when compared to macrophage cell lines like RAW 264.7 macrophages [25]. In our study, we further demonstrated the anti-inflammatory effect of SYEE by examining its impact on M1 polarization in BMDMs. To induce M1 polarization in BMDMs, a combination treatment of LPS and IFN-γ was employed, leading the development of M1-type macrophages. SYEE effectively inhibited this polarization process, as evidenced by its inhibition on M1-related markers, such as *Il1b*, *Nos2*, and *Cd86*.

M1 polarization also induced the expression of NOX1 and NOX2. As specialized reactive oxygen species (ROS), members of the NOX family can be activated by pro-inflammatory signaling cascades [26]. Although NOXs are not critical for the polarization of M1-type macrophages, their deletion leads to a dramatic decrease in ROS production in macrophages [27]. SYEE's capacity to lower *Nox1* and *Nox2* mRNA levels implies its potent intracellular antioxidant properties.

Pro-inflammatory stimuli, such as LPS, have been observed to interfere with normal cell cycle progression [28,29]. In our study, LPS treatment induced cell cycle arrest primarily in the G0/G1 phase while concurrently reducing the proportion of cells in the S and G2/M phases, indicating that LPS-induced inflammation led to cell cycle arrest in the G0/G1 phase. SYEE mitigated this LPS-induced cell cycle arrest in the G0/G1 phase, suggesting a potential role in counteracting the disruption of the cell cycle induced by LPS-mediated inflammation.

LLE was adopted in the present study to enrich the bioactive components [30]. SYEE and its hexane, chloroform, and ethyl acetate fractions obtained by LLE exhibited strong antioxidant properties. SYHF and SYCF were enriched with phenolic compounds and meroterpenoids of *S. yezoense*. SYCF presented the highest TPC as well as SHQA and SCM. The strong antioxidant capacity of SYCF may have contributed to its highest phenolic content and meroterpenoids. In another study, when the same liquid–liquid partitioning was conducted on a different species of *Sargassum*, *S. hemiphyllum*, the highest phenolic content and strongest antioxidant capacity were observed in the ethyl acetate fraction, higher than its chloroform fraction [31]. This may be attributed to the complex composition of phenolic compounds in different *Sargassum* species [32,33]. The phenolics from marine macroalgae vary from simple molecules such as phenolic acids to highly complex phlorotannins. This subgroup of tannins is formed by the polymerization of phloroglucinol units [34]. However, the profile of phenolic compounds in *S. yezoense* remains unclear. Compared to other Korean *Sagarssum* species, *S. yezoense* did not exhibit a high phenolic content and antioxidant capcity [35]. Despite the difference in extraction solvents (70% ethanol used in another study vs. 100% ethanol in the present study), the total phenolic content of SYEE was less than half of that found in *S. hemiphyllum* and *S. miyabei*.

The robust inhibition of SYCF and SYHF on the LPS-induced upregulation of proinflammatory genes was observed at concentrations as low as 2.5 µg/mL. This observation strongly supports the anti-inflammatory properties of SYHF and SYCF, indicating that LLE is an effective method for concentrating bioactive compounds with potent anti-inflammatory properties from SYEE. It is worth noting that while LLE can enhance the efficiency of extracting bioactive components, such as phenolic compounds and meroterpenoids from algae, it is important to consider the toxicity associated with the use of chloroform as a solvent.

In addition to phenolic compounds, SYCF was found to be enriched with meroterpenoids such as SHQA and SCM. Meroterpenoids are natural secondary metabolites with structures partially derived from terpenoid pathways. They have been isolated from various sources, including fungi, marine organisms, animals, and plants, displaying a wide range of structural diversity [6]. These two meroterpenoids have previously been quantified in other *Sargassum* species, such as *S. serratifolium* [36]. Our study suggests that *S. yezoense* could serve as a promoising source for SHQA extraction.

In the present study, to assess the contribution of SHQA and SCM to the anti-inflammatory effect of SYCF, a direct comparison was conducted between SYCF, SHQA, and SCM. The concentrations of SHQA and SCM were determined based on their relative abundance within SYCF. SHQA, isolated from *S. macrocarpum*, has previously demonstrated anti-inflammatory effects in LPS-stimulated RAW 264.7 macrophages at concentrations of 0.4,

0.6, and 0.8 µM [10], which aligns with the tested concentration of 0.88 µM in the current study. The significant inhibitory effect of SHQA on pro-inflammatory factors confirms its anti-inflammatory effect. It is important to note that SYCF exhibited a stronger inhibitory effect on several pro-inflammatory factors, including the mRNA of *Tnf*, *Il1b*, *Nos2*, and *Cox2*. This discrepancy was also evident in the protein expression of NOS2 and COX2 and the nuclear translocation of NF-κB.

These findings suggest that while SHQA contributes to the anti-inflammatory effects of SYCF, there are other bioactive components within SYCF that play a role in its potent anti-inflammatory properties.

SCM, derived from various *Sargassum* species, including *Sargasuum micracanthum* and *S. horneri*, has also exhibited anti-inflammatory effects in previous studies [19,37]. However, it is important to note that the doses of SCM used in other anti-inflammatory investigations are typically much higher than 0.12 µM in the current study. For instance, SCM was shown to exert protection against vascular inflammation at 10 µM [19] and against LPS-induced inflammation in RAW 264.7 macrophages at 18.3 µM [37], which is more than 80-times and 156-times the dose employed in the present study. When tested at lower doses, SCM displayed limited anti-inflammatory effects, even upregulating the mRNA expression of *Nos2*, although such an induction was not observed in the protein expression of NOS2. Given these observations, SCM may not significantly contribute to the anti-inflammatory effect of SYCF, possibly due to its low abundance in SYCF.

4. Materials and Methods

4.1. Chemicals and Reagents

S. yezoense was purchased from Para Jeju Co. (Jeju-si, Jeju Island, Republic of Korea). Phloroglucinol, ascorbic acid, Folin-ciocalteau's phenol reagent, 2,2-diphenyl-1-picrylhydrazyl (DPPH), 2,2'-azobis-(2-amidinopropane) HCl (AAPH), sodium phosphate were purchased from Sigma-Aldrich Co. (St. Louis, MO, USA); 2,2'-Azino-Bis(3-ethylbenzrhiazoline-6-sulfonic acid)diammonium (ABTS), iron(III)chloride ($FeCl_3$), 2,4,6-tris(2-pyridyl)-s-triazine (TPTZ), and ferrous sulfate ($FeSO_4$) for antioxidant assay were purchased from Roche (Roche, Basel, Switzerland).

Dulbecco's modified Eagle's medium (DMEM) was purchased from Sigma-Aldrich Co., Fetal bovine serum (FBS) and Dulbecco's phosphate-buffered saline (DPBS) were purchased from WelGENE Inc. (Daegu, Republic of Korea), and penicillin–streptomycin for cell culture was purchased from Hyclone Inc (Logan, UT, USA). Dimethylthiazol-2-yl-2,5-diphenyl, tetrazolium bromide (MTT), dimethyl sulfoxide (DMSO), and LPS were purchased from Sigma-Aldrich Co.

4.2. Preparation of Ethanol Extract of S. yezoense and Its Fractions

S. yezoense was thoroughly washed and subsequently cut into pieces of approximately 1 mm. A total mass of 1.5 kg of *S. yezoense* was then homogenized with 15 L absolute ethanol, followed by sonication in an ultrasonic apparatus at ambient temperature for 12 h. Post-sonication, the residue was subjected to a second round of homogenization and sonication. The supernatants from both stages were amalgamated and filtered using filter paper with a size of 110 mm. This filtrate was then subjected to vacuum evaporation 50 °C to obtain a concentrated extract.

The concentrated extract was dissolved in deionized water and underwent liquid–liquid extraction utilizing solvents with different polarities (Supplementary Figure S2). The aqueous crude extract underwent this extraction process three times, using an equal volume of n-hexane, chloroform, ethyl acetate, butanol, and water. Following this, the resulting fractions were concentrated once more, using a rotary vacuum evaporator. The yield obtained from each fraction was weighed after the evaporation.

4.3. Total Phenolic Content and Antioxidant Assays

4.3.1. Total Phenolic Content

The amount of total phenolic content was determined using a colorimetric method with Folin and Ciocalteu's reagent [38]. Initially, 10 µL of the diluted samples was combined with 130 µL of distilled water in a 96-well plate. Following this, 10 µL of Folin and Ciocalteu's reagent was added. After a 6 min reaction time, 100 µL of a 7% Na_2CO_3 solution was added. The mixture's absorbance at 750 nm was measured after a 90 min incubation period using a Multiscan SkyHigh Microplate Spectrophotometer (Thermo Fisher Scientific, Waltham, MA, USA). The total phenolic content is the samples was reported in mg of phloroglucinol equivalent per gram of dry weight.

4.3.2. ABTS Radical Scavenging Assay

The ABTS assay was performed to measure the antioxidant capacity of SYEE and its different, fractions with minor modifications to the method described by Kim et al. [39]. Briefly, a solution was prepared by mixing 1 mM of 2,2'-azobis(2-amidinopropane) dihydrochloride (AAPH) with 2.5 mM 2,2'-azino-bis (3-ethylbenzothiazoline-6-sulfonic acid) diammonium salt (ABTS) in 100 mL of phosphate-buffered solution (PBS). This mixture was then heated at 75 °C for 30 min in a water bath to initiate the formation of the ABTS radicals. Once formed, the ABTS radical solution was filtered using a 0.45 µm PVDF filter and subsequently diluted with PBS to achieve an absorbance reading at 734 nm with a range of 0.650 ± 0.020. To assess the antioxidant capacity, 4 µL of the diluted samples was added to 196 µL of the ABTS radical solution. The resulting solution was incubated at 37 °C for 10 min, after which the reduction in absorbance at 734 nm was measured. The antioxidant activity of the samples was quantified in terms of mg of vitamin C equivalent per gram of dry weight sample.

4.3.3. DPPH Radical Scavenging Assay

The DPPH assay was performed with minor modifications to the method described by Blois. In summary, 2,2-diphenyl-1-picrylhydrazyl (DPPH) was dissolved in 80% (v/v) aqueous methanol to achieve a 100 µM concentration. Five µL of sample was combined with 295 µL of the DPPH solution. The mixture's absorbance was measured at 510 nm following a 30 min reaction period in a dark room at ambient temperature. The capacity of samples to scavenge DPPH radicals was quantified as mg of vitamin C equivalent per gram of dry weight sample.

4.3.4. Ferric-Reducing Antioxidant Power (FRAP) Assay

The FRAP assay was modified from the method by Benzie and Strain [40]. To prepare the FRAP reagent, 10 volumes of acetate buffer (300 mM, pH 3.6) were mixed with 1 volume of 10 mM TPTZ (2,4,6-tri[2-pyridyl]-s-triazine) solution, 1 volume of 20 mM $FeCl_3$ solution, and 1.2 volumes of distilled water. In a 96-well plate, 10 µL samples were mixed with 250 µL of the FRAP reagent and incubated for 4 min at 37 °C. The absorbance of the mixture was measured at 593 nm. The reducing power of the samples was quantified as mM $FeSO_4$ equivalent per gram of dry weight of sample.

4.4. Cell Culture and Treatment

The RAW 264.7 macrophage cells were purchased from Korean Cell Line Bank (Seoul, Republic of Korea). They were cultured in DMEM supplemented with 10% fetal bovine serum (FBS) and 1% penicillin–streptomycin at 37 °C in a 5% CO_2 humidified atmosphere. For experimental procedures, cells were pretreated with SYEE or its fractions for a duration of 6 h, followed by stimulation 100 ng/mL LPS for indicated period of time.

Mouse BMDMs were harvested from 19-week-old male C57BL/6N mice. The process began with collecting femurs and tibias from euthanized mice, followed by the removal of bone ends and retrieval of bone marrow by centrifugation at $10,000 \times g$ for 15 s. The harvested bone marrow pellet was then passed through a 21 G needle and suspended in DMEM/F12 medium. Subsequently, the bone marrow pellet was incubated in Red Blood Cell Lysing Buffer for 5 min. The lysis reaction was halted with PBS, follwed by centrifugation at $500 \times g$ for 5 min. The resulting cell pellets were than seeded into 12-well plate at a density of 1×10^6 cells/well. The cells were cultured in DMEM containing 10% FBS and 100 U/mL recombinant macrophage colony-stimulating factor (M-CSF) for 6 days. By the seventh day, mature BMDMs were observed. For M1 polarization induction, the cells were treated with 100 ng/mL LPS and 10 ng/ml IFN-γ for 24 h. The animal study was conducted with the approval of the Animal Committee of Pukyong National University and in strict adherence to the ethical guidelines and principles established by the committee for animal handling and care.

4.5. Cell Viability

To investigate the impact of SYEE and its fractions on the proliferation of RAW 264.7 macrophage cells, an MTT assay was conducted as per the methodology outlined in a prevous study [31]. Briefly, cells were seeded in a 96-well plate at a density of 4×10^4 cells/well. On the following day, cells were treated with SYEE or its fractions at indicated concentrations for a duration of 24 h. Following treatment, 100 µL of MTT solution (5 mg/mL in PBS) was administered to each well. After an incubation of 2 h, 200 µL of DMSO was added to each well. The viability of the cells was quantitatively assessed by measuring the absorbance of 540 nm using a microplate reader.

4.6. Total RNA Isolation and Real-Time PCR

Cells were seeded in 12-well plates at a density of 5×10^5 cells/well. One day later, cells were pretreated with SYEE or its fractions for a duration of 6 h, followed by stimulation 100 ng/mL LPS for 24 h. Total RNA extraction from cells, cDNA synthesis, and real-time PCR was carried out as described previously [36]. In brief, macrophages were lysed using 1 mL of homemade Trizol reagent. After a 5 min incubation, 200 µL of chloroform was added, followed by centrifugation at $12,000 \times g$ for 15 min at 4 °C. The aqueous phase containing RNA was transferred to new microcentrifuge tubes, mixed with 500 µL of isopropanol, and incubated for 10 min. Subsequently, the mixture was centrifuged at $12,000 \times g$ for 10 min at 4 °C. The resulting pellets were washed with 1 mL of 75% ethanol and then dissolved in 50 µL of RNase-free water. The extracted RNA was then reverse-transcribed into cDNA using SmartGene compact cDNA synthesis kit (Smart Gene, Daejeon, Republic of Korea). Real-time PCR was subsequently performed using the SYBR Green Q-PCR Master Mix (Smart Gene, Daejeon, Republic of Korea). The amplification and detection of specific gene expression were carried out using the QuantStudio™ 1 Real-Time PCR system (Thermo Fisher Scientific). The primers used in the present study are listed in Supplementary Table S1.

4.7. Western Blot Analysis

Cells were seeded in 6-well plates at a density of 1×10^6 cells/well. One day later, cells were pretreated with SYEE or its fractions for a duration of 6 h, followed by stimulation of 100 ng/mL LPS for 24 h. Cell lysates were prepared, and Western blot analyses were conducted as described [40]. Macrophages were subjected to lysis using CETi lysis buffer (TransLab, Daejeon, Republic of Korea) to release intracellular proteins. The lysate protein concentrations were quantitatively determined utilizing the Pierce BCA Protein Assay Kit (Thermo Fisher Scientific). Protein lysates were resolved by SDS-PAGE gel, under an initial electrophoresis voltage of 60V for 30 min, followed by 120V for 1 h. Following separation, protein transfer onto a nitrocellulose membrane was achieved using the Pierce G2 Turbo Blot system (Thermo Fisher Scientific). The membranes underwent a blocking process and were incubated with primary antibodies at 4 °C overnight. The antibodies against NOS2 and COX2 (sc-650 and sc-1745, 1:1000, Santa Cruz Biotechnology, Santa Cruz, CA, USA) were used, and beta-actin (sc-47778, 1:1000, Santa Cruz Biotechnology) served as a loading control for data normalization. The following day, the membranes were incubated with corresponding secondary antibodies at ambient temperature for 1 h. Detection of the proteins was conducted using the Pierce ECL Western Blotting substrate. Images of the blots were captured using the ImageQuant LAS 500 system (GE Healthcare, Chicago, IL, USA) and analyzed using Image Studio Lite software Version 5.2 (LI-COR Biosciences, Lincoln, NE, USA).

4.8. Cell Cycle Analysis by Flow Cytometry

Following a 24 h exposure of cells to 100 ng/mL LPS, a total of 1×10^6 cells were collected through centrifugation at $300\times g$ for 5 min, rinsed once with DPBS, and subsequently subjected to fixation in 1 mL 70% cold ethanol at $-20\,°C$ for a minimum duration of 3 h. Following this fixation process, 200 µL fixed cells underwent a PBS wash and were suspended in 200 µL of Muse Cell Cycle reagent. This suspension was allowed to react for 30 min at room temperature in the absence of light. This assay utilized propidium iodide (PI)-based staining of DNA content to differentiate and quantify the proportion of cells in different phases of cell cycle (G0/G1, S, and G2/M). Cell cycle analysis was conducted using the Muse Cell Cycle Software Module on the Guava Muse cell analyzer (Luminex Co., Austin, TX, USA).

4.9. Enzyme-linked Immunosorbent Assay (ELISA)

SYEE and fraction samples were dissolved in DMSO for treatment. RAW 264.7 macrophages were pretreated with SYEE and fraction samples in FBS-free medium for 6 h, followed by simulation with 100 ng/mL of LPS for 24 h. The conditioned media were collected, and their TNF levels were quantified using an enzyme-linked immunosorbent assay employing a TNF mouse uncoated ELISA kit (Thermo Fisher Scientific) in accordance with the manufacturer's instruction.

4.10. Quantification and Isolation of SHQA and SCM

Chromatographic analysis was performed using a Dionex Summit high-performance liquid chromatograph (HPLC) equipped with UV-photodiode array (PDA) detector (Dionex Corp, Sunnyvale, CA, USA). A SUPERSIL ODS-III reversed-phase column (250 mm × 4.6 mm, 5 µm particle size) was used for analysis. Detection of SHQA and SCM was achieved at 270 nm, with a wavelength scanning range of 190–700 nm. The mobile phase consisted of deionized water with 0.1 % (v/v) formic acid (solvent A) and acetonitrile (HPLC grade) with 0.1% (v/v) formic acid (solvent B), applied in a gradient elution protocol. The flow rate was maintained at 1.0 mL/min, and the injection volume of samples or standard compounds was set at 20 µL. Column and autosampler temperatures were stabilized at $35\,°C$ and $25\,°C$, respectively. The gradient elution profile was established as follows: 0 min at 90:10 (A:B), 3 min at 90:10, 8 min at 23:77, 10 min at 23:77, 28 min at 18:82, 32 min at 0:100, 35 min at 0:100, 40 min at 90:10, 42 min at 90:10. Using the above gradient elution, the calibration curves and linear equations of peak area versus concentration were determined for the two meroterpenoids (SHQA and SCM) and expressed as mg/g dry weight. The standards of SHQA and SCM were acquired from Dr. Hyeong-rak Kim, whose samples were identified with ^{1}H and ^{13}C-NMR [8]. The elution of SHQA and SCM was monitored, and each peak corresponding to these compounds was collected and evaporated under nitrogen gas to isolate pure compounds. The isolated pure compounds were stored at $-80\,°C$ until use for cell culture study.

4.11. Immunofluorescence

The protocol for immunofluorescence staining was conducted per the guideline in reference [41]. Cells were initially seeded in 35 mm 4-well confocal dishes at a density of 2×10^5 cells/well one day prior to treatment. On the following day, the cells were pretreated with SYCF or SHQA for 6 h, followed by treatment with 100 ng/mL LPS for 2 h. Cells were rinsed with ice-cold PBS. This was followed by a fixation step involving incubation in chilled 100% methanol for 5 min. Subsequently, cells underwent a triple wash with PBS to eliminate any residual fixative. For permeabilization, cells were treated with 0.1% Triton X-100 for 10 min. Blocking of non-specific binding sites was achieved by incubating the cells in a solution of 1% bovine serum albumin (BSA) and 22.52 mg/mL glycine in PBS containing 0.1% Tween 20 (PBST) for 30 min. Cells were then exposed to the primary antibody, diluted in 1% BSA in PBST, and incubated for 1 h at room temperature. Following three PBS washes to remove unbound primary antibody, cells were incubated with a secondary antibody conjugated with Alexa Fluor 488 in PBST for 1 h in a dark environment to prevent photobleaching. Imaging of the stained cells was performed using an FV3000 confocal microscope (Olympus Life Science, Tokyo, Japan), capturing detailed cellular structures and localization of the target proteins.

4.12. Statistical Analysis

All experimental data were presented as means ± standard deviation, derived from a minimum of three independent experiments. Statistical analysis of the data was performed utilizing one-way Analysis of Variance (ANOVA), followed by Tukey's post hoc test for multiple comparisons. This analysis was conducted using GraphPad Prism software version 9.0 (GraphPad Software Inc., San Diego, CA, USA). The threshold for statistical significance was set at $p < 0.05$.

5. Conclusions

This study exhibited the robust anti-inflammatory effects of a *Sargassum yezoense* ethanol extract. It found that the chloroform fraction of the extract, enriched in phenolic content and meroterpenoids, exhibited significant anti-inflammatory and antioxidant capacities. SHQA was identified as one major contributor to the anti-inflammatory properties, while SCM had a limited role. These findings suggest that SHQA, along with other bioactive compounds, works additively in the chloroform fraction to provide potent anti-inflammatory effects.

Supplementary Materials: The following supporting information can be downloaded at: https://www.mdpi.com/article/10.3390/md22030107/s1, Figure S1: Quantification of SHQA and SCM using HPLC; Figure S2: Flow chart for the fractionation of SYEE by sequential solvent extraction; Figure S3: Western blot original blots. Table S1: List of primers used in the study.

Author Contributions: Conceptualization, M.-B.K. and S.G.L.; methodology, Y.P., L.C., S.B., S.J. and H.J.Y.; software, Y.P. and L.C.; validation, M.-B.K., S.B. and S.J.; formal analysis, Y.P. and L.C.; investigation, Y.P. and L.C.; resources, S.G.L.; data curation, Y.P., L.C., S.B., S.J. and H.J.Y.; writing—original draft preparation, L.C.; writing—review and editing, M.-B.K. and S.G.L.; visualization, Y.P. and L.C.; supervision, S.G.L.; project administration, S.G.L.; funding acquisition, S.G.L. All authors have read and agreed to the published version of the manuscript.

Funding: This study was supported by a grant from the National Institute of Fisheries science, Food safety and Processing Research Division, grant number 2024058 to H.J.Y., National Research Foundation of Korea (NRF) funded by the Ministry of Education, grant number 202202240002 to S.G.L. and the Pukyong National University Industry-university Cooperation Research Fund in 2023 (202312170001) to S.G.L.

Institutional Review Board Statement: The animal study protocol was approved by the Institutional Animal Care and Use Committee of Pukyong National University (protocol code PKNUIACUC-2023-06 and date of approval 15 February 2023).

Data Availability Statement: Data are contained within the article or Supplementary Material.

Conflicts of Interest: The authors declare no conflicts of interest.

References

1. Liu, J.; Luthuli, S.; Yang, Y.; Cheng, Y.; Zhang, Y.; Wu, M.; Choi, J.I.; Tong, H. Therapeutic and nutraceutical potentials of a brown seaweed *Sargassum fusiforme*. *Food Sci. Nutr.* **2020**, *8*, 5195–5205. [CrossRef] [PubMed]
2. Liu, L.; Heinrich, M.; Myers, S.; Dworjanyn, S.A. Towards a better understanding of medicinal uses of the brown seaweed *Sargassum* in Traditional Chinese Medicine: A phytochemical and pharmacological review. *J. Ethnopharmacol.* **2012**, *142*, 591–619. [CrossRef] [PubMed]

3. Catarino, M.D.; Silva-Reis, R.; Chouh, A.; Silva, S.; Braga, S.S.; Silva, A.M.S.; Cardoso, S.M. Applications of Antioxidant Secondary Metabolites of *Sargassum* spp. *Mar. Drugs* **2023**, *21*, 172. [CrossRef] [PubMed]
4. Hong, I.-S.; Kim, G.-A.; Park, J.-K.; Boo, .S.-M. Morphology and Phenology of *Sargassum yezoense* (Sargassaceae, Phaeophyceae). *Korean J. Nat. Conserv.* **2008**, *2*, 132–139.
5. Kim, S.N.; Choi, H.Y.; Lee, W.; Park, G.M.; Shin, W.S.; Kim, Y.K. Sargaquinoic acid and sargahydroquinoic acid from *Sargassum yezoense* stimulate adipocyte differentiation through PPARalpha/gamma activation in 3T3-L1 cells. *FEBS Lett.* **2008**, *582*, 3465–3472. [CrossRef]
6. Russo, D.; Milella, L. Analysis of meroterpenoids. In *Recent Advances in Natural Products Analysis*; Elsevier: Amsterdam, The Netherlands, 2020; pp. 477–501.
7. Fuloria, N.K.; Raheja, R.K.; Shah, K.H.; Oza, M.J.; Kulkarni, Y.A.; Subramaniyan, V.; Sekar, M.; Fuloria, S. Biological activities of meroterpenoids isolated from different sources. *Front. Pharmacol.* **2022**, *13*, 830103. [CrossRef]
8. Joung, E.-J.; Gwon, W.-G.; Shin, T.; Jung, B.-M.; Choi, J.; Kim, H.-R. Anti-inflammatory action of the ethanolic extract from *Sargassum* serratifolium on lipopolysaccharide-stimulated mouse peritoneal macrophages and identification of active components. *J. Appl. Phycol.* **2017**, *29*, 563–573. [CrossRef]
9. Jeon, Y.; Jung, Y.; Kim, M.C.; Kwon, H.C.; Kang, K.S.; Kim, Y.K.; Kim, S.N. Sargahydroquinoic acid inhibits TNFalpha-induced AP-1 and NF-kappaB signaling in HaCaT cells through PPARalpha activation. *Biochem. Biophys. Res. Commun.* **2014**, *450*, 1553–1559. [CrossRef]
10. Joung, E.J.; Cao, L.; Lee, B.; Gwon, W.G.; Park, S.H.; Kim, H.R. Sargahydroquinoic Acid, a Cyclooxygenase-2 Inhibitor, Attenuates Inflammatory Responses by Regulating NF-kappaB Inactivation and Nrf2 Activation in Lipopolysaccharide-Stimulated Cells. *Inflammation* **2021**, *44*, 2120–2131. [CrossRef] [PubMed]
11. Yoon, W.J.; Heo, S.J.; Han, S.C.; Lee, H.J.; Kang, G.J.; Kang, H.K.; Hyun, J.W.; Koh, Y.S.; Yoo, E.S. Anti-inflammatory effect of sargachromanol G isolated from *Sargassum* siliquastrum in RAW 264.7 cells. *Arch. Pharm. Res.* **2012**, *35*, 1421–1430. [CrossRef] [PubMed]
12. Jahromi, S.G. Extraction techniques of phenolic compounds from plants. In *Plant Physiological Aspects of Phenolic Compounds*; IntechOpen: London, UK, 2019; pp. 3–20.
13. Jiang, H.; Yang, S.; Tian, H.; Sun, B. Research progress in the use of liquid-liquid extraction for food flavour analysis. *Trends Food Sci. Technol.* **2023**, *132*, 138–149. [CrossRef]
14. Orzolek, B.J.; Kozlowski, M.C. Separation of Food Colorings via Liquid–Liquid Extraction: An At-Home Organic Chemistry Lab. *J. Chem. Educ.* **2021**, *98*, 951–957. [CrossRef]
15. Khatibi, S.A.; Hamidi, V.; Siahi-Shadbad, M.R. Application of Liquid-Liquid Extraction for the Determination of Antibiotics in the Foodstuff: Recent Trends and Developments. *Crit. Rev. Anal. Chem.* **2022**, *52*, 327–342. [CrossRef] [PubMed]
16. Li, H.; Sun, W.; Deng, M.; Qi, C.; Chen, C.; Zhu, H.; Luo, Z.; Wang, J.; Xue, Y.; Zhang, Y. Aspverversins A and B, Two Novel Meroterpenoids with an Unusual 5/6/6/6 Ring from the Marine-Derived Fungus Aspergillus versicolor. *Mar. Drugs* **2018**, *16*, 177. [CrossRef] [PubMed]
17. Unuvar Purcu, D.; Korkmaz, A.; Gunalp, S.; Helvaci, D.G.; Erdal, Y.; Dogan, Y.; Suner, A.; Wingender, G.; Sag, D. Effect of stimulation time on the expression of human macrophage polarization markers. *PLoS ONE* **2022**, *17*, e0265196. [CrossRef] [PubMed]
18. Murray, P.J. Macrophage Polarization. *Annu. Rev. Physiol.* **2017**, *79*, 541–566. [CrossRef] [PubMed]
19. Gwon, W.G.; Joung, E.J.; Kwon, M.S.; Lim, S.J.; Utsuki, T.; Kim, H.R. Sargachromenol protects against vascular inflammation by preventing TNF-alpha-induced monocyte adhesion to primary endothelial cells via inhibition of NF-kappaB activation. *Int. Immunopharmacol.* **2017**, *42*, 81–89. [CrossRef]
20. Vadiveloo, P.K.; Keramidaris, E.; Morrison, W.A.; Stewart, A.G. Lipopolysaccharide-induced cell cycle arrest in macrophages occurs independently of nitric oxide synthase II induction. *Biochim. Biophys. Acta* **2001**, *1539*, 140–146. [CrossRef] [PubMed]
21. Bosca, L.; Zeini, M.; Traves, P.G.; Hortelano, S. Nitric oxide and cell viability in inflammatory cells: A role for NO in macrophage function and fate. *Toxicology* **2005**, *208*, 249–258. [CrossRef] [PubMed]
22. Claria, J. Cyclooxygenase-2 biology. *Curr. Pharm. Des.* **2003**, *9*, 2177–2190. [CrossRef]
23. Muller, E.; Christopoulos, P.F.; Halder, S.; Lunde, A.; Beraki, K.; Speth, M.; Oynebraten, I.; Corthay, A. Toll-Like Receptor Ligands and Interferon-gamma Synergize for Induction of Antitumor M1 Macrophages. *Front. Immunol.* **2017**, *8*, 1383. [CrossRef] [PubMed]
24. Smith, T.D.; Tse, M.J.; Read, E.L.; Liu, W.F. Regulation of macrophage polarization and plasticity by complex activation signals. *Integr. Biol.* **2016**, *8*, 946–955. [CrossRef]
25. Ying, W.; Cheruku, P.S.; Bazer, F.W.; Safe, S.H.; Zhou, B. Investigation of macrophage polarization using bone marrow derived macrophages. *J. Vis. Exp.* **2013**, *76*, e50323. [CrossRef]
26. Ogier-Denis, E.; Mkaddem, S.B.; Vandewalle, A. NOX enzymes and Toll-like receptor signaling. *Semin. Immunopathol.* **2008**, *30*, 291–300. [CrossRef] [PubMed]
27. Xu, Q.; Choksi, S.; Qu, J.; Jang, J.; Choe, M.; Banfi, B.; Engelhardt, J.F.; Liu, Z.G. NADPH Oxidases Are Essential for Macrophage Differentiation. *J. Biol. Chem.* **2016**, *291*, 20030–20041. [CrossRef]

28. Jose, S.; Tan, S.W.; Ooi, Y.Y.; Ramasamy, R.; Vidyadaran, S. Mesenchymal stem cells exert anti-proliferative effect on lipopolysaccharide-stimulated BV2 microglia by reducing tumour necrosis factor-alpha levels. *J. Neuroinflammation* **2014**, *11*, 149. [CrossRef]
29. Gammelsrud, A.; Solhaug, A.; Dendele, B.; Sandberg, W.J.; Ivanova, L.; Kocbach Bolling, A.; Lagadic-Gossmann, D.; Refsnes, M.; Becher, R.; Eriksen, G.; et al. Enniatin B-induced cell death and inflammatory responses in RAW 267.4 murine macrophages *Toxicol. Appl. Pharmacol.* **2012**, *261*, 74–87. [CrossRef]
30. Egua, M.O.; Etuk, E.U.; Bello, S.O.; Hassan, S. Antidiabetic potential of liquid-liquid partition fractions of ethanolic seed extract of Corchorus olitorious. *J. Pharmacogn. Phytother.* **2014**, *6*, 4–9.
31. Jeong, S.; Kim, M.B.; Baek, S.; Lee, J.; Lee, H.; Cao, B.; Kim, Y.; Cao, L.; Lee, S. Suppression of Pro-Inflammatory M1 Polarization of LPS-Stimulated RAW 264.7 Macrophage Cells by Fucoxanthin-Rich *Sargassum* hemiphyllum. *Mar. Drugs* **2023**, *21*, 533. [CrossRef]
32. Wu, Y.; Gao, H.; Wang, Y.; Peng, Z.; Guo, Z.; Ma, Y.; Zhang, R.; Zhang, M.; Wu, Q.; Xiao, J.; et al. Effects of different extraction methods on contents, profiles, and antioxidant abilities of free and bound phenolics of *Sargassum* polycystum from the South China Sea. *J. Food Sci.* **2022**, *87*, 968–981. [CrossRef]
33. Shen, P.; Gu, Y.; Zhang, C.; Sun, C.; Qin, L.; Yu, C.; Qi, H. Metabolomic Approach for Characterization of Polyphenolic Compounds in Laminaria japonica, Undaria pinnatifida, *Sargassum fusiforme* and *Ascophyllum nodosum*. *Foods* **2021**, *10*, 192. [CrossRef] [PubMed]
34. Generalic Mekinic, I.; Skroza, D.; Simat, V.; Hamed, I.; Cagalj, M.; Popovic Perkovic, Z. Phenolic Content of Brown Algae (Pheophyceae) Species: Extraction, Identification, and Quantification. *Biomolecules* **2019**, *9*, 244. [CrossRef]
35. Baek, S.H.; Cao, L.; Jeong, S.J.; Kim, H.-R.; Nam, T.J.; Lee, S.G. The comparison of total phenolics, total antioxidant, and anti-tyrosinase activities of Korean *Sargassum* species. *J. Food Qual.* **2021**, *2021*, 6640789. [CrossRef]
36. Lim, S.; Choi, A.-H.; Kwon, M.; Joung, E.-J.; Shin, T.; Lee, S.-G.; Kim, N.-G.; Kim, H.-R. Evaluation of antioxidant activities of various solvent extract from *Sargassum* serratifolium and its major antioxidant components. *Food Chem.* **2019**, *278*, 178–184. [CrossRef] [PubMed]
37. Han, E.J.; Jayawardena, T.U.; Jang, J.H.; Fernando, I.P.S.; Jee, Y.; Jeon, Y.J.; Lee, D.S.; Lee, J.M.; Yim, M.J.; Wang, L.; et a. Sargachromenol Purified from *Sargassum horneri* Inhibits Inflammatory Responses via Activation of Nrf2/HO-1 Signaling in LPS-Stimulated Macrophages. *Mar. Drugs* **2021**, *19*, 497. [CrossRef] [PubMed]
38. Ainsworth, E.A.; Gillespie, K.M. Estimation of total phenolic content and other oxidation substrates in plant tissues using Folin-Ciocalteu reagent. *Nat. Protoc.* **2007**, *2*, 875–877. [CrossRef]
39. Kim, D.O.; Lee, K.W.; Lee, H.J.; Lee, C.Y. Vitamin C Equivalent Antioxidant Capacity (VCEAC) of Phenolic Phytochemicals. *J. Agric. Food Chem.* **2002**, *50*, 3713–3717. [CrossRef]
40. Benzie, I.F.; Strain, J.J. The ferric reducing ability of plasma (FRAP) as a measure of "antioxidant power": The FRAP assay. *Anal. Biochem.* **1996**, *239*, 70–76. [CrossRef]
41. Donaldson, J.G. Immunofluorescence Staining. *Curr. Protoc. Cell Biol.* **2015**, *69*, 4-3. [CrossRef]

Disclaimer/Publisher's Note: The statements, opinions and data contained in all publications are solely those of the individual author(s) and contributor(s) and not of MDPI and/or the editor(s). MDPI and/or the editor(s) disclaim responsibility for any injury to people or property resulting from any ideas, methods, instructions or products referred to in the content.

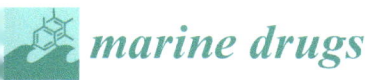

Article

Fucoidan from *Sargassum autumnale* Inhibits Potential Inflammatory Responses via NF-κB and MAPK Pathway Suppression in Lipopolysaccharide-Induced RAW 264.7 Macrophages

N. M. Liyanage [1,†], Hyo-Geun Lee [1,†], D. P. Nagahawatta [1], H. H. A. C. K. Jayawardhana [1], Kyung-Mo Song [2], Yun-Sang Choi [2], You-Jin Jeon [1,*] and Min-Cheol Kang [2,*]

[1] Department of Marine Life Sciences, Jeju National University, Jeju 63243, Republic of Korea; liyanagenm@jejunu.ac.kr (N.M.L.); hyogeunlee92@jejunu.ac.kr (H.-G.L.); pramuditha1992@jejunu.ac.kr (D.P.N.); chathuri.k.j@stu.jejunu.ac.kr (H.H.A.C.K.J.)
[2] Research Group of Process Engineering, Korea Food Research Institute, Wanju 55365, Republic of Korea; kcys0517@kfri.re.kr (Y.-S.C.)
* Correspondence: youjinj@jejunu.ac.kr (Y.-J.J.); mckang@kfri.re.kr (M.-C.K.)
† These authors contributed equally to this work.

Abstract: Fucoidans are sulfate-rich polysaccharides with a wide variety of beneficial biological activities. The present study aimed to highlight the anti-inflammatory activity of fucoidan from the brown seaweed *Sargassum autumnale* (SA) against lipopolysaccharide (LPS)-induced RAW 264.7 macrophage cells. Among the isolated fucoidan fractions, the third fraction (SAF3) showed a superior protective effect on LPS-stimulated RAW 264.7 cells. SAF3 inhibits nitric oxide (NO) production and expression of prostaglandin E-2 (PGE2) via downregulation of inducible nitric oxide synthase (iNOS) and cyclooxygenase-2 (COX2) expression in LPS-induced RAW 26.7 cells. SAF3 treatment decreased pro-inflammatory cytokines IL-1β, TNF-α, and IL-6 expression in LPS-induced cells. LPS stimulation activated NF-κB and MAPK signaling cascades in RAW 264.7 cells, while treatment with SAF3 suppressed them in a concentration-dependent manner. Existing outcomes confirm that SAF3 from *S. autumnale* possesses potent anti-inflammatory activity and exhibits good potential for application as a functional food ingredient or for the treatment of inflammation-related disorders.

Keywords: RAW 2694.7 macrophage; fucoidan; *Sargassum autumnale*; anti-inflammatory

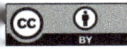

1. Introduction

Brown seaweeds are considered the main natural source of naturally occurring fucoidan [1]. The uniqueness of fucoidan compared to other polysaccharides stems from its abundant L-fucose content and sulfate groups [2]. The structure and compositional properties of fucoidans vary in different species of brown algae [3]. The structural backbone of fucoidan is made up of α-1,3-linked 1-fucopyranose residue repeats or α-1,4-linked 1-fucopyranose residues. In addition, different monosaccharide units such as mannose, galactose, and glucose can be inserted in the fucoidan backbone in place of the repeating units. Fucoidans from several brown seaweeds have been extensively studied in the past decade for their diverse biological activities, including anticoagulant, antitumor, immunomodulatory, and anti-inflammatory effects [4–6].

Inflammation is an important response of the immune system that is provoked by various stimuli and conditions, such as pathogens, particulate matter, etc. Inflammation can be acute or chronic and is considered to have the ability to protect from pathogen-induced tissue injury. Chronic inflammation is involved as part of the pathogenesis of conditions such as Alzheimer's disease, cardiovascular diseases, rheumatoid arthritis, and inflammatory bowel disease [7]. Nevertheless, the inflammatory response is a prime defensive mechanism of the human body and involves the upregulation and activation of many genes. Macrophages get activated on exposure to inflammatory stimuli, such as lipopolysaccharides (LPS). The activated cells produce inflammatory mediators such as nitric oxide (NO), prostaglandin E-2 (PGE2), and pro-inflammatory cytokines, resulting in the activation of signaling pathways such as NF-κB and MAPK [8]. It is reported that the pathogenesis of inflammatory diseases is elicited via the excess production of inflammatory mediators due to the generation of reactive oxygen species (ROS) [9]. The downregulation of pro-inflammatory factors is, therefore, considered a successful therapeutic method for curing inflammation-related diseases [10–12]. Fucoidan from brown seaweeds is extensively studied for its anti-inflammatory properties [13]. The ability of fucoidan to boost the efficiency of anti-inflammatory drugs has been studied [14]. Earlier studies have demonstrated the anti-inflammatory effects of fucoidan in a range of experimental contexts, including in vivo and in vitro [15]. However, the beneficial bioactivities of *Sargassum autumnale* have not been extensively studied.

S. autumnale is a brown alga found in tropical regions, especially in the intertidal zone of East Asian countries. *Sargassum* spp. are well-known food ingredients in East Asian countries and are also known to possess numerous important and beneficial bioactive compounds [16]. As a food ingredient, it offers a range of nutritional benefits due to its rich composition of essential nutrients, including vitamins, minerals, and antioxidants. Additionally, its unique flavor profile and versatile culinary properties make it an exciting ingredient for creative and nutritious culinary creations [17]. However, *S. autumnale* has not yet been extensively explored in terms of its physical, biological, and biochemical properties as functional ingredients such as fucoidans. A few studies have been conducted on the fucoidan isolated from *S. autumnale* for its antioxidant, antibacterial, antiviral, and anticancer properties [18–20]. In our previous study, fucoidan was isolated from *S. autumnale* and found to exhibit excellent antioxidant activity against H_2O_2-induced oxidative stress in Vero cells [21]. However, the anti-inflammatory effect of *S. autumnale* sulfated polysaccharides for the treatment of inflammatory diseases has not been explored yet to the best of our knowledge. Thus, the present study was designed as an initial study to assess the potential anti-inflammatory activity and the mechanism of action of *S. autumnale* fucoidan in vitro. The findings may boost the use of the underutilized *S. autumnale* and aid in sustainable development across a range of industries, particularly in the food and functional food sectors, as well as in pharmaceutical development.

2. Results

2.1. Chemical Composition and Structural Characterization of Isolated S. autumnale Fucoidan Fractions

The chemical composition results are reported in Table 1. Results from the current study revealed that SAP consisted mostly of polysaccharides. The DEAE chromatography resulted in three fucoidan fractions, and the purified polysaccharide fractions contained higher polysaccharide content and sulfate content, with SAF3 possessing the highest levels of sulfates (34.92 ± 0.18%) among the separated fractions. The polysaccharide content showed gradual reduction in the successive fractions while the sulfate content increased. Low protein and polyphenol contents were observed in all the fractions. These results were similar to those obtained in a previous study conducted on the antioxidant effect of sulfated polysaccharides from *Sargassum fulvellum* [22].

Table 1. Chemical composition of purified fucoidan from *S. autumnale*.

Sample	Polysaccharide%	Protein%	Polyphenol%	Sulfate%
SAP	30.25 ± 0.44	15.14 ± 0.21	10.3 ± 0.14	7.81 ± 0.24
SACP	59.34 ± 1.01	9.19 ± 0.83	8.00 ± 0.01	11.07 ± 2.09
SAF1	34.28 ± 0.50	7.99 ± 0.38	3.58 ± 0.36	21.44 ± 0.50
SAF2	24.55 ± 0.12	5.41 ± 0.14	2.91 ± 0.32	25.88 ± 0.51
SAF3	18.04 ± 0.98	2.01 ± 0.08	1.95 ± 0.18	34.92 ± 0.18

Monosaccharide and FTIR analyses of SAF3 were previously reported in our previous study [21]. Monosugar analysis identified that the *S. autumnale* polysaccharides contained five monosaccharides: fucose, rhamnose, galactose, glucose, and xylose. In addition, all the fucoidans contained higher levels of fucose (43.16%) and galactose (34.06%). The FTIR spectra of fucoidans indicated the structural similarity of *S. autumnale* fucoidan with commercial fucoidan. The common IR peak at 1035 cm^{-1} represents the stretching vibration of a glycosidic bridge (C–O–C), while the broad peak at 1220–1270 cm^{-1} represents sulfate groups. The acquired spectra had a low resolution due to the complex, heterogeneous structure of fucoidans.

2.2. Evaluation of S. autumnale Fucoidans on Macrophage Cell Viability

The effects of the three fractions of fucoidans and crude polysaccharide extract from *S. autumnale* on RAW 264.7 macrophage cells are shown in Figure 1a. Accordingly, with the treatment of SA fucoidans, the cell viability did not decrease significantly at concentrations (25, 50, 100, and 200 µg/mL), suggesting the absence of any adverse effects such as toxic effects of *S. autumnale* extracts on RAW 264.7 cells. Therefore, those concentrations were selected for future experiments. The concentration of 400 µg/mL resulted in decreased cell viability, indicating toxicity to the cells; therefore, it was removed from further experiments. The preliminary concentrations of fucoidan were selected based on previously optimized and published methods [13,23,24].

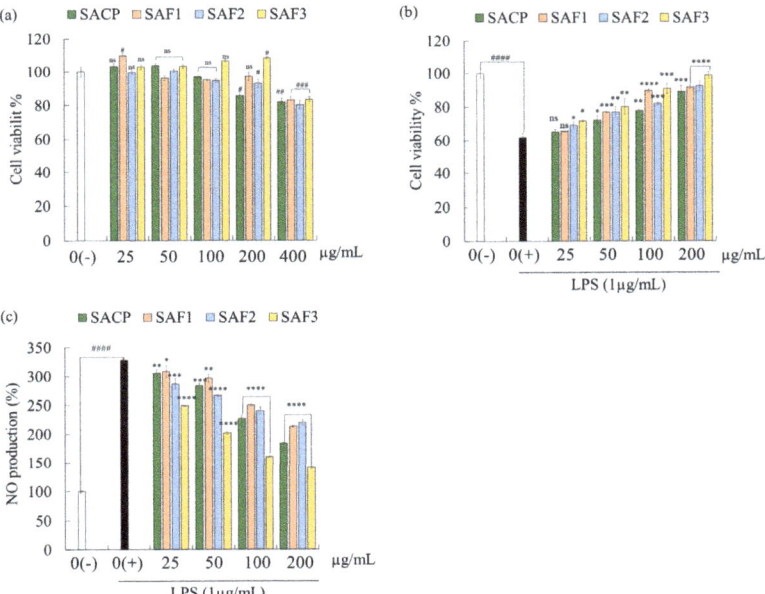

Figure 1. Determination of fucoidan fractions having superior activity. (**a**) sample toxicity, (**b**) protective effect in LPS-induced cells; and (**c**) NO production inhibition in LPS-induced cells. Experiments were performed in triplicate (n = 3), and the results are represented as means ± SD. Values are significantly different from LPS-treated group (0(+)) at * $p < 0.05$, ** $p < 0.01$, *** $p < 0.005$, and **** $p < 0.0001$ and from control group (0(−)) at # $p < 0.05$, ## $p < 0.01$, ### $p < 0.005$ and #### $p < 0.0001$. ns denotes not significant.

2.3. NO Production Inhibition by S. autumnale Fucoidan Fractions in LPS Stimulated RAW 264.7 Cells

LPS stimulation in RAW 264.7 cells resulted in a significant increase in NO production and a decrease in cell viability compared to non-stimulated cells. Interestingly, fucoidan co-treatment retracted the toxic influence of LPS on macrophage cells, leading to a recovery of cell viability (Figure 1b). NO is known as a key inflammatory mediator essential for preventing inflammation under normal physiological conditions. Nevertheless, elevated NO production under abnormal conditions can cause detrimental effects on tissues [25] On pre-treatment of cells with *S. autumnale* fucoidans, the high NO production in LPS-stimulated cells decreased in a concentration-dependent manner (Figure 1c). Based on these results, SAF3 was selected for subsequent experiments due to its superior protective activity on LPS-induced RAW 264.7 cells compared to other fractions.

2.4. Inhibition of PGE2 and Pro-Inflammatory Cytokines Secretion by SAF3

IL-1β, TNF-α, IL-6-like pro-inflammatory cytokines, and prostaglandin PGE2 play a major role in chronic inflammation due to the upregulation of their production. We tested the inhibitory effect of SAF3 against LPS-induced pro-inflammatory cytokines and PGE2 production using ELISA. As shown in Figure 2, LPS stimulation led to a higher secretion of pro-inflammatory cytokines and PGE2 in RAW 264.7 cells compared to the control group. However, pre-treatment of SAF3 (50, 100, and 200 µg/mL) resulted in a significant reduction in pro-inflammatory cytokine and PGE2 secretion compared to the LPS treated group. According to the results, PGE2 secretion decreased to 84.2% in the 200 µg/mL concentration group from that in the LPS-treated control group. To account for the variability in the data, the error associated with the mean was also determined. The standard deviation was calculated to be ±2.40. In 20 µg/mL concentration group, TNF-α, IL-6, and IL-1β secretions were lowered up to 76.56% ± 4.91, 74.84% ± 0.94, and 66.56% ± 1.24, respectively. Therefore, SAF3 was able to significantly inhibit the expression of pro-inflammatory cytokines and PGE2 during inflammation in RAW 264.7 cells induced by LPS treatment.

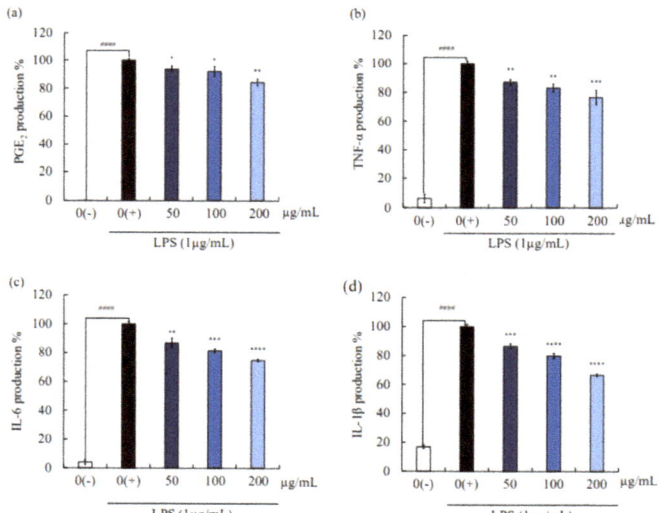

Figure 2. Effect of SAF3 on the inflammatory mediator regulation. SAF3 inhibited the production of (**a**) PGE2, (**b**) TNF-α, (**c**) IL-6, and (**d**) IL-1β pro-inflammatory cytokines. Experiments were performed in triplicate ($n = 3$), and the results are represented as means ± SD. Values are significantly different from the control (LPS treated) group at * $p < 0.05$ and ** $p < 0.001$ compared to untreated group. LPS treated group (0(+)) at * $p < 0.05$, ** $p < 0.01$, *** $p < 0.005$ and **** $p < 0.0001$ and control group (0(−)) at #### $p < 0.0001$.

2.5. Effect of SAF3 on iNOS and COX2 Protein Expression in LPS-Stimulated Cells

iNOS and COX2 play a vital role in regulating immune responses in cells [26]. The inhibitory activity of SAF3 on iNOS and COX2 expression in LPS-stimulated RAW 264.7 cells was determined using Western blot analysis. The quantitative analysis results indicated that higher expressions of the above-mentioned proteins were obtained from LPS-stimulated cells compared to un-stimulated cells (Figure 3). However, their expression was downregulated when pre-treated with SAF3 in a concentration-dependent manner, demonstrating the anti-inflammatory activity of SAF3. The highest fucoidan concentration resulted in a mean expression of iNOS of 0.087 ± 0.002, while the expression of COX2 was determined to be 0.526 ± 0.019.

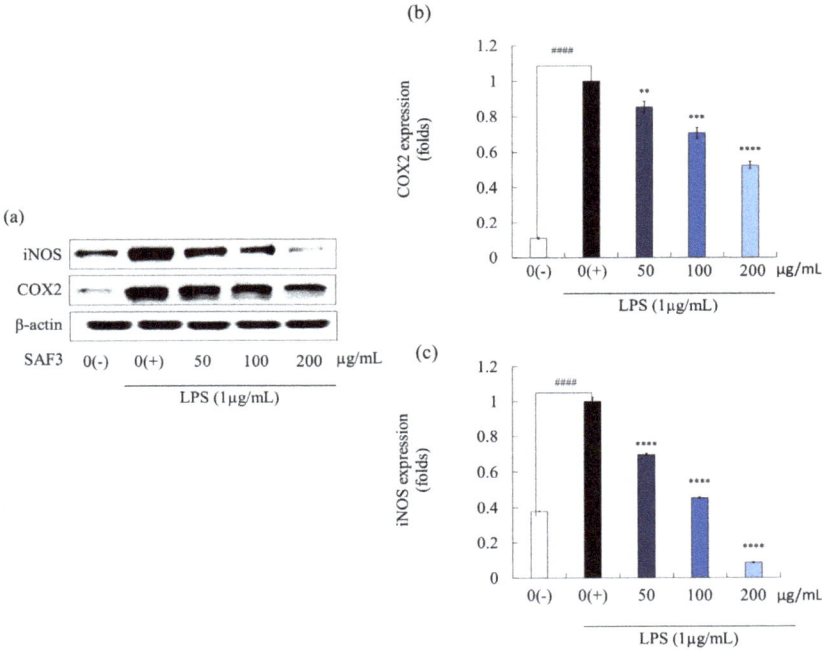

Figure 3. Effects of SAF3 on LPS-induced iNOS and COX2 protein expression in RAW 264.7 cells (**a**) Western blot image showing protein expression, (**b**) COX2, and (**c**) iNOS expression levels were quantified using western blotting after the treatment of LPS-activated macrophages with SAF3. Experiments were carried out in triplicate ($n = 3$), and the results are represented as means $\pm$ SD. ($n = 3$). Values are significantly different from the LPS treated group (0(+)) at ** $p < 0.01$, *** $p < 0.005$ and **** $p < 0.0001$ and from control group (0(−)) at #### $p < 0.0001$.

2.6. SAF3 Downregulated NF-κB/MAPK Pathway Proteins Expression

MAPK and NF-κB signaling cascades exist in eukaryotic cells and play a vital role in a wide variety of cellular functions. MAPK phosphorylation inhibition is a potential approach to curing inflammation-related diseases [27]. The effect of SAF3 on the regulation of the expression of these pathway proteins was analyzed using Western blotting. LPS stimulation initiated the activation of MAPK (Figure 4) and NF-κB (Figure 5) cascades. Stimulation of LPS resulted in the significant phosphorylation of MAPK proteins ($p < 0.05$), such as p38 and ERK; the band intensity of these proteins was higher in the un-stimulated group. Further, treatment of SAF3 interestingly downregulated this elevated expression of the phosphorylation forms of p38 and ERK.

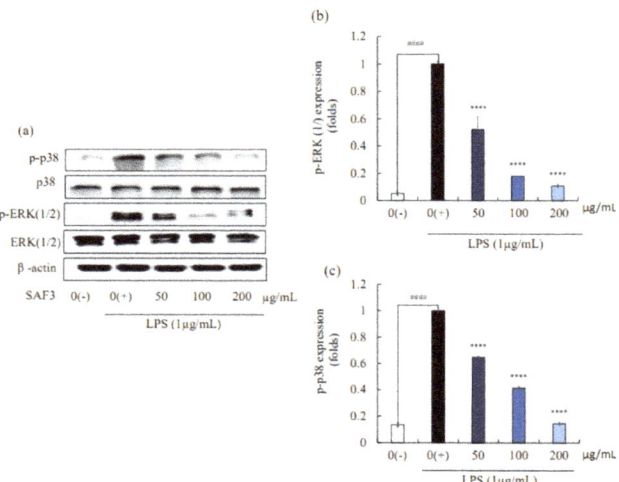

Figure 4. Inhibitory effects of SAF3 on MAPK activation in LPS-stimulated RAW 264.7 cells. (**a**) Western blot image showing protein expression; (**b**) p-ERK; and (**c**) p-p38 expression in RAW 264.7 cells. Experiments were performed in triplicate ($n = 3$), and the results are represented as means ± SD. Values are significantly different from LPS treated group (0(+)) at **** $p < 0.0001$ and from control group (0(−)) at #### $p < 0.0001$.

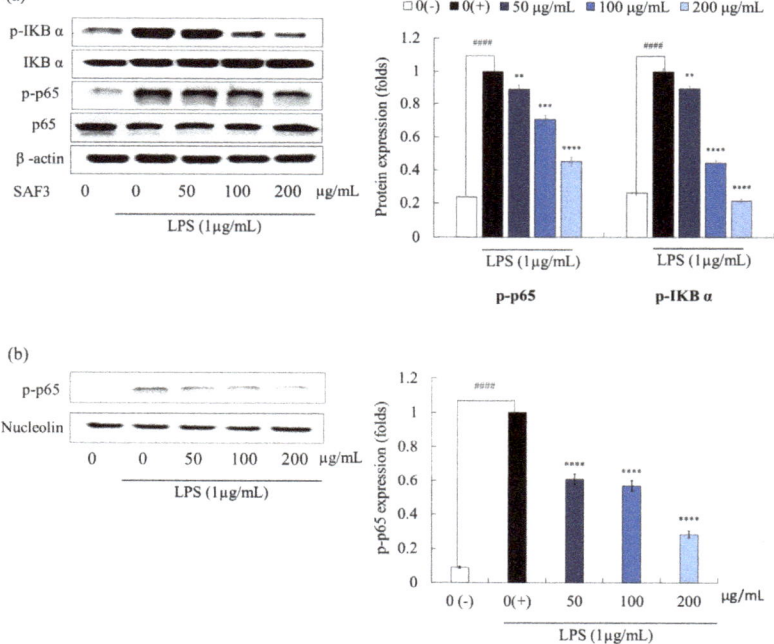

Figure 5. Inhibitory effects of SAF3 on NF-κB activation in LPS-stimulated RAW 264.7 cells. (**a**) p-p65 and p-IKBα expression in cytosol, and (**b**) p-p65 expression in nucleus. Experiments were performed in triplicate ($n = 3$), and the results are represented as means ± SD. Values are significantly different from LPS treated group (0(+)) at ** $p < 0.01$, *** $p < 0.005$ and **** $p < 0.0001$ and from control group (0(−)) at #### $p < 0.0001$.

In unstimulated cells, NF-κB, which is located in the cytoplasm, combines with IKBα-like inhibitory proteins and forms an inactive form (p50-p65-IκB). LPS stimulation of cells resulted in phosphorylation of the inactive former, allowing IκBα to be released and translocated into the nucleus [28]. According to the results obtained in our study, the phosphorylation of p65 and IKBα was enhanced by LPS stimulation in the cytosol and nucleus compared to the control group, respectively (Figure 5a,b). However, pre-incubation with SAF3 significantly reduced the phosphorylation of NF-κB proteins in a concentration-dependent manner. The mean expressions of p-p65 and p-IKBα in the cytosol were found to be 0.453 ± 0.026 and 0.215 ± 0.010 at the maximum fucoidan concentration, respectively. Moreover, the nuclear expression of p-p65 was also downregulated concentration-dependently. This solidifies the ability of SAF3 to downregulate the nuclear translocation of p65 in the NF-κB signaling pathway. These results showed that SAF3 has good anti-inflammatory activity due to the suppression of MAPK and NF-κB phosphorylation in LPS-induced RAW264.7 cells.

3. Discussion

Fucoidans represent a group of fucose-rich sulfated polysaccharides found especially in brown algae. They are mainly made of fucose and sulfate groups and contain other molecules such as uronic acid, xylose, mannose, and galactose. Fucoidans are extensively studied as they exhibit a number of biological activities such as anti-inflammatory, antiviral, antioxidant, anti-coagulant, and antitumor activities [29–32]. Experimental evidence suggests that fucoidan possesses anti-inflammatory activity and has excellent potential applications as an anti-inflammatory agent. The identification and characterization of seaweed fucoidan provide great opportunities for their development and application as functional foods and medicines for the treatment of various diseases with fewer side effects. However, the anti-inflammatory potential of fucoidan from *S. autumnale* has not yet been comprehensively studied. Therefore, in the current study, we evaluated and demonstrated the in vitro anti-inflammatory activity of fucoidan extracted from *Sargassum autumnale*.

Enzyme-assisted extraction is one of the most popular methods for extracting such important bioactive compounds from seaweed. This method is widely used in industrial extraction owing to its high effectiveness, low pollution, and low production costs [33]. In this study, enzyme-assisted extraction was used to augment the bioactive characteristics of fucoidan; the crude polysaccharide was further purified using DEAE-cellulose column chromatography, which yielded three fractions. The pooled three fractions were designated as SAF1, SAF2, and SAF3. According to the preliminary experiments, such as its cytoprotective effect and ability to downregulate NO production properties in LPS-induced macrophage cells, SAF3 showed superior activity among the other fractions. Moreover, according to the compositional analysis, SAF3 contained higher sulfate and fucose content, which is important for good anti-inflammatory activities [13]. The inclusion of differing quantities of sulfate groups, polyphenols, proteins, the structural placement of sulfated groups, structure, and molecular weight affect the biological activities of fucoidan [34]. According to several studies, having more polyphenols increases their anti-inflammatory effects [35]. However, in our investigation, the compositional analysis revealed minimal levels of proteins and polyphenols and substantially greater concentrations of polysaccharides and sulfates. Therefore, the anti-inflammatory activity of SAF3 can be identified as being mainly due to its sulfate and polysaccharide content. The lower polyphenol content in SAF3 is due to the removal of polyphenols as lipids with depigmentation. The higher sulfate and polysaccharide quantities were due to the active anion exchange column system [36]. Therefore, SAF3 was selected for further study. The FTIR analysis showed that SAF3 has a similar structure to commercial fucoidan. However, it is reported that fucoidan derived from different seaweeds exhibits significantly different levels of bioactivity. The variation in bioactivities may arise from several factors related to the seaweed's species, geographical location, environmental conditions, extraction methods, and molecular structure. According to previously published reports, different seaweed species contain distinct compositions of fucoidan, with variations in the ratio and types of monosaccharides, sulfate content, and molecular weight. These differences can influence the bioactivity of fucoidan and its interactions with biological systems [37]. Furthermore, the extraction method employed in the present study to isolate fucoidan may also affect its bioactivity. As reported in early studies, extraction techniques such as solvent selection, temperature, and time duration can impact the preservation of bioactive compounds and the structural integrity of fucoidan with varying degrees of bioactivity [38]. Therefore, although fucoidan from different seaweeds may exhibit identical or higher similarity in FTIR structure profiles, their bioactivities can differ significantly. Therefore, it is crucial to study and evaluate the bioactivity of fucoidan from *S. autumnale* to understand its potential application in different fields.

NO is a key inflammatory mediator that induces inflammation and plays a major role in pathogenesis and infectious disorders [39]. LPS exposure has been proven to increase the production and release of NO in macrophages, with the increased production of NO in cells potentially causing tissue damage [25]. Therefore, NO inhibition is important in therapeutic interventions for the treatment of inflammatory diseases [40]. The anti-inflammatory potential of fucoidan isolated from various brown seaweeds has been demonstrated in previous studies [31,34,41]. Apart from NO, PGE2 and pro-inflammatory cytokine production were also increased due to the LPS stimulation in macrophage cells. PGE2 is a principal inflammatory mediator whose production occurs in cells in response to external stimuli. Increased release of PGE2 can cause unfavorable inflammatory responses, which lead to tissue damage [42]. Immune cells such as neutrophils, macrophages, and eosinophils are also involved in the pathogenesis of inflammation through the production of inflammatory cytokines such as TNF-α, IL-6, and IL-1β. Abnormal production of the above-mentioned cytokines and PGE2 may result in the development of inflammatory lesions and pose the threat of inducing apoptosis in the cells [43]. Therefore, inhibition of their excess production is important in controlling inflammation [44].

According to our study, the LPS treatment resulted in increased release of NO, PGE2, and pro-inflammatory cytokines in RAW 264.7 cells, and the production of these compounds was significantly down-regulated by co-treatment with SAF3 concentration-dependently. Our findings are consistent with the results obtained from studies conducted on the anti-inflammatory properties of sulfated polysaccharides from *S. swartzii*, *C. minima*, and *E. cava* [5,23,45]. In addition, iNOS and COX2 expression during the inflammatory response result in NO and PGE2 production. Previous studies have demonstrated using Western blot analysis that sulfated polysaccharides such as fucoidan derived from seaweeds inhibit iNOS and COX2-like mediators in stimulated cells [10]. The key contribution to the production of NO is considered to be arginine oxidation by nitric oxide synthase (NOS), whereas PGE2 synthesis is due to the involvement of COX2 [46]. In agreement with the previous reports, COX2 and iNOS expression were repressed in our study on the treatment with SAF3 in LPS-stimulated RAW 264.7 cells. Similar results were obtained in a study on the anti-inflammatory effect of *S. swartzii* in LPS-induced RAW 264 cells [23].

It is reported that activation of complex signaling pathways such as NF-κB/MAPK results in inflammatory responses [10,47,48]. Therefore, the effect of SAF3 samples on the downstream signaling of these pathways was further examined. The NF-κB transcription factor family contains c-Rel, RelB, p50, p65, and p52 proteins. The NF-κB transcription factor resides in the cytosol under normal conditions, and it is translocated into the nucleus in its phosphorylated form due to the stimulation of macrophages [48,49]. This results in the transcription of inflammatory-related genes such as iNOS and COX2, as well as genes encoding pro-inflammatory cytokines [50]. This study revealed that the LPS stimulation promoted IKBα and p65 phosphorylation, consequently activating the NF-κB pathway. Nonetheless, down-regulation of the phosphorylation of NF-κB transcription factors and their nuclear translocation was achieved by concentration-dependent treatment with fucoidan. These results were also observed downstream of the MAPK signaling cascade. MAPK plays a major role in the release of inflammatory chemokines and the activation of pro-inflammatory cytokines [51,52]. Among the three important MAPKs (p38, JNK, and ERK (1/2)), p38 is involved in regulating the synthesis of inflammatory regulators [53,54]. With LPS-stimulation, the phosphorylation of p38 and ERK (1/2) was observed to increase, which was downregulated with the treatment with fucoidan (SAF3). Therefore, inhibition of protein expression linked with NF-κB/MAPK signaling can be considered a promising target for the treatment of inflammation-related diseases. Our study findings corroborate those of other research on the anti-inflammatory properties of fucoidan isolated from *E. maxima, C. minima,* and *S. horneri* [41]. The current study improves our understanding of cellular mechanisms related to LPS-induced inflammation. Overall, the observations obtained from the current study verify the potential of SAF3 against chronic inflammatory conditions. This also encourages further studies to confirm the relationship between the anti-inflammatory activity of *S. autumnale* fucoidan and TLR-mediated NF-κB/MAPK signaling pathways using pharmacological inhibitors.

This manuscript represents a pioneering research article focused on investigating the anti-inflammatory activity of fucoidan derived from *S. autumnale*. It stands as the first of its kind to comprehensively explore the potential therapeutic effects of fucoidan specifically sourced from *S. autumnale* in the context of inflammation. By filling this crucial research gap, the obtained results of the study have paved the way for a deeper understanding of the anti-inflammatory properties of *S. autumnale* fucoidan and its potential applications in the field of medicine. This highlights the importance of studying the unique characteristics and bioactivity of fucoidan from different sources. The findings presented will serve as a valuable foundation for future studies and inspire further exploration of the therapeutic potential of *S. autumnale* fucoidan in the treatment and management of inflammatory conditions.

4. Materials and Methods

4.1. Chemicals and Reagents

Protomax enzyme, Polysaccharide standards (fucoidan), and 3-(4,5-dimethylthiazol-2 yl)-2,5-diphenyltetrazolium bromide (MTT) were obtained from Sigma-Aldrich (St. Louis, MO, USA). The murine macrophage cell line RAW 264.7 was purchased from the American Type Culture Collection (Rockville, MD, USA). Dulbecco's modified Eagle's medium (DMEM), fetal bovine serum (FBS), and penicillin-streptomycin were purchased from Gibco/BRL (Burlington, ON, Canada). Enzyme-linked immunosorbent assay kits for PGE2, IL-6, and IL-1β were acquired from R & D Systems Inc. (Minneapolis, MN, USA). Carbohydrate-degrading enzymes were donated by Novozymes (China) Biotechnology Co., Ltd. (Tianjin, China). Ethanol, 2-propanol, the BCA protein assay kit, and chloroform were purchased from Sigma–Aldrich. Primary and secondary antibodies were purchased from Santa Cruz Biotechnology (Dallas, TX, USA). An enhanced chemiluminescence reagent was obtained from Amersham (Arlington Heights, IL, USA). All other chemicals and solvents used in this study were of analytical grade.

4.2. Sample Collection, Enzyme Assisted Extraction, and Enrichment of Fucoidan

Sargassum autumnale was collected from the coast of Jeju Island, Republic of Korea, in March 2018. The seaweed was cleaned thoroughly with water for the removal of epiphytes and other impurities and dried using a Goodle dryer [18]. Dried seaweed was then ground into a fine powder. The powder (10 g) was dissolved in 1 L of distilled water (DW) and treated with Protomax (Omax, Kent, WA, USA) (pH 6.0, 40 °C) for 24 h. The enzyme was then inactivated by heat treatment at 100 °C for 10 min, and the pH was adjusted to 7 (SAP). Precipitation of polysaccharides was done by addition of 95% ethanol and stored at 4 °C for 8 h for the precipitation of polysaccharides. Precipitated polysaccharides were recovered by centrifugation and washed with 95% ethanol by homogenizing and centrifugation. Finally, a *S. autumnale* crude polysaccharide (SACP) sample was freeze-dried and used for further experiments.

4.3. Anion Exchange Chromatography for Separation and Purification of Fucoidan

A crude polysaccharide solution was prepared in sodium acetate buffer and loaded onto a DEAE cellulose column [21]. Fucoidan fractions were separated using ion-exchange chromatography by eluting with a linear gradient of sodium chloride (50–2000 mM). Separated fucoidan fractions (SAF1, SAF2, and SAF3) were collected, dialyzed, and finally lyophilized.

4.4. Chemical Composition Analysis

Estimates of the polysaccharide, protein, polyphenol, and sulfate contents of the fractions were made using accepted techniques described in publications by the Association of Official Agricultural Chemists [21]. In order to ascertain the polysaccharide and polyphenol contents, respectively, the phenol-sulfuric and Folin–Ciocalteu procedures were applied. The amount of protein was determined using Lowry protein assays, while the amount of sulfate was determined using the barium sulfate precipitation technique.

4.5. Cell Culture

Murine macrophage cell line RAW 264.7 was purchased from the American Type Culture Collection (ATCC) (TIB-71) and maintained in DMEM with 10% FBS and 1% penicillin/streptomycin mixture at 37 °C in a 5% CO_2 humidified atmosphere. Cells were subjected to a periodic subculture, and cells showing exponential growth were used for further experiments. LPS stock solution was prepared using PBS solution, and it was diluted when necessary. *S. autumnale* extracts were dissolved in PBS solutions and diluted to prepare working concentrations.

4.6. Cell Viability and NO Production

Cell viability was evaluated by an MTT assay to measure the cytotoxicity of samples [13,24]. In brief, RAW 264.7 cells were seeded in a 96-well plate and incubated for 24 h in a CO_2 incubator prior to the treatment of SACP and *S. autumnale* fucoidan (25, 50, 100, 200, and 400 µg/mL). The sample concentrations were selected based on previously published results [55]. The MTT assay was carried out after 24 h incubation. For the analysis of the cytoprotective effect of samples against LPS stimulation, *S. autumnale* extracts were applied to the cells (25, 50, 100, and 200 µg/mL), and after 1 h, cells were stimulated with LPS (final concentration 1 µg/mL). Following the incubation, MTT reagent was added to the wells and incubated for another 2 h in a humidified incubator. Finally, MTT was removed after 2 h, and 100 µL of DMSO solution was added; absorbance was measured at 570 nm after 10 min [10].

The Griess assay was employed to determine the ability of *S. autumnale* fucoidan to inhibit NO production in LPS-stimulated RAW 264.7 cells. Briefly, the seeded cells were incubated for 24 h prior to the application of *S. autumnale* extracts at different concentrations. After 24 h of stimulation with LPS, the cell culture medium and Griess reagent were mixed in equal amounts, and absorbance was measured at 540 nm after 10 min on an ELISA plate reader (BioTek Instruments, Inc., Winooski, VT, USA). The fucoidan fraction SAF3 showed excellent NO inhibition activity and cytoprotective activity against LPS. Therefore, it was selected for further experiments [13,31].

4.7. Assessment of PGE2 and Pro-Inflammatory Cytokines Expression Levels

For the assessment of prostaglandin and pro-inflammatory cytokine levels, we cultured RAW 264.7 cells were treated with different concentrations of SAF3 (50, 100, and 200 µg/mL). After 1 h, LPS was applied to the cells and further incubated for 24 h. PGE2, IL-6, IL-1β, and TNF-α were quantified in the cell-free supernatant with the help of competitive enzyme immunoassay kits (R & D Systems Inc.) [41].

4.8. Western Blot Analysis

The effect of SAF3 on the expression levels of iNOS, COX2, NF-κB, and MAPK pathway proteins was analyzed using Western blotting [24]. In brief, seeded RAW 264.7 cells were treated with SAF3 (50, 100, and 200 μg/mL) for 2 h, followed by LPS stimulation of the cells for 24 h. Harvested cells were processed for protein extraction, and the BCA protein assay kit was used to determine protein concentration. The proteins were then separated on a 12% SDS-PAGE gel under denaturing conditions and transferred onto a nitrocellulose membrane. The membrane was blocked with 5% skim milk prior to the incubation with primary antibodies. Membranes were incubated with primary antibodies overnight at 4 °C, followed by incubation with secondary antibodies for 2 h at room temperature. Chemiluminescent substrate (Cyanagen Srl, Bologna, Italy) was used for the development of signals, and the bands were photographed using the FUSION SOLO Vilber Lourmat system. The ImageJ program (version 1.50i, Wayne Rasband, National Institute of Health, Bethesda, ML, USA) was aided in the quantification of band intensities [56].

4.9. Statistical Analysis

All the cell experiments were triplicated, and all data are expressed as means ± SD. Significant differences among data values were determined with the Kruskal–Wallis test, Mann–Whitney U test. All statistical analyses were performed using the GraphPad Prism 9 statistical analysis package (GraphPad Software Inc., San Diego, CA, USA). A p-value < 0.05 is considered significant.

5. Conclusions

In summary, this study reveals the potential anti-inflammatory activity of purified fucoidan (SAF3) from *S. autumnale* against LPS-induced inflammation. SAF3 significantly inhibited the release of NO, PGE2, and pro-inflammatory cytokines such as TNF-α, IL-6, and IL-1β in RAW 264.7 macrophage cells. The study also exhibited that the anti-inflammatory activity was related to the downregulation of iNOS and COX2 and signaling pathways such as NF-κB and MAPK. Thus, the fucoidan isolated from *S. autumnale* can be developed as a broad-spectrum anti-inflammatory drug or other health product.

Furthermore, the research findings provide an understanding of the continuous exploitation of compounds from marine algae for the prevention and mediation of inflammatory diseases. Further in vivo experiments are needed to test the anti-inflammatory properties of *S. autumnale* fucoidan before it can be developed into a human-consumable product.

Author Contributions: Conceptualization, N.M.L.; methodology, N.M.L. and H.-G.L.; software, H.-G.L., D.P.N., K.-M.S. and Y.-S.C.; validation, N.M.L., D.P.N. and H.-G.L.; formal analysis, N.M.L.; investigation, N.M.L., D.P.N. and H.-G.L.; resources, D.P.N., H.H.A.C.K.J., K.-M.S. and Y.-S.C.; data curation, N.M.L.; writing—original draft preparation, N.M.L.; writing—review and editing, N.M.L., Y.-J.J. and M.-C.K.; visualization, N.M.L.; supervision, Y.-J.J.; project administration, M.-C.K.; funding acquisition, M.-C.K. All authors have read and agreed to the published version of the manuscript.

Funding: This research was supported by the Main Research Program (E0211200-03) of the Korea Food Research Institute (KFRI), funded by the Ministry of Science and ICT.

Institutional Review Board Statement: Not applicable.

Data Availability Statement: Data will be made available upon request.

Conflicts of Interest: The authors declare no conflict of interest.

References

1. Chevolot, L.; Foucault, A.; Chaubet, F.; Kervarec, N.; Sinquin, C.; Fisher, A.-M.; Boisson-Vidal, C. Further data on the structure of brown seaweed fucans: Relationships with anticoagulant activity. *Carbohydr. Res.* **1999**, *319*, 154–165. [CrossRef] [PubMed]
2. Li, B.; Lu, F.; Wei, X.; Zhao, R. Fucoidan: Structure and bioactivity. *Molecules* **2008**, *13*, 1671–1695. [CrossRef] [PubMed]
3. Bilan, M.I.; Grachev, A.A.; Ustuzhanina, N.E.; Shashkov, A.S.; Nifantiev, N.E.; Usov, A.I. Structure of a fucoidan from the brown seaweed *Fucus evanescens* C.Ag. *Carbohydr. Res.* **2002**, *337*, 719–730. [CrossRef]

4. Liyanage, N.M.; Nagahawatta, D.P.; Jayawardena, T.U.; Jeon, Y.-J. The Role of Seaweed Polysaccharides in Gastrointestinal Health: Protective Effect against Inflammatory Bowel Disease. *Life* **2023**, *13*, 1026. [CrossRef]
5. Liyanage, N.M.; Nagahawatta, D.P.; Jayawardhana, H.H.A.C.K.; Jayawardena, T.U.; Kim, Y.-S.; Lee, H.-G.; Park, Y.-J.; Jeon, Y.-J. Therapeutic effect of *Sargassum swartzii* against urban particulate matter–induced lung inflammation via toll-like receptor-mediated NF-κB pathway inhibition. *Algal Res.* **2023**, *71*, 103045. [CrossRef]
6. Nagahawatta, D.P.; Liyanage, N.M.; Je, J.-G.; Jayawardhana, H.H.A.C.K.; Jayawardena, T.U.; Jeong, S.-H.; Kwon, H.-J.; Choi, C.S.; Jeon, Y.-J. Polyphenolic Compounds Isolated from Marine Algae Attenuate the Replication of SARS-CoV-2 in the Host Cell through a Multi-Target Approach of 3CLpro and PLpro. *Mar. Drugs* **2022**, *20*, 786. [CrossRef]
7. Hou, C.; Chen, L.; Yang, L.; Ji, X. An insight into anti-inflammatory effects of natural polysaccharides. *Int. J. Biol. Macromol.* **2020**, *153*, 248–255. [CrossRef]
8. Jeong, J.W.; Hwang, S.J.; Han, M.H.; Lee, D.S.; Yoo, J.S.; Choi, I.W.; Cha, H.J.; Kim, S.; Kim, H.S.; Kim, G.Y.; et al. Fucoidan inhibits lipopolysaccharide-induced inflammatory responses in RAW 264.7 macrophages and zebrafish larvae. *Mol. Cell. Toxicol.* **2017**, *13*, 405–417. [CrossRef]
9. Kauppinen, A.; Suuronen, T.; Ojala, J.; Kaarniranta, K.; Salminen, A. Antagonistic crosstalk between NF-κB and SIRT1 in the regulation of inflammation and metabolic disorders. *Cell Signal.* **2013**, *25*, 1939–1948. [CrossRef]
10. Park, H.Y.; Han, M.H.; Park, C.; Jin, C.-Y.; Kim, G.-Y.; Choi, I.-W.; Kim, N.D.; Nam, T.-J.; Kwon, T.K.; Choi, Y.H. Anti-inflammatory effects of fucoidan through inhibition of NF-κB, MAPK and Akt activation in lipopolysaccharide-induced BV2 microglia cells. *Food Chem. Toxicol.* **2011**, *49*, 1745–1752. [CrossRef] [PubMed]
11. Seok, J.; Kim, T.S.; Kwon, H.J.; Lee, S.P.; Kang, M.H.; Kim, B.J.; Kim, M.N. Efficacy of *Cistanche Tubulosa* and *Laminaria Japonica* Extracts (MK-R7) Supplement in Preventing Patterned Hair Loss and Promoting Scalp Health. *Clin. Nutr. Res.* **2015**, *4*, 124–131 [CrossRef]
12. Phull, A.-R.; Majid, M.; Haq, I.-U.; Khan, M.R.; Kim, S.J. In vitro and in vivo evaluation of anti-arthritic, antioxidant efficacy of fucoidan from *Undaria pinnatifida* (Harvey) Suringar. *Int. J. Biol. Macromol.* **2017**, *97*, 468–480. [CrossRef] [PubMed]
13. Liyanage, N.M.; Lee, H.-G.; Nagahawatta, D.P.; Jayawardhana, H.H.A.C.K.; Ryu, B.; Jeon, Y.-J. Characterization and therapeutic effect of *Sargassum coreanum* fucoidan that inhibits lipopolysaccharide-induced inflammation in RAW 264.7 macrophages by blocking NF-κB signaling. *Int. J. Biol. Macromol.* **2022**, *223*, 500–510. [CrossRef]
14. Haggag, Y.A.; Abd Elrahman, A.A.; Ulber, R.; Zayed, A. Fucoidan in Pharmaceutical Formulations: A Comprehensive Review for Smart Drug Delivery Systems. *Mar. Drugs* **2023**, *21*, 112. [CrossRef] [PubMed]
15. Apostolova, E.; Lukova, P.; Baldzhieva, A.; Delattre, C.; Molinié, R.; Petit, E.; Elboutachfaiti, R.; Nikolova, M.; Iliev, I.; Murdjeva, M.; et al. Structural Characterization and In Vivo Anti-Inflammatory Activity of Fucoidan from *Cystoseira crinita* (Desf.) Borry. *Mar. Drugs* **2022**, *20*, 714. [CrossRef]
16. Watanabe, K.; Homma, Y.; Karakisawa, H.; Ishikawa, R.; Uwai, S.J.P.R. Haplotypic differentiation between seasonal populations of *Sargassum horneri* (Fucales, Phaeophyceae) in Japan. *Phycol. Res.* **2019**, *67*, 59–64. [CrossRef]
17. Yoshiie, T.; Maeda, M.; Kimura, M.; Hama, Y.; Uchida, M.; Kimura, Y. Structural Features of N-Glycans of Seaweed Glycoproteins Predominant Occurrence of High-Mannose Type N-Glycans in Marine Plants. *Biosci. Biotechnol. Biochem.* **2012**, *76*, 1996–1998. [CrossRef] [PubMed]
18. Nagahawatta, D.P.; Sanjeewa, K.K.A.; Jayawardena, T.U.; Kim, H.-S.; Yang, H.-W.; Jiang, Y.; Je, J.-G.; Lee, T.-K.; Jeon, Y.-J. Drying seaweeds using hybrid hot water Goodle dryer (HHGD): Comparison with freeze-dryer in chemical composition and antioxidan activity. *Fish. Aquat. Sci.* **2021**, *24*, 19–31. [CrossRef]
19. Maneesh, A.; Chakraborty, K. Previously undescribed *fridooleanenes* and oxygenated labdanes from the brown seaweed *Sargassum wightii* and their protein tyrosine phosphatase-1B inhibitory activity. *Phytochemistry* **2017**, *144*, 19–32. [CrossRef] [PubMed]
20. Arisawa, M.; Hayashi, K.; Nikaido, T.; Koike, K.; Fujita, D.; Nunomura, N.; Tanaka, M.; Sasaki, T. Screening of Some Marine Organism Extracts for cAMP Phosphodiesterase Inhibition, Cytotoxicity, and Antiviral Activity against HSV-1. *Int. J. Pharmacogr.* **1997**, *35*, 6–11. [CrossRef]
21. Lee, H.G.; Jayawardena, T.U.; Liyanage, N.M.; Song, K.-M.; Choi, Y.-S.; Jeon, Y.-J.; Kang, M.-C. Antioxidant potential of low molecular weight fucoidans from *Sargassum autumnale* against H2O2-induced oxidative stress in vitro and in zebrafish models based on molecular weight changes. *Food Chem.* **2022**, *384*, 132591. [CrossRef]
22. Wang, L.; Oh, J.Y.; Hwang, J.; Ko, J.Y.; Jeon, Y.-J.; Ryu, B. In Vitro and In Vivo Antioxidant Activities of Polysaccharides Isolated from Celluclast-Assisted Extract of an Edible Brown Seaweed, *Sargassum fulvellum*. *Antioxidants* **2019**, *8*, 493. [CrossRef] [PubMed]
23. Jayawardena, T.U.; Sanjeewa, K.K.A.; Nagahawatta, D.P.; Lee, H.-G.; Lu, Y.-A.; Vaas, A.P.J.P.; Abeytunga, D.T.U.; Nanayakkara, C.M.; Lee, D.-S.; Jeon, Y.-J. Anti-Inflammatory Effects of Sulfated Polysaccharide from *Sargassum swartzii* in Macrophages via Blocking TLR/NF-Kb Signal Transduction. *Mar. Drugs* **2020**, *18*, 601. [CrossRef]
24. Nagahawatta, D.P.; Liyanage, N.M.; Jayawardhana, H.H.A.C.K.; Lee, H.-G.; Jayawardena, T.U.; Jeon, Y.-J. Anti-Fine Dust Effect of Fucoidan Extracted from *Ecklonia maxima* Laves in Macrophages via Inhibiting Inflammatory Signaling Pathways. *Mar. Drugs* **2022**, *20*, 413. [CrossRef]
25. Heo, S.-J.; Yoon, W.-J.; Kim, K.-N.; Ahn, G.-N.; Kang, S.-M.; Kang, D.-H.; Affan, A.; Oh, C.; Jung, W.-K.; Jeon, Y.-J. Evaluation of anti-inflammatory effect of fucoxanthin isolated from brown algae in lipopolysaccharide-stimulated RAW 264.7 macrophages. *Food Chem. Toxicol.* **2010**, *48*, 2045–2051. [CrossRef]

26. Koh, W.; Shin, J.-S.; Lee, J.; Lee, I.-H.; Lee, S.K.; Ha, I.-H.; Chung, H.-J. Anti-inflammatory effect of *Cortex Eucommiae* via modulation of the toll-like receptor 4 pathway in lipopolysaccharide-stimulated RAW 264.7 macrophages. *J. Ethnopharmacol.* **2017**, *209*, 255–263. [CrossRef]
27. Li, K.K.; Shen, S.S.; Deng, X.; Shiu, H.T.; Siu, W.S.; Leung, P.C.; Ko, C.H.; Cheng, B.H. Dihydrofisetin exerts its anti-inflammatory effects associated with suppressing ERK/p38 MAPK and Heme Oxygenase-1 activation in lipopolysaccharide-stimulated RAW 264.7 macrophages and carrageenan-induced mice paw edema. *Int. Immunopharmacol.* **2018**, *54*, 366–374. [CrossRef] [PubMed]
28. Zha, X.-Q.; Lu, C.-Q.; Cui, S.-H.; Pan, L.-H.; Zhang, H.-L.; Wang, J.-H.; Luo, J.-P. Structural identification and immunostimulating activity of a *Laminaria japonica* polysaccharide. *Int. J. Biol. Macromol.* **2015**, *78*, 429–438. [CrossRef] [PubMed]
29. Serafini, M.; Peluso, I.; Raguzzini, A. Flavonoids as anti-inflammatory agents. *Proc. Nutr. Soc.* **2010**, *69*, 273–278. [CrossRef]
30. Thuy, T.T.T.; Ly, B.M.; Van, T.T.T.; Van Quang, N.; Tu, H.C.; Zheng, Y.; Seguin-Devaux, C.; Mi, B.; Ai, U. Anti-HIV activity of fucoidans from three brown seaweed species. *Carbohydr. Polym.* **2015**, *115*, 122–128. [CrossRef]
31. Rewerski, W.; Wysokowski, J. Kinetics of the process of metabolism, absorption and breakdown of drug in the organism. *Pol. Tyg. Lek.* **1965**, *20*, 735–737. [CrossRef]
32. Hayashi, K.; Lee, J.-B.; Nakano, T.; Hayashi, T.J.M. Infection, Anti-influenza A virus characteristics of a fucoidan from sporophyll of *Undaria pinnatifida* in mice with normal and compromised immunity. *Microbes Infect.* **2013**, *15*, 302–309. [CrossRef] [PubMed]
33. Wijesinghe, W.A.J.P.; Jeon, Y.-J. Biological activities and potential industrial applications of fucose rich sulfated polysaccharides and fucoidans isolated from brown seaweeds: A review. *Carbohydr. Polym.* **2012**, *88*, 13–20. [CrossRef]
34. Shanura Fernando, I.P.; Asanka Sanjeewa, K.K.; Samarakoon, K.W.; Kim, H.-S.; Gunasekara, U.K.D.S.S.; Park, Y.-J.; Abeytunga, D.T.U.; Lee, W.W.; Jeon, Y.-J. The potential of fucoidans from *Chnoospora minima* and *Sargassum polycystum* in cosmetics: Antioxidant, anti-inflammatory, skin-whitening, and antiwrinkle activities. *J. Appl. Phycol.* **2018**, *30*, 3223–3232. [CrossRef]
35. Mhadhebi, L.; Mhadhebi, A.; Robert, J.; Bouraoui, A. Antioxidant, Anti-inflammatory and Antiproliferative Effects of Aqueous Extracts of Three Mediterranean Brown Seaweeds of the *Genus Cystoseira*. *Iran. J. Pharm. Res.* **2014**, *13*, e125413. [CrossRef]
36. Wang, J.; Zhang, Q.; Zhang, Z.; Song, H.; Li, P. Potential antioxidant and anticoagulant capacity of low molecular weight fucoidan fractions extracted from *Laminaria japonica*. *Int. J. Biol. Macromol.* **2010**, *46*, 6–12. [CrossRef]
37. Ale, M.T.; Mikkelsen, J.D.; Meyer, A.S. Important Determinants for Fucoidan Bioactivity: A Critical Review of Structure-Function Relations and Extraction Methods for Fucose-Containing Sulfated Polysaccharides from Brown Seaweeds. *Mar. Drugs* **2011**, *9*, 2106–2130. [CrossRef] [PubMed]
38. Ale, M.T.; Meyer, A.S. Fucoidans from brown seaweeds: An update on structures, extraction techniques and use of enzymes as tools for structural elucidation. *RSC Adv.* **2013**, *3*, 8131–8141. [CrossRef]
39. Moncada, S.; Higgs, A. The L-Arginine-Nitric Oxide Pathway. *N. Engl. J. Med.* **1993**, *329*, 2002–2012. [CrossRef] [PubMed]
40. Sharma, J.N.; Al-Omran, A.; Parvathy, S.S. Role of nitric oxide in inflammatory diseases. *Inflammopharmacology* **2007**, *15*, 252–259. [CrossRef] [PubMed]
41. Sanjeewa, K.K.A.; Fernando, I.P.S.; Kim, E.-A.; Ahn, G.; Jee, Y.; Jeon, Y.-J. Anti-inflammatory activity of a sulfated polysaccharide isolated from an enzymatic digest of brown seaweed *Sargassum horneri* in RAW 264.7 cells. *Nutr. Res. Pract.* **2017**, *11*, 3. [CrossRef]
42. Dubois, R.N.; Abramson, S.B.; Crofford, L.; Gupta, R.A.; Simon, L.S.; Van De Putte, L.B.; Lipsky, P.E. Cyclooxygenase in biology and disease. *FASEB J.* **1998**, *12*, 1063–1073. [CrossRef] [PubMed]
43. George, L.; Ramasamy, T.; Sirajudeen, K.N.S.; Manickam, V. LPS-induced Apoptosis is Partially Mediated by Hydrogen Sulphide in RAW 264.7 Murine Macrophages. *Immunol. Investig.* **2019**, *48*, 451–465. [CrossRef] [PubMed]
44. Lee, S.-H.; Ko, C.-I.; Ahn, G.; You, S.; Kim, J.-S.; Heu, M.S.; Kim, J.; Jee, Y.; Jeon, Y.-J. Molecular characteristics and anti-inflammatory activity of the fucoidan extracted from *Ecklonia cava*. *Carbohydr. Polym.* **2012**, *89*, 599–606. [CrossRef]
45. Fernando, I.P.S.; Sanjeewa, K.K.A.; Samarakoon, K.W.; Lee, W.W.; Kim, H.-S.; Kang, N.; Ranasinghe, P.; Lee, H.-S.; Jeon, Y.-J. A fucoidan fraction purified from *Chnoospora minima*; a potential inhibitor of LPS-induced inflammatory responses. *Int. J. Biol. Macromol.* **2017**, *104*, 1185–1193. [CrossRef]
46. Clancy, R.M.; Abramson, S.B. Nitric oxide: A novel mediator of inflammation. *Proc. Soc. Exp. Biol. Med.* **1995**, *210*, 93–101. [CrossRef]
47. Kang, J.S.; Yoon, Y.D.; Lee, K.H.; Park, S.-K.; Kim, H.M. Costunolide inhibits interleukin-1β expression by down-regulation of AP-1 and MAPK activity in LPS-stimulated RAW 264.7 cells. *Biochem. Biophys. Res. Commun.* **2004**, *313*, 171–177. [CrossRef] [PubMed]
48. Jayawardena, T.U.; Kim, H.-S.; Asanka Sanjeewa, K.K.; Han, E.J.; Jee, Y.; Ahn, G.; Rho, J.-R.; Jeon, Y.-J. Loliolide, isolated from *Sargassum horneri*; abate LPS-induced inflammation via TLR mediated NF-κB, MAPK pathways in macrophages. *Algal Res.* **2021**, *56*, 102297. [CrossRef]
49. Shawish, H.B.; Wong, W.Y.; Wong, Y.L.; Loh, S.W.; Looi, C.Y.; Hassandarvish, P.; Phan, A.Y.L.; Wong, W.F.; Wang, H.; Paterson, I.C.; et al. Nickel(II) Complex of Polyhydroxybenzaldehyde N4-Thiosemicarbazone Exhibits Anti-Inflammatory Activity by Inhibiting NF-κB Transactivation. *PLoS ONE* **2014**, *9*, e100933. [CrossRef]
50. Li, Q.; Verma, I.M. NF-κB regulation in the immune system. *Nat. Rev. Immunol.* **2002**, *2*, 725–734. [CrossRef]
51. Sanjeewa, K.A.; Jayawardena, T.U.; Kim, H.-S.; Kim, S.-Y.; Ahn, G.; Kim, H.-J.; Fu, X.; Jee, Y.; Jeon, Y.-J. Ethanol extract separated from *Sargassum horneri* (Turner) abate LPS-induced inflammation in RAW 264.7 macrophages. *Fish. Aquat. Sci.* **2019**, *22*, 6. [CrossRef]
52. Akira, S.J. Toll-like Receptors and Innate Immunity. *Adv. Immunol.* **2001**, *78*, 1–56. [CrossRef]

53. Kaminska, B. MAPK signalling pathways as molecular targets for anti-inflammatory therapy—From molecular mechanisms to therapeutic benefits. *Biochim. Biophys. Acta (BBA) Proteins Proteom.* **2005**, *1754*, 253–262. [CrossRef] [PubMed]
54. Madrid, L.V.; Wang, C.-Y.; Guttridge, D.C.; Schottelius, A.J.G.; Baldwin, A.S.; Mayo, M.W. Akt Suppresses Apoptosis by Stimulating the Transactivation Potential of the RelA/p65 Subunit of NF-κB. *Mol. Cell. Biol.* **2000**, *20*, 1626–1638. [CrossRef] [PubMed]
55. Jayawardhana, H.H.A.C.K.; Lee, H.-G.; Liyanage, N.M.; Nagahawatta, D.P.; Ryu, B.; Jeon, Y.-J. Structural characterization and anti-inflammatory potential of sulfated polysaccharides from *Scytosiphon lomentaria*; attenuate inflammatory signaling pathways. *J. Funct. Foods* **2023**, *102*, 105446. [CrossRef]
56. Jeong, G.-S.; Lee, D.-S.; Li, B.; Byun, E.; Kwon, D.-Y.; Park, H.; Kim, Y.-C. Protective effect of sauchinone by upregulating heme oxygenase-1 via the P38 MAPK and Nrf2/ARE pathways in HepG2 cells. *Planta Med.* **2010**, *76*, 41–47. [CrossRef] [PubMed]

Disclaimer/Publisher's Note: The statements, opinions and data contained in all publications are solely those of the individual author(s) and contributor(s) and not of MDPI and/or the editor(s). MDPI and/or the editor(s) disclaim responsibility for any injury to people or property resulting from any ideas, methods, instructions or products referred to in the content.

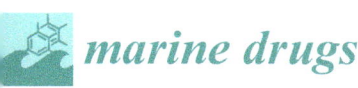

Article

Photoprotective and Anti-Aging Properties of the Apical Frond Extracts from the Mediterranean Seaweed *Ericaria amentacea*

Serena Mirata [1,2], Valentina Asnaghi [3,4], Mariachiara Chiantore [3,4], Annalisa Salis [1], Mirko Benvenuti [1], Gianluca Damonte [1] and Sonia Scarfì [2,3,4,*]

1. Department of Experimental Medicine (DIMES), Biochemistry Section, University of Genova, 16132 Genova, Italy; serena.mirata@edu.unige.it (S.M.); annalisa.salis@unige.it (A.S.); mirko.benvenuti@edu.unige.it (M.B.); gianluca.damonte@unige.it (G.D.)
2. Centro 3R, Interuniversity Center for the Promotion of the Principles of the 3Rs in Teaching and Research, 56122 Pisa, Italy
3. Department of Earth, Environment and Life Sciences (DISTAV), University of Genova, 16132 Genova, Italy; valentina.asnaghi@unige.it (V.A.); mariachiara.chiantore@unige.it (M.C.)
4. National Biodiversity Future Center (NBFC), 90133 Palermo, Italy
* Correspondence: soniascarfi@unige.it; Tel.: +0039-010-3350227

Abstract: There is a growing interest in using brown algal extracts thanks to the bioactive substances they produce for adaptation to the marine benthic environment. We evaluated the anti-aging and photoprotective properties of two types of extracts (50%-ethanol and DMSO) obtained from different portions, i.e., apices and thalli, of the brown seaweed, *Ericaria amentacea*. The apices of this alga, which grow and develop reproductive structures during summer when solar radiation is at its peak, were postulated to be rich in antioxidant compounds. We determined the chemical composition and pharmacological effects of their extracts and compared them to the thallus-derived extracts. All the extracts contained polyphenols, flavonoids and antioxidants and showed significant biological activities. The hydroalcoholic apices extracts demonstrated the highest pharmacological potential, likely due to the higher content of meroditerpene molecular species. They blocked toxicity in UV-exposed HaCaT keratinocytes and L929 fibroblasts and abated the oxidative stress and the production of pro-inflammatory cytokines, typically released after sunburns. Furthermore, the extracts showed anti-tyrosinase and anti-hydrolytic skin enzyme activity, counteracting the collagenase and hyaluronidase degrading activities and possibly slowing down the formation of uneven pigmentation and wrinkles in aging skin. In conclusion, the *E. amentacea* apices derivatives constitute ideal components for counteracting sunburn symptoms and for cosmetic anti-aging lotions.

Keywords: *Ericaria amentacea*; *Cystoseira amentacea*; antioxidant; anti-collagenase; anti-hyaluronidase; anti-tyrosinase; polyphenols; meroditerpenes; inflammation

1. Introduction

Macroalgae, the multicellular algae, are large aquatic photosynthetic organisms classified into three classes based on their photosynthetic pigments, the depth in which they live and their ability to absorb sunlight: the green, brown and red algae [1]. The uses of algae in the world go far beyond their simple food consumption; indeed, their anti-cancer (e.g., Liu et al. [2]), anti-inflammatory and immune system strengthening effects (e.g., Apostolova et al. [3]) have been repeatedly reported. The Mediterranean Sea represents a biodiversity hotspot for the brown algae belonging to the genus *Cystoseira sensu lato* (order Fucales). Chemical investigations of members of this genus led to the discovery of various bioactive secondary metabolites [4,5]. These isolated metabolites are very interesting, both for their biological activity and for their structural complexity. There is also a growing interest in the use of brown algal extracts for their beneficial effects on skin care. Since some of these algae thrive in very shallow waters, they produce bioactive substances that are natural photoprotective agents [6]. These photoprotective substances include amino acids, sulphated polysaccharides, carotenoids and polyphenols. They exhibit a wide range of biological activities, such as the absorption of ultraviolet (UV) rays, inhibition of metalloproteases, and anti-aging, antioxidant and immunomodulatory activities [7]. Indeed, both the oral intake and topical use of brown algae or their extracts demonstrated the ability to reduce the harmful effects of dermal exposure to UV-B rays. It has also been demonstrated that the polyphenols contained in brown algae are able to reduce the proliferation of cancer cells and the volume of UV-B exposure-derived tumors developed in mouse models [8]. Phlorotannins, the phloroglucinol-based polyphenols commonly found in brown algae, appear to be active in the treatment of arthritis [9] and have been reported as effective tyrosinase inhibitors [10] without side effects [11]. Free radicals (i.e., superoxide, nitric oxide and hydroxyl radicals) and other reactive species (i.e., hydrogen peroxide, peroxynitrite and hypochlorous acid) are naturally produced in the human organism, mainly because of aerobic metabolism. They can also be produced due to external factors Oxidative stress, which often results from the imbalance of the body's antioxidant status, has been implicated in aging and reactions leading to the generation of reactive oxygen species (ROS) in the skin and is one of the most interesting subjects of cosmetic research because they are involved in various skin diseases and skin aging processes, including atypical pigmentation, wrinkles, thinning, loss of elasticity and last but not least, cancer [12] Since UV rays promote the generation of ROS in cells, skin aging is usually related to UV exposure [13]. UV rays from the sun, exposure to cigarette smoke and pollutants, and the natural cellular aging process all contribute to the generation of free radicals and ROS. UV rays cause the depletion of cellular antioxidants and antioxidant enzymes (SOD, catalase) initiate DNA damage leading to thymine dimer formation and activate the neuroendocrine system with the release of neuroendocrine mediators. All this leads to the increased synthesis and release of pro-inflammatory mediators from both epidermal and dermal cells [14] Pro-inflammatory mediators increase capillary permeability, leading to the infiltration and activation of neutrophils and other phagocytic cells. Proteases, such as elastase and metalloproteases, are also released during the inflammatory process, and they are responsible for the degradation of many extracellular matrices (ECM) proteins, which together provide the structural and functional support for the skin tissue, ensuring skin tone, resistance elasticity and hydration. Therefore, with their hyperactivation, metalloproteases contribute to undermining the skin microarchitecture, favoring premature skin aging [15].

The re-integration of antioxidants in the skin, though exogenous administration, is an extremely valid approach that limits the skin damage induced by ROS caused by UV radiation. These exogenous antioxidants can be both synthetic and natural, and in this second case, the marine environment, thanks to its great biodiversity, can be an important source of these substances to be taken into consideration for the replacement of synthetic antioxidants, which their use is sometimes limited due to the toxic side effects [16,17]. Among all marine organisms, brown macroalgae are an inexhaustible source of these substances, and some of them are, in fact, already used in the field of cosmetics in skin care, sun protection products and anti-aging creams [18].

In this study, we evaluated the anti-inflammatory, photoprotective, antioxidant and hydrolytic enzyme-inhibitory activities on skin cells of two organic extracts obtained from different portions (apices and thalli) of the brown seaweed, *Ericaria amentacea*. Indeed, some bioactive properties of this Mediterranean brown seaweed have already been demonstrated in recent works [19–24]. *E. amentacea* is a protected species (listed as "of community interest" according to the European Union's Habitat Directive 92/43/EEC, under surveillance by the IUCN (International Union for Conservation of Nature), the Berne Convention—Council of Europe, 1979, and the Barcelona Convention—UNEP/MAP, 2009) and its indiscriminate collection, even for pharmaceutical purposes, is undesirable. Although it has been demonstrated that the collection of small apical portions of *E. amentacea* thalli is not harmful to its populations [25], it would be desirable to obtain extracts from laboratory-grown algae or from dedicated seaweed maricultures. Techniques for culturing *E. amentacea* have been refined in recent years [26,27], although obtaining large quantities of biomass from lab cultures is still an issue. Presently, a great deal of effort is dedicated to scaling up laboratory production, mainly with the aim of restoring endangered and damaged natural populations; however, the results of these efforts will also be useful for the future set up of macroalgal mariculture to exploit these precious bioactive molecules.

The apical component of this brown alga, which grows and develops reproductive structures in late spring/early summer, when solar radiation is maximum, is expected to be particularly rich in antioxidants [28] and, therefore, it is interesting to investigate their beneficial effect on the cells of the epidermis and dermis in comparison to extracts from the rest of the thallus (primary and secondary branches without apices) of the same seaweed. Additionally, 50%-ethanolic (hydroalcoholic) and 100%-dimethyl sulfoxide (DMSO) extracts of the two *E. amentacea* portions were obtained from algae collected in the Ligurian Sea (the Northwestern Mediterranean) in July, and their multifactorial anti-aging properties were studied in two cellular models of keratinocytes and fibroblasts. The final goal was to investigate the potential use of *E. amentacea* derivatives as lenitive and/or anti-aging cosmetics or as antioxidant nutraceutical additives.

2. Results and Discussion

2.1. TPC and TFC in E. amentacea Extracts

The total phenolic (TPC) and flavonoid (TFC) contents of the extracts obtained from the *E. amentacea* apices and thalli (Scheme 1) using two different solvents, DMSO and a hydroalcoholic solution (50% EtOH), were quantified.

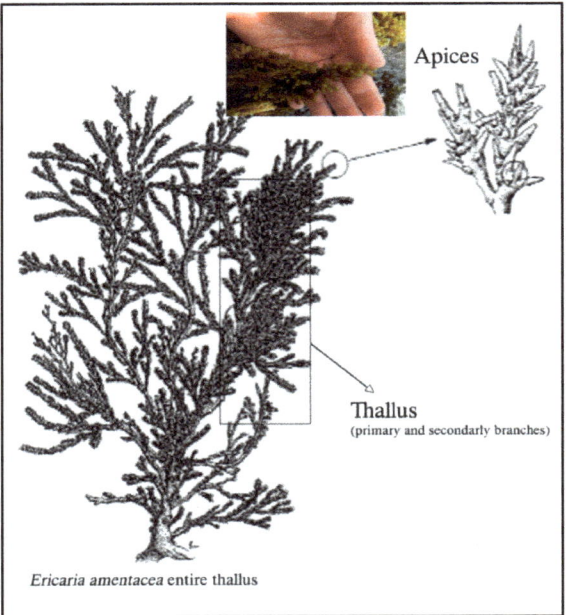

Scheme 1. Schematic representation of *E. amentacea* seaweed body parts.

The results in Table 1 show that the EtOH extraction retrieved 2.6-folds higher TPC from the apices of the seaweed compared to the thalli; meanwhile, the DMSO extraction allowed to retrieve 1.4-folds more TPC from the thalli compared to the apices.

Table 1. TPC and TFC of E. amentacea extracts.

Extract	TPC (µg/mg extr)	TFC (µg/mg extr)
EtOH Apex	48.32 ± 0.54	5.60 ± 0.66
EtOH Thallus	18.47 ± 3.49	2.28 ± 0.27
DMSO Apex	39.40 ± 1.94	2.433 ± 0.35
DMSO Thallus	55.52 ± 6.08	4.45 ± 0.19

Quantification of the total phenolic content (TPC) and total flavonoid content (TFC) by the Folin–Ciocalteu and AlCl3 colorimetric assays, respectively.

In the various extracts, the TFC percentage, compared to their respective TPCs, was higher in the EtOH samples compared to the DMSO ones. In particular, the TFCs of the EtOH apices and thalli extracts were 11.5% and 12.3% of the respective TPC, while the TFC of the DMSO apices and thalli extracts accounted for 6.1% and 8% of the respective TPC. These results indicate that the apices and the thalli are both rich in polyphenols but qualitatively different since the apices provide high yields of hydroalcoholic soluble polyphenols, while the thalli provide more organic soluble molecular species of the same family. This is entirely possible, however, since polyphenols are a very large and heterogenous family of compounds [29], going from a single phenol moiety (i.e., gallic acid) in the molecule to multiple covalently linked phenol rings (i.e., ellagitannin), which can prefer organic solvent extraction. Therefore, these results could suggest that the fast summer growth of the fronds, and especially of the apices carrying the reproductive structures, may favor a higher synthesis of the hydroalcoholic soluble as compared to the soluble organic species, and then, when the seaweed continues growing, more organic soluble species are produced and are retrievable from the thalli. Similarly, van Alstyne et al. [30] found an intra-thallus distribution of TPC, usually more concentrated in the meristematic zones i.e., the distal extremities, while Mannino et al. [22] observed the highest TPC values for the *E. amentacea* ethanol extracts in summer when higher protection to solar radiation is needed, in particular, in the most sensitive portions of the thallus (i.e., the newly sprouted branches and the developing reproductive structures).

The TPC values obtained by the thalli extraction with the two solvents are also in line with the results obtained in our previous paper [23], where *E. amentacea* total fronds collected during the summer season in the Ligurian Sea, with no separation between the apices and thalli, were extracted via the same protocols. Since the apical fronds are only 2–3 cm long compared to the whole thallus (usually more than 10–15 cm), it is likely that the total fronds' extraction values, obtained in the previous work, were close to those of the thalli obtained in this work and significantly different from the values of the apices of the seaweed. These values are also significantly higher than those obtained by the Atlantic *Cystoseira abies-marina* innovative extraction methods, i.e., by ultrasound or microwave-assisted extraction [31], but are in line with the results from the Mediterranean *Cystoseira compressa* microwave-assisted extraction [32], and from the Mediterranean *Cystoseira sensu lato* species traditional extraction [33]. Both the results from the *Cystoseira compressa* [32] and *Cystoseira sensu lato* [33] analyses notate the seasonal chemical composition differences of the investigated seaweeds, while conversely, our data report, for the first time, the differences in chemical composition and bioactive properties of the extracts from the reproductive portion of the alga compared to the whole yet recently produced thallus, highlighting interesting and promising features.

Furthermore, the EtOH solvent extraction of *E. amentacea* fronds allowed a higher recovery (close to double) of the flavonoid fraction with respect to the DMSO. In this case, no remarkable differences were observed between the extract of the apical fronds and of the thallus with the same solvent, likely indicating, for this class of molecules, a constant synthesis throughout the year, not affected by the seasonal growth of the seaweed nor by the reproductive vs. structural portions of the thallus. This is also an important result, given that flavonoids have demonstrated a protective effect from UV radiation and, consequently, in inhibiting oxidative damage and mitigating skin aging processes [34,35].

Thus, a significant fraction of flavonoids within the extracts make them optimal ingredients for sunburn lotions and anti-aging concoctions.

2.2. In Chemico Antioxidant Activity

The antioxidant properties of the four *E. amentacea* extracts were measured by means of several in chemico assays, namely by measuring the DPPH, hydroxyl and nitric oxide radical scavenging abilities, as well as the Fe-reducing power (Figure 1).

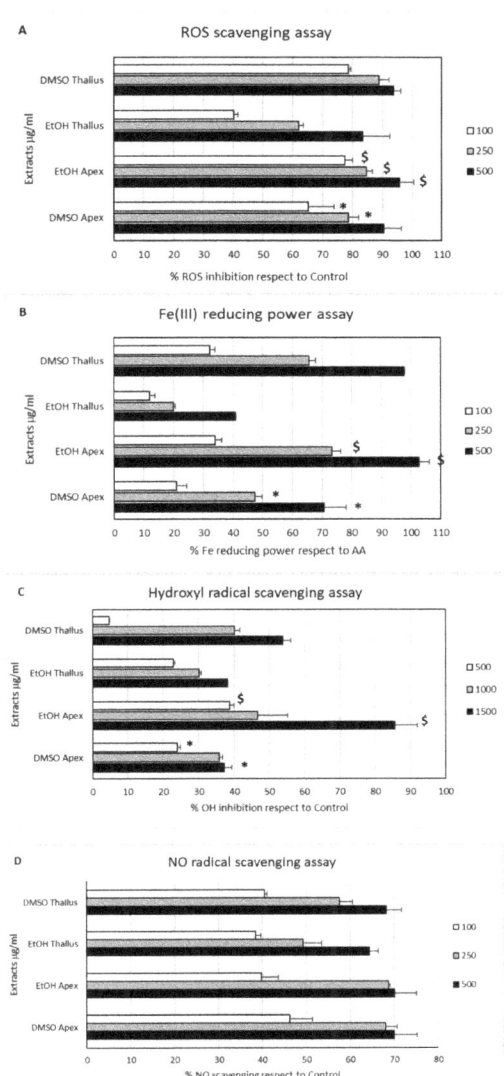

Figure 1. Antioxidant activity of *E. amentacea* extracts in spectrophotometric tests. (**A**) ROS scavenging activity by the DPPH assay. Data are expressed as a percentage of scavenging of the DPPH radical with respect to the absorbance of the DPPH radical alone (control). Symbols indicate significance in paired Tukey test (ANOVA $p < 0.0001$; Tukey of DMSO apex vs. DMSO thallus' respective concentration, * $p < 0.05$; Tukey of EtOH apex vs. EtOH thallus' respective concentration, $ $p < 0.05$)

(**B**) Fe (III)-reducing power assay, measured by the potassium ferricyanide method. Data are expressed as a percentage of reducing power compared to the Fe reduction of ascorbic acid (AA, concentration 30 µg/mL) positive control. Symbols indicate significance in paired Tukey test (ANOVA $p < 0.000001$; Tukey of DMSO apex vs. DMSO thallus' respective concentration, * $p < 0.05$; Tukey of EtOH apex vs. EtOH thallus' respective concentration, $ $p < 0.005$). (**C**) OH radical scavenging activity by Mohr's salt assay. Data are expressed as a percentage of inhibition of OH radical production with respect to the absorbance of the OH radical-producing solution alone (Control). Symbols indicate significance in paired Tukey (ANOVA $p < 0.0001$; Tukey of DMSO apex vs. DMSO thallus' respective concentration, * $p < 0.05$; Tukey of EtOH apex vs. EtOH thallus' respective concentration, $ $p < 0.05$). (**D**) NO radical scavenging activity was measured by the sodium nitroprusside method coupled with the Griess assay. Data are expressed as a percentage of inhibition of NO production with respect to the absorbance of the NO radical-producing solution alone (Control).

The DPPH scavenging assay, quantifying the whole ROS scavenging activity (Panel A), provided remarkable dose-dependent antioxidant properties. Based on the inhibition values obtained in the range of the tested concentrations, we extrapolated the DPPH EC75 values of each extract. In particular, we measured EC75 activities of 233.7 and 45.4 µg/mL for the DMSO apices and thalli extracts and 41.9 and 404.1 µg/mL for the EtOH apices and thalli extracts, respectively. These data indicate the retrieval of significant amounts of antioxidant molecular species from both the apices and thalli of the seaweed with both solvents but with some differences, with the highest concentrations obtained by EtOH solvent extraction in the apices and, conversely, by the DMSO solvent extraction in the thalli. This result probably reflects what was already observed for the TPC and TFC of the same extracts. The Fe-reducing power assay (Panel B) revealed a similar dose-dependent behavior of the extracts. The extrapolated EC75 activities for the extracts were 512.5 and 343.1 µg/mL for the DMSO apices and thalli extracts and 311.6 and 970.2 µg/mL for the EtOH apices and thalli extracts, respectively. In a similar way to the DPPH, in the Fe-reducing power assay, the highest activity was found in the EtOH apices extract, followed by the DMSO thalli extract. These results confirm the high antioxidant potential of the four *E. amentacea* extracts that were to be expected from the TPC and TFC analyses of the same extracts reported in Table 1. These are in line with the results from the Mediterranean *C. compressa* extracts [32] and are significantly higher than those obtained from the Atlantic *C. abies-marina* extracts [31]. The lower TPC yields and antioxidant activities of the latter could also be due to the different location of the seaweed, the Atlantic Ocean, with respect to the other *Cystoseira* spp. studies from different locations in the Mediterranean Sea, i.e., the Ligurian Sea in our case and the Adriatic Sea in the Cagalj et al. study [32].

The two final assays were performed to quantify the ability of the extracts to specifically scavenge the biologically relevant hydroxyl (OH) and nitric oxide (NO) radicals. These highly reactive molecules are produced in large quantities in states of cellular oxidative stress and during immune responses as second messengers and defense mechanisms; however, they can seriously damage cell integrity and survival in severe situations [12]. The highest OH radical scavenging activity (Panel C) was again measured for the EtOH apices extract. For this extract, we extrapolated an EC50 of 869.2 µg/mL, followed by the values of the other extracts, which were all above the 1 mg/mL EC50 threshold, with the DMSO thalli extract being 1326.5 µg/mL and, lastly, the DMSO apices and the EtOH thalli having an EC50 of 2097 and 2291.6 µg/mL, respectively. Finally, the potential to scavenge the highly reactive NO radical provided very close EC50-calculated values for all four extracts (Panel D), with the DMSO apices and thalli extracts measuring 163.9 and 207.9 µg/mL, while the EtOH apices and thalli retrieved the values of 234.2 and 272.8 µg/mL, respectively. Overall, these results indicate that the apices of the seaweed in summer possess higher quantities of ROS scavenging molecules and that, in the apices of the fronds growing in summer, i.e., the younger and reproductive parts of the seaweed, *E. amentacea* preferably produces higher quantities of water-soluble antioxidant molecules as compared to the arsenal of molecules with a similar activity present in the already grown thalli. Conversely, both solvent treatments, independently of the section of seaweed extracted (apices or thalli), were able to extract molecules with similar EC50 NO scavenging activities. This is an indication of the production of NO counteracting molecular species with good solubility in both hydroalcoholic and organic solvents, with no significant production increase in the growing apices during the summer season. The various scavenging activities by the extracts shown here also confirm the wide diversity of molecules and secondary metabolites with bioactive properties produced by this brown seaweed, which are already partly reported in the literature [4].

2.3. Cell Proliferation and Rescue from Stressful Stimuli

Before assessing the pharmacological and/or cosmetic properties of the four *E. amentacea* extracts in humans, their biocompatibility was analyzed by measuring the cell viability on two skin-derived cell lines, L929 fibroblasts and HaCaT keratinocytes. The results projected a good perspective on their biocompatibility, given that neither of the four extracts showed significant cytotoxicity on both cell lines (Figure 2).

Conversely, significant cell growth-promoting activity (up to 1.4-folds increase) was revealed upon treatment of the fibroblasts with both the EtOH and DMSO extracts, with no relevant differences between the apices and thalli, especially at the highest concentration tested (Panels A and B, respectively). In the case of human keratinocyte treatment with the extracts, neither significant cytotoxicity nor a remarkable cell growth-promoting effect was observed, except for a slight cell decrease in the highest apices' EtOH extract concentration and a slight increase in the lowest thalli DMSO concentration (Panels C and D, respectively). These results suggest a safe use of the *E. amentacea* extracts in cosmetic formulations for skincare products, also highlighting a potential dermal thickening effect due to the fibroblast cell growth-promoting effect observed in these experiments. Indeed, with aging, the turnover of epidermal cells decreases, and this explains why the wound healing time increases and desquamation becomes less effective. The dermis also becomes atrophic with a reduced number of fibroblasts [13]. Thus, a product promoting fibroblast proliferation is a really coveted property in cosmetic formulations since the appearance of wrinkles is primarily due to the insufficient proliferation and ECM deposition of these cells in the dermal layer. These results are surprisingly different from others reported in the literature on the cytotoxic and antitumor activity of different *Cystoseira* spp. extracts, i.e., those of *C. tamariscifolia* [36] and *C. barbata* [37], to cite a few. Although, in many cases, the extracts were obtained in more aggressive conditions (heating) by use of strong organic solvents, such as hexane and diethyl ether for *C. tamariscifolia* and acetone for *C. barbata*, respectively. Thus, even if we cannot exclude the presence of cytotoxic/antitumor secondary metabolites in *E. amentacea* seaweed, we can confirm that the molecular species retrieved by the extraction procedures used in this paper, i.e., DMSO and hydroalcoholic, can be considered safe for human use.

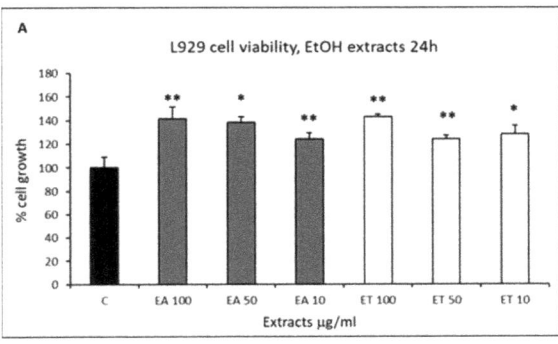

Figure 2. *Cont.*

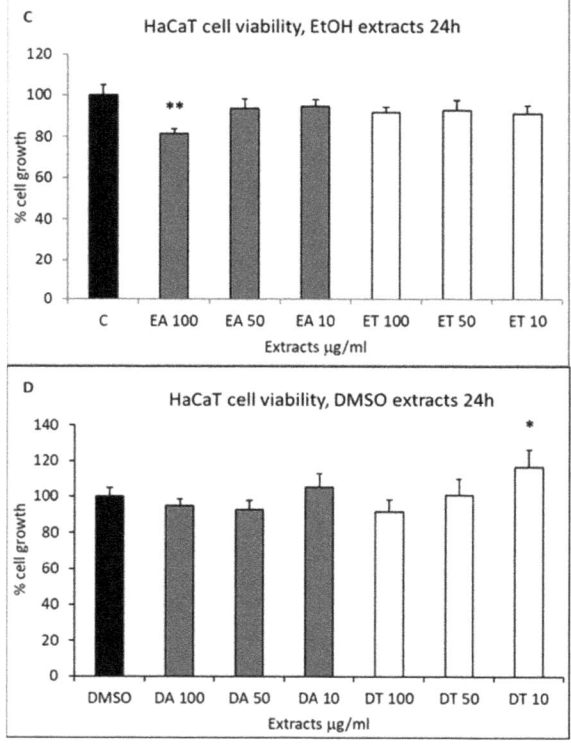

Figure 2. Cell viability evaluation. (**A,B**) L929 fibroblast cell growth evaluation by MTT test at 24 h in the presence of increasing concentrations of *E. amentacea* 50%-ethanol (**A**) and DMSO (**B**) extracts—gray bars, apices extracts; white bars, thallus extracts, respectively. Results are expressed as cell percentages with respect to the control. Asterisks indicate significance in paired Tukey test (ANOVA, $p < 0.00005$; Tukey of respective bar vs. C: * $p < 0.01$ and ** $p < 0.005$). (**C,D**) HaCaT keratinocyte cell growth evaluation by MTT test at 24 h in the presence of increasing concentrations of *E. amentacea* 50%-ethanol (**A**) and DMSO (**B**) extracts (ANOVA, $p < 0.000001$; Tukey of respective bar vs. C: * $p < 0.05$ and ** $p < 0.005$).

The extract's beneficial properties on skin cell survival in stressful conditions were also tested. Fibroblasts and keratinocytes were challenged with UV-B to mimic the sun's dangerous radiation effects and with hydrogen peroxide to mimic cell damage by oxidative stress (Figures 3 and 4, respectively).

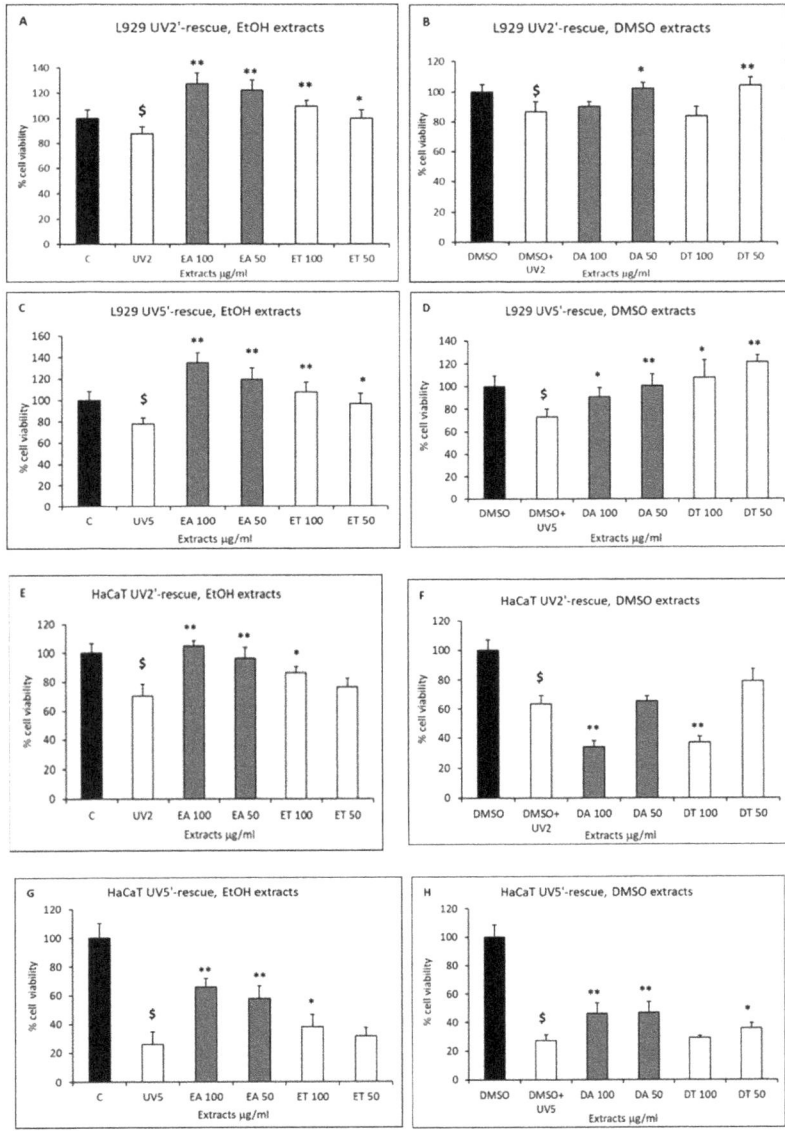

Figure 3. Cell death rescue evaluation after UV challenge. (**A–D**) Cell death rescue from 2 min UV (**A,B**) and 5 min UV (**C,D**) challenge of L929 fibroblasts in the presence of 50%-ethanol and DMSO extracts, evaluated by MTT test 24 h after the stimulus. Gray bars, apices extracts; white bars, thallus extracts, respectively. Results are expressed as a cell percentage with respect to control, untreated cells. Symbols indicate significance in paired Tukey test (ANOVA, $p < 0.0005$ in all panels; Tukey of UV2 or UV5 vs. C $ $p < 0.005$; Tukey of respective bar vs. UV2: * $p < 0.05$ and ** $p < 0.001$; Tukey of respective bar vs. UV5: * $p < 0.05$ and ** $p < 0.0005$). (**E–H**) Cell death rescue from 2 min UV (**E,F**) and 5 min UV (**G,H**) challenge of HaCaT keratinocytes in the presence of 50%-ethanol and DMSO extracts, evaluated by MTT test 24 h after the stimulus (ANOVA, $p < 0.000001$ in all panels; Tukey of UV2 or UV5 vs. C $ $p < 0.0001$; Tukey of respective bar vs. UV2: * $p < 0.01$ and ** $p < 0.0005$; Tukey of respective bar vs. UV5: * $p < 0.05$ and ** $p < 0.005$).

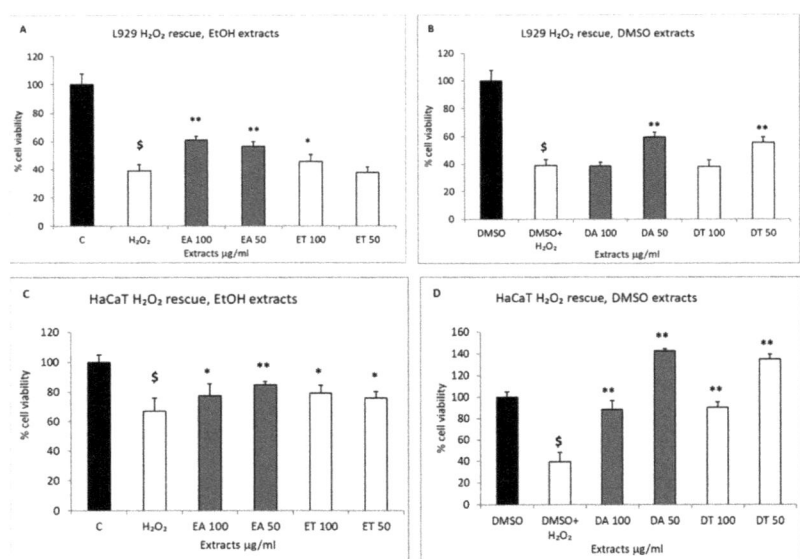

Figure 4. Cell death rescue evaluation after H_2O_2-challenge. (**A,B**) Cell death rescue from 200 μM H_2O_2-challenge of L929 fibroblasts in the presence of 50%-ethanol and DMSO extracts, evaluated by MTT test 24 h after the stimulus. Gray bars, apices extracts; white bars, thallus extracts, respectively. Results are expressed as cell percentages with respect to control, untreated cells. Symbols indicate significance in paired Tukey test (ANOVA, $p < 0.000001$; Tukey of H_2O_2 vs. C, \$ $p < 0.0001$; Tukey of respective bar vs. H_2O_2: * $p < 0.05$ and ** $p < 0.001$). (**C,D**) Cell death rescue from 500 μM H_2O_2-challenge of HaCaT keratinocytes in the presence of 50%-ethanol and DMSO extracts, evaluated by MTT test 24 h after the stimulus (ANOVA, $p < 0.0005$; Tukey of H_2O_2 vs. C, \$ $p < 0.0005$; Tukey of respective bar vs. H_2O_2: * $p < 0.05$ and ** $p < 0.0005$).

The results show that in both cases, the extracts were able to rescue, partially or totally, the detrimental effects of the two stressful stimuli. In detail, UV-B radiation for 2 or 5 min induced, respectively, 13% or 26% cell death in the L929 fibroblasts compared to the control cells (Figure 3A,B and C,D, respectively).

The apices and thalli EtOH extracts were able to nullify the induced cell death, both in the UV 2′-exposure (Panel A) and the 5′-exposure (Panel C) at both concentrations tested (50 and 100 μg/mL). In addition, the apices extract (gray bars) showed cell growth values significantly exceeding those of the control—the untreated cells—in a dose-dependent way. Conversely, the apices and thalli DMSO extracts were more effective at the lowest concentration tested, which, also in this case, counteracted the UV-induced cell death both after the 2′ and 5′ radiation (Panels B and D, respectively). No significant differences were observed between the apices and thalli DMSO extract rescuing effects. UV-B radiation in the HaCaT keratinocytes led to higher cell death percentages as compared to the fibroblasts and amounted to 30% and 75% for the 2′ and 5′ exposures, respectively (Figure 3E,F and G,H). In the case of the EtOH extracts, only the apices (gray bars) were able to effectively counteract the UV-induced toxicity by completely restoring the cell viability in the 2′ UV exposure (Panel E) and partially in the 5′ UV exposure (+40% cell rescue, Panel G). The DMSO extracts exerted a different effect on the UV-exposed keratinocytes; none of them were able to rescue the 2′ UV-induced cell death (Panel F), and only the apices extract (gray bars) was able to partially counteract the 5′ UV-induced cell death (+20% cell rescue, Panel H).

As far as the hydrogen peroxide-induced cell death (60%) in the L929 fibroblasts (Figure 4A,B) was concerned, the cell damage was partially rescued by the EtOH apices extract in a dose-dependent way (Panel A, gray bars), and by both the apices and thalli DMSO extracts at the lowest concentration tested (Panel B, gray and white bars, respectively).

Conversely, HaCaT keratinocyte cell death, induced by hydrogen peroxide, was partially rescued by both apices and thalli EtOH extracts (Panel C) and completely by both apices and thalli DMSO extracts (Panel D) at both concentrations tested. These results indicate a prevalent rescuing effect of the apices extracts compared to the thalli, although also in the latter, a significant retrieval of molecules with a beneficial effect is clearly obtained by the two extracting solvents, as indicated by the higher survival rates when compared to the UV- and H_2O_2-treated positive controls. These results demonstrate that the growth-promoting effects of the extracts also expand to stressful conditions of the skin, such as in the case of UV exposure and oxidative stress, enhancing the chances of survival of the damaged epidermal and dermal cells and thus slowing down the skin aging process. The percentages of cell survival upon UV radiation and after *E. amentacea* extract administration demonstrate significant and possibly preventive effects, even higher than those observed on the same cellular model (fibroblast cells) with the use of purified phlorotannins from other brown algae administered at µmolar concentrations (from 10 to 250 µM), as reported by Heo et al. [38]. In our case, the single bioactive molecules that are present in the extracts likely have significantly lower concentrations than those used by Heo et al. since, in the cellular setting, they are always used at a 100 µg/mL final concentration. Thus, our results probably show an additive and/or synergic effect of the heterogenous antioxidant and vitaminic compounds exerting such a dramatic effect. This points out the possibility that the polyphenol and meroditerpenes concoctions, as those present in our extracts (see Section 2.7 and De La Fuente et al. [23]), at lower concentrations, perform better than the single-molecule concentrated solutions in counteracting UV damage in skin cells, probably acting at different cellular levels instead of targeting single chemical pathways. However, we must remark that our experimental conditions only demonstrate a preventive action of the extracts on the UV stressful stimulus at the cellular level. In fact, since the extracts were administered to cells before UV exposure, thus mimicking the application of sunscreen, the rescue results likely reflect the sum of both the extracellular UV direct screening effect and the increase in survival due to an intracellular rescuing activity. Further experiments will help us to elucidate the contribution of each effect to the increased cell survival, for example, by the administration of the extracts after UV exposure, which would enable us to discriminate only the intracellular effect on cell survival.

2.4. Intracellular Antioxidant Activity

It is well known that most of the cell-damaging effects of UV radiation and acute inflammation are due to the production of high amounts of ROS [12], with the consequent oxidation and deterioration of fundamental cellular components (proteins, nucleic acids, lipids). Therefore, we evaluated the four extracts' ability to scavenge UV- and H_2O_2-derived ROS production (Figure 5), which would explain the cell death-reversing effect of the extracts described in the previous paragraph.

Indeed, the UV-B-stimulated fibroblasts and keratinocytes (Panels A–B and C–D, respectively) produced remarkable amounts of ROS after a 3 min exposure, as compared to the control cells (from a 15- to 21-fold increase in fibroblasts, Panels A–B, and from a 6- to 7-fold increase in keratinocytes, Panels C–D, respectively). In fibroblasts, the apices EtOH extracts showed a higher percentage of ROS inhibition with respect to the thalli (Panel A, 31% vs. 22% scavenging effect, respectively), while a similar rate of inhibition was observed for the two DMSO extracts (Panel B, ~30%). In the HaCaT keratinocytes, the EtOH extracts from the apices showed the highest rate of ROS inhibition (Panel C, gray bars, 64%) compared to the EtOH extracts from the thalli (Panel C, white bars, 38%) and to both the apices and thalli DMSO extracts (Panel D, 30–32% ROS lowering). Considering the extremely high levels of ROS produced by UV radiation in both cell types, the intracellular scavenging results obtained by the *E. amentacea* extracts, especially the EtOH apices, are indeed significant. These experiments clearly demonstrate the extreme degree of damage that UV radiation can cause by ROS production at the cellular level and the possibility of rapidly assessing the photoprotective activity of compounds in a simple in vitro setting on skin cells, as described here.

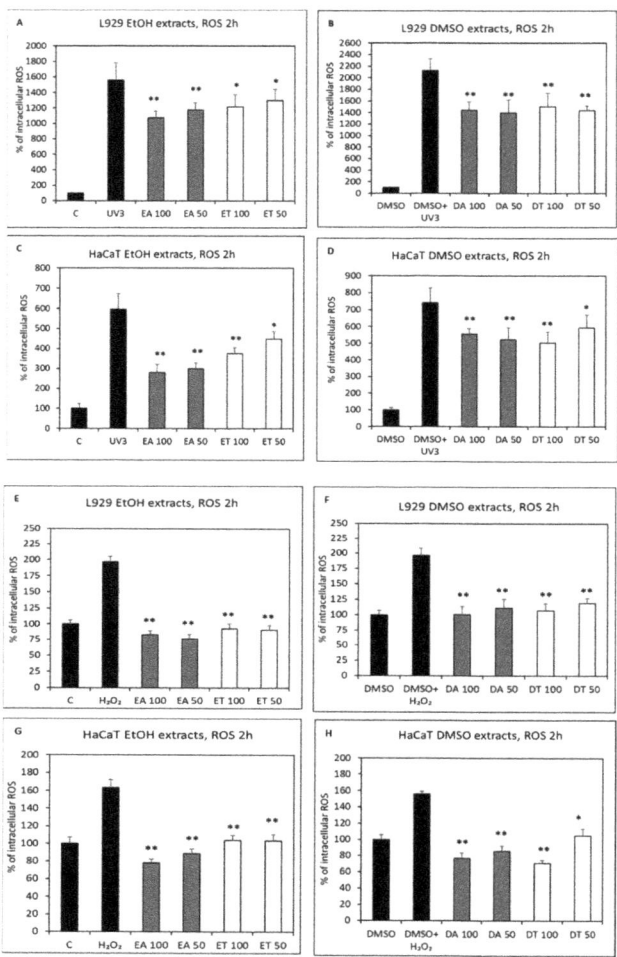

Figure 5. ROS scavenging activity in cellular assays. (**A,B**) Intracellular ROS production, measured by DCF fluorometric analysis in L929 fibroblasts incubated for 2 h in the presence or absence of 50 and 100 µg/mL of 50%-ethanol (**A**) or DMSO (**B**) extracts, respectively, after a 3 min UV challenge. Gray bars, apices extracts; white bars, thallus extracts, respectively. Results are expressed as a percentage of ROS production with respect to control, untreated cells. Asterisks indicate significance in the Tukey test (ANOVA $p < 0.000001$; Tukey of respective bar vs. UV3, * $p < 0.05$ and ** $p < 0.005$). (**C,D**) Intracellular ROS production in HaCaT keratinocytes incubated with 50 and 100 µg/mL of 50%-ethanol (**C**) or DMSO (**D**) extracts after a 3 min UV challenge (ANOVA $p < 0.000001$; Tukey of respective bar vs. UV3, * $p < 0.05$ and ** $p < 0.005$). (**E,F**) Intracellular ROS production in L929 fibroblasts incubated for 2 h with 200 µM H_2O_2 in the presence or absence of 50 and 100 µg/mL of 50%-ethanol (**E**) or DMSO (**F**) extracts (ANOVA $p < 0.000001$; Tukey of respective bar vs. H_2O_2, ** $p < 0.0001$). (**G,H**) Intracellular ROS production in HaCaT keratinocytes incubated for 2 h with 200 µM H_2O_2 with 50 and 100 µg/mL of 50%-ethanol (**G**) or DMSO (**H**) extracts (ANOVA $p < 0.00001$; Tukey of respective bar vs. H_2O_2, * $p < 0.001$ and ** $p < 0.0001$).

The H$_2$O$_2$-challenged cells showed a lower intracellular ROS stimulation compared to the UV-B exposure (with a 2-fold increase in fibroblasts, Panels E–F, and a 1.6-fold increase in keratinocytes, Panels G–H, respectively). In both cell types, all four extracts were able to inhibit the ROS production completely; in particular, in the case of the EtOH extract from the apices, the values were even below those of the control cells in both fibroblasts and keratinocytes (Panels E and G, gray bars). Furthermore, in the HaCaT cells, the two DMSO extracts were also able to reduce the H$_2$O$_2$-induced ROS production below the values of the control cells (Panel H). These data clearly indicate the potent antioxidant and photoprotective activity of the four *E. amentacea* extracts on skin cells, with the hydroalcoholic apices extract again showing the highest pharmacological effect. Moreover, in this case, as already observed in the cell death rescue experiments, the beneficial, antioxidant effect of the extracts is higher than that observed using single purified molecules, as in the case of phlorotannins [38] in a very similar cellular setting, indicating an additive/synergistic effect of the compounds contained in the *E. amentacea* extracts (see Section 2.7). The strong antioxidant activity of the extracts is likely the main mechanism that allows cell survival and growth in the fibroblast and keratinocyte cells after UV and hydrogen peroxide noxious stimuli administration.

2.5. Skin Hydrolytic Enzyme Inhibition

Skin aging is characterized by the loss of dermal thickness and hydration, wrinkle formation and dyspigmentation with the appearance of unsightly sunspots due to uneven melanin production by melanocytes [13]. These features are mainly due to photo-induced oxidative stress [14], reduced fibroblast proliferation and an imbalance between the synthesis and degradation of important ECM components, such as collagen and hyaluronic acid. Both the number and diameter of collagen fibers are reduced, and the ratio between type III and type I collagen is increased [13]. The approaches to restore dermal thickness span from a daily intake of marine collagen hydrolysate nutraceuticals [39] to hyaluronic acid subcutaneous injections [40] and/or the application of collagen- and/or hyaluronic acid-based cosmetic creams [41,42] and skincare products containing oxidative stress-counteracting vitamins, such as vitamin A-derived retinol, vitamin E and C [43]. The latter has an important double role in skin homeostasis since it is also directly involved in the synthesis and deposition of collagen [44]. An alternative approach to improve dermal thickness is based on the use of the enzymatic inhibitors of collagenases and hyaluronidases to increase the ECM components' stability [45]. Thus, the four *E. amentacea* extracts were tested for possible anti-collagenase and anti-hyaluronidase activities in spectrophotometric enzymatic tests. The results shown in Figure 6 highlight the presence of molecules with such activities in almost all extracts, although with differences in their efficacy.

A 45–50% inhibition of collagenase activity (Panel A) was obtained in the presence of the two apices extracts, while a slightly higher effect was observed with the two thalli extracts (65% inhibition). No significant differences were observable between the two extraction solvents (EtOH and DMSO), indicating a collagenase inhibitory activity with promiscuous solubility that is more concentrated in the older part of the seaweed fronds. These results show higher anti-collagenase properties for the *E. amentacea* extracts compared to other seaweeds of the same family, as, for instance, *Cystoseira abies-marina*, whose extracts were obtained by ultrasound or microwave-assisted technologies and never exceeded a 50% enzymatic inhibitory effect [31].

The highest inhibition of enzymatic activity was obtained against the hyaluronidase (Panel B), reaching values close to 80% by the two DMSO extracts and was slightly lower in the presence of the two EtOH extracts, again indicating the presence of inhibitory molecules with promiscuous solubility and no substantial differences between the concentration of the activity in the apices as compared to the thalli. These results show a high hyaluronidase inhibitory potential of the *E. amentacea* extracts, probably due to an additive effect of the various molecular species present in the seaweed. It is known that phlorotannins can exert this effect [46], as demonstrated by the purified molecules from four different algae belonging to the same order of *E. amentacea*, i.e., Fucales; however, their effective concentration is in the order of more than 1 mg/mL of purified molecules. Since, in our case, the highest inhibitory effect was obtained with 50 µg/mL of extracts, we can conclude that probably other types of polyphenols are contributing to the anti-hyaluronidase effect of *E. amentacea*. In addition, the inhibition of collagenase, also known as MMP1, and hyaluronidase can be considered an important antitumor activity since these enzymes are usually overexpressed in spreading cancers, favoring tumor cell proliferation and migration by degrading connective tissue ECM components [46–48].

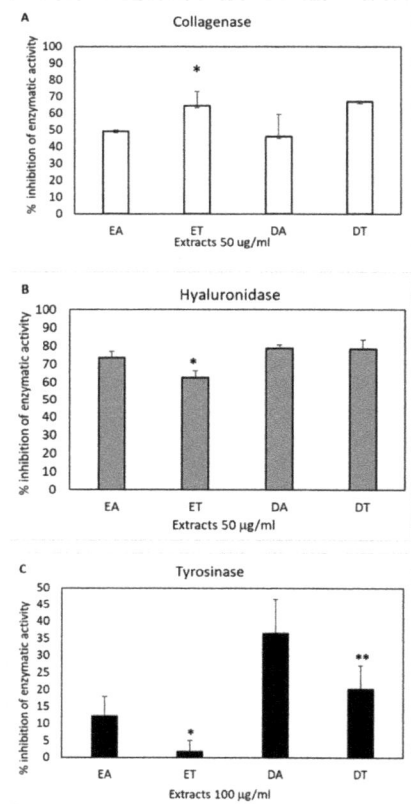

Figure 6. Counteraction of skin hydrolytic enzyme activity. (**A**) Inhibition of collagenase (from *C. histolyticum*) by enzymatic kinetic assay, measured as a reduced degradation of FALGPA, a synthetic peptide that mimics the collagen structure, in the presence of 50 µg/mL of algal extracts as compared to the activity of the control enzyme (in the presence of the respective vehicle solvents). EA and ET, apices and thallus 50%-ethanol extracts; DA and DT, apices and thallus DMSO extracts, respectively. Asterisks indicate significance in paired Tukey test (ANOVA $p < 0.0005$, Tukey of ET vs. EA, * $p < 0.05$). (**B**) Inhibition of hyaluronidase (from bovine testes) by enzyme kinetic assay measured as a reduced degradation of hyaluronic acid in the presence of 50 µg/mL algal extracts as compared to the control enzyme activity (in the presence of the respective vehicle solvents). Asterisks indicate significance in paired Tukey test (ANOVA $p < 0.0005$, Tukey of ET vs. EA, * $p < 0.05$). (**C**) Inhibition of mushroom tyrosinase by the relative enzyme kinetic assay, measured as a reduced conversion of L-Dopa to Dopachrome in the presence of 100 µg/mL of algal extracts as compared to the activity of the control enzyme (in the presence of the respective vehicle solvents). Asterisks indicate significance in paired Tukey test (ANOVA $p < 0.0005$, Tukey of ET vs. EA, * $p < 0.05$; Tukey of DT vs. DA, ** $p < 0.01$).

The anti-tyrosinase activity was also tested, given that this enzyme was responsible for the uneven production of melanin from the tyrosine precursor in sunspots. Not all UV rays can affect our skin; UV-C, in fact, is filtered by the ozone layer. UV-A and UV-B, on the other hand, are not completely filtered and, therefore, can cause phenomena such as tanning, wrinkles and hyperpigmentation once absorbed by the layers of the skin. Hyperpigmentation is usually a harmless form of skin pigmentation in which the skin patches become darker than the surrounding normal skin due to the overproduction and accumulation of melanin. Melanogenesis is controlled by the enzyme tyrosinase, a glycoprotein located in the membrane of melanocytes that catalyzes the conversion of L-tyrosine into melanin [49]. A different efficacy was observed in the four extracts in terms of their ability to inhibit the tyrosinase enzyme (Panel C). In particular, at 100 µg/mL, the DMSO extract of the apices showed the highest percentage of inhibition (36%), followed by the thalli DMSO extract (20% inhibition). As far as the EtOH extracts are concerned, while the apices still showed a slight inhibitory activity (12%), the thalli were practically ineffective. Therefore, this enzymatic inhibitory activity seems to be more concentrated in the apices of the seaweed and more compatible with organic solvents. It has been reported that polyphenols belonging to the phlorotannin group show very high anti-tyrosinase activity [6]. As compared with the literature, *E. amentacea* does not seem to possess better properties in this specific activity, compared to other brown algae extracts, i.e., *C. abies-marina* and *E. stolonifera*, showing more significant whitening performances [31,50].

2.6. Skin Anti-Inflammatory Effect

In the skin, direct sun exposure leads to photo-aging over time and to an inflammatory response called erythema or sunburn immediately after irradiation [12]. Pharmacological topical creams or cosmetic lenitive skincare products are thought to quench or reduce the symptoms of this very common condition. Here, we tested the ability of the extracts to significantly reduce the gene expression of the relevant inflammatory cytokines produced by UV-exposed keratinocytes and fibroblasts, demonstrating their efficiency in counteracting the inflammatory process from the beginning. Indeed, the pro-inflammatory cytokines IL1-β, IL-6 and IL-8, which their expression is known to be significantly induced in the skin by UV irradiation [51], were inhibited in keratinocytes, as revealed by the analysis of their expression profile 6 h after exposure (Figure 7).

The four extracts showed different efficacies in inhibiting the three UV-induced cytokines in human keratinocytes. IL1-β was significantly inhibited by all four extracts (Panel A), with the apices EtOH extract showing a slightly higher efficiency (82% inhibition) compared to the others (58–77% inhibition). IL-6 showed a remarkable, comparable inhibition after treatment with both the EtOH and DMSO apices extracts (Panel B, 73% and 77% inhibition, respectively) and a partial but significant inhibition by the thalli DMSO extract. Finally, IL-8's enhanced gene expression was efficiently inhibited by the apices EtOH extract (78% inhibition) and only partially by the thalli EtOH extract (Panel C). In fibroblasts, the gene expression analysis was performed in the same conditions after UV irradiation on the IL1-β, IL-6 and CXCL5 cytokines (Figure 8).

The latter was chosen because it is well known that the mouse genome does not contain an IL-8 homologue; therefore, we analyzed the CXCL5 cytokine, which is recognized as the functional homologue of human IL-8 [52], being L929 fibroblasts of murine origin. In this case, the IL1-β UV-induced rise was completely inhibited by the apices EtOH extract and by both DMSO extracts (Panel A), while the IL-6 rise was inhibited by all extracts (Panel B) and CXCL5 was only partially inhibited by all four extracts (Panel C) with a slightly higher efficiency by the two DMSO extracts (35% inhibition). The anti-inflammatory mechanism of action on the two cell types likely depends on the strong ROS-inhibitory effect exerted by the *E. amentacea* extracts. In fact, it is well known that ROSs are one of the main triggers of pro-inflammatory NF-κB transcription factor activation, which in turn, in skin cells, stimulates IL-1β, IL-6, IL-8, TNF-α and MMP1 production, among others [12]. The contribution of meroditerpene molecular species should also be considered since this class of molecules has demonstrated anti-inflammatory properties [53] and because our analyses confirmed a higher content of these compounds in the apices hydroalcoholic extracts (see Section 2.7). Thus, considering the inhibitory effects in the two cell lines of all the three cytokines analyzed, these data indicate that the EtOH extract from the apices displays the highest skin anti-inflammatory properties, confirming our hypothesis that the apical seaweed portion collected during the summer season contains remarkable bioactive molecules that counteract several oxidative and inflammatory symptoms caused by UV radiation and enhance the lenitive effect of those already present in the lower body part (thallus) of the *E. amentacea* seaweed.

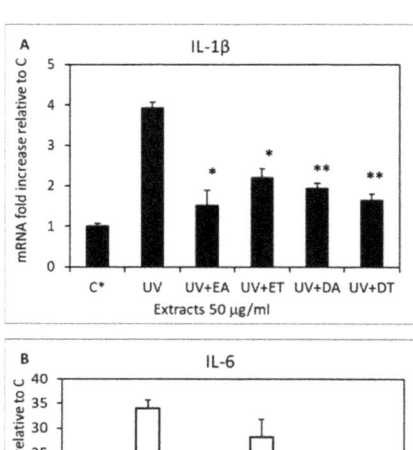
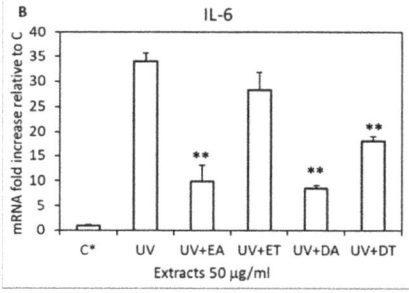
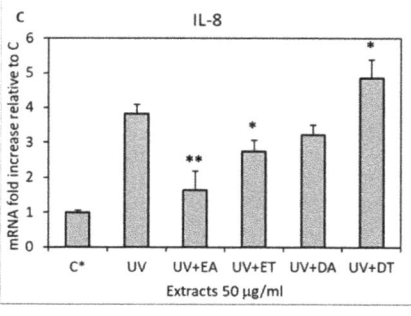

Figure 7. Inhibition of gene expression in UV-challenged HaCaT human keratinocytes. Gene expression was measured by qPCR analyses of IL-1β (**A**), IL-6 (**B**), and IL-8 (**C**) at 6 h, after a 3 min UV challenge and in the presence of 50 μg/mL algal extracts. EA and ET, apices and thallus 50%-ethanol extracts; DA and DT, apices and thallus DMSO extracts, respectively. Data are normalized on the HPRT-1 housekeeping gene and expressed as mRNA-fold increase compared to control cells. Asterisks indicate significance in Tukey test (IL-1β ANOVA $p < 0.000001$, Tukey of respective bar vs. UV, * $p < 0.0005$ and ** $p < 0.0001$, respectively; IL-6 ANOVA $p < 0.000001$, Tukey of respective bar vs. UV, ** $p < 0.0005$; IL-8 ANOVA $p < 0.000001$, Tukey of respective bar vs. UV, * $p < 0.05$ and ** $p < 0.005$).

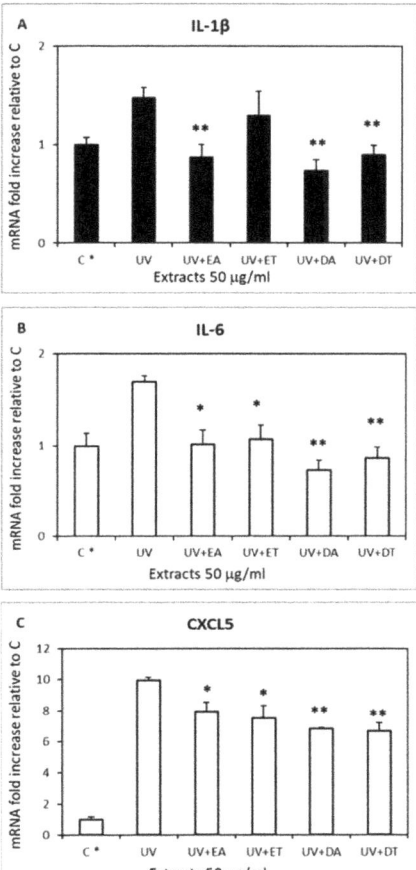

Figure 8. Inhibition of gene expression in UV-challenged L929 murine fibroblasts. Gene expression was measured by qPCR analyses of IL-1β (**A**), IL-6 (**B**), and CXCL5 (**C**) at 6 h, after a 3 min UV challenge and in the presence of 50 μg/mL algal extracts. EA and ET, apices and thallus ethanol extracts; DA and DT, apices and thallus DMSO extracts, respectively. Data are normalized on the GAPDH housekeeping gene and expressed as mRNA-fold increase compared to control, untreated cells. Asterisks indicate significance in the Tukey test (IL-1β ANOVA $p < 0.0005$, Tukey of respective bar vs. UV, ** $p < 0.005$; IL-6 ANOVA $p < 0.00005$, Tukey of respective bar vs. UV, * $p < 0.005$ and ** $p < 0.0005$; CXCL5 ANOVA $p < 0.000001$, Tukey of respective bar vs. UV, * $p < 0.05$ and ** $p < 0.001$).

2.7. Chemical Characterization of E. amentacea Apices and Thalli Extracts

As reported in the present work (see the Result paragraphs above), significant functional differences in the biological effects of the extracts were observed, mainly between the apices and thalli hydroalcoholic extracts (EtOH), with the correspondent DMSO extracts showing essentially comparable effects between them. The molecular characterization of the whole thallus of the *E. amentacea* EtOH and DMSO extracts was already obtained in our previous work [23]. Thus, we decided to perform more accurate HPLC-MS/MS analyses on the two apices and thalli EtOH extracts with the aim of identifying the main molecular components responsible for the different biological effects between the extracts of the two algal parts. The analysis is shown in Figure 9, highlighting the molecular species identified in the EtOH apices (Panel A) and in the EtOH thalli (Panel B), respectively.

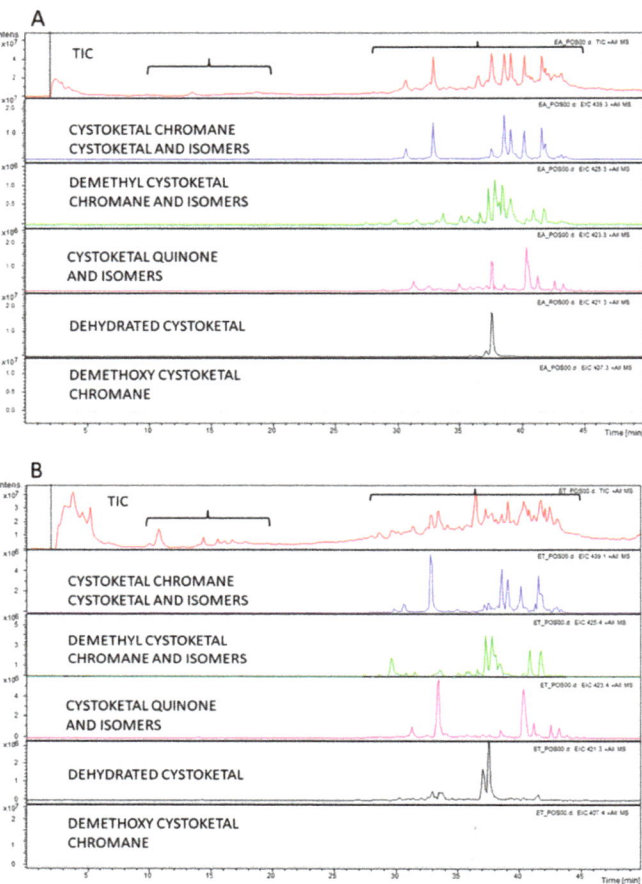

Figure 9. HPLC/MS analyses of the EtOH extracts. Total ion current (TIC) and extracted ion chromatograms (EIC) obtained by full-scan MS/MS analysis coupled to HPLC separation of an aliquot of the *E. amentacea* apices hydroalcoholic (**A**) and thalli (**B**) extracts at a starting dilution of 2.5 mg/mL (injection volume, 8 µL), acquiring the most abundant species under each peak. The red chromatogram in both panels represents the TIC of each extract, while the following blue, green, pink, black and gray chromatograms in both panels represent the EICs of the molecules indicated in the respective panels. The acquisition was performed on negative and positive ions in the 100–1000 mass range and analyzed using integrated software.

In detail, the two MS chromatograms in red (the total ion chromatogram in the first inserts in both Panels A and B) show a group of peaks in the timeframe between a 10- and 20-minute retention time, which the MS analysis ascribed to the polyphenol family, and a second, more significant group of peaks, starting from the 28-minute retention time, belongs to the meroditerpene family. The heights of the peaks in the two chromatograms show that the meroditerpenes species are more abundant in the apices (Panel A) as compared to the thalli (Panel B). Thus, we focused on their characterization to ascribe the functional differences between the extracts from the two body parts of the seaweed. We observed that the two seaweed body parts contained the same meroditerpenes compounds. In fact, both panels reporting the extracted ion chromatograms (EIC) of the same identified molecules show the following species: cystoketal, cystoketal chromane and their related isomers (blue EIC in both panels, *m/z* 439.3), dimethyl cystoketal chromane and their related isomers (green EIC in both panels, m/z 425.3), cystoketal quinone and their related isomers (pink EIC in both panels, m/z 423.3), dehydrated cystoketal (black EIC in both panels, m/z 421.3) and dimethoxy cystoketal chromane (gray EIC in both panels, m/z 407.3). Indeed, the presence of meroditerpene-like structures has already been described in the same genus, and some of their biological effects have also been investigated [4,5,36,53–58]. Furthermore, the main molecular structures—although without the characterization of the isomers—were also identified in our previous work, both for the EtOH and DMSO extracts of the total fronds of the seaweed [23]. The main chemical structures of the molecules are shown in Table 2, which also reports the literature on the up-to-date investigated pharmacological properties of the listed species.

Table 2. Chemical structure of the identified compounds. The main meroditerpenes molecules identified in *E. amentacea* apices and thalli hydroalcoholic extracts and references related to reported biological activities.

Molecular Structure	Name	References
	Cystoketal	[56,57]
	Cystoketal Chromane	
	Cystoketal quinone	[58]
	Demethyl cystoketal chromane	
	Demethoxy cystoketal chromane	[4,36]
	Dehydrated cystoketal	

In our analysis, we can also show that there is a quantitative difference in the abundance of the abovementioned molecules between the apices and thalli, i.e., the younger/reproductive and the slightly older/structural parts of the seaweed fronds, respectively. Table 3 reports a relative quantitative comparison between the abundance of the meroditerpenes species in the two extracts retrievable from the EIC of each molecule. From this analysis, we can formulate the hypothesis that the enhanced biological effects shown by the apices hydroalcoholic extracts, as compared to the thalli, probably are ascribable to the higher amounts of cystoketal, cystoketal chromane and their relative isomers as well as to the dehydrated cystoketal molecules, which are significantly much more present in the apices extracts respectively to the thalli. Future HPLC extraction and purification of these molecules and further analyses of their biological effects will enable the validation of this hypothesis.

Table 3. Compounds' relative abundance in the apices and thalli hydroalcoholic (EtOH) extracts.

Identified Compounds	Abundance in Apices	Abundance in Thalli
Cystoketal, cystoketal chromane and isomers	++++	+
Demethyl cystoketal chromane, and isomers	+	+++
Cystoketal quinone, and isomers	+	+++
Dehydrated cystoketal	++++	+
Demethoxy cystoketal chromane	+	++

Indication of the relative abundance of the main meroditerpenes identified in the apices and thalli hydroalcoholic (EtOH) extracts obtained by the comparative analysis of the respective extracted ion chromatogram for each molecule in the two extracts. The plus signs, from + to ++++, indicate an increasing degree of abundance of the respective molecule.

3. Materials and Methods

3.1. Chemicals

All the reagents were acquired from Sigma-Aldrich (Milan, Italy) unless otherwise stated.

3.2. Algae Collection

In the Ligurian Sea (Northwestern Mediterranean), fronds of *Ericaria amentacea* were collected in the midlittoral zone, on exposed rocky shores, at Bogliasco, Genoa (NW Italy, 44°22′40.37″ N—9°4′35.14″ E). The collection was performed in July, in the summer of 2020, when the sea temperature values ranged between 25 and 26 °C. After the collection, the fronds were stored in plastic bags, kept in cold conditions, and immediately transported to the laboratory at the University of Genova. No specific permits were required for collecting the specimens. Additionally, non-destructive sampling was performed, as only the upper branches were collected without harming the individual organisms, let alone the whole population. Figure 10 shows the *E. amentacea* photographs from the site of collection in the Ligurian Sea (panel A) and of freshly collected fronds (panel B).

3.3. Production of Extracts from E. amentacea

E. amentacea fronds were washed with deionized water. The apical parts (with a 3 cm maximum length, referred to in the text as "apices"), distinguishable for the presence of reproductive structures and by a lighter brown color, were cut from the rest of the thallus. Both the apices and thallus fragments (i.e., the primary and secondary branches, devoid of the apical part, referred to in the text as "thalli"; Scheme 1) were air-dried, cut into tiny pieces using a blender and then dried in a lyophilizer. The extracts were obtained by incubation in mild conditions for 48 h in the dark in a rotary disk shaker at 30 °C, as already reported [23]. Briefly, aliquots of 2 g of the lyophilized apices or thalli of the seaweed were extracted in 20 mL of either dimethyl sulfoxide (DMSO) or ethanol: water 1:1 (EtOH). At the end of the incubation, four different extracts were obtained: seaweed apices in DMSO (DA extract) or in EtOH (EA extract), seaweed thalli in DMSO (DT extract) or in EtOH (ET extract). After filtration with a strainer, the aliquots were lyophilized and weighted to determine the yield of the extraction with the two solvents, and finally, the four extracts were diluted to a starting concentration of 25 mg/mL and frozen at −20 °C until further use. The solvent selection was chosen to ensure a higher yield of polyphenol and meroditerpene species extraction since these molecules show remarkable pharmacological activities and seem particularly abundant in the brown algae of the *Ericaria* genre and in this seaweed, as shown in Figure 9 and Table 2. Thus, since these molecular species show both hydrophobic (i.e., phenolic) as well as hydrophilic (i.e., hydroxyl) moieties, the choice of the solvent was a 50% hydroalcoholic solution to attempt to meet the abovementioned compound solubility needs. The DMSO solvent was also chosen because of its broad range of solubility capacity.

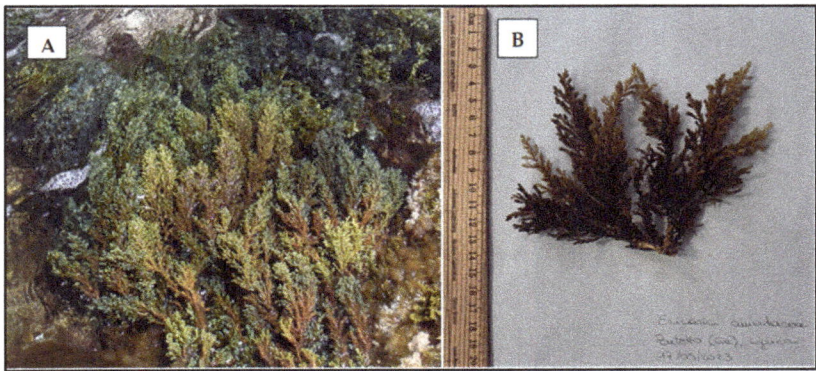

Figure 10. *E. amentacea* specimen. (**A**) Photograph from the site of collection in the Ligurian Sea, in the lower intertidal zone; (**B**) photograph of freshly collected seaweed thalli with a scale bar.

3.4. Total Phenolic and Flavonoid Contents

The total phenolic content (TPC) was evaluated using the Folin–Ciocalteu assay, as previously reported by Biju et al. [59]. The four *E. amentacea* extracts were quantified at a concentration of 500 µg/mL of the raw extracts, to which the reagents necessary for the TPC quantification were added. The phenolic concentration was obtained by comparison with a calibration curve of gallic acid (from 0.05 to 20 µg/mL final concentrations), and the TPC was expressed as mg of gallic acid equivalents (GAE).

The total flavonoid content (TFC) was assessed employing the $AlCl_3$ colorimetric method, as described by Biju et al. [59]. The four *E. amentacea* extracts were quantified at a concentration of 1 mg/mL of the raw extracts, to which the reagents necessary for the TFC quantification were added. The flavonoid concentration was calculated by comparison with a calibration curve of quercetin (from 1.5 to 30 µg/mL final concentrations), and the TFC was expressed as mg of quercetin equivalents (QE). The TPC and TFC quantifications were performed two times in duplicate.

3.5. In Chemico Antioxidant Activity

3.5.1. DPPH Assay

To estimate the total radical scavenging activity of the four *E. amentacea* extracts, the DPPH assay was performed as previously reported [60]. The four *E. amentacea* extracts were tested at 500, 250 and 100 µg/mL final concentrations. Moreover, a negative control with water replacing the extracts and a positive control with ascorbic acid (a 500 µg/mL final concentration) were prepared. The antioxidant activity of the extracts was obtained by estimating the quenching of the DPPH radical with respect to the negative control after subtracting the extracts' intrinsic absorbance at 517 nm due to their natural color, which was measured in a sample containing only the extracts in water: methanol 1:3. The assay was performed two times in duplicate.

3.5.2. Reducing Fe (III) Power Assay, Hydroxyl Radical and NO Scavenging Activities

The evaluation of the four *E. amentacea* extracts potential to reduce Fe (III) was carried out, as already reported in De La Fuente et al. [23]. The four extracts were tested at 500, 250 and 100 µg/mL final concentrations. Moreover, a negative control with water replacing the extracts and a positive control with ascorbic acid (a 30 µg/mL final concentration) were prepared. Thus, the reducing Fe (III) power of the extracts was calculated as a percentage with respect to the maximum activity of the ascorbic acid positive control. The assay was performed two times in duplicate.

The hydroxyl radical scavenging activity of the extracts was measured employing Mohr's salt method, according to De La Fuente et al. [23]. The four extracts were tested at 1.5, 1.0 and 0.5 mg/mL final concentrations. In addition, a negative control with water substituting the extracts and a positive control with gallic acid (a 0.5 mg/mL final concentration) were prepared. The test was performed two times in duplicate.

To assess the NO scavenging activity exerted by the extracts, the assay was carried out by De La Fuente et al. [23] by the sodium nitroprusside assay, followed by nitrite quantification through the Griess assay. The four extracts were tested at 500, 250 and 100 µg/mL final concentrations. The NO scavenging activity was calculated as a percentage with respect to a positive control of the sodium nitroprusside solution alone, generating the NO radical by light exposure. For the Griess assay, a calibration curve based on the $NaNO_2$ scalar concentrations was used (from 1 to 50 µM). The assay was performed two times in duplicate.

3.6. Tyrosinase, Collagenase and Hyaluronidase Inhibition

The tyrosinase inhibition was estimated using the colorimetric assay [61]. An increase in Dopachrome, a highly colored substance obtained by the catalytic conversion of L-Dopa, is proportional to tyrosinase enzymatic activity. Thus, the samples comprised *E. amentacea* extracts (a 100 µg/mL final concentration) in 300 µL of 50 mM Na_2HPO_4 (pH 6.8) and 200 µL of L-Dopa solution (25 mM in 50 mM Na_2HPO_4, pH 6.8). After 20 µL of mushroom tyrosinase (starting concentration 2500 U/mL) was added to the mixture, the absorbance (ABS) of the sample was immediately recorded at 475 nm for 10 min at 15-second intervals using a Beckman spectrophotometer (DU640). The tyrosinase inhibition was then calculated as a percentage of the activity (activity = speed/min = (ABS at t10'−ABS at t0')/10) of the positive control (in the presence of the respective vehicle solvents), prepared with 300 µL of 50 mM Na_2HPO_4, 200 µL of L-Dopa solution and 20 µL of the enzyme.

The evaluation of the collagenase inhibition was performed according to van Wart and Steinbrink [62]. The inhibition of the collagenase catalytic activity was evidenced by a reduced depletion of FALGPA, a synthetic peptide that mimics the collagen structure. In this enzymatic test, both FALGPA and collagenase were prepared in a reaction buffer made with 50 mM Tricine, 10 mM $CaCl_2$ and 400 mM NaCl in deionized water (pH 7.5). After the *E. amentacea* extracts (a 50 µg/mL final concentration) were dissolved in 40 µL of 1 mM FALGPA, 10 µL of collagenase from Clostridium histolyticum (20 U/mL) was added to the sample and its absorbance was immediately recorded at 345 nm for 15 min at intervals of 15 s using a Beckman spectrophotometer (DU640). The collagenase inhibition was obtained by comparison to a positive control (in the presence of the respective vehicle solvents) containing only 40 µL of 1 mM FALGPA and 10 µL of collagenase.

Hyaluronidase activity was assessed using the turbidimetric method described by Bralley et al. [63]. This assay measures the absorbance of the complex between hyaluronan and CTAB (cetyltrimethylammonium bromide) after incubation with the enzyme so that the absorbance is proportional to the remaining amount of undigested hyaluronan. Thus, an absorbance increase is correlated to a hyaluronidase inhibitory effect. For this assay, both hyaluronic acid and hyaluronidase were dissolved in an acetate buffer (0.15 M NaCl in 0.2 M sodium acetate–acetic acid, pH 6.0). Briefly, the test solution comprised *E. amentacea* extracts (50 µg/mL final concentration), 6.6 µL of hyaluronic acid (3 mg/mL), 1.5 µL of hyaluronidase from bovine testes (3000 U/mL) and acetate buffer up to the final volume of 50 µL. The samples were incubated for 15 min at 37 °C before adding 200 µL of the CTAB solution (2.5% CTAB and 2% NaOH in deionized water, pH 12). After 10 more minutes, the optical density was read at 405 nm on an AMR-100 Microplate Reader against a blank with 50 µL of acetate buffer and 200 µL of CTAB. Moreover, since the extracts showed an intrinsic absorbance at 405 nm due to the presence of phenolic compounds, their absorbance values were then subtracted from the value recorded after the enzymatic assay. The hyaluronidase inhibition was obtained by comparison with a positive control containing the enzyme and the reaction substrate without the extracts (in the presence of the respective vehicle solvents). The experiments were performed two times in duplicate.

3.7. Cell Cultures

The choice of the mouse fibroblast L929 and the human keratinocyte HaCaT cell lines was made since these are widely used biological systems in a very high number of cytotoxicity as well as cosmetic studies [64–67]. Concerning the L929 non-human fibroblasts, they were used because of the reproducibility of the past results obtained in several studies from our lab for cosmetic/pharmacological purposes [23,60,68–70] and because the use of the same cell line allowed for comparisons with previous results using similar extracts of the same seaweed [23].

The mouse fibroblast L929 cell line and the human keratinocyte HaCaT cell line used in this study were obtained, respectively, from the American Type Culture Collection (LGC Standards srl, Milan, Italy) and the Cell Lines Service (CLS GmbH, Eppelheim, Germany). Both cell lines were cultured at 37 °C in a humidified 5% CO_2 atmosphere in high glucose DMEM with 2 mM L-glutamine (Euroclone, Milan, Italy), supplemented with 10% FBS (Euroclone) and penicillin/streptomycin as the antibiotics (Corning Inc, Corning, NY, USA).

3.8. Cell Toxicity and Rescue from UV and H_2O_2 Treatment

The potential cytotoxicity of the *E. amentacea* extracts was estimated in both the L929 fibroblasts and HaCaT keratinocytes. In fact, after the cells were seeded in 96-well plates at a density of 10,000 cells/well and allowed to adhere overnight, they were treated with different extracts (100, 50 and 10 µg/mL final concentrations). The plates were incubated for 24 h at 37 °C, and at the end of the experiments, the cell viability was measured with the MTT assay, as previously reported in Pozzolini et al. [68]. The results are the means ± SD of three independent experiments, in which each condition was tested eight times, including the solvents alone (1% final dilutions).

The extracts' efficiency in reducing the H_2O_2- or the UV-induced cytotoxicity was assessed in the L929 fibroblasts and HaCaT keratinocytes, which were plated in 96-well plates at 10,000 cells/well and allowed to adhere overnight in a complete medium. The cells were then alternatively challenged with H_2O_2 200 µM or irradiated for 2 or 5 min under a UV lamp (Sanikyo Denki G20T10) at a 20 cm distance (90 mJ/cm^2 and 227 mJ/cm^2 total radiation doses, respectively), in the presence or absence of the *E. amentacea* extracts (100, 50 and 10 µg/mL concentrations). After 24 h of incubation, the cell viability was assayed by the MTT test and compared to the control—the untreated cells. Data are the means ± SD of three independent experiments in which each condition was tested eight times. Preliminary experiments were previously performed on these two cell lines to establish the suitable radiation doses that were able to induce significant cell death while still allowing us to measure the eventual rescue of cell viability, both mimicking a milder rate and a more severe exposure rate (90 mJ/cm^2 and 227 mJ/cm^2, respectively). These radiation values were based on the previous papers [71,72] mainly applied in the in vivo studies. Furthermore, the same conditions used in this work are already reported in our previous study, where the same cell lines and experimental settings were satisfactorily used [68].

3.9. Inhibition of Intracellular ROS Production

L929 fibroblasts and HaCaT keratinocytes were seeded in 96-well plates at a density of 10,000 cells/well, and on the following day, the assay was performed according to Pozzolini et al. [73]. Briefly, after being washed once with Hank's Balanced Salt Solution (HBSS), the cells were incubated for 45 min at 37 °C with 10 µM 2′,7′-dichlorodihydrofluorescein diacetate dye in HBSS (Life Technologies). Once washed with HBSS to remove the excess dye, the cells were either UV-irradiated for 3 min or challenged with 200 µM H_2O_2 and then treated with the *E. amentacea* extracts (the 100 µg/mL or 50 µg/mL final concentrations). Following 2 h of incubation, the plates were read on the Fluostar Optima BMG at 485/520 excitation/emission wavelengths. Data are the means ± SD of three independent experiments in which each condition was tested eight times.

3.10. Gene Expression Analyses

After being seeded in the 6-well plates at 300,000 cells/well and allowed to adhere overnight, the L929 fibroblasts were UV-irradiated for 5 min and treated with 50 µg/mL of the *E. amentacea* extracts. The gene expressions of interleukin-1β (IL-1β), interleukin-6 (IL-6) and chemokine (C-X-C motif) ligand 5 (CXCL5) were quantified by qPCR after 6 h. Alternatively, the HaCaT keratinocytes, seeded on the previous day in 6-well plates at a density of 300,000 cells/well, were UV-irradiated for 2 min and treated with 50 µg/mL of the extracts. The gene expressions of interleukin-1β (IL-1β), interleukin-6 (IL-6) and interleukin-8 (IL-8) were measured by qPCR after 6 h. At the end of the incubation, the RNA was extracted using the NucleoSpin RNA Mini kit (MACHEREY-NAGEL, Dueren, Germany) and subsequently analyzed using a NanoDrop spectrophotometer (Nanodrop Technologies, Wilmington, DE, USA). The cDNA was synthesized from 1 µg RNA using the iScript cDNA Synthesis Kit (Bio-Rad Laboratories, Milan, Italy). The PCR reaction (10 µL volume) contained: 4 × master mixes (Biotechrabbit GmbH, Hennigsdorf, Germany), 0.2 µM primers and 5 ng of cDNA. The analysis was performed in triplicate for each sample. The thermal conditions were: 3 min at 95 °C for the initial denaturation, followed by 45 cycles with 15 s at 95 °C for denaturation and 60 s at 60 °C for annealing and elongation. The samples were normalized on GAPDH and HPRT-1 (housekeeping gene) mRNAs for the L929 fibroblasts and HaCaT keratinocytes, respectively. The primer pair design (Table 4) was obtained using the Beacon Designer 7.0 software (Premier Biosoft International, Palo Alto, CA, USA) and synthesized by TibMolBiol (Genova, Italy). Data analyses were obtained using the DNA Engine Opticon 3 Real-Time Detection System Software program (3.03 version, Bio-Rad, Milan, Italy). The experiments were performed two times in triplicate.

Table 4. List of primers used in qPCR experiments.

GENE	GenBank (a.n.)	Forward	Reverse	Size (bp)
Human:				
IL-1β	NM_008361.4	gCAgCACATCAACAAgAg	CAgCAggTTATCATCATCAT C	184
IL-6	NM_031168.2	ACCTgTCTATACCACTTC	gCATCATCgTTgTTCATA	117
IL-8	NM_000584.4	AATTCATTCTCTgTggTATC	CCAGGAATCTTgTATTgC	127
HPRT-1	NM_000194.3	ggTCAggCAgTATAATCCAAAg	TTCATTATAgTCAAgggCATATCC	144
Murine:				
CXCL5	NM_009141.3	TgCTTAACCgTAACTCCAA	ATCCAgACAgACCTCCTT	129
IL-1b	NM_008361.4	gCAgCACATCAACAAgAg	CAgCAggTTATCATCATCATC	184
IL-6	NM_031168.2	ACCTgTCTATACCACTTC	gCATCATCgTTgTTCATA	117
GAPDH	NM_001289726.1	TCTCCCTCACAATTTCCATCCCAg	gggTgCAGCgAACTT TATTgATgg	99

3.11. HPLC/MS Analyses

The chromatographic separation of the two extracts was carried out using the Agilent 1100 µHPLC equipped with an automatic micro-sampler and an XSelect C18 column (300 Å pore size, 5 µm particle size, 1 mm, internal diameter, ×150 mm, length, respectively) maintained at 30 °C. The injection volume was 8 µL (with a starting concentration of

2.5 mg/mL). The chromatographic method comprised the following gradient of 45 min: 0–5 min 8% B, 5–40 min from 8% to 100% B, 40–45 min 100% B, at a flow rate of 30 µL/min, where A was H_2O containing 0,1% formic acid (FOA) and B was acetonitrile 0.05% FOA. The detector was set at 220/280 nm. Finally, the HPLC was coupled with the mass spectrometer (HPLC-ESI-MS) to qualitatively evaluate the compounds in the extract.

The instrument used was a mass spectrometer with an electrospray ion source (ESI) and a high-capacity ion trap (Agilent 1100 MSD XCT ion trap). All parameters were established to obtain the best ionization of the components. The analysis was performed in an ion-charge mode control with a target selected at 100,000 and an accumulation time of 300 ms. The operating parameters were as follows: capillary voltage, 3.6 V; nebulizer pressure, 20 psi; drying gas, 10 L/min; dry temperature, 350 °C; moving averages, 3; fragmentation width, 1 V, respectively. All mass spectra were acquired in full-scan and MS-MS mode, acquiring the most abundant species under each peak. The acquisition was performed on negative and positive ions in the 100–1000 mass range and analyzed using the integrated Agilent Data Analysis software (LC/MSD Trap software 5.3).

3.12. Statistical Analyses

Statistical analyses were performed using one-way ANOVA plus Tukey's post-test (GraphPad Prism Software 5.0, Inc., San Diego, CA, USA). The significance level of the tests was set at 0.05.

4. Conclusions

The data obtained in this study demonstrate the remarkable photoprotective and anti-aging effects of the hydroalcoholic and DMSO extracts from two portions of the Mediterranean seaweed *E. amentacea* (i.e., algal apices and thalli) by molecular and cellular analyses, highlighting the significantly stronger beneficial effects from the extracts of the apical portions. We were able to demonstrate the postulate that because during summer, the apical portions grow and hold reproductive structures, and given that in this season, the algae are subjected to the highest solar UV radiation, these upper seaweed portions would be particularly enriched in antioxidant and photoprotective molecules which can counteract the detrimental effects of UV-B radiation on the cellular skin models. In fact, although all the extracts were enriched in polyphenols, flavonoids and ROS scavenging molecules and showed significant biological activities, the apices extracts, and those retrieved by hydroalcoholic extraction, demonstrated the highest pharmacological potential, likely due to the abundance of meroditerpenes structures, such as cystoketal, dehydrated cystoketal, cystoketal chromane and some of their related isomers. The extracts showed cell rescue, antioxidant and anti-inflammatory abilities in the UV-exposed keratinocyte and fibroblast cellular models. They ultimately restored cell viability in both cell types, abated the intracellular oxidative stress and significantly reduced the production of important mediators that propagate and exacerbate the inflammatory process, i.e., IL-1β, IL-6 and IL-8, which are typically released after sunburns and contribute to erythema formation and pain. Furthermore, the algal extracts showed important in vitro hydrolytic skin enzyme inhibition abilities by significantly reducing collagenase and hyaluronidase degrading activities and anti-sunspot formation properties by partially blocking the tyrosinase enzymatic activity. Thus, a good biocompatibility and cell growth-promoting effect in the skin in the in vitro models was clearly demonstrated, alongside remarkable multifactorial anti-aging properties, which were particularly concentrated in the apical portions of the seaweed. Therefore, the *E. amentacea* algal extracts may constitute ideal additives to cosmetic and/or phyto-pharmaceutical products for lenitive and photoprotective treatments to cure UV-derived skin inflammatory states and to promote skin renovation in elders.

Author Contributions: Conceptualization, S.S., V.A. and M.C.; Methodology, S.S., V.A., M.C. and A.S.; Investigation, S.S., S.M., V.A., M.C., A.S., M.B. and G.D.; Data curation, S.S., S.M. and A.S.; Writing, S.S., M.C., V.A. and S.M.; Writing—review and editing, S.S., M.C. and V.A.; Supervision, S.S.; Funding acquisition, S.S., M.C., V.A. and G.D. All authors have read and agreed to the published version of the manuscript.

Funding: This research was funded by grants from the University of Genova to S.S. and M.C. and from the EU-funded project ROCPOP-Life (LIFE16 NAT/IT/000816 ROCPOP.Life). This work was also supported by the Project National Biodiversity Future Center (NBFC), funded under the National Recovery and Resilience Plan (NRRP), Mission 4 Component 2 Investment 1.4—Call for tender No. 3138 of 16 December 2021, rectified by Decree n.3175 of 18 December 2021 of the Italian Ministry of University and Research, funded by the European Union, NextGenerationEU, Project code CN_00000033, Concession Decree No. 1034 of 17 June 2022, adopted by the Italian Ministry of University and Research, CUP D33C22000960007.

Institutional Review Board Statement: Not applicable.

Data Availability Statement: Data sharing is not applicable to this article.

Conflicts of Interest: The authors declare no conflict of interest.

References

1. Guiry, M.D. How Many Species of Algae Are There? *J. Phycol.* **2012**, *48*, 1057–1063. [CrossRef]
2. Liu, Z.; Gao, T.; Yang, Y.; Meng, F.; Zhan, F.; Jiang, Q.; Sun, X. Anti-Cancer Activity of Porphyran and Carrageenan from Red Seaweeds. *Molecules* **2019**, *24*, 4286. [CrossRef]
3. Apostolova, E.; Lukova, P.; Baldzhieva, A.; Katsarov, P.; Nikolova, M.; Iliev, I.; Peychev, L.; Trica, B.; Oancea, F.; Delattre, C.; et al. Immunomodulatory and Anti-Inflammatory Effects of Fucoidan: A Review. *Polymers* **2020**, *12*, 2338. [CrossRef]
4. de Sousa, C.B.; Gangadhar, K.N.; Macridachis, J.; Pavão, M.; Morais, T.R.; Campino, L.; Varela, J.; Lago, J.H.G. *Cystoseira* algae (Fucaceae): Update on their chemical entities and biological activities. *Tetrahedron Asymmetry* **2017**, *28*, 1486–1505. [CrossRef]
5. Gaysinski, M.; Ortalo-Magné, A.; Thomas, O.P.; Culioli, G. Extraction, purification, and NMR analysis of terpenes from brown algae. In *Methods in Molecular Biology Book Series*; Humana Press: Clifton, NJ, USA, 2015; Volume 1308, pp. 207–223.
6. Jesumani, V.; Du, H.; Aslam, M.; Pei, P.; Huang, N. Potential Use of Seaweed Bioactive Compounds in Skincare—A Review. *Mar. Drugs* **2019**, *17*, 688. [CrossRef]
7. Pangestuti, R.; Siahaan, E.A.; Kim, S.-K. Photoprotective Substances Derived from Marine Algae. *Mar. Drugs* **2018**, *16*, 399. [CrossRef]
8. Hwang, H.; Chen, T.; Nines, R.G.; Shin, H.-C.; Stoner, G.D. Photochemoprevention of UVB-induced skin carcinogenesis in SKH-1 mice by brown algae polyphenols. *Int. J. Cancer* **2006**, *119*, 2742–2749. [CrossRef]
9. Kang, K.; Hye, J.H.; Dong, H.H.; Park, Y.; Seong, H.K.; Bong, H.L. Antioxidant and antiinflammatory activities of ventol, a phlorotannin-rich natural agent derived from *Ecklonia cava*, and its effect on proteoglycan degradation in cartilage ex-plant culture. *Res. Commun. Mol. Pathol. Pharmacol.* **2004**, *115–116*, 77–95.
10. Manandhar, B.; Wagle, A.; Seong, S.H.; Paudel, P.; Kim, H.-R.; Jung, H.A.; Choi, J.S. Phlorotannins with Potential Anti-Tyrosinase and Antioxidant Activity Isolated from the Marine Seaweed Ecklonia stolonifera. *Antioxidants* **2019**, *8*, 240. [CrossRef]
11. Kim, M.-M.; Kim, S.-K. Effect of phloroglucinol on oxidative stress and inflammation. *Food Chem. Toxicol.* **2010**, *48*, 2925–2933. [CrossRef]
12. Nakai, K.; Tsuruta, D. What Are Reactive Oxygen Species, Free Radicals, and Oxidative Stress in Skin Diseases? *Int. J. Mol. Sci.* **2021**, *22*, 10799. [CrossRef] [PubMed]
13. Masaki, H. Role of antioxidants in the skin: Anti-aging effects. *J. Dermatol. Sci.* **2010**, *58*, 85–90. [CrossRef] [PubMed]
14. Ichihashi, M.; Ueda, M.; Budiyanto, A.; Bito, T.; Oka, M.; Fukunaga, M.; Tsuru, K.; Horikawa, T. UV-induced skin damage. *Toxicology* **2003**, *189*, 21–39. [CrossRef] [PubMed]
15. McCullough, J.L.; Kelly, K. Prevention and Treatment of Skin Aging. *Ann. N. Y. Acad. Sci.* **2006**, *1067*, 323–331. [CrossRef]
16. Yan, X.; Nagata, T.; Fan, X. Antioxidative activities in some common seaweeds. *Plant Foods Hum. Nutr.* **1998**, *52*, 253–262. [CrossRef]
17. Hirose, Y.; Yoshimi, N.; Suzui, M.; Kawabata, K.; Tanaka, T.; Mori, H. Expression of bcl-2, bax, and bcl-XL proteins in azoxymethane-induced rat colonic adenocarcinomas. *Mol. Carcinog.* **1997**, *19*, 25–30. [CrossRef]
18. Ariede, M.B.; Candido, T.M.; Jacome, A.L.M.; Velasco, M.V.R.; De Carvalho, J.C.M.; Baby, A.R. Cosmetic attributes of algae—A review. *Algal Res.* **2017**, *25*, 483–487. [CrossRef]
19. Stanoikovic, T.P.; Konic-Ristic, A.; Kljajic, Z.; Grozdanic-Stanisavljevic, N.; Srdic-Rajic, T.; Zdunic, G.; Savikin, K. Antioxidant, antiplatelet and cytotoxic activity of extract of *Cystoseira amentacea* from the coast of Montenegro (South-east Adriatic Sea). *Digest J. Nanomat. Biostruct.* **2014**, *9*, 869–880.
20. Ruberto, G.; Baratta, M.T.; Biondi, D.M.; Amico, V. Antioxidant activity of extracts of the marine algal genus *Cystoseira* in a micellar model system. *J. Appl. Phycol.* **2001**, *13*, 403–407. [CrossRef]

21. De La Fuente, G.; Pinteus, S.; Silva, J.; Alves, C.; Pedrosa, R. Antioxidant and antimicrobial potential of six Fucoids from the Mediterranean Sea and the Atlantic Ocean. *J. Sci. Food Agric.* **2022**, *102*, 5568–5575. [CrossRef]
22. Mannino, A.M.; Vaglica, V.; Oddo, E. Seasonal variation in total phenolic content of *Dyctiopteris polypodioides* (Dictyotaceae) and *Cystoseira amentacea* (Sargassacee) from the Sicilian coast. *Flora Mediterr.* **2014**, *24*, 39–50. [CrossRef]
23. De La Fuente, G.; Fontana, M.; Asnaghi, V.; Chiantore, M.; Mirata, S.; Salis, A.; Damonte, G.; Scarfì, S. The Remarkable Antioxidant and Anti-Inflammatory Potential of the Extracts of the Brown Alga *Cystoseira amentacea* var. *stricta*. *Mar. Drugs* **2021**, *19*, 2. [CrossRef] [PubMed]
24. Goutzourelas, N.; Kevrekidis, D.P.; Barda, S.; Malea, P.; Trachana, V.; Savvidi, S.; Kevrekidou, A.; Assimopoulou, A.N.; Goutas, A.; Liu, M.; et al. Antioxidant Activity and Inhibition of Liver Cancer Cells' Growth of Extracts from 14 Marine Macroalgae Species of the Mediterranean Sea. *Foods* **2023**, *12*, 1310. [CrossRef]
25. Falace, A.; Kaleb, S.; De La Fuente, G.; Asnaghi, V.; Chiantore, M. Ex situ cultivation protocol for *Cystoseira amentacea* var. stricta (Fucales, Phaeophyceae) from a restoration perspective. *PLoS ONE* **2018**, *13*, e0193011. [CrossRef]
26. De La Fuente, G.; Chiantore, M.; Asnaghi, V.; Kaleb, S.; Falace, A. First ex situ outplanting of the habitat-forming seaweed *Cystoseira amentacea* var. stricta from a restoration perspective. *PeerJ* **2019**, *7*, e7290. [CrossRef] [PubMed]
27. Clausing, R.J.; De La Fuente, G.; Falace, A.; Chiantore, M. Accounting for environmental stress in restoration of intertidal foundation species. *J. Appl. Ecol.* **2023**, *60*, 305–318. [CrossRef]
28. Celis-Plá, P.S.M.; Bouzon, Z.L.; Hall-Spencer, J.M.; Korbee, N.; Figueroa, F.L. Seasonal biochemical and photophysiological responses in the intertidal macroalga *Cystoseira tamariscifolia* (Ochrophyta). *Mar. Environ. Res.* **2016**, *115*, 89–97. [CrossRef]
29. Manach, C.; Scalbert, A.; Morand, C.; Rémésy, C.; Jiménez, L. Polyphenols: Food sources and bioavailability. *Am. J. Clin. Nutr.* **2004**, *79*, 727–747. [CrossRef]
30. Van Alstyne, K.; McCarthy, J.J.; Hustead, C.L.; Kearns, L.J. Phlorotannin allocation among tissues of northeastern pacific kelps and rockweeds. *J. Phycol.* **1999**, *35*, 483–492. [CrossRef]
31. Rosa, G.P.; Peixoto, A.F.; Barreto, M.C.; Seca, A.M.L.; Pinto, D.C.G.A. Bio-Guided Optimization of *Cystoseira abiesmarina* Cosmeceuticals Extraction by Advanced Technologies. *Mar. Drugs* **2023**, *21*, 35. [CrossRef]
32. Čagalj, M.; Skroza, D.; Razola-Díaz, M.D.C.; Verardo, V.; Bassi, D.; Frleta, R.; Mekinić, I.G.; Tabanelli, G.; Šimat, V. Variations in the Composition, Antioxidant and Antimicrobial Activities of *Cystoseira compressa* during Seasonal Growth. *Mar. Drugs* **2022**, *20*, 64. [CrossRef] [PubMed]
33. Mannino, A.M.; Micheli, C. Ecological Function of Phenolic Compounds from Mediterranean Fucoid Algae and Seagrasses: An Overview on the Genus *Cystoseira sensu lato* and *Posidonia oceanica* (L.) Delile. *J. Mar. Sci. Eng.* **2020**, *8*, 19. [CrossRef]
34. Kootstra, A. Protection from UV-B-induced DNA damage by flavonoids. *Plant Mol. Biol.* **1994**, *26*, 771–774. [CrossRef] [PubMed]
35. Stahl, W.; Sies, H. Carotenoids and Flavonoids Contribute to Nutritional Protection against Skin Damage from Sunlight. *Mol. Biotechnol.* **2007**, *37*, 26–30. [CrossRef] [PubMed]
36. Vizetto-Duarte, C.; Custódio, L.; Acosta, G.; Lago, J.H.G.; Morais, T.R.; Bruno de Sousa, C.; Gangadhar, K.N.; Rodrigues, M.J.; Pereira, H.; Lima, R.T.; et al. Can macroalgae provide promising anti-tumoral compounds? A closer look at *Cystoseira tamariscifolia* as a source for antioxidant and anti-hepatocarcinoma compounds. *PeerJ* **2016**, *4*, e1704. [CrossRef] [PubMed]
37. Trifan, A.; Vasincu, A.; Luca, S.V.; Neophytou, C.; Wolfram, E.; Opitz, S.E.; Sava, D.; Bucur, L.; Cioroiu, B.I.; Miron, A.; et al. Unravelling the potential of seaweeds from the Black Sea coast of Romania as bioactive compounds sources. Part I: *Cystoseira barbata* (Stackhouse) C. Agardh. *Food Chem. Toxicol.* **2019**, *134*, 110820. [CrossRef]
38. Heo, S.-J.; Ko, S.-C.; Cha, S.-H.; Kang, D.-H.; Park, H.-S.; Choi, Y.-U.; Kim, D.; Jung, W.-K.; Jeon, Y.-J. Effect of phlorotannins isolated from *Ecklonia cava* on melanogenesis and their protective effect against photo-oxidative stress induced by UV-B radiation. *Toxicol. Vitr.* **2009**, *23*, 1123–1130. [CrossRef]
39. De Luca, C.; Mikhal'chik, E.V.; Suprun, M.V.; Papacharalambous, M.; Truhanov, A.I.; Korkina, L.G. Skin Antiageing and Systemic Redox Effects of Supplementation with Marine Collagen Peptides and Plant-Derived Antioxidants: A Single-Blind Case-Control Clinical Study. *Oxid. Med. Cell. Longev.* **2016**, *2016*, 4389410. [CrossRef]
40. Bukhari, S.N.A.; Roswandi, N.L.; Waqas, M.; Habib, H.; Hussain, F.; Khan, S.; Sohail, M.; Ramli, N.A.; Thu, H.E.; Hussain, Z. Hyaluronic acid, a promising skin rejuvenating biomedicine: A review of recent updates and pre-clinical and clinical investigations on cosmetic and nutricosmetic effects. *Int. J. Biol. Macromol.* **2018**, *120*, 1682–1695. [CrossRef]
41. Venkatesan, J.; Anil, S.; Kim, S.-K.; Shim, M.S. Marine Fish Proteins and Peptides for Cosmeceuticals: A Review. *Mar. Drugs* **2017**, *15*, 143. [CrossRef]
42. Bravo, B.; Correia, P.; Junior, J.E.G.; Sant'Anna, B.; Kerob, D. Benefits of topical hyaluronic acid for skin quality and signs of skin aging: From literature review to clinical evidence. *Dermatol. Ther.* **2022**, *35*, 15903. [CrossRef] [PubMed]
43. Neves, J.R.; Grether-Beck, S.; Krutmann, J.; Correia, P.; Gonçalves, J.E.; Sant'anna, B.; Kerob, D. Efficacy of a topical serum containing L-ascorbic acid, neohesperidin, pycnogenol, tocopherol, and hyaluronic acid in relation to skin aging signs. *J. Cosmet. Dermatol.* **2022**, *21*, 4462–4469. [CrossRef] [PubMed]
44. Pullar, J.M.; Carr, A.C.; Vissers, M.C.M. The Roles of Vitamin C in Skin Health. *Nutrients* **2017**, *9*, 866. [CrossRef] [PubMed]
45. Zhang, S.; Duan, E. Fighting against Skin Aging: The Way from Bench to Bedside. *Cell Transplant.* **2018**, *27*, 729–738. [CrossRef]
46. Ferreres, F.; Lopes, G.; Gil-Izquierdo, A.; Andrade, P.B.; Sousa, C.; Mouga, T.; Valentão, P. Phlorotannin Extracts from Fucales Characterized by HPLC-DAD-ESI-MS^n: Approaches to Hyaluronidase Inhibitory Capacity and Antioxidant Properties. *Mar. Drugs* **2012**, *10*, 2766–2781. [CrossRef]

47. Li, Y.-X.; Wijesekara, I.; Kim, S.-K. Phlorotannins as bioactive agents from brown algae. *Process. Biochem.* **2011**, *46*, 2219–2224. [CrossRef]
48. Joe, M.-J.; Kim, S.-N.; Choi, H.-Y.; Shin, W.-S.; Park, G.-M.; Kang, D.-W.; Kim, Y.K. The Inhibitory Effects of Eckol and Dieckol from *Ecklonia stolonifera* on the Expression of Matrix Metalloproteinase-1 in Human Dermal Fibroblasts. *Biol. Pharm. Bull.* **2006**, *29*, 1735–1739. [CrossRef]
49. Pillaiyar, T.; Manickam, M.; Namasivayam, V. Skin whitening agents: Medicinal chemistry perspective of tyrosinase inhibitors. *J. Enzyme Inhib. Med. Chem.* **2017**, *32*, 403–425. [CrossRef]
50. Kang, H.S.; Kim, H.R.; Byun, D.S.; Son, B.W.; Nam, T.J.; Choi, J.S. Tyrosinase inhibitors isolated from the edible brown algaEcklonia stolonifera. *Arch. Pharmacal. Res.* **2004**, *27*, 1226–1232. [CrossRef]
51. Zhao, H.-C.; Xiao, T.; Chen, Y.-J. Ultraviolet-Induced Skin Inflammation. *Int. J. Dermatol. Venereol.* **2021**, *4*, 229–235. [CrossRef]
52. Hol, J.; Wilhelmsen, L.; Haraldsen, G. The murine IL-8 homologues KC, MIP-2, and LIX are found in endothelial cytoplasmic granules but not in Weibel-Palade bodies. *J. Leukoc. Biol.* **2010**, *87*, 501–508. [CrossRef] [PubMed]
53. de los Reyes, C.; Ortega, M.J.; Zbakh, H.; Motilva, V.; Zubía, E. *Cystoseira usneoides*: A Brown Alga Rich in Antioxidant and Anti-inflammatory Meroditerpenoids. *J. Nat. Prod.* **2016**, *79*, 395–405. [CrossRef] [PubMed]
54. Valls, R.; Mesguiche, V.; Piovetti, L.; Prost, M.; Peiffer, G. Meroditerpenes from the brown alga *Cystoseira amentacea* var. stricta collected off the French mediterranean coast. *Phytochemistry* **1996**, *41*, 1367–1371. [CrossRef]
55. Mesguiche, V.; Valls, R.; Piovetti, L.; Banaigs, B. Meroditerpenes from *Cystoseira amentacea* var. stricta collected off the French Mediterranean coasts. *Phytochemistry* **1997**, *45*, 1489–1494. [CrossRef]
56. Rahman, M.; Biswas, S.; Islam, K.J.; Paul, A.S.; Mahato, S.K.; Ali, A.; Halim, M.A. Antiviral phytochemicals as potent inhibitors against NS3 protease of dengue virus. *Comput. Biol. Med.* **2021**, *134*, 104492. [CrossRef]
57. Laird, D.W.; van Altena, I.A. Tetraprenyltoluquinols from the brown alga *Cystophora fibrosa*. *Phytochemistry* **2006**, *67*, 944–955. [CrossRef]
58. Ainane, T.A.; Fatouma, A.A.; Ayoub, A.; Ayoub, R.; Ahmed, B.; Abdelmjid, A. Methoxycystoketal Quinone: Natural Compound from Bioactive Diethyl Ether Extract of Brown Seaweed *Cystoseira tamariscifolia*. *Pharmacol. Online Arch.* **2021**, *2*, 583–589. Available online: https://pharmacologyonline.silae.it/files/archives/2021/vol2/PhOL_2021_2_A066_AINANE.pdf (accessed on 9 May 2023).
59. Biju, J.; Sulaiman, C.T.; Sateesh, G.; Reddy, V.R.K. Total phenolics and flavonoids in selected medicinal plants in Kerala. *Int. J. Pharm. Pharm. Sci.* **2014**, *6*, 406–408.
60. Pozzolini, M.; Scarfì, S.; Gallus, L.; Castellano, M.; Vicini, S.; Cortese, K.; Gagliani, M.C.; Bertolino, M.; Costa, G.; Giovine, M. Production, Characterization and Biocompatibility Evaluation of Collagen Membranes Derived from Marine Sponge *Chondrosia reniformis* Nardo, 1847. *Mar. Drugs* **2018**, *16*, 111. [CrossRef]
61. Chan, E.W.C.; Lim, Y.Y.; Wong, L.F.; Lianto, F.S.; Wong, S.K.; Lim, K.K.; Joe, C.E.; Lim, T.Y. Antioxidant and tyrosinase inhibition properties of leaves and rhizomes of ginger species. *Food Chem.* **2008**, *109*, 477–483. [CrossRef]
62. Van Wart, H.E.; Steinbrink, D. A continuous spectrophotometric assay for *Clostridium histolyticum* collagenase. *Anal. Biochem.* **1981**, *113*, 356–365. [CrossRef] [PubMed]
63. Bralley, E.; Greenspan, P.; Hargrove, J.L.; Hartle, D.K. Inhibition of Hyaluronidase Activity by *Vitis rotundifolia*. (Muscadine) Berry Seeds and Skins. *Pharm. Biol.* **2007**, *45*, 667–673. [CrossRef]
64. Cannella, V.; Altomare, R.; Leonardi, V.; Russotto, L.; Di Bella, S.; Mira, F.; Guercio, A. In Vitro Biocompatibility Evaluation of Nine Dermal Fillers on L929 Cell Line. *BioMed Res. Int.* **2020**, *2020*, 8676343. [CrossRef] [PubMed]
65. Kozlova, T.O.; Popov, A.L.; Kolesnik, I.V.; Kolmanovich, D.D.; Baranchikov, A.E.; Shcherbakov, A.B.; Ivanov, V.K. Amorphous and crystalline cerium(iv) phosphates: Biocompatible ROS-scavenging sunscreens. *J. Mater. Chem. B* **2022**, *10*, 1775–1785. [CrossRef]
66. Mebert, A.M.; Baglole, C.J.; Desimone, M.F.; Maysinger, D. Nanoengineered silica: Properties, applications and toxicity. *Food Chem. Toxicol.* **2017**, *109*, 753–770. [CrossRef]
67. Pavelkova, R.; Matouskova, P.; Hoova, J.; Porizka, J.; Marova, I. Preparation and characterisation of organic UV filters based on combined PHB/liposomes with natural phenolic compounds. *J. Biotechnol.* **2020**, *324*, 100021. [CrossRef]
68. Pozzolini, M.; Millo, E.; Oliveri, C.; Mirata, S.; Salis, A.; Damonte, G.; Arkel, M.; Scarfì, S. Elicited ROS scavenging activity, photoprotective, and wound-healing properties of collagen-derived peptides from the marine sponge *Chondrosia reniformis*. *Mar. Drugs* **2018**, *16*, 465. [CrossRef]
69. Dodero, A.; Scarfì, S.; Mirata, S.; Sionkowska, A.; Vicini, S.; Alloisio, M.; Castellano, M. Effect of Crosslinking Type on the Physical-Chemical Properties and Biocompatibility of Chitosan-Based Electrospun Membranes. *Polymers* **2021**, *13*, 831. [CrossRef]
70. Dodero, A.; Donati, I.; Scarfì, S.; Mirata, S.; Alberti, S.; Lova, P.; Comoretto, D.; Alloisio, M.; Vicini, S.; Castellano, M. Effect of sodium alginate molecular structure on electrospun membrane cell adhesion. *Mater. Sci. Eng. C* **2021**, *124*, 112067. [CrossRef]
71. Chen, T.; Hou, H. Protective effect of gelatin polypeptides from Pacific cod (*Gadus macrocephalus*) against UV irradiation-induced damages by inhibiting inflammation and improving transforming growth factor-β/Smad signaling pathway. *J. Photochem. Photobiol. B Biol.* **2016**, *162*, 633–640. [CrossRef]

72. Hou, H.; Li, B.; Zhang, Z.; Xue, C.; Yu, G.; Wang, J.; Bao, Y.; Bu, L.; Sun, J.; Peng, Z.; et al. Moisture absorption and retention properties, and activity in alleviating skin photodamage of collagen polypeptide from marine fish skin. *Food Chem.* **2012**, *135*, 1432–1439. [CrossRef] [PubMed]
73. Pozzolini, M.; Vergani, L.; Ragazzoni, M.; Delpiano, L.; Grasselli, E.; Voci, A.; Giovine, M.; Scarfi, S. Different reactivity of primary fibroblasts and endothelial cells towards crystalline silica: A surface radical matter. *Toxicology* **2016**, *361–362*, 12–23. [CrossRef] [PubMed]

Disclaimer/Publisher's Note: The statements, opinions and data contained in all publications are solely those of the individual author(s) and contributor(s) and not of MDPI and/or the editor(s). MDPI and/or the editor(s) disclaim responsibility for any injury to people or property resulting from any ideas, methods, instructions or products referred to in the content.

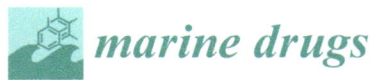

Article

Protective Effects of an Oligo-Fucoidan-Based Formula against Osteoarthritis Development via iNOS and COX-2 Suppression following Monosodium Iodoacetate Injection

Yi-Fen Chiang [1,†], Ko-Chieh Huang [1,†], Kai-Lee Wang [2], Yun-Ju Huang [3], Hsin-Yuan Chen [1], Mohamed Ali [4,5], Tzong-Ming Shieh [6,*] and Shih-Min Hsia [1,7,8,9,10,*]

[1] School of Nutrition and Health Sciences, College of Nutrition, Taipei Medical University, Taipei 110301, Taiwan
[2] Department of Nursing, Deh Yu College of Nursing and Health, Keelung 203301, Taiwan
[3] Department of Biotechnology and Food Technology, Southern Taiwan University of Science and Technology, Tainan 710301, Taiwan
[4] Department of Obstetrics and Gynecology, University of Chicago, Chicago, IL 60637, USA; mohamed.ali@bsd.uchicago.edu
[5] Clinical Pharmacy Department, Faculty of Pharmacy, Ain Shams University, Cairo 11566, Egypt
[6] School of Dentistry, China Medical University, Taichung 404328, Taiwan
[7] Graduate Institute of Metabolism and Obesity Sciences, College of Nutrition, Taipei Medical University, Taipei 11031, Taiwan
[8] School of Food and Safety, Taipei Medical University, Taipei 11031, Taiwan
[9] Nutrition Research Center, Taipei Medical University Hospital, Taipei 11031, Taiwan
[10] TMU Research Center for Digestive Medicine, Taipei Medical University, Taipei 11031, Taiwan
* Correspondence: tmshieh@mail.cmu.edu.tw (T.-M.S.); bryanhsia@tmu.edu.tw (S.-M.H.); Tel.: +886-4-2205-3366-6 (ext. 2316) (T.-M.S.); +886-2-2736-1661 (ext. 6558) (S.-M.H.)
† These authors contributed equally to this work.

Abstract: Osteoarthritis (OA) is a debilitating joint disorder characterized by cartilage degradation and chronic inflammation, accompanied by high oxidative stress. In this study, we utilized the monosodium iodoacetate (MIA)-induced OA model to investigate the efficacy of oligo-fucoidan-based formula (FF) intervention in mitigating OA progression. Through its capacity to alleviate joint bearing function and inflammation, improvements in cartilage integrity following oligo-fucoidan-based formula intervention were observed, highlighting its protective effects against cartilage degeneration and structural damage. Furthermore, the oligo-fucoidan-based formula modulated the p38 signaling pathway, along with downregulating cyclooxygenase-2 (COX-2) and inducible nitric oxide synthase (iNOS) expression, contributing to its beneficial effects. Our study provides valuable insights into targeted interventions for OA management and calls for further clinical investigations to validate these preclinical findings and to explore the translational potential of an oligo-fucoidan-based formula in human OA patients.

Keywords: osteoarthritis; oligo-fucoidan-based formula; oxidative stress; inflammatory

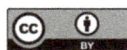

1. Introduction

Osteoarthritis (OA), also known interchangeably as degenerative joint disease or osteoarthrosis, represents the predominant form of joint pathology. Its primary manifestations include joint pain, stiffness, swelling, and structural malformation. Additionally, abnormal joint sounds, notably crepitus, may accompany movements. In the early stages of the disease, individuals typically experience pain during routine activities such as squatting, kneeling, ascending stairs, or transitioning from seated to standing positions. As the condition progresses, this discomfort may persist during both walking and periods of rest. Moreover, prolonged immobilization in fixed postures, such as extended periods of sitting or standing, or even during nocturnal rest, may contribute to knee discomfort [1,2].

The pathogenesis of osteoarthritis (OA) involves the loss of proteoglycans and type II collagen within the articular cartilage, alongside the degradation of the extracellular matrix (ECM) [3]. This degradation leads to the deterioration of the articular cartilage, resulting in increased friction between bones, inflammation, and severe pain. Consequently, joint mobility becomes compromised, potentially leading to joint disability [4]. Accumulating evidence has demonstrated that secreted inflammatory cytokines play a central role as mediators of pathology in the progression of OA [5,6]. Interleukin-1 beta (IL-1β), tumor necrosis factor-alpha (TNF-α), and IL-6 are major factors involved in and associated with cartilage degradation. These cytokines perpetuate an inflammatory cascade, contributing to the destruction of cartilage and perpetuation of the disease process [7].

The modulation of inflammatory cytokines may occur via inducible nitric oxide synthase (iNOS) and cyclooxygenase-2 (COX-2), which can exacerbate the progression of OA by impairing cartilage function, triggering apoptosis, and worsening the disease [8].

Currently, the treatment for osteoarthritis (OA) primarily relies on medication to alleviate pain. Nonsteroidal anti-inflammatory drugs (NSAIDs) such as acetaminophen, celecoxib, and aspirin are commonly used to reduce pain and inflammation [9]. However, studies have shown that the prolonged use of NSAIDs may inhibit proteoglycan synthesis, hastening the deterioration of OA [10]. Therefore, there is a need to identify effective compounds capable of delaying proteoglycan degradation, preventing extracellular matrix (ECM) loss, and alleviating inflammatory responses.

Exploring alternative therapeutic approaches that target specific pathways involved in OA pathogenesis, such as iNOS and COX-2, could offer promising avenues for the development of more targeted and efficacious treatments. Additionally, research into natural compounds with anti-inflammatory and chondroprotective properties may provide novel therapeutic options with fewer adverse effects compared with traditional NSAIDs. Ultimately, a multifaceted approach that addresses both pain relief and disease modification is essential in effectively managing OA and improving the quality of life for affected individuals.

Previous studies have revealed the anti-inflammatory properties of low-molecular-weight fucoidan derived from brown algae extracts [11]. Fucoidan, a sulfated polysaccharide found in various species of brown seaweed, has garnered attention for its diverse biological activities, including anti-inflammatory, antioxidative, and immunomodulatory properties [12,13]. These characteristics make it an attractive candidate for exploring its efficacy in OA treatment. However, despite numerous studies highlighting its beneficial effects, the specific mechanisms by which fucoidan exerts its actions in the context of OA are not yet fully characterized. By establishing an oligo-fucoidan-based formula and determining its potential in relieving OA symptoms, we are evaluating its efficacy in mitigating OA-related pathology. By elucidating the molecular pathways through which the oligo-fucoidan-based formula exerts its protective effects on OA-affected knee joints, this study aims to provide valuable insights into its therapeutic mechanisms. These findings have the potential to inform the development of novel fucoidan-based therapies for OA management, offering new hope for patients suffering from this debilitating condition. Ultimately, a deeper understanding of the therapeutic properties of fucoidan may pave the way for personalized approaches to OA treatment that are tailored to individual patient needs.

2. Results

2.1. Formula Selection thorugh Examination of iNOS Expression (In Vitro Study)

To determine whether the formula has a greater effect than its individual components, we measured the iNOS expression in response to the oligo-fucoidan-based formula (FF) and its individual components, including the formula without oligo-fucoidan, oligo-fucoidan, and UC-II. Experimenting with Raw264.7 cells induced with LPS, we observed that the FF displayed superior inhibition of iNOS production compared with the individual fucoidan and UC-II components, which exhibited only partial inhibition abilities (Figure 1).

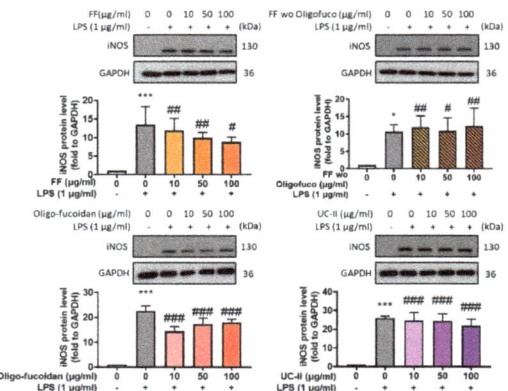

Figure 1. iNOS expression modulation by FF and FF-related components. Raw 264.7 cells were treated with the oligo-fucoidan-based formula (FF) and its related components and then induced by LPS for 24 h. Western blot was used to evaluate the iNOS expression. * $p < 0.05$; *** $p < 0.001$ compared with the control group. # $p < 0.05$; ## $p < 0.01$; ### $p < 0.001$ compared with the LPS-induced group.

2.2. Protective Effect of the Oligo-Fucoidan-Based Formula (FF) on Joint Swelling Induced by MIA-Induced Osteoarthritis

The flow chart of procedures was shown in Figure 2A. Three weeks after intervention with the oligo-fucoidan-based formula, the width of the knee joint in the hind limbs was measured using a caliper. The results demonstrated that intervention with the oligo-fucoidan-based formula effectively reduced the occurrence of joint swelling induced by MIA (Figure 2B,C).

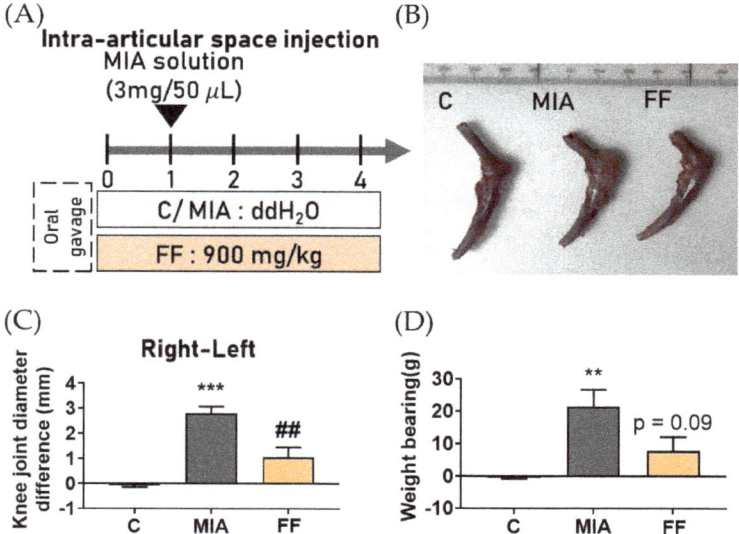

Figure 2. The effects of oligo-fucoidan-based formula intervention on the symptoms of OA. (**A**) Flow chart of the procedure. (**B**) Knee appearance after treatment. (**C**) Knee diameter difference. (**D**) Weight bearing ability. The experimental groups were the following: C, control group; MIA, MIA-induced group; FF, oligo-fucoidan-based formula (FF) 900 mg/kg + MIA-induced group. Statistical significance is denoted as ** $p < 0.01$; *** $p < 0.001$ compared with the control group, and ## $p < 0.01$ compared with the MIA-induced group.

The data obtained from the incapacitance tester were calculated using the following formula: the pressure ratio between the non-induced side and the MIA-induced side was determined to assess the difference in hind-limb pressure [14]. The results indicated a significant transfer of pressure to the non-induced side in the MIA-induced group, while the groups treated with the oligo-fucoidan-based formula exhibited a trend t restoring joint function (Figure 2D). These results indicated that the oligo-fucoidan-based formula has a potential protective effect on MIA-induced osteoarthritis symptoms.

2.3. Oligo-Fucoidan-Based Formula Toxicity Evaluation

Changes in organ weight are recognized as highly sensitive indicators of organ damage in determining compound toxicity [15]. The results revealed that following 4 weeks of treatment, the administration of the oligo-fucoidan-based formula had no distinct effect on body weight or on the weight changes of other major organs, including the heart, liver, spleen, kidneys, and testes. These findings suggest that prolonged intervention with the oligo-fucoidan-based formula would not cause any toxicity (Figure 3).

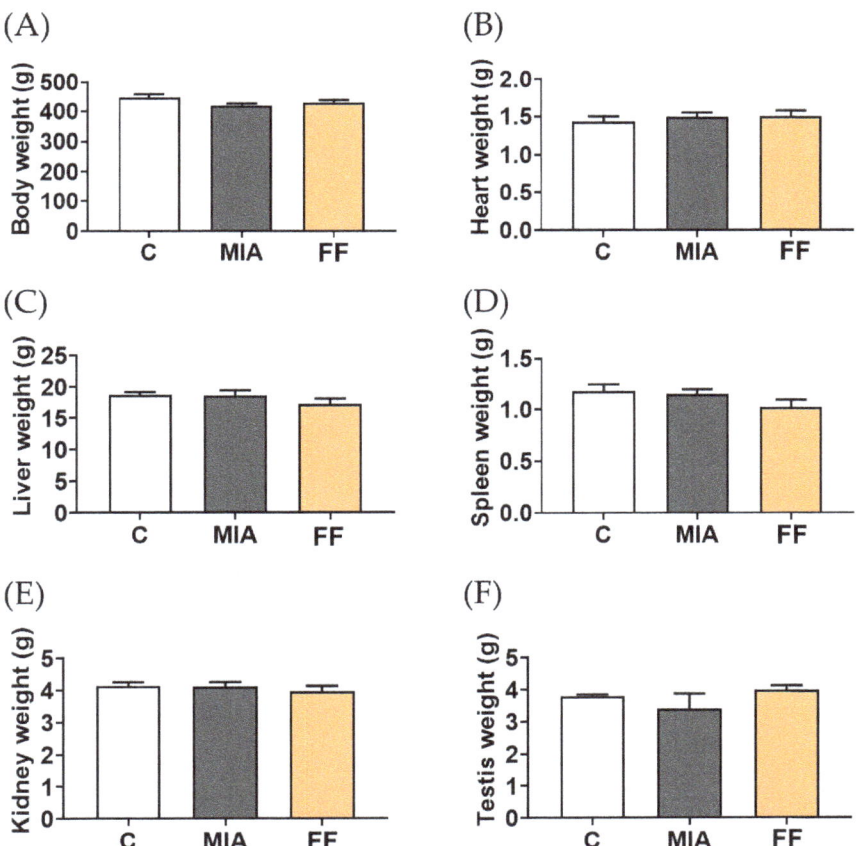

Figure 3. The toxicity evaluation of oligo-fucoidan-based formula intervention. The examination of body weight (**A**), heart (**B**), liver (**C**), spleen (**D**), kidney (**E**), and testis weight (**F**) showed no significant differences after the intervention. The experimental groups were the following: C, control group; MIA, MIA-induced group; FF, oligo-fucoidan-based formula (FF) 900 mg/kg + MIA-induced group.

2.4. Cytokine Secretion and Malondialdehyde (MDA) Concentration

Due to the inflammatory cytokines induced by MIA playing a critical role as mediators of pathology in the progression of OA, it was essential to explore whether the oligo-fucoidan-based formula could alleviate cytokine secretion. The serum level of the inflammatory cytokine IL-6 was analyzed for this purpose. The results showed that MIA-induced osteoarthritis significantly increased the IL-6 content, enhancing its inflammatory response. However, after three weeks of intervention with the oligo-fucoidan-based formula, the inflammatory response induced by MIA was significantly restored, indicating its potential to delay joint pain and swelling, possibly through reducing inflammation (Figure 4A).

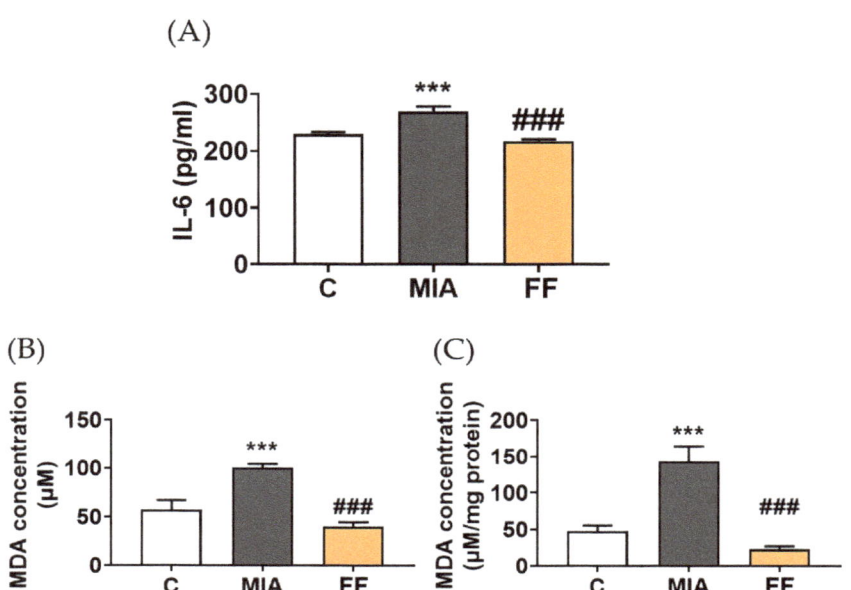

Figure 4. Cytokine secretion and oxidative stress evaluation. (**A**) IL-6 levels were evaluated after the intervention. (**B**) The serum MDA concentration and (**C**) tissue MDA concentration were evaluated by the TBARS assay. The experimental groups were the following: C, control group; MIA, MIA-induced group; FF, oligo-fucoidan-based formula (FF) 900 mg/kg + MIA-induced group. Statistical significance is denoted as *** indicating $p < 0.001$ compared with the control group, and ### indicating $p < 0.001$ compared with the MIA-induced group.

Elevated levels of IL-6 may induce the production of reactive oxygen species (ROS), leading to the degradation of the cartilage extracellular matrix and subsequent joint dysfunction [16]. To understand the effect of the oligo-fucoidan-based formula on ROS release, the measurement of malondialdehyde (MDA) was conducted, revealing a potential oxygen radical activity that is indicative of an inflammatory status [17]. As shown in Figure 4B,C, the generation of MDA was observed in the MIA group both in serum and tissue, while oligo-fucoidan-based formula intervention successfully decreased the MDA concentration. The results suggest that the oligo-fucoidan-based formula had a preventive ability on MIA-induced osteoarthritis via the inhibition of inflammation and oxidative stress.

2.5. Histological Assessment

Next, in order to understand the histology of cartilage integrity and to explore whether the oligo-fucoidan-based formula could have a recovery effect on MIA-induced osteoarthritis, we utilized histological assessment by employing hematoxylin and eosin (H&E) staining and Masson's trichrome staining in the articular cartilage. In the MIA group, the articular cartilage displayed surface irregularities (as shown by the red arrow), accompanied by extracellular matrix leakage (as shown by the yellow arrow), compared with the control group (Figure 5). These observations suggest the initiation of cartilage degeneration and structural damage caused by MIA.

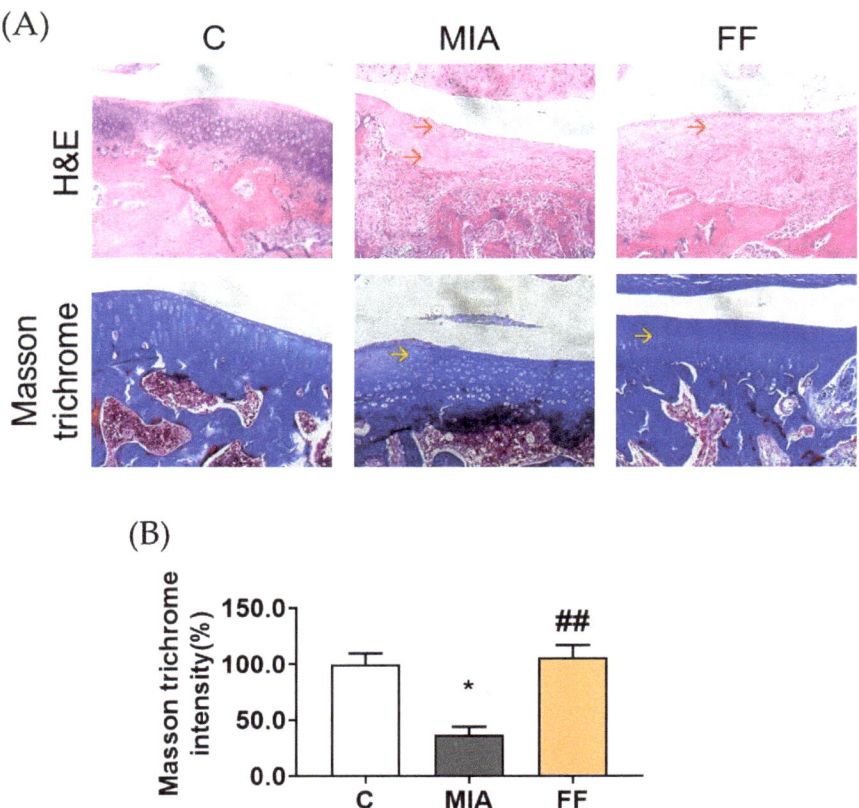

Figure 5. Histological appearance of the articular cartilage after the intervention. (**A**) Histological image after staining with H&E and Masson trichrome. (**B**) Quantification of the Masson trichrome intensity. The experimental groups were the following: C, control group; MIA, MIA-induced group; FF, oligo-fucoidan-based formula (FF) 900 mg/kg + MIA-induced group. Red arrow: articular cartilage showing some irregularities on the surface. Yellow arrow: extracellular matrix leakage. Statistical significance is denoted as * indicating $p < 0.05$ compared with the control group, and ##, indicating $p < 0.01$ compared with the MIA-induced group.

In contrast, there was an opposite consequence in the oligo-fucoidan-based formula group; the articular cartilage appeared more preserved, with fewer surface irregularities and reduced extracellular matrix leakage as shown in the quantitative results (Figure 5). This observation suggests that oligo-fucoidan-based formula intervention may help mitigate cartilage degeneration and maintain structural integrity, potentially contributing to improved joint health.

2.6. Modulation of Related Pathways

To comprehensively examine the potential modulation effects and molecular pathways influenced by the oligo-fucoidan-based formula in MIA-induced osteoarthritis, the protein expression of key markers, including phosphorylated p38 (p-p38), inducible nitric oxide synthase (iNOS), and cyclooxygenase-2 (COX-2), were assessed using Western blot analysis.

The results revealed that in the MIA model group, there was a notable increase in the protein expression of phosphorylated p38, iNOS, and COX-2, while oligo-fucoidan-based formula intervention demonstrated a significant reduction in p-p38 signaling, along with decreased protein expression of downstream targets such as iNOS and COX-2. These findings suggest that the oligo-fucoidan-based formula may exert its effects by modulating these pathways, thereby potentially contributing to its anti-inflammatory and protective properties in the context of joint health (Figure 6).

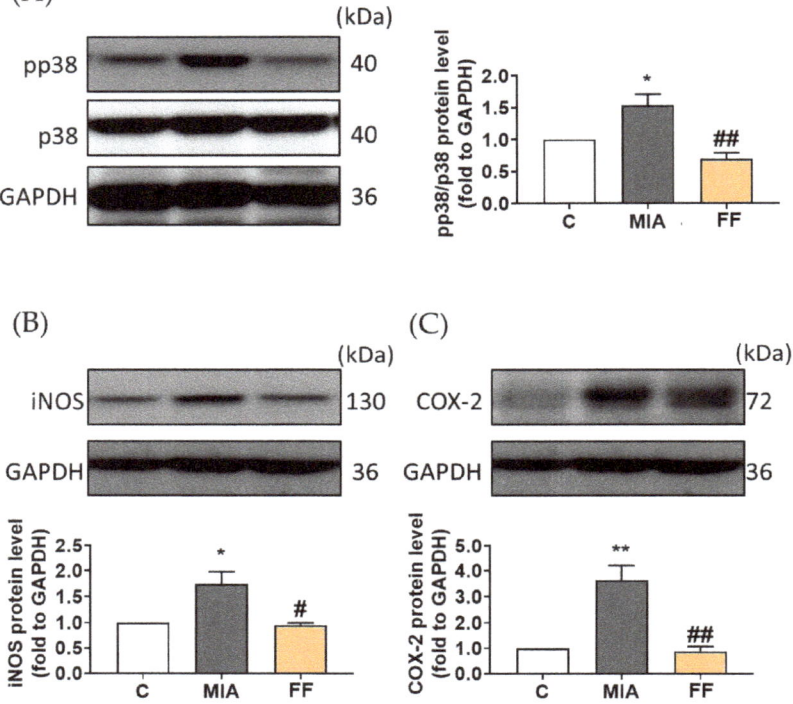

Figure 6. Related pathway modulation in oligo-fucoidan-based formula modulation. (**A**) pp38/p38, (**B**) iNOS, and (**C**) COX-2 protein expression was examined by Western blotting. The experimental groups were the following: C, control group; MIA, MIA-induced group; FF, oligo-fucoidan-based formula (FF) 900 mg/kg + MIA-induced group. Statistical significance is denoted as * $p < 0.05$; ** $p < 0.01$ compared with the control group, and # $p < 0.05$; ## $p < 0.01$ compared with the MIA-induced group.

3. Discussion

Here, we present evidence supporting the protective role of an oligo-fucoidan-based formula in the progression of osteoarthritis (OA). The oligo-fucoidan-based formula acts by modulating the p38 signaling pathway and reducing the expression of COX-2 and iNOS, which enables it to alleviate joint burden and inflammation. This indicates its potential to mitigate OA progression by targeting key inflammatory pathways and processes involved in joint degeneration.

Excessive oxidative stress production may occur during the progression of OA due to the relatively low oxygen supply in cartilage [18]. This imbalance between the production of reactive oxygen species (ROS) and antioxidative defense mechanisms in the joint tissue can lead to oxidative damage and contribute to the pathogenesis of OA. In the context of OA pathology, situations such as ischemia–reperfusion phenomena can trigger oxygen responses, further exacerbating ROS production. ROS, including superoxide anions, hydrogen peroxide, and hydroxyl radicals, are highly reactive molecules that can cause damage to cellular components [19]. This oxidative damage can disrupt the normal functioning of chondrocytes, leading to cartilage degradation and joint dysfunction. Additionally, ROS can stimulate inflammatory responses by activating signaling pathways involved in the production of pro-inflammatory cytokines and mediators [20]. Thus, the interplay between oxidative stress and inflammation accelerates and participates in the crucial pathogenesis of OA, highlighting the importance of targeting ROS-mediated pathways for therapeutic intervention in OA management.

Clinical treatments for OA are divided into medication and dietary supplementation. Medications commonly prescribed for OA management include the non-steroidal anti-inflammatory drugs (NSAIDs), acetaminophen, and serotonin–norepinephrine reuptake inhibitors (SNRIs). However, it is crucial to acknowledge the potential side effects associated with these medications [21]. Acetaminophen, while effective in managing pain, carries the risk of causing liver damage, elevating transient liver enzymes, and inducing hepatotoxicity [22]. NSAIDs, often used to alleviate pain and inflammation, can lead to gastrointestinal discomfort and may exacerbate pre-existing kidney conditions [23]. SNRIs, which are primarily indicated for treating depression and mood disorders, can result in adverse effects such as fatigue and sexual dysfunction [24].

These side effects underscore the need for alternative treatment options with fewer adverse reactions. Natural compounds with antioxidative properties have shown advantages in alleviating OA progression through animal studies. Resveratrol, a natural polyphenol compound, has demonstrated the ability to restore chondrocyte apoptosis, alleviate oxidative stress, and improve disease progression [25,26]. Galangin, a bioactive flavonoid, has been shown to minimize ROS production, elevate antioxidative enzyme levels, and reduce inflammatory cytokines related to OA. These effects contribute to an improvement in OA performance [27]. By harnessing the therapeutic potential of nature's resources, we can provide patients with OA relief while minimizing the risk of adverse reactions, ultimately improving their quality of life.

Fucoidan, a prominent component of the oligo-fucoidan-based formula, has garnered attention for its multifaceted biological properties. Studies have revealed its ability to regulate key signaling pathways such as the MAPK pathway, which plays a pivotal role in mediating cellular responses to various stimuli, including inflammation and oxidative stress. The MAPK pathway encompasses a cascade of protein kinase reactions that ultimately regulate gene expression, cell proliferation, differentiation, and apoptosis. By modulating the MAPK signaling transduction, fucoidan can exert antioxidative effects, thereby mitigating tissue damage and promoting cellular resilience. Moreover, fucoidan has been demonstrated to attenuate ROS generation, further enhancing its protective capabilities against oxidative damage. While ROS play essential roles in cellular signaling and host defense mechanisms, excessive ROS production can lead to oxidative stress, resulting in damage to lipids, proteins, and DNA. In the context of osteoarthritis (OA), oxidative stress contributes to cartilage degradation, inflammation, and joint tissue damage [28]. Fucoidan's ability to scavenge ROS and modulate antioxidative enzyme activity helps maintain the redox balance within the joint microenvironment, thereby alleviating OA symptoms and slowing disease progression. These properties of fucoidan extend beyond joint health, as evidenced by its efficacy in protecting against retinal harm. Oxidative stress in the retina contributes to the development and progression of various eye disease, including age-related macular degeneration (AMD), diabetic retinopathy, and glaucoma [29]. Fucoidan's antioxidative properties help mitigate retinal oxidative damage, thereby preserving retinal function and preventing the vision loss associated with these conditions [30].

In OA, the expression of inducible nitric oxide synthase (iNOS) and cyclooxygenase-2 (COX-2) is regulated by the MAPK signaling pathway, which is modulated by cytokines and the breakdown of the extracellular matrix. In our study, we observed that oligo-fucoidan-based formula intervention suppressed inflammation and downregulated the expression of phosphorylated p38 (p-p38), iNOS, and COX-2 [31]. These findings suggest a modulatory role for the oligo-fucoidan-based formula in attenuating OA-associated inflammation and ECM degradation through the regulation of the MAPK signaling pathway.

Moreover, pain associated with OA could be exacerbated by the presence of ROS, which activate MAPK signaling and modulate COX-2 expression. MIA, acting as an inhibitor of glyceraldehyde-3-phosphate dehydrogenase, induces cartilage degradation, leading to ROS accumulation and inflammation. This pathological mechanism closely resembles the progression of OA, where cartilage degradation, ROS accumulation, and inflammation contribute to the development and exacerbation of pain symptoms [32].

With the observation of the downregulation of p-p38, inducible nitric oxide synthase (iNOS), and COX-2 expression after oligo-fucoidan-based formula treatment, potential improvement by the oligo-fucoidan-based formula in the monosodium iodoacetate (MIA)-induced animal model was suggested. This was accompanied by modulation of the MAPK pathway and the regulation of inflammatory cytokine release. These findings demonstrate the potential role of the oligo-fucoidan-based formula as a therapeutic agent in OA management.

Previous studies have demonstrated the multifaceted modulatory capabilities of fucoidan, including its formulation's role in reducing COX-2 expression and cytokine secretion [33]. Through its modulation of iNOS expression and IL-6 secretion and its reduction of MAPK signaling, fucoidan exhibits promising potential in relieving symptoms associated with OA [34]. These findings underscore the broad therapeutic potential of fucoidan in addressing the complex pathophysiology of OA and highlight its role as a promising candidate for the development of OA-relieving interventions.

The remaining 70% of the oligo-fucoidan-based formula consists of UC-II®, undenatured type II collagen, hyaluronic acid, chondroitin, calcium carbonate, glucosamine, and excipients. These components have been reported to have potential effectiveness in OA progression. Among them, UC-II has been found to be the most effective and is one of the most commonly used supplements on the market [35]. Additionally, a study demonstrated inflammatory alleviation and pain relief by UC-II in combination with glucosamine hydrochloride and chondroitin sulfate during a 150-day treatment period [36]. However, due to commercial confidentiality and the limitations in these studies, we cannot conclusively determine the effectiveness and synergistic effect of UC-II or of oligo-fucoidan. Nevertheless, it is worth noting that the oligo-fucoidan-based formula may offer enhanced antioxidative and anti-inflammatory abilities, potentially contributing to improved OA progression. Nevertheless, further studies are warranted to fully elucidate its efficacy and potential benefits in clinical settings.

This study highlights the potential functional efficacy of the oligo-fucoidan-based formula for osteoarthritis, underscoring its role as a promising substance. Given the multifactorial nature of OA, which involves many mechanisms, there is a growing interest in exploring novel treatment approaches using advanced "omics" tools, including genomics, proteomics, metabolomics, and transcriptomics. Building upon these findings, further studies employing multi-omics technologies will be crucial in investigating the underlying mechanisms of action of the oligo-fucoidan-based formula in OA treatment, thereby offering valuable insights into its therapeutic potential [37,38].

4. Materials and Methods

4.1. Reagents

The oligo-fucoidan-based formula (FF) provided by HiQ Marine Biotech (Taipei, Taiwan) and branded as Joint-free®, comprises UC-II® and undenatured type II collagen, along with food-grade effective hyaluronic acid, high-purity chondroitin, oligo-fucoidan (OliFuco®), calcium carbonate, and glucosamine. Its key ingredient is oligo-fucoidan (comprising more than 30% of the formula), derived from naturally dried oceanic brown seaweed; specifically, Laminaria japonica.

In brief, the preparation of oligo-fucoidan involves subjecting the crude extract of Laminaria japonica to elution with a sodium chloride gradient using a DEAE (diethylaminoethyl)-Sephadex A-25 column. The fucose- and sulfate-enriched fraction is then preserved by hydrolyzing it with glycolytic enzymes [39] to an average MW of 1.2 kDa (~90.1%) [40]. The components of oligo-fucoidan have been reported to consist of sulfate and neutral monosaccharides comprising fucose, glucose, galactose, myo-inositol, mannose, xylose, and rhamnose [40].

4.2. Cell Culture and Treatment

Raw264.7 cells were kindly provided by Professor Yong-Han Hong (National Taiwan Normal University, Taipei, Taiwan). These were cultured in DMEM(HG) (Gibco, Life Technologies, Carlsbad, CA, USA) supplemented with 10% fetal bovine serum (FBS) (Corning, New York, NY, USA) and a 1% Antibiotic-Antimycotic (Corning) solution in a 5% CO_2, 37 °C incubator. The aim was to evaluate the formula and the related components' ability in suppressing iNOS expression. The FF, FF without oligo-fucoidan, oligo-fucoidan, and UC-II supplied from Hi-Q were co-treated with 1 µg/mL of lipopolysaccharides from Escherichia coli O111:B4 (Sigma Aldrich, St. Louis, MO, USA), based on a previous study [41].

4.3. Animal Osteoarthritis Model and Evaluation

Four-week-old Wistar rats were used in this study. Osteoarthritis was induced by the intra-articular injection of 3 mg of monosodium iodoacetate (MIA, Sigma-Aldrich, St. Louis, MO, USA) dissolved in 50 µL of 0.9% saline into the ligament of the right knees using a 29-gauge, 0.5-inch needle, while the control group received saline injections [42,43]. Body weight and knee joint width were measured prior to injection to establish baseline values. All animal procedures were approved by the IAUAC (No: LAC-2021-0308). The experimental group received the oligo-fucoidan-based formula (FF group), which was administered orally via oral gavage (0.9 mL/rat dissolved in ddH_2O) for 4 weeks, beginning one week before the injection and continuing starting the day after injection, while the control group received standard care. Body weight and knee joint width were monitored weekly post-injection to assess disease progression. Bilateral weight-bearing pressure distribution was evaluated every two weeks using the incapacitance test to measure pain and functional impairment.

4.4. Bilateral Weight-Bearing Test

The bilateral weight-bearing test is employed to quantify weight distribution during the hind-limb stance and serves as an indicator for assessing joint pain and discomfort in animals. In physiological conditions, rats typically exhibit an equitable weight distribution across their hind limbs, resulting in a bilateral pressure difference approaching zero. Conversely, unilateral knee joint injury in rats necessitates the non-injured hind limb to support a greater portion of the body weight, leading to an elevation in the bilateral pressure difference attributable to pain sensation. The Incapacitance tester (Ugo Basile Biological Instruments, Gemonio, Italy), designed specifically for this purpose, facilitates the measurement of hind-limb weight distribution. Rats undergo preliminary training to stand on their hind limbs within a force plate box outfitted with a 65° inclined plane. Subsequently, during formal testing, this force plate box is positioned atop the bilateral weight-bearing test apparatus, enabling rats to autonomously assume a hind-limb stance. The bilateral weight-bearing test apparatus then records and analyzes the pressure difference between the two hind limbs individually. Following five repetitions of this procedure, the average pressure difference is computed to derive a representative value.

4.5. Measurement of Knee Joint Width

Knee joint width was measured from both right and left knees using an electronic digital caliper.

4.6. IL-6 Level Measurement

The evaluation of serum levels of the inflammatory cytokine IL-6 was performed using a commercially available enzyme-linked immunosorbent assay (ELISA) kit obtained from Abcam (Cambridge, UK). The procedure was conducted following the manufacturer's instructions.

4.7. Thiobarbituric Acid-Reactive Substances (TBARS) Assay

The assessment of malondialdehyde (MDA) concentration was conducted using a commercially available assay kit obtained from Cayman Chemical (Ann Arbor, MI, USA). The procedure was carried out according to the manufacturer's instructions. Briefly, samples were treated with sodium dodecyl sulfate (SDS), followed by the addition of sodium hydroxide (NaOH) and 2-thiobarbituric acid (TBA). The mixture was then subjected to boiling at 95 °C for 1 h. Absorbance measurements were performed at the 532 nm wavelength.

4.8. Histological Examination

Following sacrifice, knee joints were harvested and fixed in 10% formalin solution for 48 h. Subsequently, the samples underwent dehydration with ethanol, embedding in paraffin, and sectioning into 4 μm slices for staining. Hematoxylin and eosin (H&E), as well as Masson's trichrome staining procedures, were conducted by Bio-Check Laboratories Ltd. (Taipei, Taiwan). Masson's trichrome staining marks collagen via blue staining, and Image J was used for quantifying the blue area [44].

4.9. Western Blot

The hind-limb knee joints were excised and lysed using lysis buffer containing RIPA supplemented with phosphatase and protease inhibitors (Roche, Basel, Switzerland). The tissue was homogenized using a homogenizer. Protein quantification was performed using the BCA assay (T-Pro Biotechnology, New Taipei City, Taiwan). Subsequently, sodium dodecyl sulfate polyacrylamide gel electrophoresis (SDS-PAGE) was utilized for protein separation, followed by transfer to a polyvinylidene fluoride (PVDF) membrane (Millipore Sigma, Billerica, MA, USA) using a Bio-Rad equivalent system (Bio-Rad, Hercules, USA). Blocking was carried out using 5% BSA (Biomax, Taipei, Taiwan). The primary antibodies against pp38 and p38 from Cell Signaling (Boston, MA, USA) and against iNOS, COX-2, and GAPDH from Proteintech (Rosemont, IL, USA) were incubated overnight at 4 °C. After washing thrice for 10 min each with TBST (T-Pro), an HRP-conjugated goat anti-rabbit IgG secondary antibody (Jackson ImmunoResearch Laboratories, West Grove, PA, USA) was applied for 2 h at room temperature. Signal capture was performed using the eBlot Touch Imager™ (eBlot Photoelectric Technology, Shanghai, China), and quantification was conducted using Image J software (Version 1.53t, NIH, Bethesda, MD, USA).

4.10. Statistical Analysis

The data are presented as the mean ± standard error of the mean (SEM). Statistical analyses were performed using GraphPad Prism, version 9.0. The student's t-test and one-way analysis of variance (ANOVA) followed by Tukey's post hoc test were employed for comparisons. Results with a p-value of less than 0.05 were considered statistically significant.

5. Conclusions

In conclusion, our study underscores the efficacy of oligo-fucoidan-based formula (FF) intervention in mitigating the progression of OA. Through its ability to alleviate joint burden and inflammation, the oligo-fucoidan-based formula shows promise as a therapeutic intervention. Histological assessments revealed substantial improvements in cartilage integrity following oligo-fucoidan-based formula intervention, indicating its protective effects against cartilage degeneration and structural damage. Furthermore, the modulation of the p38 signaling pathway, coupled with the downregulation of COX-2 and iNOS expression, sheds light on the mechanistic insights underlying oligo-fucoidan-based formula's beneficial effects. These findings underscore the therapeutic potential of the oligo-fucoidan-based formula in mitigating OA-associated joint dysfunction and inflammation, offering new avenues for targeted interventions in OA management. Further clinical investigations are warranted to validate these preclinical findings and to explore the translational potential of the oligo-fucoidan-based formula in OA patients.

Author Contributions: Conceptualization, Y.-F.C. and S.-M.H.; methodology, Y.-F.C., K.-C.H. and K.-L.W.; software, Y.-J.H., H.-Y.C. and M.A.; validation, Y.-F.C. and S.-M.H.; formal analysis, Y.-F.C. and K.-C.H.; investigation, Y.-F.C.; resources, K.-L.W., Y.-J.H. and S.-M.H.; data curation, Y.-F.C. and K.-C.H.; writing—original draft preparation, Y.-F.C.; writing—review and editing, S.-M.H.; visualization, Y.-F.C., K.-C.H. and S.-M.H.; supervision, T.-M.S. and S.-M.H.; project administration, S.-M.H.; funding acquisition, S.-M.H. All authors have read and agreed to the published version of the manuscript.

Funding: This research was funded by the grants NSTC111–2811-B-038-022, NSTC111-2314-B-038-006, NSTC111-2628-B-038-019, 112-2320-B-038-010-MY3 and NSTC112-2811-B-038-044 from the National Science and Technology Council, Taiwan.

Institutional Review Board Statement: The animal study protocol was approved by the Ethics Committee of Taipei Medical University IAUAC (No: LAC-2021-0308), approved on 3 November 2021.

Informed Consent Statement: Not applicable.

Data Availability Statement: The data presented in this study are available on request from the corresponding author.

Conflicts of Interest: The authors declare no conflicts of interest. The funders had no role in the design of the study; in the collection, analyses, or interpretation of the data; in the writing of the manuscript; or in the decision to publish the results.

References

1. Tonge, D.P.; Pearson, M.J.; Jones, S.W. The hallmarks of osteoarthritis and the potential to develop personalised disease-modifying pharmacological therapeutics. *Osteoarthr. Cartil.* **2014**, *22*, 609–621. [CrossRef]
2. Philp, A.M.; Davis, E.T.; Jones, S.W. Developing anti-inflammatory therapeutics for patients with osteoarthritis. *Rheumatology* **2017**, *56*, 869–881. [CrossRef] [PubMed]
3. Tekari, A.; Luginbuehl, R.; Hofstetter, W.; Egli, R.J. Chondrocytes expressing intracellular collagen type ii enter the cell cycle and co-express collagen type i in monolayer culture. *J. Orthop. Res.* **2014**, *32*, 1503–1511. [CrossRef]
4. Cicuttini, F.M.; Wluka, A.E. Osteoarthritis: Is oa a mechanical or systemic disease? *Nat. Rev. Rheumatol.* **2014**, *10*, 515–516. [CrossRef]
5. Molnar, V.; Matišić, V.; Kodvanj, I.; Bjelica, R.; Jeleč, Ž.; Hudetz, D.; Rod, E.; Čukelj, F.; Vrdoljak, T.; Vidović, D.; et al. Cytokines and chemokines involved in osteoarthritis pathogenesis. *Int. J. Mol. Sci.* **2021**, *22*, 9208. [CrossRef]
6. Kapoor, M.; Martel-Pelletier, J.; Lajeunesse, D.; Pelletier, J.P.; Fahmi, H. Role of proinflammatory cytokines in the pathophysiology of osteoarthritis. *Nat. Rev. Rheumatol.* **2011**, *7*, 33–42. [CrossRef]
7. Shin, M.R.; Lee, J.A.; Kim, M.J.; Park, H.J.; Park, B.W.; Seo, S.B.; Roh, S.S. Protective effects of *Phellinus linteus* mycelium on the development of osteoarthritis after monosodium iodoacetate injection. *Evid. Based Complement. Alternat. Med.* **2020**, *2020*, 7240858. [CrossRef]
8. Lee, Y.T.; Yunus, M.H.M.; Ugusman, A.; Yazid, M.D. Natural compounds affecting inflammatory pathways of osteoarthritis. *Antioxidants* **2022**, *11*, 1722. [CrossRef]
9. Bijlsma, J.W.; Berenbaum, F.; Lafeber, F.P. Osteoarthritis: An update with relevance for clinical practice. *Lancet* **2011**, *377*, 2115–2126. [CrossRef] [PubMed]
10. Brandt, K.D. Effects of nonsteroidal anti-inflammatory drugs on chondrocyte metabolism in vitro and in vivo. *Am. J. Med.* **1987**, *83*, 29–34. [CrossRef] [PubMed]
11. Park, H.Y.; Han, M.H.; Park, C.; Jin, C.Y.; Kim, G.Y.; Choi, I.W.; Kim, N.D.; Nam, T.J.; Kwon, T.K.; Choi, Y.H. Anti-inflammatory effects of fucoidan through inhibition of nf-κb, mapk and akt activation in lipopolysaccharide-induced bv2 microglia cells. *Food Chem. Toxicol. Int. J. Publ. Br. Ind. Biol. Res. Assoc.* **2011**, *49*, 1745–1752. [CrossRef] [PubMed]
12. Chau, Y.T.; Chen, H.Y.; Lin, P.H.; Hsia, S.M. Preventive effects of fucoidan and fucoxanthin on hyperuricemic rats induced by potassium oxonate. *Mar. Drugs* **2019**, *17*, 343. [CrossRef] [PubMed]

13. Vasarri, M.; Barletta, E.; Degl'Innocenti, D. Marine migrastatics: A comprehensive 2022 update. *Mar. Drugs* **2022**, *20*, 273. [CrossRef]
14. Di Cesare Mannelli, L.; Micheli, L.; Zanardelli, M.; Ghelardini, C. Low dose native type ii collagen prevents pain in a rat osteoarthritis model. *BMC Musculoskelet. Disord.* **2013**, *14*, 228. [CrossRef]
15. Lazic, S.E.; Semenova, E.; Williams, D.P. Determining organ weight toxicity with bayesian causal models: Improving on the analysis of relative organ weights. *Sci. Rep.* **2020**, *10*, 6625. [CrossRef] [PubMed]
16. Ansari, M.Y.; Ahmad, N.; Haqqi, T.M. Oxidative stress and inflammation in osteoarthritis pathogenesis: Role of polyphenols. *Biomed. Pharmacother.* **2020**, *129*, 110452. [CrossRef]
17. Cherian, D.A.; Peter, T.; Narayanan, A.; Madhavan, S.S.; Achammada, S.; Vynat, G.P. Malondialdehyde as a marker of oxidative stress in periodontitis patients. *J. Pharm. Bioallied Sci.* **2019**, *11*, S297–S300. [CrossRef]
18. Blake, D.R.; Merry, P.; Unsworth, J.; Kidd, B.L.; Outhwaite, J.M.; Ballard, R.; Morris, C.J.; Gray, L.; Lunec, J. Hypoxic-reperfusion injury in the inflamed human joint. *Lancet* **1989**, *1*, 289–293. [CrossRef]
19. Koike, M.; Nojiri, H.; Ozawa, Y.; Watanabe, K.; Muramatsu, Y.; Kaneko, H.; Morikawa, D.; Kobayashi, K.; Saita, Y.; Sasho, T.; et al. Mechanical overloading causes mitochondrial superoxide and sod2 imbalance in chondrocytes resulting in cartilage degeneration. *Sci. Rep.* **2015**, *5*, 11722. [CrossRef]
20. Mathy-Hartert, M.; Deby-Dupont, G.P.; Reginster, J.Y.; Ayache, N.; Pujol, J.P.; Henrotin, Y.E. Regulation by reactive oxygen species of interleukin-1beta, nitric oxide and prostaglandin e(2) production by human chondrocytes. *Osteoarthr. Cartil.* **2002**, *10*, 547–555. [CrossRef]
21. Zhang, W.; Robertson, W.B.; Zhao, J.; Chen, W.; Xu, J. Emerging trend in the pharmacotherapy of osteoarthritis. *Front. Endocrinol.* **2019**, *10*, 431. [CrossRef]
22. Hochberg, M.C.; Altman, R.D.; April, K.T.; Benkhalti, M.; Guyatt, G.; McGowan, J.; Towheed, T.; Welch, V.; Wells, G.; Tugwell, P. American college of rheumatology 2012 recommendations for the use of nonpharmacologic and pharmacologic therapies in osteoarthritis of the hand, hip, and knee. *Arthritis Care Res.* **2012**, *64*, 465–474. [CrossRef] [PubMed]
23. Bally, M.; Dendukuri, N.; Rich, B.; Nadeau, L.; Helin-Salmivaara, A.; Garbe, E.; Brophy, J.M. Risk of acute myocardial infarction with nsaids in real world use: Bayesian meta-analysis of individual patient data. *BMJ* **2017**, *357*, j1909. [CrossRef] [PubMed]
24. da Costa, B.R.; Nüesch, E.; Reichenbach, S.; Jüni, P.; Rutjes, A.W. Doxycycline for osteoarthritis of the knee or hip. *Cochrane Database Syst. Rev.* **2012**, *11*, Cd007323. [CrossRef]
25. Wang, J.; Gao, J.S.; Chen, J.W.; Li, F.; Tian, J. Effect of resveratrol on cartilage protection and apoptosis inhibition in experimental osteoarthritis of rabbit. *Rheumatol. Int.* **2012**, *32*, 1541–1548. [CrossRef] [PubMed]
26. Wei, Y.; Jia, J.; Jin, X.; Tong, W.; Tian, H. Resveratrol ameliorates inflammatory damage and protects against osteoarthritis in a rat model of osteoarthritis. *Mol. Med. Rep.* **2018**, *17*, 1493–1498. [CrossRef]
27. Su, Y.; Shen, L.; Xue, J.; Zou, J.; Wan, D.; Shi, Z. Therapeutic evaluation of galangin on cartilage protection and analgesic activity in a rat model of osteoarthritis. *Electron. J. Biotechnol.* **2021**, *53*, 8–13. [CrossRef]
28. Lepetsos, P.; Papavassiliou, A.G. Ros/oxidative stress signaling in osteoarthritis. *Biochim. Biophys. Acta* **2016**, *1862*, 576–591. [CrossRef]
29. Wang, K.; Chen, Y.S.; Chien, H.W.; Chiou, H.L.; Yang, S.F.; Hsieh, Y.H. Melatonin inhibits naio(3)-induced arpe-19 cell apoptosis via suppression of hif-1α/bnip3-lc3b/mitophagy signaling. *Cell Biosci.* **2022**, *12*, 133. [CrossRef]
30. Li, X.; Zhao, H.; Wang, Q.; Liang, H.; Jiang, X. Fucoidan protects arpe-19 cells from oxidative stress via normalization of reactive oxygen species generation through the ca^{2+}-dependent erk signaling pathway. *Mol. Med. Rep.* **2015**, *11*, 3746–3752. [CrossRef]
31. Meng, X.; Sun, L.; Meng, X.; Bi, Q. The protective effect of ergolide in osteoarthritis: In vitro and in vivo studies. *Int. Immunopharmacol.* **2024**, *127*, 111355. [CrossRef]
32. Zahan, O.M.; Serban, O.; Gherman, C.; Fodor, D. The evaluation of oxidative stress in osteoarthritis. *Med. Pharm. Rep.* **2020**, *93*, 12–22. [CrossRef] [PubMed]
33. Manikandan, R.; Parimalanandhini, D.; Mahalakshmi, K.; Beulaja, M.; Arumugam, M.; Janarthanan, S.; Palanisamy, S.; You, S.; Prabhu, N.M. Studies on isolation, characterization of fucoidan from brown algae turbinaria decurrens and evaluation of it's in vivo and in vitro anti-inflammatory activities. *Int. J. Biol. Macromol.* **2020**, *160*, 1263–1276. [CrossRef] [PubMed]
34. Apostolova, E.; Lukova, P.; Baldzhieva, A.; Katsarov, P.; Nikolova, M.; Iliev, I.; Peychev, L.; Trica, B.; Oancea, F.; Delattre, C.; et al. Immunomodulatory and anti-inflammatory effects of fucoidan: A review. *Polymers* **2020**, *12*, 2338. [CrossRef] [PubMed]
35. Gencoglu, H.; Orhan, C.; Sahin, E.; Sahin, K. Undenatured type ii collagen (uc-ii) in joint health and disease: A review on the current knowledge of companion animals. *Animals* **2020**, *10*, 697. [CrossRef]
36. Gupta, R.C.; Canerdy, T.D.; Lindley, J.; Konemann, M.; Minniear, J.; Carroll, B.A.; Hendrick, C.; Goad, J.T.; Rohde, K.; Doss, R.; et al. Comparative therapeutic efficacy and safety of type-ii collagen (uc-ii), glucosamine and chondroitin in arthritic dogs: Pain evaluation by ground force plate. *J. Anim. Physiol. Anim. Nutr.* **2012**, *96*, 770–777. [CrossRef]
37. Gonzalez-Alvarez, M.E.; Sanchez-Romero, E.A.; Turroni, S.; Fernandez-Carnero, J.; Villafañe, J.H. Correlation between the altered gut microbiome and lifestyle interventions in chronic widespread pain patients: A systematic review. *Medicina* **2023**, *59*, 256. [CrossRef]
38. Kraus, V.B.; Reed, A.; Soderblom, E.J.; Moseley, M.A.; Hsueh, M.F.; Attur, M.G.; Samuels, J.; Abramson, S.B.; Li, Y.J. Serum proteomic panel validated for prediction of knee osteoarthritis progression. *Osteoarthr. Cartil. Open* **2024**, *6*, 100425. [CrossRef]

39. Liao, C.H.; Lai, I.C.; Kuo, H.C.; Chuang, S.E.; Lee, H.L.; Whang-Peng, J.; Yao, C.J.; Lai, G.M. Epigenetic modification and differentiation induction of malignant glioma cells by oligo-fucoidan. *Mar. Drugs* **2019**, *17*, 525. [CrossRef]
40. Chen, L.M.; Yang, P.P.; Al Haq, A.T.; Hwang, P.A.; Lai, Y.C.; Weng, Y.S.; Chen, M.A.; Hsu, H.L. Oligo-fucoidan supplementation enhances the effect of olaparib on preventing metastasis and recurrence of triple-negative breast cancer in mice. *J. Biomed. Sci.* **2022**, *29*, 70. [CrossRef]
41. Cao, Y.; Chen, J.; Ren, G.; Zhang, Y.; Tan, X.; Yang, L. Punicalagin prevents inflammation in lps-induced raw264.7 macrophages by inhibiting foxo3a/autophagy signaling pathway. *Nutrients* **2019**, *11*, 2794. [CrossRef] [PubMed]
42. Takahashi, I.; Matsuzaki, T.; Kuroki, H.; Hoso, M. Induction of osteoarthritis by injecting monosodium iodoacetate into the patellofemoral joint of an experimental rat model. *PLoS ONE* **2018**, *13*, e0196625. [CrossRef] [PubMed]
43. Pitcher, T.; Sousa-Valente, J.; Malcangio, M. The monoiodoacetate model of osteoarthritis pain in the mouse. *J. Vis. Exp.* **2016**, *16*, 53746.
44. Chen, Y.; Yu, Q.; Xu, C.-B. A convenient method for quantifying collagen fibers in atherosclerotic lesions by imagej software. *Int. J. Clin. Exp. Med.* **2017**, *10*, 14927–14935.

Disclaimer/Publisher's Note: The statements, opinions and data contained in all publications are solely those of the individual author(s) and contributor(s) and not of MDPI and/or the editor(s). MDPI and/or the editor(s) disclaim responsibility for any injury to people or property resulting from any ideas, methods, instructions or products referred to in the content.

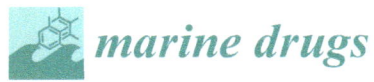

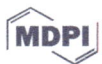

Article

Mining Xanthine Oxidase Inhibitors from an Edible Seaweed *Pterocladiella capillacea* by Using In Vitro Bioassays, Affinity Ultrafiltration LC-MS/MS, Metabolomics Tools, and In Silico Prediction

Yawen Wang [1,†], Longjian Zhou [1,2,3,†], Minqi Chen [1], Yayue Liu [1,2,3], Yu Yang [1], Tiantian Lu [1], Fangfang Ban [1], Xueqiong Hu [1], Zhongji Qian [1,2], Pengzhi Hong [1,2,3] and Yi Zhang [1,2,3,*]

1. Guangdong Provincial Key Laboratory of Aquatic Product Processing and Safety, Guangdong Provincial Engineering Laboratory for Marine Biological Products, Guangdong Provincial Center for Modern Agricultural Scientific Innovation, Shenzhen Institute of Guangdong Ocean University, Zhanjiang Municipal Key Laboratory of Marine Drugs and Nutrition for Brain Health, Research Institute for Marine Drugs and Nutrition, College of Food Science and Technology, Guangdong Ocean University, Zhanjiang 524088, China; yavin_wang@163.com (Y.W.); zhoulongjian@gdou.edu.cn (L.Z.); katelyn@outlook.com (M.C.); yayue_liu@163.com (Y.L.); yangyu515900@163.com (Y.Y.); lutiantiana@163.com (T.L.); banfangfang@126.com (F.B.); hxw247@163.com (X.H.); zjqian78@163.com (Z.Q.); hongpengzhi@126.com (P.H.)
2. Southern Marine Science and Engineering Guangdong Laboratory (Zhanjiang), Zhanjiang 524088, China
3. Collaborative Innovation Center of Seafood Deep Processing, Dalian Polytechnic University, Dalian 116034, China
* Correspondence: hubeizhangyi@163.com or zhangyi@gdou.edu.cn; Tel.: +86-759-239-6046
† These authors contributed equally to this work.

Abstract: The prevalence of gout and the adverse effects of current synthetic anti-gout drugs call for new natural and effective xanthine oxidase (XOD) inhibitors to target this disease. Based on our previous finding that an edible seaweed *Pterocladiella capillacea* extract inhibits XOD, XOD-inhibitory and anti-inflammatory activities were used to evaluate the anti-gout potential of different *P. capillacea* extract fractions. Through affinity ultrafiltration coupled with liquid chromatography tandem mass spectrometry (LC-MS/MS), feature-based molecular networking (FBMN), and database mining of multiple natural products, the extract's bioactive components were traced and annotated. Through molecular docking and ADMET analysis, the possibility and drug-likeness of the annotated XOD inhibitors were predicted. The results showed that fractions F4, F6, F4-2, and F4-3 exhibited strong XOD inhibition activity, among which F4-3 reached an inhibition ratio of 77.96% ± 4.91% to XOD at a concentration of 0.14 mg/mL. In addition, the *P. capillacea* extract and fractions also displayed anti-inflammatory activity. Affinity ultrafiltration LC-MS/MS analysis and molecular networking showed that out of the 20 annotated compounds, 8 compounds have been previously directly or indirectly reported from seaweeds, and 4 compounds have been reported to exhibit anti-gout activity. Molecular docking and ADMET showed that six seaweed-derived compounds can dock with the XOD activity pocket and follow the Lipinski drug-like rule. These results support the value of further investigating *P. capillacea* as part of the development of anti-gout drugs or related functional foods.

Keywords: *Pterocladiella capillacea*; xanthine oxidase inhibitors; anti-inflammatory; affinity ultrafiltration LC-MS/MS; molecular networking

Citation: Wang, Y.; Zhou, L.; Chen, M.; Liu, Y.; Yang, Y.; Lu, T.; Ban, F.; Hu, X.; Qian, Z.; Hong, P.; et al. Mining Xanthine Oxidase Inhibitors from an Edible Seaweed *Pterocladiella capillacea* by Using In Vitro Bioassays, Affinity Ultrafiltration LC-MS/MS, Metabolomics Tools, and In Silico Prediction. *Mar. Drugs* 2023, *21*, 502. https://doi.org/10.3390/md21100502

Academic Editors: Donatella Degl'Innocenti and Marzia Vasarri

Received: 20 August 2023
Revised: 16 September 2023
Accepted: 18 September 2023
Published: 22 September 2023

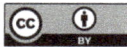

Copyright: © 2023 by the authors. Licensee MDPI, Basel, Switzerland. This article is an open access article distributed under the terms and conditions of the Creative Commons Attribution (CC BY) license (https://creativecommons.org/licenses/by/4.0/).

1. Introduction

Hyperuricemia is a chronic metabolic disease characterized by elevated serum uric acid levels due to long-term purine metabolic disorder or decreased uric acid excretion in the body [1,2]. The long-term high concentration of serum uric acid leads to the crystallization of uric acid in joints and soft tissues in the body, causing damage to connective tissues and triggering gout [3,4]. In acute gouty arthritis, the interaction between urate crystals and phagocytes (such as macrophages and infiltrating white blood cells) induces the secretion of various inflammatory mediators, including cytokines, chemokines, and interleukin, triggering typical inflammatory reactions [5,6]. Therefore, the usual means of treating gout aim to inhibit the production of uric acid and promote the excretion of uric acid. Xanthine oxidase (XOD, EC 1.17.3.2) is the key enzyme involved in the metabolism of human purines into uric acid. It exists in the liver, intestine, serum, and lactating breast, catalyzing the gradual hydroxylation of hypoxanthine into xanthine, and then into uric acid [7]. Its activity directly determines the rate of uric acid formation to a certain extent. Therefore, this target enzyme has received much attention in the treatment of or intervention in cases of hyperuricemia and gout.

Studies have shown that inhibiting the catalytic activity of xanthine oxidase can effectively reduce the production of uric acid, making this an important means to relieve and treat hyperuricemia and gout in the clinic [8]. Allopurinol [9], febuxostat [10], and topiroxostat [11] are the most commonly used xanthine oxidase inhibitors in clinical practice for hyperuricemia and gout. However, these synthetic inhibitors are associated with strong side effects in clinical use, including varying degrees of liver damage, neurological adverse effects, and others. Allopurinol may even cause 'allopurinol hypersensitivity syndrome' [12,13]. Therefore, it is of great significance to find new XOD inhibitors from natural sources, with strong activity and low toxicity, for the development of new antigout functional foods or drugs. Currently, natural xanthine oxidase inhibitors such as apigenin [14,15], quercetin [15,16], galangin [17,18], and myricetine [19,20] have been reported, most of which are found in terrestrial plants. However, their xanthine oxidase inhibition activity is lower than that of positive drugs, which may hinder their further research and development.

The ocean is a vast treasury of medicinal and edible biological resources, among which seaweeds have the advantage of a huge biomass and cultivability for sustainable development. Till now, there have been several reports on anti-gout active substances including XOD inhibitors derived from seaweeds. For instance, vine alkaloid isolated from *Caulerpa prolifera* has an irreversible XOD-inhibitory effect with an IC_{50} value of 26.92 μM [21]. The fucoidan from *Laminaria japonica* was found to completely reverse the negative changes induced by adenine in mice, restoring the activities of adenosine deaminase (ADA) and XOD in the liver to normal levels [22], which can effectively reduce the serum uric acid content and blood uric acid content of hyperuricemia mice and rats [23]. The *Enteromorpha prolifera* polysaccharide significantly reduced serum uric acid (UA), serum blood urea nitrogen, and serum and hepatic XOD, and also improved histological parameters in hyperuricemic mice [24]. These findings suggest that seaweeds are a meaningful avenue for XOD inhibitor exploration.

For highly efficient discovery of enzyme inhibitors, affinity ultrafiltration mass spectrometry (UF-LC/MS) is a powerful tool that has been increasingly used in screening of bioactive compounds from natural products. In the process of biological affinity ultrafiltration, the ligand–enzyme complexes are retained by the ultrafiltration membrane from the mixture, and then, the ligands released from the complex in the next step of treatment are further identified and quantified using high-performance liquid chromatography–mass spectrometry (HPLC-MS) analysis to achieve rapid identification of bioactive molecules from complex mixtures. Compared with the traditional separation-dependent procedure of active ingredients discovery from natural medicinal plants, UF-LC/MS greatly reduces the cost in terms of time, samples, and expensive reagents [25]. Furthermore, several metabolomics tools have been developed to automate secondary metabolite identification such as MSDAIL [26], MSFINDER [27], Global Natural Products Social Molecular Networking (GNPS) [28], and its updated version, feature-based molecular networking (FBMN) [29,30]. Previously, we presented a combined strategy named Bio-LCMS-GNPS to connect UF-LC/MS and GNPS, which provided a new approach to enzyme inhibitor discovery from terrestrial and marine bioresources [31].

Pterocladiella capillacea (S.G. Gmelin) belongs to the family of Pterocladiaceae, the order of Gelidiales, and the Phylum of Rhodophyta. It is mainly found in tropical and sub-tropical waters and partially inhabits temperate zones. As an edible seaweed plant, *P. capillacea* has been traditionally used as a source of jelly production in eastern Asian countries [32]. Currently, reports have appeared on the antibacterial [33], antioxidant [34], and bacterial cell agglutination potential [35] of *P. capillacea*. In a preliminary study based on local seaweeds in Zhanjiang, China, the crude extracts of *P. capillacea* exhibited strong xanthine oxidase-inhibitory activity. To explore the value of this edible seaweed as anti-gout drugs or functional foods, we further evaluated the XOD-inhibitory and anti-inflammatory activities of its fractions, traced the possible XOD inhibitors via UF-LC-MS/MS, annotated them using metabolomics tools including MSDIAL, MSFINDER, and FBMN, and predicted the action mechanism and drug-likeness of the annotated XOD inhibitors via molecular docking and ADMET, as described in this paper.

2. Results

2.1. Evaluation of XOD Inhibition Activity

The *P. capillacea* samples were collected along the seashore of Naozhou Island, Zhanjiang, China (see voucher specimens in Figure 1a). Its crude extract was prepared by anhydrous ethanol extraction using an air-dried seaweed sample. Then, the extract was fractioned by a silica gel column to produce twelve primary fractions F1–F12, as shown in the thin-layer chromatography (TLC) images (Figure 1b,c). The XOD inhibition activity screening indicated that fractions F4 and F6 ranked as the top two for activity (Figure 1f). Considering the relative simplicity of the fingerprint and the relatively higher amount of F4 compared with F6, this fraction was preferentially chosen for further study. The separation of F4 on Sephadex LH-20 gel column yielded four secondary fractions, F4-1 to F4-4 (Figure 1d,e). Among them, F4-2 and F4-3 displayed the top two highest XOD inhibition ratios (IRs: $66.47\% \pm 7.96\%$ and $77.96\% \pm 4.91\%$, respectively) at the final concentration of 0.14 mg/mL (Figure 1g). At the same dose, the positive control, allopurinol showed an IR of $92.21\% \pm 3.38\%$.

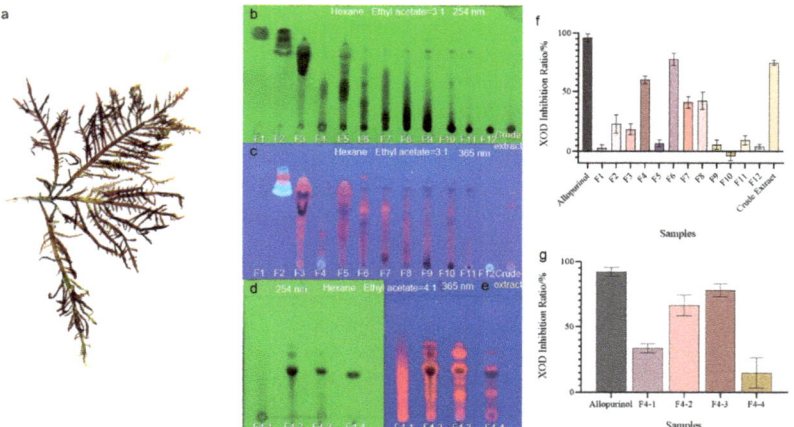

Figure 1. The TLC fingerprints and XOD-inhibitory activity of the crude extract and fractions of *Pterocladiella capillacea*. (**a**) The image of the seaweed material *P. capillacea*. (**b–e**) The TLC images of fractions F1–F12, F4-1–F4-4, and crude extract detected under 254 nm and 365 nm UV light, respectively (sample numbers are marked below the start line). (**f,g**) The XOD inhibition rates of fractions F1–F12, F4-1–F4-4, crude extract, and allopurinol.

2.2. Evaluation of Anti-Inflammatory Activity

Since xanthine oxidase catalyzes the production of urea from xanthine and hypoxanthine, generating a large amount of hydrogen peroxide and superoxide anion, it is possible that substances with xanthine oxidase-inhibitory activity may also exhibit anti-inflammatory activity, and many studies have confirmed this hypothesis [36–38]. Considering that inflammation can severely influence the progress of gout, the XOD-inhibitory samples F4 and F6, and the crude extracts found in the preliminary screening, were also evaluated for their anti-inflammatory activity.

As shown in Figure 2a, the NO production in the RAW264.7 cells of the control group (C) significantly increased compared with the blank group (B) ($p < 0.001$) under the stimulus of lipopolysaccharide (LPS), while samples F4 and F6, and the crude extract can significantly decrease the NO production at a dose of 20 µg/mL. Meanwhile, F4, F6, and the crude extract did not show toxicity to the cells at this dose (Figure 2b). This result was consistent with that of XOD inhibition activity, indicating that these samples also possess anti-inflammatory activity.

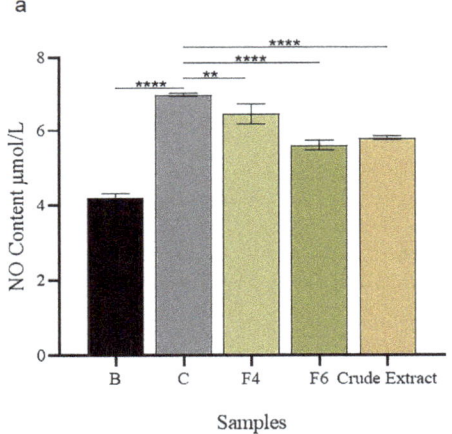
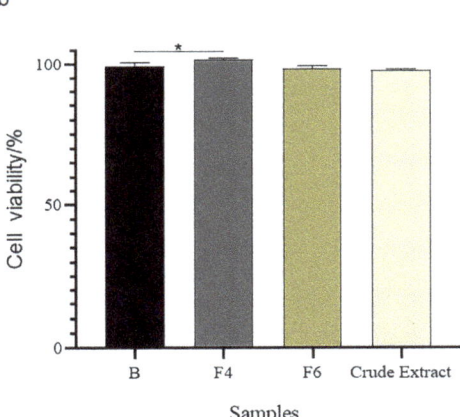

Figure 2. Anti-inflammatory activity and cell viability of XOD-inhibitory samples including F4, F6, and the crude extract. (**a**) The control group (C) was RAW264.7 cells stimulated with lipopolysaccharide (LPS). The sample groups (F4, F6, and crude extract) were RAW264.7 cells stimulated with LPS (dose: 1 µg/mL) and treated with the samples (dose: 20 µg/mL). (**b**) The blank group (B) was cells with viability of RAW 264.7 without treatment. The sample groups (F4, F6, and crude extract) were cells with viability of RAW 264.7 and treated with the samples (dose: 20 µg/mL). Data were expressed as mean ± SD ($n = 3$). **** $p < 0.001$, vs. control; ** $p < 0.01$, vs. control; * $p < 0.05$, vs. blank.

2.3. UF-LC-MS Screening of XOD Ligands in P. capillacea Extract

To trace the active molecules targeting XOD in active secondary fractions F4-2 and F4-3, affinity ultrafiltration-LC-MS/MS analyses were performed.

After the affinity ultrafiltration treatment, a preliminary HPLC analysis was conducted to check the capturing effect of the enzyme on the possible ligands contained in the samples. This was based on the hypothesis that compounds specifically bound to XOD should exhibit higher peaks in the process groups (P) incubated with XOD than in the corresponding blank groups (B) which were incubated with the inactivated enzyme. Indeed, larger peaks of the captured ligands were observed in the chromatograms of both F4-2 and F4-3 after affinity ultrafiltration treatment.

Among them, the peak heights of peak 1, peak 2, peak 5, and peak 8 of F4-2 in the process group 4-2(P) after affinity ultrafiltration treatment were remarkably higher than those of the inactivated enzyme blank group 4-2(B) (Figure 3a). More dramatically, in sample F4-3, more peaks, including peaks 5, 6, 7, 8, 9, 10, 11, and 12, were observed in the process group 4-3(P), with much stronger intensity than in the blank group 4-3(B) (Figure 3b). The peaks were assumed to be the substances in *P. capillacea* that specifically interact with xanthine oxidase.

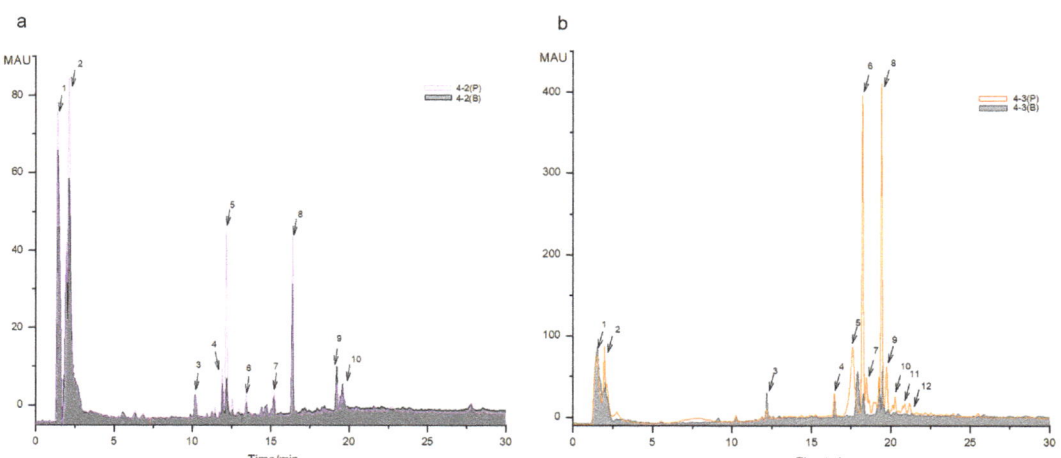

Figure 3. The comparison of HPLC traces of the ultrafiltration membrane-retained samples after incubation with XOD or inactivated XOD ultrafiltration (the chromatograms were monitored under 290 nm). (**a**) The comparison of affinity ultrafiltration process group (4-2(P)) and inactivated enzyme blank group (4-2(B)) for sample F4-2. (**b**) The comparison of affinity ultrafiltration process group (4-3(P)) and inactivated enzyme blank group (4-3(B)) for sample F4-3. The numbers associated with arrows marked the main peaks.

2.4. Comparison of Metabolite Profiles by LC-MS/MS and Multiple Database Mining

To further characterize the possible XOD ligands in F4-2 and F4-3, the above samples for groups 4-2(B), 4-2(P), 4-3(B), and 4-3(P) were analyzed using Orbitrap LC-MS/MS. The data were aligned via MS-DIAL to accurately localize the XOD ligands based on peak area comparison between different treatment groups, obtain their chromatographic and mass spectroscopic information (retention times, molecular weights, molecular formulae, and MS/MS spectra), and annotate them via FBMN, MSDIAL, and MSFINDER. In addition, the sources of compounds were manually screened by searching open and accessible natural product databases, including PubChem, Natural Product Dictionary (DNP), NPASS, LOTUS, COCONUT, and The Natural Products Atlas. As shown in Figure 4 and Tables 1 and 2, a total of 20 compounds from fractions F4-2 and F4-3 were identified as XOD ligands based on their much higher peak areas in the affinity ultrafiltration process groups ("P" groups) than in the corresponding enzyme inactivated blank groups ("B" groups). Compounds **1–11** were from F4-2, compounds **12–20** were from F4-3, and compounds **7–8** were from both (Figure 4).

Table 1. The annotation of bioactive molecules in fraction F4-2 through UF-LC-MS/MS combined with metabolomics tools and bioresource searching.

Number	Average Retention Time (min)	Average M/Z	Adduct Ion Name	Area Ratio (4-2F/4-2B)	Predicted Formula	Compound Name	Annotation Method	MS/MS Matched (Y/N)	Bioresource	Reports on Anti-Gout or Anti-Inflammatory Activities
Compound 1	19.92	233.1533	[M+H]⁺	—(Area of 4-2B is 0)	C₁₅H₂₂O₃	Chondroterpene C	MW-MF searching	N	P. capillacea symbiotic fungus	effectively inhibits the production of NO in BV-2 cells stimulated by LPS [39]
Compound 2	11.28	247.1686	[M+H]⁺	—(Area of 4-2B is 0)	C₁₆H₂₄O₃	Chondroterpene H	MW-MF searching	N	P. capillacea symbiotic fungus [39]	-
Compound 3	14.97	637.3047	[M+H]⁺	23.67	C₂₉H₄₈O₁₅	[6-[4-acetyloxy-3-hydroxy-2,5-bis(hydroxymethyl)oxolan-2-yl]oxy-2-(hydroxymethyl)-4,5-difipentanoyloxyoxan-3-yl] pentanoate	MW-MF searching, MS/MS matching (MSDIAL, FBMN)	Y	Nicotiana tabacum [40]	-
Compound 4	17.17	223.2052	[M+H]⁺	23.02	C₁₅H₂₆O	unknown	MW-MF searching, MS/MS matching (MSDIAL, FBMN)	Y	Euglena gracilis [41]	-
Compound 5	11.98	373.1336	[M+H]⁺	12.85	C₂₀H₂₀O₇	Sinensetin	MW-MF searching, MS/MS matching (MSDIAL, FBMN)	Y	Citrus tamlan, Citrus keraji [42]	anti-inflammatory and anti-oxidative activities [43]
Compound 6	15.97	277.2161	[M+H]⁺	9.39	C₁₈H₂₈O₂	Octadeca-2,4,6,8-tetraenoic acid	MW-MF searching, MS/MS matching (MSDIAL, MSFINDER, FBMN)	Y	Cnidoscolum purpureum [44]	-
Compound 7	14.96	243.1008	[M+H]⁺	7.73	C₁₅H₁₄O₃	Fenoprofen	MW-MF searching, MS/MS matching (MSDIAL, FBMN)	N	unknown	non-steroidal drug used for acute pain and chronic arthritis [45]
Compound 8	17.39	274.2743	[M+H-H₂O]⁺	1.91	C₁₆H₃₂O₂	Palmitic acid	MW-MF searching, MS/MS matching (MSDIAL, FBMN)	Y	Ulva lactuca [46] Pterocladiella tenuis [47]	palmitic acid in propolis exhibits XO-inhibitory activity [47]
Compound 9	14.89	263.1275	[M+H]⁺	1.77	C₁₅H₁₈O₄	Chondroterpene B	MW-MF searching	N	P. capillacea symbiotic fungus [39]	-
Compound 10	0.72	235.1689	[M+H]⁺	1.31	C₁₅H₂₄O₃	Chondroterpene E	MW-MF searching	Y	P. capillacea symbiotic fungus [39]	-
Compound 11	14.97	338.0263	[M+H]⁺	1.55	C₁₃H₁₁N₃O₄S₂	Tenoxicam	MW-MF searching, MS/MS matching (MSDIAL, MSFINDER, FBMN)	Y	unknown	used as drug to treat pain and inflammation in osteoarthritis and rheumatoid arthritis [48]

Note: MW-MF searching: molecular weight (MW) and molecular formula (MF) searching in multiple natural product databases. Y: Yes; N: No. The structures of these compounds are presented in Figure 5.

Table 2. The annotation of bioactive molecules in fraction F4-3 through UF-LC-MS/MS combined with metabolomics tools and bioresource searching.

Number	Average Retention Time (min)	Average M/Z	Adduct Ion Name	Area Ratio (4-2F/4-2B)	Predicted Formula	Compound Name	Annotation Method	MS/MS Matched (Y/N)	Bioresource	Reports on Anti-Gout or Anti-Inflammatory Activities
Compound 12	12.86	300.2905	[M+H]⁺	35.22	C₁₈H₃₇NO₂	C₁₈-sphingosine	MW-MF searching, MS/MS matching (MSDIAL, MSFINDER, FBMN)	Y	Amansia glomerata, Laurrencia nidifica [49]	anti-inflammatory activity [50]
Compound 13	0.91	221.1241	[M+H]⁺	21.12	C₁₃H₁₆O₃	Precocene ii	MW-MF searching, MS/MS matching (MSDIAL, MSFINDER, FBMN)	Y	Artemisia capillaris, Boenninghausenia albiflora (LOTUS)	antibacterial and antioxidant activities [51,52]
Compound 14	11.97	385.0913	[M+Na]⁺	20.07	C₁₈H₁₈O₈	Methyl Asterrate	MW-MF searching, MS/MS matching (MSDIAL, MSFINDER, FBMN)	Y	Ruprechtia tangarana (COCONUT)	-
Compound 15	11.97	577.1323	[M+K]⁺	16.89	C₂₅H₃₀O₁₃	Grandifloroside	MW-MF searching, MS/MS matching (MSDIAL, MSFINDER, FBMN)	Y	Nauclea sessilifolia (PubChem)	used in traditional medicine to treat gout [53]
Compound 16	15.02	670.3364	[2M+ACN+H]⁺	6950.76	unknown	unknown	MW-MF searching, MS/MS matching (MSFINDER)	N	unknown	-
Compound 17	14.99	295.1728	[M+Na]⁺	13.80	C₁₈H₂₄O₂	Estradiol	MW-MF searching, MS/MS matching (MSDIAL, MSFINDER, FBMN)	Y	Punica granatum (LOTUS)	reduces serum urate levels [54]
Compound 18	15.11	241.1587	[M+Na]⁺	11.67	C₁₅H₂₂O	Germacrone	MW-MF searching, MS/MS matching (MSDIAL, FBMN)	Y	Curcuma amada, Curcuma aeruginosa (COCONUT)	reduces serum uric acid levels in mice in diabetes-related studies [53] shows a defensive mechanism against oxidative stress and neuroinflammation by inhibiting the NF-κB pathway [56]
Compound 19	13.27	369.1823	[M+Na]⁺	9.99	C₁₉H₂₂O₆	Cynaropicrin	MW-MF searching, MS/MS matching (MSDIAL, FBMN)	Y	Centaurea scoparia (NPASS)	-
Compound 20	17.17	258.2422	[M+NH₄]⁺	23.02	C₁₅H₂₈O₂	Proximadiol	MW-MF searching, MS/MS matching (MSDIAL, MSFINDER, FBMN)	Y	Euglena gracilis (LOTUS)	-
Compound 7	12.18	243.1013	[M+H]⁺	1.88	C₁₅H₁₄O₃	Fenoprofen	MW-MF searching, MS/MS matching (MSDIAL, MSFINDER, FBMN)	Y	unknown	non-steroidal drug used for acute pain and chronic arthritis [45]
Compound 8	12.60	274.2735	[M+H-H₂O]⁺	1.91	C₁₆H₃₂O₂	Palmitic acid	MW-MF searching, MS/MS matching (MSDIAL, FBMN)	Y	Ulva lactuca (LOTUS)	palmitic acid in propolis exhibits XOD-inhibitory activity [47]

Note: MW-MF searching: molecular weight (MW) and molecular formula (MF) searching in multiple natural product databases. Y: Yes; N: No. The structures of these compounds are presented in Figure 6.

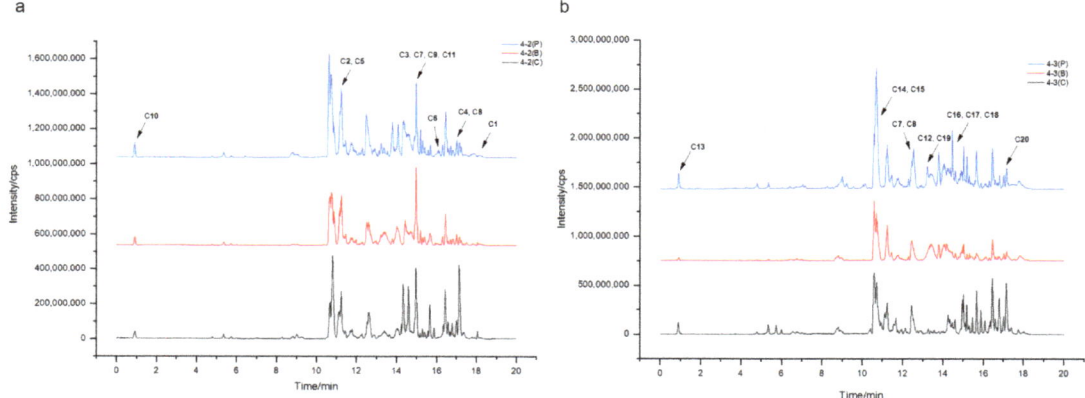

Figure 4. The LC-MS traces (base peak chromatographies, BPC) for the fraction samples 4-2 and 4-3 under positive ion mode of the ultrafiltration membrane-retained samples after incubation with XOD or inactivated XOD ultrafiltration (the chromatograms were monitored under 290 nm). (**a**) The comparison of affinity ultrafiltration process group (4-2(P)), inactivated enzyme blank group (4-2(B)), and crude sample group (4-2(C)) for sample F4-2. (**b**) The comparison of affinity ultrafiltration process group (4-3(P)), inactivated enzyme blank group (4-3(B)), and crude sample group (4-3(C)) for sample F4-3.

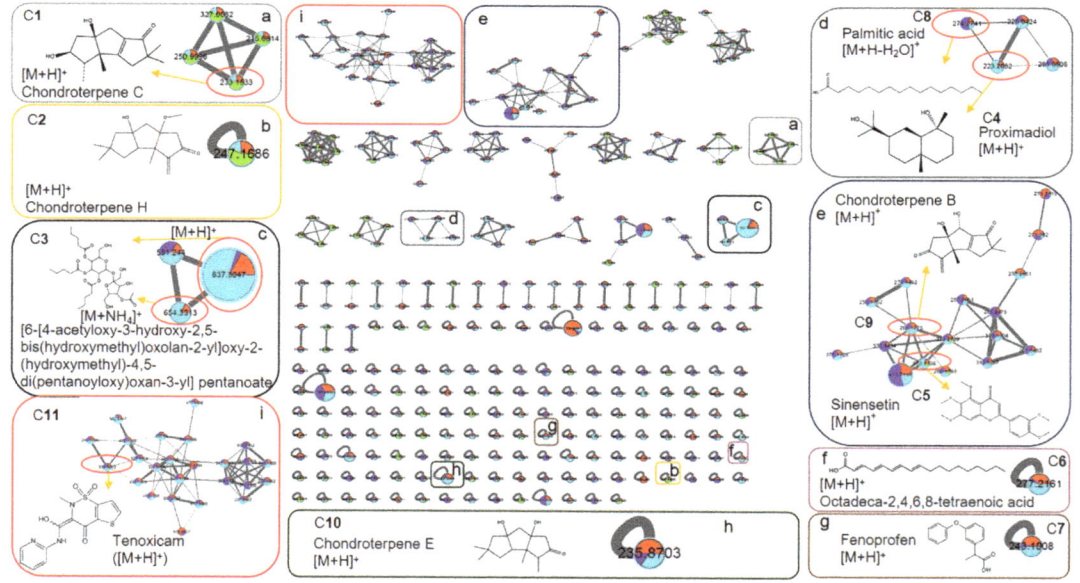

Figure 5. The FNMB molecular network for the fraction sample 4-2 based on positive ion MS/MS spectral similarity. Sub-figures (**a**–**i**) show the details of the amplified clusters including the annotated compounds 1–11 (C1–C11), respectively. The nodes display the measured average masses of the molecular ions with identical MS/MS spectra. The sizes of the nodes reflect the relative amount of the corresponding compounds. The different colors of sections in the nodes represent different sample groups, i.e., ■ ■ ■ : 4-2(C) (Group1), 4-2(B) (Group 2), 4-2(P) (Group 3), and Blank (Group 4).

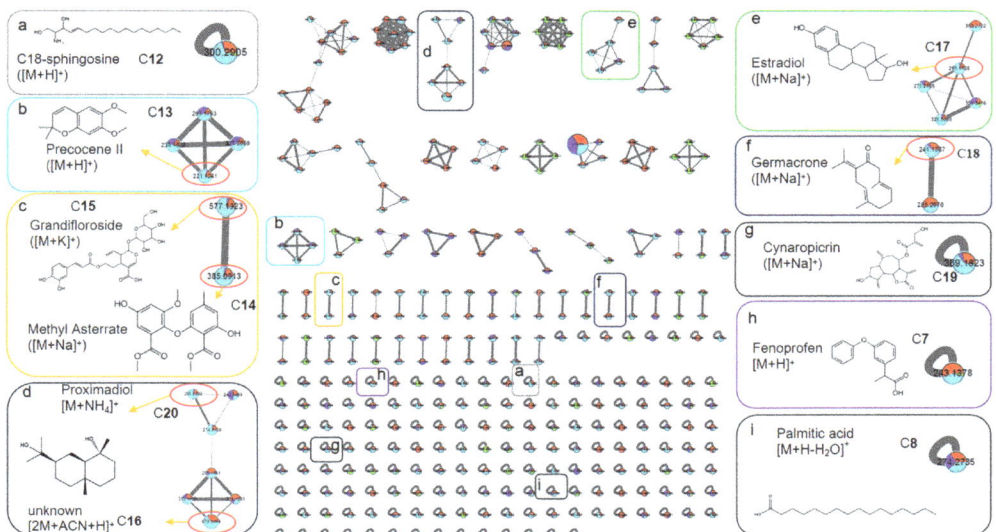

Figure 6. The FBMN molecular network for the fraction sample 4-3 based on positive ion MS/MS spectral similarity. Sub-figures (**a**–**i**) show the details of the amplified clusters including the annotated compounds **7**, **8**, and **12**–**20** (C7, C8, and C12–C20), re-spectively. The nodes display the measured average masses of the molecular ions with identical MS/MS spectra. The sizes of the nodes reflect the relative amount of the corresponding compounds. The different colors of sections in the nodes represent different sample groups, i.e., ■ ■ ■ ■ : 4-3(C) (Group 1), 4-3(B) (Group 2), 4-3(P) (Group 3), and Blank (Group 4).

For these ligands, the MSDIAL-MSFINDER-FBMN pipeline provided some annotated structures through MS/MS matching. However, manual searching in natural product databases showed that most of these structures were not from taxonomically close sources (Order of Gelidiales or Phylum of *Rhodophyta*). It was deduced that the MS/MS spectral libraries of MSDIAL, MSFINDER, and FBMN had not indexed a sufficient amount of records from this taxon. Thus, the molecular weight (MW) and molecular formula (MF) information of the annotations were used to search the natural product databases as well. And the taxonomical range was restricted to the Order of Gelidiales to obtain the most relevant hits. Finally, 15 compounds were annotated through MS/MS matching combined with MW-MF searching, 4 compounds were annotated through MW-MF searching, and 1 compound remained unknown (compound **16**). The annotation details, including metabolite information, results, methods, biological sources, and reports on anti-gout or anti-inflammatory related activities, are summarized in Tables 1 and 2 and Figures 5 and 6. The MS/MS spectra of these compounds are provided in the (Supporting Information Figures S1–S21).

Among the 20 annotated compounds (XOD ligands), 8 are natural products derived from seaweeds, including 4 from *P. capillacea* endophytic fungus, and 10 (compounds **1**, **5**, **7**, **8**, **11**, **12**, **15**, **17**, **18**, and **19**) have been reported for anti-gout-related or anti-inflammatory activities, providing scientific support for the XOD-inhibitory and anti-inflammatory activity of the extract and fractions of *P. capillacea*.

Based on MS/MS spectral similarity, the FBMN molecular networks were visualized to display the metabolites in fractions F4-2 (Figure 5 presents ligands **1**–**11**) and F4-3 (Figure 6 presents ligands **7**, **8**, **12**–**20**).

2.5. Molecular Docking and ADMET Analysis

Seven annotated compounds with seaweed-related origins but without reports of anti-gout-related activity were predicted to have an affinity for XOD using molecular docking and were then subjected to ADMET drug-likeness analysis. The Molybdopterin domain is the catalytic center of XOD [57], which is used for docking the treated ligand compound and calculate the minimum binding affinity. The lower the minimum binding affinity, the stronger the affinity between ligand and XOD, and the higher the binding stability. The molecular docking scoring results are shown in Table 3.

Table 3. The docking results of 7 annotated compounds with XOD crystal structure (PDB ID: 3nvw).

PubChem ID	Compound Name	Hydrogen-Bonding Residues	Minimum Binding Affinity (kcal/mol)
139589725	Chondroterpene B	THR-1083, SER-1080, SER-1082	−8.4
139589728	Chondroterpene E	SER-1080, THR-1083, SER-1082, GLN-1040	−7.8
165258	Proximadiol	GLN-1194	−7.5
11778225	Octadeca-2,4,6,8-tetraenoic acid	ARG-880, THR-1010	−7.4
139589726	Chondroterpene C	TRY-735, ILE-698	−6.8
139589731	Chondroterpene H	HIS-1212	−6.3
1104	Sphingosine	—	—

The ranking of the minimum binding affinity shows that the XOD protein binds most stably to Chondroterpene B, followed by Chondroterpene E, Proximadiol, and Octadeca-2,4,6,8-tetraenoic acid. The docking diagram showed that Chondroterpene B enters deeply into the XOD active pocket and forms one hydrogen bond with residues SER-1080 and THR-1083 of the XOD protein and two hydrogen bonds with residue SER-1082, respectively (Figure 7a). Chondroterpene E enters deeply into the XOD active pocket and forms one hydrogen bond with residues SER-1080 and SER-1082 and forms two hydrogen bonds with residues GLN-1040 and THR-1083 each, respectively (Figure 7b). Proximadiol enters deeply into the XOD active pocket and forms a hydrogen bond with residue GLN-1194 of the XOD protein (Figure 7c). Octadeca-2,4,6,8-tetraenoic acid enters into the XOD active pocket and forms two hydrogen bonds with residues ARG-880 and THR-1010 each, respectively (Figure 7d). In addition, the docking results showed that all of the seven compounds except sphingosine enter the XOD activity pocket.

The ADMET properties of a drug are the absorption, distribution, metabolism, excretion, and toxicity of the drug in the human body, and these are key factors used to evaluate whether a compound can become a drug or not. To validate the drug-likeness of the compounds annotated in the active fractions of *P. capillacea*, they were subjected to online ADMET prediction, and the results are shown in Table 4.

Table 4. The results of ADMET analysis of the annotated compounds.

Name	Chondroterpene C	Chondroterpene H	Proximadiol	Octadeca-2,4,6,8-Tetraenoic Acid	Chondroterpene B	Chondroterpene E	C_{18}-Sphingosine
MW	250.160	264.170	240.210	276.210	254.190	252.170	299.280
LogS	−2.596	−3.083	−1.99	−3.054	−2.835	−1.967	−4.193
HIA	0.019	0.023	0.006	0.019	0.029	0.045	0.314
PPB	62.65%	64.28%	84.36%	95.56%	58.72%	38.63%	98.30%
BBB	0.932	0.859	0.875	0.013	0.982	0.969	0.167
CYP1A2-inhibitor	0.017	0.008	0.022	0.459	0.021	0.007	0.317
CYP2C19-inhibitor	0.038	0.139	0.028	0.26	0.013	0.049	0.249
CYP2C9-inhibitor	0.02	0.108	0.107	0.588	0.03	0.049	0.103
CYP2D6-inhibitor	0.007	0.011	0.009	0.849	0.003	0.006	0.483
CL	9.426	11.781	8.425	0.957	13.004	11.913	3.769
H-HT	0.283	0.221	0.049	0.449	0.332	0.246	0.358
DILI	0.048	0.148	0.026	0.552	0.039	0.091	0.02
Skin Sensitization	0.041	0.297	0.096	0.959	0.061	0.061	0.928
Lipinski Rule	Accepted	Accepted	Accepted	Accepted	Accepted	Accepted	Accepted
Pfizer Rule	Accepted	Accepted	Rejected	Rejected	Accepted	Accepted	Rejected
GSK Rule	Accepted	Accepted	Accepted	Rejected	Accepted	Accepted	Rejected
Golden Triangle	Accepted	Accepted	Accepted	Accepted	Accepted	Accepted	Accepted

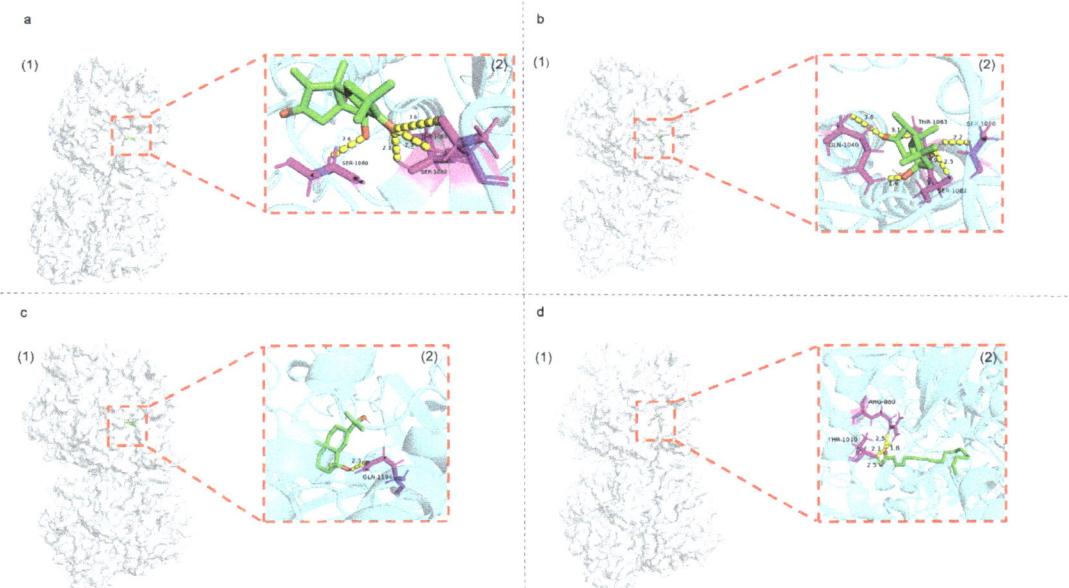

Figure 7. Molecular docking results of Chondroterpene B (**a**), Chondroterpene E (**b**), Proximadiol (**c**), and Octadeca-2,4,6,8-tetraenoic acid (**d**), respectively, with XOD. Docking pose (1) and ligand interaction (2) diagrams of different ligands and XOD are presented for each docking result. Yellow dotted lines indicate hydrogen bonds.

Likewise, the seven annotated compounds, except the C_{18}-sphingosine, showed suitable water solubility ($-4 <$ LogS < 0.5), excellent absorption in the human small intestine (HIA < 0.3), and low effect on drug metabolism (CYP inhibitor). Octadeca-2,4,6,8-tetraenoic acid and Sphingosine have poor oral bioavailability (PPB $> 90\%$) and may also cross the blood–brain barrier, while the other five compounds have low blood–brain barrier penetration (BBB > 0.7) and therefore do not cause side effects on the central nervous system. Moreover, Chondroterpene C, Chondroterpene H, Proximadiol, and Chondroterpene E may have improved safety characteristics, since they may not cause hepatotoxicity, liver damage, or skin sensitization (H-HT, DILI, Skin Sensitization < 0.3). Generally, all the seven compounds meet the five principles of Lipinski's rule for oral drugs [58].

3. Discussion

In the present study, two extract fractions (F4 and F6) from edible seaweed *P. capillacea* were discovered to have strong XOD-inhibitory and anti-inflammatory activities. From F4, with relatively simple components, two active subfractions, F4-2 and F4-3, were obtained and exhibited remarkable XOD-inhibitory activity. By using UF-LC-MS/MS, metabolomics tools, multiple natural product database mining, molecular docking, and ADMET analysis, 20 plausible XOD ligands in the active subfractions were localized and annotated, and 7 annotated seaweed-derived compounds were further predicted to have binding affinity with XOD and drug-likeness. Among them, Chondroterpene C, Chondroterpene E, and Proximadiol displayed strong XOD affinity and good drug-likeness properties.

Hyperuricemia and gout have become increasingly prevalent globally, while current clinical drugs like allopurinol have severe side effects including triggering 'allopurinol hypersensitivity syndrome' [13]. Therefore, there is a need for new effective drugs and functional foods to cope with this issue. *P. capillacea*, a globally spread seaweed that is traditionally eaten in eastern Asia, has not been reported for its anti-gout activity. In this study, potent fractions and subfractions from *P. capillacea* have been found to inhibit XOD activity and inflammation. The potency of *P. capillacea* fractions and subfractions is generally comparable to the control allopurinol at the same dose. Furthermore, the fractions did not show cytotoxicity to macrophage cells. Since XOD is the key target in hyperuricemia and gout, and inflammation also plays an important role in the development of gout [36], *P. capillacea*, as an edible seaweed with huge biomass, may have great potential as a new source for the development of anti-hyperuricemia and anti-gout drugs or functional foods.

Preliminary UF-LC-MS/MS tracing, annotating, and predictive investigations located the active peaks and suggested 20 compounds as plausible XOD inhibitors in *P. capillacea*, including 8 compounds with seaweed and *P. capillacea*-related origins, and 9 compounds with XOD-inhibitory or anti-inflammatory reports. Furthermore, molecular docking of seven compounds with seaweed and seaweed-related origins and no reported anti-gout effects showed that six of them enter the XOD activity pocket and dock with XOD by forming hydrogen-bonding forces with amino acid residues. Three compounds, Chondroterpene C, Chondroterpene E, and Proximadiol, displayed strong XOD affinity and good drug-likeness properties. To some extent, the above results have provided reasonable explanations for the XOD-inhibitory and anti-inflammatory activity of *P. capillacea* extracts and useful clues for future studies on natural product research for anti-gout treatments using this seaweed.

In addition, it is intriguing that compounds **1** (Chondroterpene C), **2** (Chondroterpene H), **10** (Chondroterpene B), and **11** (Chondroterpene E) are hirsutane-type sesquiterpenes, which are reported to be isolated from *P. capillacea* endophytic fungus *Chondrostereum* sp NTOU4196 [39]. Until now, all reported hirsutane-type sesquiterpenes have been identified from terrestrial and marine Basidiomycotina, especially from Agaricomycetes including genera/species like *Stereum hirsutum* [59,60], *Chondrostereum* sp. [61,62], *Cerrena* sp. [63], etc. Seaweed *P. capillacea* has been reported to be a rich source of endophytic fungi, including four genera belonging to Agaricomycetes, i.e., *Chondrostereum* sp., *Cerrena* sp., *Bjerkandera* sp., and *Grammothele* sp. [64], two of which are reported to be hirsutane-producing genera. Considering the fact that many natural plant products like Taxol, Camptothecin, and Quinine are produced by the endophytic fungi [65], it is reasonable to suggest that the plausible Chondroterpenes detected in *P. capillacea* are possibly produced by its endophytes.

UF-LC-MS/MS has been increasingly used in enzyme inhibitor discovery, where the LC-MS profile of an affinity-treated enzyme group is usually compared with that of the blank group without enzyme incubation to recognize the ligands specifically binding with the enzyme [66–68]. In the blank group, the molecules absorbed by the ultrafiltration membrane are taken as non-specific binders. However, it is not easy to discriminate the molecules absorbed by the surface of the proteins using this method. In this study, the authors used heat-inactivated enzymes for the incubation treatment as a blank group instead of only ultrafiltration membrane, by which the small molecular ligands that specifically interact with the target enzyme may be more accurately recognized from complex natural product mixtures. Although LC-MS/MS can provide rich information about the samples, in this study, a preliminary HPLC-DAD analysis was performed for the ultrafiltration experimental samples before formal LC-MS/MS analysis. This measurement can not only verify the effect of ultrafiltration experiments, but also provide more spectrometric information on the active peaks, in addition to mass spectra for further natural product purification, since HPLC-DAD is a more frequently used approach in regular analytic tasks.

Bioactivity-coupled molecular networking analysis can rationalize natural product isolation and help in deduplication before time-consuming isolation tasks. Compared with our previously reported "Bio-LCMS-GNPS" strategy used in acetylcholinesterase inhibitors and antioxidants mining [31], improvements have been made in two aspects of the present study. Firstly, FBMN has been used to construct molecular networks instead of classical GNPS, and more metabolomics tools and multiple natural product databases are utilized to annotate ligands together. Since high-resolution mass spectrometry-based FBMN provides molecular formulae, more accurate peak area integration, and improved retention times for the features, and recognize different adduct ions of the same substance [69], it has an advantage in comparing peak areas of ligands between different groups and providing molecular formulae for library searching over classical GNPS. FBMN combined with MSDIAL, MSFINDER, and natural products databases, also provides more comprehensive annotation than GNPS individually. Secondly, following the annotation, in silico molecular docking and ADMET were performed to evaluate the possibility of annotated compounds as enzyme ligands and their drug-likeness, which is more reliable than mere metabolomics annotation. Therefore, this updated bioactivity-coupled mass spectrometric metabolomics pipeline is named "Bio-LCMS-Metabolomic-in silico Prediction".

The application of this pipeline to the discovery of XOD inhibitors in *P. capillacea* has not only provided plausible explanations for the bioactivity of samples, but has also located the XOD ligands in the samples. The feature information, including retention time, molecular weights, MS/MS spectra, and UV spectra, will guide future compound isolation and elucidation. As with all the MS metabolomics-based studies, the isolation, structural elucidation, and bioactivity study of isolated pure compounds is the final verification and "golden criterion" for the annotated results. This study and ongoing similar processes on fraction F6 will guide our in-depth chemistry and biology studies on the anti-gout constituents of *P. capillacea* for drugs and functional foods purposes.

In conclusion, the present study has revealed the great potential of the edible seaweed *P. capillacea* for developing anti-hyperuricemia and anti-gout drugs and functional foods. Furthermore, it has established a new bioactivity-coupled metabolomics investigating pipeline "Bio-LCMS-Metabolomic-in silico Prediction" for bioactive natural product discovery.

4. Materials and Methods

4.1. Materials and Chemicals

P. capillacea was harvested from Naozhou Island, Zhanjiang, China, in July of 2020. The seaweed was identified by an algologist, Prof. Enyi Xie, at Guangdong Ocean University, and a voucher specimen was deposited in our laboratory with number ZJNZ2020-2. Xanthine oxidase (EC 1.17.3.2, 5 U, Sigma, Saint Louis, MO, USA), allopurinol (98% purity, 25 g, Aladdin, Shanghai, China), xanthine (analytical purity, 1 g, Solabao, Beijing, China), Tris-HCL (pH 8.7, 0.5 mmol/L, Solabao, Beijing, China), 96-well UV plate (Model 3635, Corning, Kennebunk, ME, USA), ultrafiltration centrifuge tube (0.5 mL, 100 Kd, Millipore, Billerica, MA, USA), nitric oxide detection kit (Beyotime, Shanghai, China), Cell Counting Kit-8 (CCK-8, Zeta Life, Menlo Park, NJ, USA) and RAW264.7 cell line (Cell Bank of Chinese Academy of Sciences, Shanghai, China) were used in the bioassays. All organic mobile-phase solvents used for LC-MS and the thin-layer chromatographic plate (silica gel 60 F254) were from Merck (Darmstadt, Germany). The materials for column chromatography (CC) included silica gel (100–200 mesh, Qingdao Marine Chemistry Co., Ltd., Qingdao, China) and Sephadex LH-20 (GE Healthcare Biosciences AB, Stockholm, Sweden). All other reagents were of analytical purity.

An Agilent 1200 high-performance liquid chromatography and a Thermo Orbitrap Fusion LUMOS Tribrid liquid chromatography–mass spectrometer (Orbitrap LC-MS/MS, Thermo Fisher Scientific, Waltham, MA, USA) were used to analyze the samples. A 96-well microplate reader (Bio-Tek Epoch 2, Bio Tek Instruments, Winooski, VT, USA) was used for spectrophotometric measurements. An Allegra X-30R high-speed centrifugator (Beckman Coulter, Brea, CA, USA) was used for ultrafiltration experiment.

4.2. Preparation of Crude Extracts of P. capillacea

The air-dried *P. capillacea* (3 kg) was crushed and soaked in anhydrous ethanol for 24 h with a ratio (g:mL) of 1:10, extracted three times, filtered, and concentrated to dryness below 40 °C with a rotary evaporator to obtain the crude extract, and then stored at -20 °C.

4.3. Separation of the Crude Extract

First, 13 g of crude extract was separated with a silica gel column (200–300 mesh) which was eluted stepwise using n-hexane/ethyl acetate (1:0 to 0:1) and ethyl acetate/methanol

(1:0 to 0:1); the eluates were detected via HPTLC. Twelve primary fractions (F1 to F12) were obtained. The fraction F4 showing strong XOD-inhibitory activity in bioassay and was further separated using a Sephadex LH-20 gel filtration column, eluted with methanol/dichloromethane = 2:1 solution to yield four secondary fractions (F4-1 to F4-4) for further study.

4.4. In Vitro Determination of XOD-Inhibitory Activity

The in vitro XOD-inhibitory activities were evaluated with UV transparent 96-well microwell plates using a modified method based on Andriana's report [70], in which the enzyme activity was reflected by the UV absorbance of uric acid derived from xanthine.

The reaction mixture contained 17.5 µL XOD solution (20 U/L, in phosphate-buffered solution (PBS) containing 0.014 mol/L KH_2PO_4, 0.061 mol/L $K_2HPO_4 \cdot 3H_2O$, and 0.111 mol/L EDTA-Na_2 with pH 7.4), 119.5 µL PBS, 3 µL sample solution (10 mg/mL in DMSO), and 70 µL xanthine (0.4 mmol/L in PBS). The microwell plates were incubated at 37°C for 10 min before absorbance was measured (OD_1) at 295 nm. For control, the sample was replaced by DMSO (OD_2). For sample background subtraction, XOD was replaced by PBS (OD_3). For the blank sample, XOD and sample were replaced by PBS (OD_4). Allopurinol (10 mg/mL in 0.1 mol/L NaOH) was taken as positive control. All samples were tested in triplicate. The inhibition ratios were calculated using the following formula:

$$I(\%) = (1 - \frac{OD_1 - OD_3}{OD_2 - OD_4}) \times 100\%, \tag{1}$$

4.5. Cellular Anti-Inflammatory Activity Assay

The content of NO in cells and cell survival rate were determined in accordance with a previously reported method [71]. In accordance with the manufacturer's protocol, the NO level of RAW264.7 cells treated with or without lipopolysaccharide and P. capillacea extracts (crude extract, F4 and F6) was evaluated using the Griess reagent system. The viability of RAW264.7 cells treated with or without P. capillacea extracts (crude extract, F4 and F6) was evaluated via CCK-8.

RAW264.7 cells were seeded in a 24-well plate at a density of 5×10^4 cells/well. In all the test groups, the cells were treated with the extracts (crude extract, F4 and F6) of P. capillacea with a concentration of 20 µg/mL. Subsequently, they were activated with LPS (1 µg/mL) for 24 h, except for the blank group. Finally, NO production was estimated via spectrophotometry at 540 nm.

Cell viability assay: RAW264.7 cells were inoculated in 96-well plates at a density of 5×10^4 cells/well for 24 h. P. capillacea extract (crude extract, F4 and F6) was added to reach a final concentration of 20 µg/mL and incubated for 24 h. After 10 µL of CCK-8 solution was added to each well for 1 h, absorbance values were measured at 450 nm.

4.6. UF-LC-MS/MS

4.6.1. Affinity Ultrafiltration Treatment

First, 10 mg of sample (in 100 µL methanol) was applied onto a reverse SPE column, eluted with 1 mL pure water to remove salts, and then with 1 mL methanol to collect the eluent. This eluent solution was then filtrated through 0.22 µm membrane, dried completely, and finally dissolved in 20 µL of DMSO plus 80 µL of water to form the sample solution used for affinity ultrafiltration. For the process group (P), 50 µL of sample solution, 50 µL of 0.5 U/mL of XOD solution, and 100 µL of Tris-HCL buffer were added to a 1.5 mL centrifuge tube and incubated at 37 °C for 30 min. Afterwards, the unbound small molecules were removed by centrifugation at 11,200× g for 10 min and repeatedly washed using Tris-HCL buffer and centrifugation 3 times. Then, the ligands were released from the retained ligand–enzyme complexes on the ultrafiltration membrane using 100 µL of methanol-water (4:1) (centrifugation at 11,200× g for 10 min, repeated 3 times). The eluate was dried and dissolved in 1 mL of LC-MS pure methanol for HPLC and Orbitrap LC-MS/MS analyses. For the blank group (B), the difference was that the XOD solution was denatured at 100 °C for 30 min before use. For the crude sample group (C), the sample was prepared directly to 5 mg/mL after desalting, without ultrafiltration.

4.6.2. HPLC Preliminary Analysis

The HPLC analyses of samples were performed on an Agilent 1200 HPLC instrument connected with a diode array detector (DAD). The columns were Phenomenex Kinetex C18 100A (Phenomenex, Torrance, CA, USA) reversed-phase columns (100 × 4.60 mm, 5 μm). The injection volume was 20 μL. The gradient mobile phase was: 30% MeCN/H_2O for 2 min, 30% MeCN/H_2O to 95% in 12 min, 95% MeCN/H_2O for 15 min, 95% MeCN/H_2O to 30% MeCN/H_2O in 0.2 min, and finally 30% MeCN/H_2O for 2.8 min with a flow rate of 0.6 mL/min. The MeCN was added with 0.1% HCOOH.

4.6.3. LC-MS/MS Analysis

LC–MS/MS analysis was performed on a Thermo Orbitrap Fusion LUMOS Tribrid liquid chromatography–mass spectrometer, and a Waters Acquity UPLC BEH C18 column (1.7 μm, 2.1 × 100 mm, Waters, Milford, CT, USA) was used for analysis. The injection volume was 10 μL. The gradient mobile phase was: 10% MeCN/H_2O for 1 min, 10% MeCN/H_2O to 60% in 9 min, 60% MeCN/H_2O to 90% in 3 min, 90% MeCN/H_2O for 3 min, then 90% MeCN/H_2O to 10% MeCN/H_2O in 0.2 min, and finally 10% MeCN/H_2O for 3.8 min with a flow rate of 0.3 mL/min. Both the water and the MeCN contained 0.1% HCOOH. Mass spectra were recorded in positive ESI mode (m/z 200–2000) and with an automated fully dependent MS/MS scan enabled.

4.7. Annotation of the Bioactive Molecules Using Metabolomics Tools

The standard pipeline of feature-based molecular networking (FBMN) with MS-DIAL was performed by referring to a previous report [29] and following the instructions on the webpage of the GNPS platform (https://ccms-ucsd.github.io/GNPSDocumentation/featurebasedmolecularnetworking-with-ms-dial/, accessed on 17 December 2022). The parameters for clustering and compound matching were set as follows: minimum matching fragment of 6; minimum cluster size of 2; cosine threshold of 0.7; and search database range of the entire GNPS library. Data visualization was performed using Cytoscape 3.7.2 software. In addition, the annotation of compounds was also performed via MS-DIAL database matching and MS-FINDER matching with all its indexed natural product databases [72,73].

Furthermore, to retrieve the biological source of the annotated compounds, the following open access natural product databases were searched manually: the PubChem (https://pubchem.ncbi.nlm.nih.gov/, accessed on 15 August 2023), the Dictionary of Natural Products (DNP) (http://dnp.chemnetbase.com/, accessed on 15 August 2023), the NPASS (http://bidd.group/NPASS/, accessed on 15 August 2023), the Natural Product Atlas (https://www.npatlas.org/, accessed on 15 August 2023), and the COCONUT (https://coconut.naturalproducts.net/, accessed on 15 August 2023).

4.8. Molecular Docking and ADMET Analysis

The sdf structures of ligands were downloaded from the PubChem database and were batch processed into pdbqt files suitable for molecular docking using openbabel 2.3.2. The crystal structure of XOD protein was obtained from the Protein Database Bank (PDB ID: 3nvw). Water molecules and guanine ligands were removed from the protein using Pymol 2.5.4 software and the protein was exported to pdb format. Then, the protein was hydrogenated and structurally optimized using Autodock vina 1.5.7, and finally exported to pdbqt format. Molecular docking of all ligands to XOD was performed using Autodock vina 1.5.7 and the docking results are visualized using Pymol 2.5.4.

ADMET analysis was performed online on the ADMETlab prediction website (https://admetmesh.scbdd.com/, accessed on 2 April 2023) to predict the adsorption, distribution, metabolism, excretion, and toxicity characteristics of compounds by entering the SMILES codes of the compounds.

4.9. Statistical Analysis

All experiments and analyses were performed at least in triplicate, and the obtained results were expressed as "mean ± standard deviation". Statistical differences of mean values were evaluated using Duncan's multiple range test using GraphPad Prism 8.0.1 software (San Diego, CA, USA). A probability of less than 5% ($p < 0.05$) was considered significant.

Supplementary Materials: The following supporting information can be downloaded at: https://www.mdpi.com/article/10.3390/md21100502/s1, Figure S1: The MS/MS spectrum of compound 1 captured by the affinity ultrafiltration from fraction F4-2(P); Figure S2: The MS/MS spectrum of compound 2 captured by the affinity ultrafiltration from fraction F4-2(P); Figure S3: The MS/MS spectrum of the [M+NH4]+ ion of compound 3 captured by the affinity ultrafiltration from fraction F4-2(P); Figure S4: The MS/MS spectrum of the [M+H]+ ion of compound 3 captured by the affinity ultrafiltration from fraction F4-2(P); Figure S5: The MS/MS spectrum of compound 4 captured by the affinity ultrafiltration from fraction F4-2(P); Figure S6: The MS/MS spectrum of compound 5 captured by the affinity ultrafiltration from fraction F4-2(P); Figure S7: The MS/MS spectrum of compound 6 captured by the affinity ultrafiltration from fraction F4-2(P); Figure S8: The MS/MS spectrum of compound 7 captured by the affinity ultrafiltration from fractions F4-2(P) and F4-3(P); Figure S9: The MS/MS spectrum of compound 8 captured by the affinity ultrafiltration from fractions F4-2(P) and F4-3(P); Figure S10: The MS/MS spectrum of compound 9 captured by the affinity ultrafiltration from fraction F4-2(P); Figure S11: The MS/MS spectrum of compound 10 captured by the affinity ultrafiltration from fraction F4-2(P); Figure S12: The MS/MS spectrum of compound 11 captured by the affinity ultrafiltration from fraction F4-2(P); Figure S13: The MS/MS spectrum of compound 12 captured by the affinity ultrafiltration from fraction F4-3(P); Figure S14: The MS/MS spectrum of compound 13 captured by the affinity ultrafiltration from fraction F4-3(P); Figure S15: The MS/MS spectrum of compound 14 captured by the affinity ultrafiltration from fraction F4-3(P); Figure S16: The MS/MS spectrum of compound 15 captured by the affinity ultrafiltration from fraction F4-3(P); Figure S17: The MS/MS spectrum of compound 16 captured by the affinity ultrafiltration from fraction F4-3(P); Figure S18: The MS/MS spectrum of compound 17 captured by the affinity ultrafiltration from fraction F4-3(P); Figure S19: The MS/MS spectrum of compound 18 captured by the affinity ultrafiltration from fraction F4-3(P); Figure S20: The MS/MS spectrum of compound 19 captured by the affinity ultrafiltration from fraction F4-3(P); Figure S21: The MS/MS spectrum of compound 20 captured by the affinity ultrafiltration from fraction F4-3(P).

Author Contributions: Y.W., L.Z., M.C., Y.L., Y.Y., T.L. and F.B. performed the experiments. Y.W. wrote the paper. X.H., Z.Q. and P.H. provided advice on the research. Y.Z. conceived, designed, and supervised the experiments. Y.Z. and L.Z. revised the manuscript. All authors have read and agreed to the published version of the manuscript.

Funding: This research was funded by the Guangdong Provincial Natural Science Foundation under Grant 2022A1515010783, the Guangdong Provincial Special Project in Science and Technology under Grant 2021A05240, the National Natural Science Foundation under Grant 21807015, the Special project in key fields of Guangdong provincial higher education institutions (Biomedicine and health care) under Grant 2021ZDZX2064, the Basic Research Project of Shenzhen Science and Technology Innovation Commission under Grants JCYJ20220530162014032 and JCYJ20190813105005619, the Zhanjiang Marine Youth Talent Innovation Project under Grant 2022E05010, the Shenzhen Dapeng New District Scientific and Technological Research and Development Fund under Grant KJYF202001-07, the Science and Technology Development Special Fund Competitive Allocation Project of Zhanjiang City under Grant 2020A01030, the Program for Scientific Research Start-up Funds of Guangdong Ocean University under Grants R18008 and 060302042201, and the Graduate Student Education Innovation Project of Guangdong Ocean University under Grant 202232.

Institutional Review Board Statement: Not applicable for studies not involving humans or animals.

Data Availability Statement: All data are provided in full in the results section and Supplementary Materials of this paper.

Conflicts of Interest: The authors declare no conflict of interest.

References

1. Kwon, H.C.; Ahn, S.S.; Yoo, B.W.; Yoo, J.; Jung, S.M.; Song, J.J.; Park, Y.B.; Lee, S.W. Hyperuricemia is associated with decreased renal function and occurrence of end-stage renal disease in patients with microscopic polyangiitis and granulomatosis with polyangiitis: A retrospective study. *Rheumatol. Int.* **2020**, *40*, 1089–1099. [CrossRef] [PubMed]
2. So, A.K.; Martinon, F. Inflammation in gout: Mechanisms and therapeutic targets. *Nat. Rev. Rheumatol.* **2017**, *13*, 639–647. [CrossRef] [PubMed]
3. Choi, H.K.; Mount, D.B.; Reginato, A.M. Pathogenesis of Gout. *Ann. Intern. Med.* **2005**, *143*, 499–516. [CrossRef] [PubMed]
4. Wang, Y.T.; Zhang, W.L.; Qian, T.T.; Sun, H.; Xu, Q. Reduced renal function may explain the higher prevalence of hyperuricemia in older people. *Sci. Rep.* **2021**, *11*, 1302–1308. [CrossRef]
5. Ruiz-Miyazawa, K.W.; Borghi, S.M.; Pinho-Ribeiro, F.A.; Staurengo-Ferrari, L.; Fattori, V.; Fernandes, G.S.A.; Casella, A.M.; Alves-Filho, J.C.; Cunha, T.M.; Cunha, F.Q.; et al. Quercetin inhibits gout arthritis in mice: Induction of an opioid-dependent regulation of inflammasome. *Inflammopharmacology* **2017**, *25*, 555–570. [CrossRef]
6. Barros, C.H.; Matosinhos, R.C. *Lychnophora pinaster*'s effects on inflammation and pain in acute gout. *J. Ethnopharmacol.* **2021**, *280*, 114460. [CrossRef]
7. Hille, R.; Hall, J.; Basu, P. The mononuclear molybdenum enzymes. *Chem. Rev.* **1996**, *96*, 2757–2816. [CrossRef]
8. Zhao, M.M. In Vitro and In Vivo studies on adlay-derived seed extracts: Phenolic profiles, antioxidant activities, serum uric acid suppression, and xanthine oxidase inhibitory effects. *J. Agric. Food Chem.* **2014**, *62*, 7771–7778. [CrossRef]
9. Lee, B.E.; Toledo, A.H.; Anaya-Prado, R.; Roach, R.R.; Toledo-Pereyra, L.H. Allopurinol, xanthine oxidase, and cardiac ischemia. *J. Investig. Med. Off. Publ. Am. Fed. Clin. Res.* **2009**, *57*, 902–909. [CrossRef]
10. Bruce, S.P. Febuxostat: A selective xanthine oxidase inhibitor for the treatment of hyperuricemia and gout. *Ann. Pharmacother.* **2006**, *40*, 2187–2194. [CrossRef]
11. Takashi, N.; Takayo, M.; Mai, N.; Nobutaka, M.; Naoki, A.; Takashi, I.; Ryusuke, S. Effects of topiroxostat and febuxostat on urinary albumin excretion and plasma xanthine oxidoreductase activity in dbidb mice. *Eur. J. Pharmacol. Int. J.* **2016**, *780*, 224–231.
12. Gliozzi, M.; Malara, N.; Muscoli, S.; Mollace, V. The treatment of hyperuricemia. *Int. J. Cardiol.* **2016**, *213*, 23–27. [CrossRef]
13. Badve, S.V.; Pascoe, E.M.; Tiku, A.; Boudville, N.; Brown, F.G.; Cass, A.; Clarke, P.; Dalbeth, N.; Day, R.O.; Zoysa, J.R.d.; et al. Effects of Allopurinol on the Progression of Chronic Kidney Disease. *N. Engl. J. Med.* **2020**, *382*, 2504–2513. [CrossRef] [PubMed]
14. Yao, F.F.; Zhang, R.; Fu, R.J.; Chen, J.; He, W. Effect and mechanism study of the same doses of Quercetin and Apigenin on hyperuricemic rats. *Mod. Prev. Med.* **2012**, *39*, 1365–1367.
15. Zhu, J.X.; Wang, Y.; Kong, L.D.; Yang, C.; Zhang, X. Effects of *Biota orientalis* extract and its flavonoid constituents, quercetin and rutin on serum uric acid levels in oxonate-induced mice and xanthine dehydrogenase and xanthine oxidase activities in mouse liver. *J. Ethnopharmacol.* **2004**, *93*, 133–140. [CrossRef]
16. Shin-Ichi, A.; Mifuyu, O.; Shinji, K.; Kazumi, Y. Comparative effects of quercetin, luteolin, apigenin and their related polyphenols on uric acid production in cultured hepatocytes and suppression of purine bodies-induced hyperuricemia by rutin in mice. *Cytotechnology* **2021**, *73*, 343–351.
17. Ou, R.R.; Lin, L.Z.; Zhao, M.M.; Xie, Z.Q. Action mechanisms and interaction of two key xanthine oxidase inhibitors in galangal: Combination of In Vitro and in silico molecular docking studies. *Int. J. Biol. Macromol.* **2020**, *162*, 1526–1535. [CrossRef] [PubMed]
18. Zhang, C.; Zhang, G.W.; Pan, J.H.; Gong, D.M. Galangin competitively inhibits xanthine oxidase by a ping-pong mechanism. *Food Res. Int.* **2016**, *89*, 152–160. [CrossRef] [PubMed]
19. Liang, Q.C.; Shen, G.Z.; Wei, T.; Wu, D.M. Study on interaction between myricetin and XO via spectroscopy. *J. Harbin Univ. Commer. Nat. Sci. Ed.* **2011**, *27*, 279–281.
20. Zhang, C.; Zhang, G.W.; Liao, Y.J. Myricetin inhibits the generation of superoxide anion by reduced form of xanthine oxidase. *Food Chem.* **2017**, *221*, 1569–1577. [CrossRef]
21. Cengiz, S.; Yurdakoc, K.; Aksu, S. Inhibition of xanthine oxidase by Caulerpenyne from *Caulerpa prolifera*. *Turk. J. Biochem.* **2012**, *37*, 445–451. [CrossRef]
22. Zhang, D.Y.; Liu, H.Z.; Luo, P.; Li, Y.Q. Production Inhibition and Excretion Promotion of Urate by Fucoidan from *Laminaria japonica* in Adenine-Induced Hyperuricemic Mice. *Mar. Drugs* **2018**, *16*, 472. [CrossRef] [PubMed]
23. Zhang, Y.; Tan, X.H.; Lin, Z.; Liu, H.Z.; Shang, J.H. Fucoidan from *Laminaria japonica* inhibits expression of GLUT9 and URAT1 via PI3K/Akt, JNK and NF-κB pathways in uric acid-exposed HK-2 Cells. *Mar. Drugs* **2021**, *19*, 238. [CrossRef] [PubMed]
24. Li, X.Q.; Gao, X.X. The anti-hyperuricemic effects of green alga *Enteromorpha prolifera* polysaccharide via regulation of the uric acid transporters In Vivo. *Food Chem. Toxicol.* **2021**, *158*, 112630. [CrossRef] [PubMed]
25. Chen, G.L.; Guo, M.Q. Rapid screening for α-Glucosidase inhibitors from *Gymnema sylvestre* by Affinity Ultrafiltration–HPLC-MS. *Front. Pharmacol.* **2017**, *8*, 228. [CrossRef] [PubMed]
26. Tsugawa, H.; Cajka, T.; Kind, T.; Ma, Y. MS-DIAL: Data-independent MS/MS deconvolution for comprehensive metabolome analysis. *Nat. Methods* **2015**, *12*, 523–526. [CrossRef]
27. Tsugawa, H. Computational MS/MS fragmentation and structure elucidation using MS-FINDER software. *Compr. Nat. Prod. III* **2020**, *7*, 189–210.
28. Oppong-Danquah, E.; Parrot, D.; Bluemel, M.; Labes, A.; Tasdemir, D. Molecular networking-based metabolome and bioactivity analyses of marine-adapted fungi co-cultivated with phytopathogens. *Front. Microbiol.* **2018**, *9*, 2072. [CrossRef]

29. Nothias, L.F.; Petras, D.; Schmid, R.; Dührkop, K.; Rainer, J. Feature-based Molecular Networking in the GNPS analysis environment. *Nat. Methods* **2020**, *17*, 905–908. [CrossRef]
30. Remy, S.; Solis, D.; Silland, P.; Neyts, J.; Roussi, F.; Touboul, D.; Litaudon, M. Isolation of phenanthrenes and identification of phorbol ester derivatives as potential anti-CHIKV agents using FBMN and NAP from *Sagotia racemosa*. *Phytochemistry* **2019**, *167*, 112101. [CrossRef]
31. Nie, Y.Y.; Yang, W.C.; Liu, Y.Y.; Yang, J.M.; Lei, X.L.; Gerwick, W.H.; Zhang, Y. Acetylcholinesterase inhibitors and antioxidants mining from marine fungi: Bioassays, bioactivity coupled LC–MS/MS analyses and molecular networking. *Mar. Life Sci. Technol.* **2020**, *2*, 386–397. [CrossRef]
32. Patarra, R.F.; Iha, C.; Pereira, L.; Neto, A.I. Concise review of the species *Pterocladiella capillacea* (S.G. Gmelin) Santelices & Hommersand. *J. Appl. Phycol.* **2020**, *32*, 787–808.
33. Cavalli, P.A.; Wanderlind, E.H.; Hemmer, J.V.; Gerlach, O.M.S.; Emmerich, A.K.; Bella-Cruz, A.; Tamanahae, M.r.; Almerindo, G.I. *Pterocladiella capillacea*-stabilized silver nanoparticles as a green approach toward antibacterial biomaterials. *New J. Chem.* **2021**, *45*, 3382–3386. [CrossRef]
34. Alencar, D.B.D.; Diniz, J.C.; Rocha, S.A.S.; Pires-Cavalcante, K.M.S.; Lima, R.L.D.; Sousa, K.C.D.; Freitas, J.O.; Bezerra, R.M.; Baracho, B.M.; Sampaio, A.H.; et al. Fatty acid composition from the marine red algae *Pterocladiella capillacea* (S. G. Gmelin) Santelices & Hommersand 1997 and *Osmundaria obtusiloba* (C. Agardh) R. E. Norris 1991 and its antioxidant activity. *An. Acad. Bras. Ciências* **2018**, *90*, 449–459.
35. Alencar, D.B.d.; Carvalho, F.C.T.d.; Rebouças, R.H.; Santos, D.R.D.; Pires-Cavalcante, K.M.D.S.; Lima, R.L.d.; Baracho, B.M.; Bezerra, R.M.; Viana, F.A.; Vieira, R.H.S.D.F.; et al. Bioactive extracts of red seaweeds *Pterocladiella capillacea* and *Osmundaria obtusiloba* (Floridophyceae:Rhodophyta) with antioxidant and bacterial agglutination potential. *Asian Pac. J. Trop. Med.* **2016**, *9*, 372–379. [CrossRef]
36. Bou-Salah, L.; Benarous, K.; Linani, A.; Rabhi, F.; Chaib, K.; Chine, I.; Bensaidane, H.; Yousfi, M. Anti-inflammatory drugs as new inhibitors to xanthine oxidase: In vitro and in silico approach. *Mol. Cell. Probes* **2021**, *58*, 101733. [CrossRef]
37. Nile, S.H.; Ko, E.Y.; Kim, D.H.; Keum, Y.-S. Screening of ferulic acid related compounds as inhibitors of xanthine oxidase and cyclooxygenase-2 with anti-inflammatory activity. *Rev. Bras. Farmacogn.* **2015**, *26*, 50–55. [CrossRef]
38. Preethi, J.; Chitra, L.; Ancy, I.; Kumaradhas, P.; Palvannan, T. S-allyl cysteine as potent anti-gout drug: Insight into the xanthine oxidase inhibition and anti-inflammatory activity. *Biochimie* **2018**, *154*, 1–9.
39. Hsiao, G.; Chi, W.C.; Pang, K.L.; Chen, J.; Kuo, Y. Hirsutane-Type sesquiterpenes with inhibitory activity of microglial nitric oxide production from the red alga-derived fungus *Chondrostereum* sp. NTOU4196. *J. Nat. Prod.* **2017**, *80*, 1615–1622. [CrossRef]
40. Tsugawa, H.; Nakabayashi, R.; Mori, T.; Yamada, Y.; Takahashi, M. A cheminformatics approach to characterize metabolomes in stable-isotope-labeled organisms. *Nat. Methods* **2019**, *16*, 295–298. [CrossRef]
41. He, J.Y.; Liu, C.C.; Du, M.Z.; Zhou, X.Y.; Hu, Z.L.; Lei, A.P.; Wang, J.X. Metabolic responses of a model green microalga *Euglena gracilis* to different environmental stresses. *Front. Bioeng. Biotechnol.* **2021**, *9*, 662655. [CrossRef] [PubMed]
42. Chen, J.; Montanari, A.M.; Widmer, W.W. Two new polymethoxylated flavones, a class of compounds with potential anticancer activity, isolated from cold pressed dancy tangerine peel oil solids. *J. Agric. Food Chem.* **1997**, *45*, 364–368. [CrossRef]
43. Yang, D.; Yang, R.G.; Shen, J.Y.; Huang, L.; Men, S.; Wang, T.C. Sinensetin attenuates oxygen-glucose deprivation/reperfusion-induced neurotoxicity by MAPK pathway in human cerebral microvascular endothelial cells. *J. Appl. Toxicol. JAT* **2021**, *42*, 683–693. [CrossRef]
44. Findwy, J.A.; Patil, A.D. Antibacterial constituents of the red alga *Cystoclonium purpureum*. *Phytochemistry* **1986**, *25*, 548–550. [CrossRef]
45. Useini, L.; Mojić, M.; Laube, M.; Lönnecke, P.; Mijatović, S. Carborane analogues of Fenoprofen exhibit Improved antitumor activity. *ChemMedChem* **2023**, *18*, e202200583. [CrossRef] [PubMed]
46. Ashry, E.S.H.E.; Atta-ur-Rahman; Choudhary, M.I.; Kandil, S.H.; Nemr, A.E.; Gulzar, T.; Shobier, A.H. Studies on the constituents of the green alga *Ulva lactuca*. *Chem. Nat. Compd.* **2011**, *47*, 335–338. [CrossRef]
47. Naik, R.R.; Shakya, A.K.; Oriquat, G.A.; Katekhaye, S. Fatty acid analysis, chemical constituents, biological activity and pesticide residues screening in jordanian propolis. *Molecules* **2021**, *26*, 5076. [CrossRef]
48. Elakkad, Y.E.; Younis, M.K.; Allam, R.M.; Mohsen, A.F.; Khalil, I.A. Tenoxicam loaded hyalcubosomes for osteoarthritis. *Int. J. Pharm.* **2021**, *601*, 120483. [CrossRef]
49. Ardellina, J.H.; Moore, R.E. Sphingosine derivatives from red algae of the ceramiales. *Phytochemistry* **1978**, *17*, 554–555. [CrossRef]
50. Verstockt, B.; Vetrano, S.; Salas, A.; Nayeri, S.; Duijvestein, M.; Casteele, N.V. Sphingosine 1-phosphate modulation and immune cell trafficking in inflammatory bowel disease. *Nat. Rev. Gastroenterol. Hepatol.* **2022**, *19*, 351–366. [CrossRef]
51. Furukawa, T.; Sakamoto, N.; Suzuki, M.; Kimura, M.; Nagasawa, H.; Sakuda, S. Precocene II, a trichothecene production inhibitor, binds to voltage-dependent anion channel and increases the superoxide level in mitochondria of *Fusarium graminearum*. *PLoS ONE* **2015**, *10*, e0135031. [CrossRef] [PubMed]
52. Sukmawan, Y.P.; Anggadiredja, K.; Adnyana, I.K. Anti-neuropathic pain mechanistic study on *A. conyzoides* essential oil, Precocene II, Caryophyllene, or Longifolene as single agents and in combination with pregabalin. *CNS Neurol. Disord.—Drug Targets* **2023**, *22*, 924–931. [CrossRef] [PubMed]
53. Anyanwu, G.O.; Nisar-ur-Rehman; Onyeneke, C.E.; Rauf, K. Medicinal plants of the genus *Anthocleista*—A review of their ethnobotany, phytochemistry and pharmacology. *J. Ethnopharmacol.* **2015**, *175*, 648–667. [CrossRef] [PubMed]

54. Liu, L.; Zhao, T.Y.; Shan, L.Z.; Cao, L.; Zhu, X.X.; Xue, Y. Estradiol regulates intestinal ABCG2 to promote urate excretion via the PI3K/Akt pathway. *Nutr. Metab.* **2021**, *18*, 63–73. [CrossRef]
55. Wang, Y.G.; Feng, F.F.; He, W.F.; Sun, L.F.; He, Q.; Jin, J. MiR-188-3p abolishes germacrone-mediated podocyte protection in a mouse model of diabetic nephropathy in type I diabetes through triggering mitochondrial injury. *Bioengineered* **2022**, *13*, 774–788. [CrossRef]
56. Jin, T.; Leng, B. Cynaropicrin averts the oxidative stress and neuroinflammation in ischemic/reperfusion injury through the modulation of NF-κB. *Appl. Biochem. Biotechnol.* **2023**, *195*, 5424–5438. [CrossRef]
57. Yamaguchi, Y.; Matsumura, T.; Ichida, K.; Okamoto, K.; Nishino, T. Human xanthine oxidase changes its substrate specificity to aldehyde oxidase type upon mutation of amino acid residues in the active site: Roles of active site residues in binding and activation of purine substrate. *J. Biochem.* **2007**, *141*, 513–524. [CrossRef]
58. Lipinski, C.A.; Lombardo, F.; Dominy, B.W.; Feeney, P.J. Experimental and computational approaches to estimate solubility and permeability in drug discovery and development settings. *Adv. Drug Deliv. Rev.* **2001**, *46*, 3–26. [CrossRef]
59. Ma, K.; Bao, L.; Han, J.J.; Jin, T.; Yang, X.L.; Zhao, F.; Li, S.F.; Song, F.H.; Liu, M.M.; Liu, H.W. New benzoate derivatives and hirsutane type sesquiterpenoids with antimicrobial activity and cytotoxicity from the solid-state fermented rice by the medicinal mushroom *Stereum hirsutum*. *Food Chem.* **2014**, *143*, 239–245. [CrossRef]
60. Qi, Q.Y.; Bao, L.; Ren, J.W.; Han, J.J.; Zhang, Z.Y.; Li, Y.; Yao, Y.J.; Cao, R.; Liu, H.W. Sterhirsutins A and B, two new heterodimeric sesquiterpenes with a new skeleton from the culture of *Stereum hirsutum* collected in Tibet Plateau. *Org. Lett.* **2014**, *16*, 5092–5095. [CrossRef]
61. Huang, L.; Lan, W.J.; Li, H.J. Two new hirsutane-type sesquiterpenoids chondrosterins N and O from the marine fungus *Chondrostereum* sp. *Nat. Prod. Res.* **2018**, *32*, 1578–1582. [CrossRef]
62. Huang, L.; Lan, W.J.; Deng, R.; Feng, G.K.; Xu, Q.Y.; Hu, Z.Y. Additional new cytotoxic triquinane-type sesquiterpenoids chondrosterins K–M from the marine fungus *Chondrostereum* sp. *Mar. Drugs* **2016**, *14*, 157. [CrossRef] [PubMed]
63. Liu, H.X.; Tan, H.B.; Chen, K.; Chen, Y.C.; Li, S.N.; Li, H.H.; Zhang, W.M. Cerrenins A–C, cerapicane and isohirsutane sesquiterpenoids from the endophytic fungus *Cerrena* sp. *Fitoterapia* **2018**, *129*, 173–178. [CrossRef] [PubMed]
64. Cha, H.J.; Chiang, M.W.L.; Guo, S.Y.; Lin, S.M.; Pang, K.L. Culturable fungal community of *Pterocladiella capillacea* in Keelung, Taiwan: Effects of surface sterilization method and isolation medium. *J. Fungi* **2021**, *7*, 651. [CrossRef] [PubMed]
65. Tiwari, P.; Bae, H. Endophytic Fungi: Key insights, emerging prospects, and challenges in natural product drug discovery. *Microorganisms* **2022**, *10*, 360. [CrossRef] [PubMed]
66. Tang, P.; Si, S.; Liu, L. Analysis of bovine serum albumin ligands from *Puerariae flos* using ultrafiltration combined with HPLC-MS. *J. Chem.* **2015**, *2015*, 648361. [CrossRef]
67. Wang, J.; Liu, S.; Ma, B.; Chen, L. Rapid screening and detection of XOD inhibitors from *S. tamariscina* by ultrafiltration LC-PDA-ESI-MS combined with HPCCC. *Anal. Bioanal. Chem.* **2014**, *406*, 7379–7387. [CrossRef]
68. Chen, G.L.; Huang, B.X.; Guo, M.Q. Current advances in screening for bioactive components from medicinal plants by affinity ultrafiltration mass spectrometry. *Phytochem. Anal. PCA* **2018**, *29*, 375–386. [CrossRef]
69. Wang, M.X.; Carver, J.J.; Phelan, V.V.; Sanchez, L.M. Sharing and community curation of mass spectrometry data with Global Natural Products Social Molecular Networking. *Nat. Biotechnol.* **2016**, *34*, 828–837. [CrossRef]
70. Andriana, Y.; Xuan, T.D.; Quy, T.N.; Minh, T.N.; Van, T.M.; Viet, T.D. Antihyperuricemia, Antioxidant, and Antibacterial Activities of *Tridax procumbens* L. *Foods* **2019**, *8*, 21. [CrossRef]
71. Chen, M.Q.; Liang, J.Y.; Wang, Y.; Liu, Y.; Zhou, C.X.; Hong, P.Z.; Zhang, Y.; Qian, Z.J. A new benzaldehyde from the coral-derived fungus *Aspergillus* terreus C23-3 and its anti-Inflammatory effects via suppression of MAPK signaling pathway in RAW264.7 cells. *J. Zhejiang Univ.-Sci. B Biomed. Biotechnol.* **2022**, *23*, 230–240. [CrossRef] [PubMed]
72. Sun, Y.; Liu, W.C.; Shi, X.; Zheng, H.Z.; Zheng, Z.; Lu, X.H.; Xing, Y. Inducing secondary metabolite production of *Aspergillus sydowii* through microbial co-culture with *Bacillus subtilis*. *Microb. Cell Factories* **2021**, *20*, 42–57. [CrossRef] [PubMed]
73. Triastuti, A.; Haddad, M.; Barakat, F.; Mejia, K.; Rabouille, G.; Fabre, N.; Amasifuen, C.; Jargeat, P.; Vansteelandt, M. Dynamics of chemical diversity during co-cultures: An integrative time-scale metabolomics study of fungal Endophytes *Cophinforma mamane* and *Fusarium solani*. *Chem. Biodivers.* **2021**, *18*, e2000672. [CrossRef] [PubMed]

Disclaimer/Publisher's Note: The statements, opinions and data contained in all publications are solely those of the individual author(s) and contributor(s) and not of MDPI and/or the editor(s). MDPI and/or the editor(s) disclaim responsibility for any injury to people or property resulting from any ideas, methods, instructions or products referred to in the content.

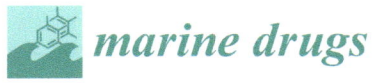 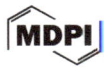

Article

Zeaxanthin epoxidase 3 Knockout Mutants of the Model Diatom *Phaeodactylum tricornutum* Enable Commercial Production of the Bioactive Carotenoid Diatoxanthin

Cecilie Græsholt [1], Tore Brembu [1], Charlotte Volpe [2], Zdenka Bartosova [1], Manuel Serif [1], Per Winge [1] and Marianne Nymark [1,2,*]

[1] Department of Biology, Norwegian University of Science and Technology, 7491 Trondheim, Norway; tore.brembu@ntnu.no (T.B.); zdenka.bartosova@ntnu.no (Z.B.); manuel.serif@ntnu.no (M.S.); per.winge@ntnu.no (P.W.)

[2] Department of Fisheries and New Biomarine Industry, SINTEF Ocean, 7010 Trondheim, Norway; charlotte.volpe@sintef.no

* Correspondence: marianne.nymark@sintef.no

Abstract: Carotenoids are pigments that have a range of functions in human health. The carotenoid diatoxanthin is suggested to have antioxidant, anti-inflammatory and chemo-preventive properties. Diatoxanthin is only produced by a few groups of microalgae, where it functions in photoprotection. Its large-scale production in microalgae is currently not feasible. In fact, rapid conversion into the inactive pigment diadinoxanthin is triggered when cells are removed from a high-intensity light source, which is the case during large-scale harvesting of microalgae biomass. Zeaxanthin epoxidase (ZEP) 2 and/or ZEP3 have been suggested to be responsible for the back-conversion of high-light accumulated diatoxanthin to diadinoxanthin in low-light in diatoms. Using CRISPR/Cas9 gene editing technology, we knocked out the *ZEP2* and *ZEP3* genes in the marine diatom *Phaeodactylum tricornutum* to investigate their role in the diadinoxanthin–diatoxanthin cycle and determine if one of the mutant strains could function as a diatoxanthin production line. Light-shift experiments proved that *ZEP3* encodes the enzyme converting diatoxanthin to diadinoxanthin in low light. Loss of ZEP3 caused the high-light-accumulated diatoxanthin to be stable for several hours after the cultures had been returned to low light, suggesting that *zep3* mutant strains could be suitable as commercial production lines of diatoxanthin.

Keywords: bioactive carotenoid; diatoxanthin; *Phaeodactylum tricornutum*; CRISPR/Cas9 gene editing; zeaxanthin epoxidase; commercial production line

Citation: Græsholt, C.; Brembu, T.; Volpe, C.; Bartosova, Z.; Serif, M.; Winge, P.; Nymark, M. *Zeaxanthin epoxidase 3* Knockout Mutants of the Model Diatom *Phaeodactylum tricornutum* Enable Commercial Production of the Bioactive Carotenoid Diatoxanthin. *Mar. Drugs* **2024**, *22*, 185. https://doi.org/10.3390/md22040185

Academic Editors: Donatella Degl'Innocenti and Marzia Vasarri

Received: 29 March 2024
Revised: 14 April 2024
Accepted: 15 April 2024
Published: 19 April 2024

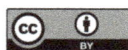

Copyright: © 2024 by the authors. Licensee MDPI, Basel, Switzerland. This article is an open access article distributed under the terms and conditions of the Creative Commons Attribution (CC BY) license (https:// creativecommons.org/licenses/by/ 4.0/).

1. Introduction

Carotenoids are a diverse group of pigments produced by plants, algae and photosynthetic bacteria that have crucial roles in photosynthesis and protection from photodamage [1]. In humans, carotenoids can have health benefits mainly through their antioxidant effects and are emerging as molecules of vital importance that might offer protection against a variety of chronic diseases like cancer, obesity, cataracts, cardiovascular diseases and neurodegenerative diseases [2–5]. Additionally, carotenoids like α-carotene and β-carotene are dietary precursors of vitamin A, essential for human eye health and vision. The main applications of these compounds are as dietary supplements, fortified foods, food colours, animal feed, nutraceuticals, pharmaceuticals and cosmetics [6–8]. Today, only a few carotenoids are commercially produced, including carotenes (β-carotene and lycopene) and xanthophylls (astaxanthin, canthaxanthin, capsanthin, lutein, zeaxanthin (Zx) and fucoxanthin (Fx)) [9].

Fx is one of the most valuable carotenoids present in the marine environment (market price 40,000–80,000 USD/kg), and it can be extracted from certain groups of marine microalgae or brown seaweed [6,10–13]. Applications of Fx currently extend from use in the pharma- and nutraceutical industries to animal feed and cosmetic products [6,10]. In algae cells, the main role of Fx is in light harvesting, and low light (LL) conditions increase the production of this carotenoid [10,14,15]. Recent research has highlighted the pronounced bioactivity of another marine carotenoid, diatoxanthin (Dtx), outperforming commercially available carotenoids as potential disease-preventing agents [16–19]. Antioxidant and anti-inflammatory abilities have been reported, with Dtx found to lower the production of reactive oxygen species (ROS) and pro-inflammatory cytokines in vitro [16–18]. Dtx has also been suggested as a potential therapeutic agent in the treatment and/or prevention of the severe inflammatory syndrome related to the SARS-CoV-2 infection [18]. These findings highlight Dtx as a new marine antioxidant and an anti-inflammatory agent of commercial interest.

Dtx is a low-abundance xanthophyll exclusively found in diatoms and a few other groups of microalgae, including dinophytes and haptophytes [20]. Dtx, together with diadinoxanthin (Ddx), comprise the xanthophyll cycle, which is crucial for regulating the flow of energy to photosystem II (PSII) in these algae [20]. The Ddx–Dtx cycle is equivalent to the xanthophyll cycle in higher plants and green algae, where violaxanthin (Vx) is converted to zeaxanthin (Zx) via the intermediate antheraxanthin by violaxanthin de-epoxidase (VDE) [20]. The reverse reaction is catalysed by zeaxanthin epoxidase (ZEP). In diatoms, the qE component (pH- or energy-dependent component) of the photoprotective mechanism non-photochemical quenching (NPQ) of chlorophyll (Chl) *a* fluorescence depends on the high-light (HL)-induced buildup of a transthylakoidal ΔpH, the de-epoxidation of Ddx to Dtx and the presence of specific light-harvesting complex (LHC) proteins of the LHCX class [20,21]. The reverse reaction takes place in low LL. The interconversion between the pigments of the xanthophyll cycle in diatoms is a rapid process, and relaxation of NPQ, including back-conversion of Dtx to Ddx, takes place within minutes after a shift from HL to LL conditions [20,21]. The rapid loss of accumulated Dtx in LL will hamper industrial-scale production of this potentially valuable carotenoid because Dtx will be converted to Ddx during the lengthy harvesting process of the algae biomass. A possible solution is to knock out the gene encoding the enzyme responsible for the epoxidation of Dtx to Ddx, thereby stabilising HL-accumulated Dtx. Transgene-free CRISPR/Cas9 gene editing is possible in the diatom *Phaeodactylum tricornutum*, and this alga is already being produced commercially, making it an obvious choice for studies of genes involved in the Ddx–Dtx cycle [22–24]. Enzymes catalysing several of the reactions in the multi-step carotenoid synthesis pathway leading to the formation of Fx, Ddx and Dtx are still unknown, despite great progress in this research area during the last couple of years [25–27]. The genome of *P. tricornutum* encodes three proteins belonging to the ZEP family: ZEP1–3 [28,29]. *ZEP1* has recently been found to encode an enzyme essential for the synthesis of Fx [26], whereas *ZEP2* and/or *ZEP3* are candidate genes for encoding the epoxidase converting Dtx to Ddx [26,29,30]. A transmembrane region is predicted to be in the C-terminal domain of ZEP3, which has been hypothesised to be involved in the localisation and/or regulation of the enzyme [20,29]. The roles of ZEP2 and ZEP3 have not yet been confirmed in diatoms, and one or both of these enzymes might also be responsible for an earlier step in the Fx synthesis pathway converting Zx to Vx [26]. Identification of the ZEP responsible for the epoxidation of Dtx to Ddx will be not only of academic interest, filling an important knowledge gap in the carotenoid synthesis pathway of diatoms, but also of commercial interest. A mutant strain where accumulated Dtx remains stable in the cells can facilitate large-scale production of the pigment.

In this context, we created CRISPR/Cas9-mediated knockout mutants of *ZEP2* and *ZEP3* in *P. tricornutum*, aiming to identify the gene encoding the epoxidase responsible for the conversion of Dtx to Ddx. We exposed the mutants to shifts between different light intensities that would trigger the interconversion between the xanthophyll pigments. The carotenoid content, growth, NPQ induction/relaxation and other photosynthetic parameters were compared between *zep* mutants and wild-type (WT) as a response to light treatments. The role of ZEP3 in the Ddx–Dtx cycle was successfully determined, and HL-accumulated Dtx was stabilised.

2. Results and Discussion

2.1. Phylogenetic and Structural Study of ZEP Genes

The *ZEP* genes are widely distributed in plants and algae, but in terrestrial plants and green algae, they are often represented by a single gene, such as in *Arabidopsis thaliana* (*ZEP/ABA1*) or *Chlamydomonas reinhardtii* (*ZEP1*). In marine algae, the *ZEP* genes have diversified, and several distinct groups have evolved through gene duplications in different phyla [26,31]. In diatoms, most species have three distinct ZEP paralogs: ZEP1, 2 and 3. The *P. tricornutum* gene pairs *ZEP1/VDE-like2* and *ZEP3/VDE* are located next to each other in the genome due to segmental gene duplications. Structurally, the diatom ZEP proteins are similar, but ZEP1 and ZEP2 differ from ZEP3 by having three insert regions that are not found in ZEP3 (Figure 1). In addition, ZEP1 has a conserved N-terminal alpha-helical domain not found in ZEP2 and ZEP3. Some species of Ochrophyta have only one *ZEP* gene, such as the brown algae *Ectocarpus siliculosus* and the raphidophyte *Chattonella subsalsa* (Supplementary File S1). What is common for all single-copy ZEP homologs is that they are structurally more related to ZEP3 proteins. In our search for *ZEP* genes, we also discovered a novel ZEP family in diatoms, named ZEP4 in the phylogenetic tree presented in Figure 2, that may have evolved from a ZEP1-like ancestor. Similar to the ZEP1 proteins, they have a conserved N-terminal domain, which is predicted to form an alpha helix, and they lack the C-terminal alpha-helical part found in ZEP2 and ZEP3. The ZEP4 family has a sparse distribution and is missing in many diatoms, such as *P. tricornutum*, but can be found in several species from the Naviculales, Rhizosoleniales and Thalassiosirales orders. Accession numbers for the ZEP proteins/genes and the distribution of ZEP proteins in various marine phyla are shown in a table in Supplementary File S1.

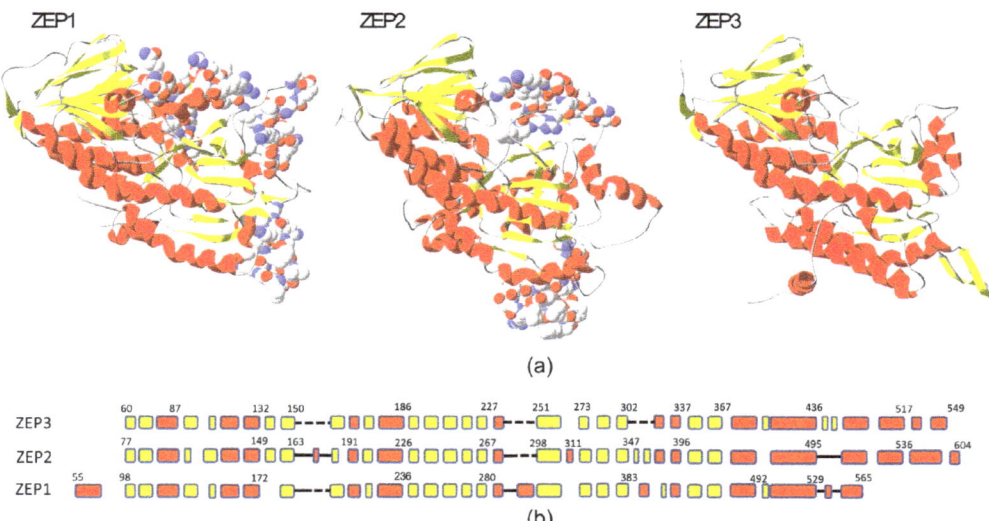

Figure 1. Structural comparison of *P. tricornutum* ZEP proteins. (**a**) The 3D structures of *P. tricornutum* ZEP1, ZEP2 and ZEP3. The protein regions of ZEP1 and ZEP2 that are missing in ZEP3 are shown with side chains in space fill in the ZEP1 and ZEP2 3D models. (**b**) An alignment of the conserved core structure of the ZEP proteins shows the similarities and differences, including the regions missing in ZEP3. The alpha helixes are shown in red, the beta sheets are shown in yellow, and the dashed lines show the missing regions in ZEP3. A solid line indicates loop regions. The numbers indicate amino acid positions at some of the junctions.

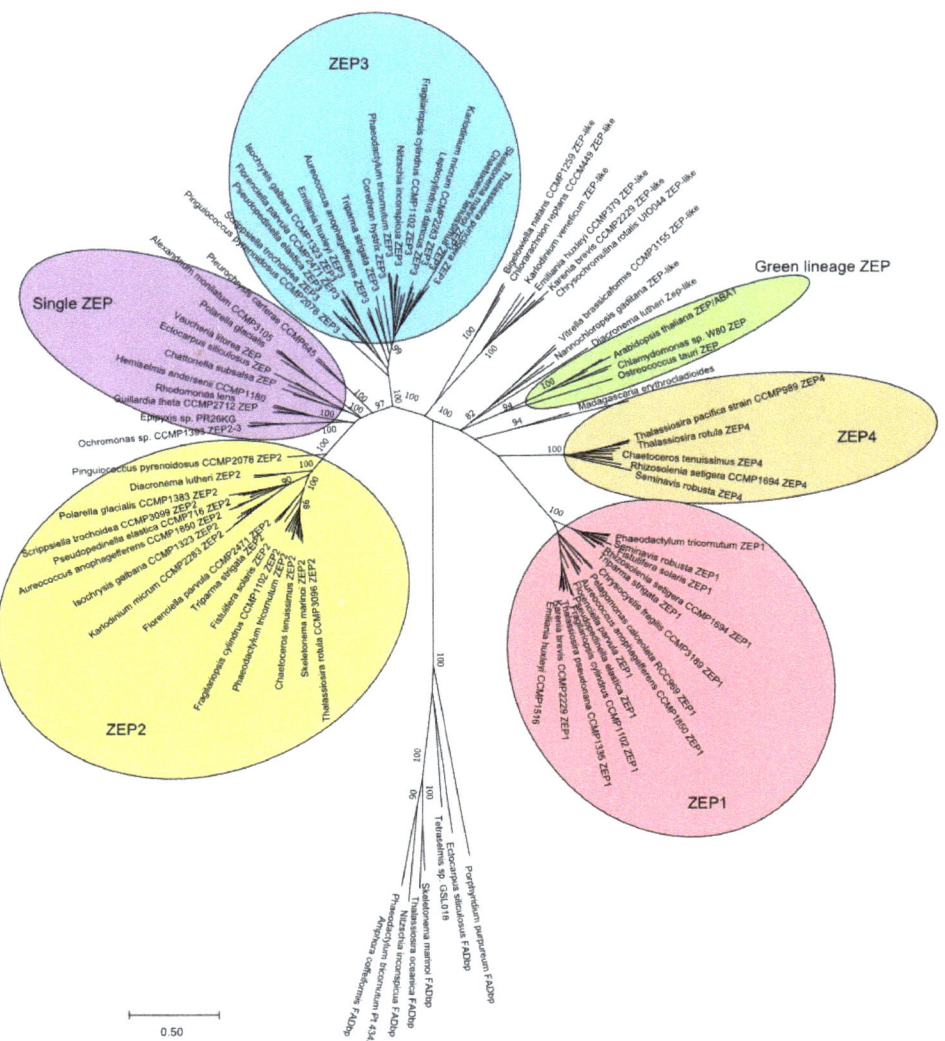

Figure 2. Phylogenetic tree of ZEP proteins. A neighbour-joining (N–J) tree was constructed based on a protein alignment of 158 full-length ZEP proteins. Bootstrap numbers for main clusters with high confidence are shown in the tree. All positions with less than 80% site coverage were eliminated.

2.2. CRISPR/Cas9-Generated zep2 and zep3 Knockout Mutants

Vectors expressing Cas9 and gRNAs targeting either the *ZEP2* or *ZEP3* gene were introduced into *P. tricornutum* cells by bacterial conjugation [22]. Conjugative transformation allows the vector to be maintained as an episome in the diatom cells, avoiding permanent integration of vector DNA into the genome and possible disruption of genetic elements [22,32]. This method also enables the creation of transgene-free mutants because the removal of selection pressure after identification of the mutations of interest causes the cells to lose the CRISPR/Cas9 vector [22]. Mutants containing no foreign DNA might not be legally viewed as GMOs, depending on the individual countries' gene technology legislation. These mutants are likely to have a higher level of customer acceptance, and the use of the biomass will be subject to fewer restrictions. Most countries outside the

EU do not regulate transgene-free gene-edited organisms as GMOs [33], and the EU is currently establishing a new regulatory framework for this type of mutant [34]. Screening of transformants for CRISPR/Cas9-induced mutations resulted in the identification of two *zep2* and two *zep3* knockout lines containing indels of different sizes causing frameshift mutations (Figure 3). Amplification of the two *ZEP* genes by PCR and Sanger sequencing of the PCR products revealed a lack of polymorphism in the sequence for three out of four mutants, indicating that only one allele had been amplified for these mutant lines. This phenomenon is typically caused by large indels or mitotic gene conversion affecting the target site, as observed previously [35,36]. No background signal indicating the presence of a non-mutated WT sequence was observed in any of the mutants where only one allele was amplified by PCR.

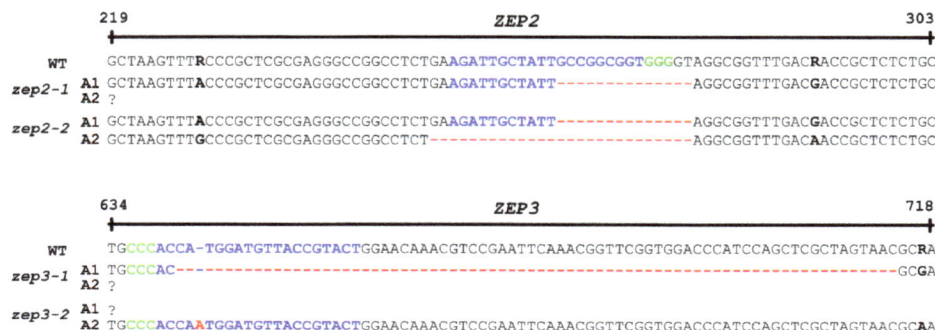

Figure 3. Overview of indels in the two alleles (A1 and A2) of the *ZEP2* and *ZEP3* genes. Blue characters: target sequences; red characters/dashed lines: indels; black characters in bold: polymorphisms; green characters: protospacer adjacent motifs (PAMs). The PAM for *ZEP3* is located on the reverse strand.

2.3. Loss of ZEP3 Blocks the Back-Conversion of Diatoxanthin to Diadinoxanthin in Low Light

Fx is responsible for the golden-brown colour of diatoms. Green phenotypes have been reported for diatom mutants of the carotenoid synthesis pathway being completely devoid of Fx, and for mutants with strongly reduced levels of Fx as a result of lowered levels of pigment-binding proteins [26,27,37,38]. An initial examination of the *zep2* and *zep3* mutant cultures did not reveal a colour change from brown to green in either mutant (Figure 4a), indicating that Fx synthesis was not affected and that neither ZEP2 nor ZEP3 are essential for the conversion of Zx to Vx (Figure 4b). To determine the effect of knocking out the *ZEP2* and *ZEP3* genes on the carotenoid synthesis in *P. tricornutum*, LL-acclimated WT and mutant cells were exposed to HL for 2 h before being returned to LL (rLL) for 0.5 h. Material harvested at the different time points was subjected to high-performance liquid chromatography (HPLC) analyses to determine the pigment content. The analyses showed that the Fx and Chl concentrations were at WT levels in both mutants, confirming the visual impression of the mutant lines (Figures 5a and S1). In contrast, significant and mutant-specific differences were identified for Ddx and Dtx when compared to WT (Figure 5b,c). The Ddx and Dtx concentrations in *zep2* mutants were consistently lower than WT at all light treatments, resulting in a smaller pool of photoprotective pigments. However, the *zep2* mutants displayed a close to identical de-epoxidation state (DES) index (Dtx/(Dtx+Ddx)) pattern as WT as a response to the shifts in light intensities (Figure 5d), indicating that the cyclic interconversion between Ddx and Dtx is unaffected by the loss of ZEP2. Despite the *zep2* mutants displaying WT levels of Fx and a functional Ddx–Dtx cycle, the reduced pool of Dtx+Ddx still implies that ZEP2 plays a role in the synthesis of carotenoids in diatoms. The mild *zep2* phenotype might be explained by ZEP3 being able to compensate for the loss of ZEP2 by catalysing the Zx to Vx reaction, although with a lower efficiency than ZEP2.

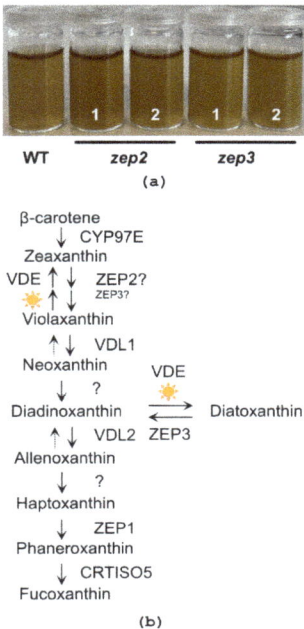

Figure 4. Culture colour and schematic model of the carotenoid biosynthetic pathway. (**a**) Culture colour of low-light (LL)-acclimated WT, *zep2* and *zep3* knockout lines concentrated to 15 million cells, mL^{-1}. (**b**) The schematic model of the carotenoid biosynthetic pathway is modified from Bai et al. [26] and Cao et al. [27] and updated with findings from this study described in the main text. The sun symbols indicate reactions taking place under HL conditions. The presence of ZEP3 is necessary for the back-conversion of diatoxanthin (Dtx) to diadinoxanthin (Ddx), and ZEP3 might possibly compensate for a lack of ZEP2 in the zeaxanthin (Zx)–violaxanthin (Vx) reaction step. Abbreviations: CYP97: cytochrome P450 97 family; VDE: violaxanthin de-epoxidase; VDL: violaxanthin de-epoxidase-like; ZEP: zeaxanthin epoxidase; CRTISO5: carotenoid isomerase-like protein 5.

In contrast to the *zep2* strains, the *zep3* strains show higher Dtx and higher DES index levels than WT throughout the experiments and, most strikingly, an inability to back-convert Dtx accumulated during the HL treatment to Ddx when returned to LL conditions (Figure 5b–d). In *zep3* mutants, Dtx is already abundant in LL conditions. In green algae, where Zx and Vx comprise the xanthophyll cycle, a similar phenotype has been reported for *zep* knockout mutants, where Zx accumulates in all light conditions [39,40]. To further investigate the stability of accumulated Dtx in the *zep3* strains, an additional experiment was performed, where material was harvested 1, 2 and 6 h after the cultures had been returned to LL (Figure 5e–h). These results corroborated our initial findings that ZEP3 is the enzyme responsible for the epoxidation of Dtx to Ddx (Figure 5f–h). The Dtx concentration in the *zep3* strains remained at HL levels after 1 and 2 h of rLL (Figure 5g) and was ten times higher than in the WT at the same time points. The maximum Dtx concentrations in the *zep3* strains in our study were also five times higher than the concentrations reported using transgenic *P. tricornutum* double (*Vde*/*Vde-related* (*Vdr*)) and triple (*Vde*/*Vdr*/*Zep3*) overexpression lines (light intensity: 90 µmol photons m^{-2} s^{-1}) [41]. An average decline in Dtx levels of approximately 40% could, however, be observed at the 6 h rLL time point compared to HL levels (Figure 5g), but the decline coincided with a similar increase in cell number, suggesting that Dtx had been distributed between daughter cells. The above-described results suggest that the yield of Dtx produced from a *zep3* mutant culture will stay high during harvesting of the biomass in an industrial setting.

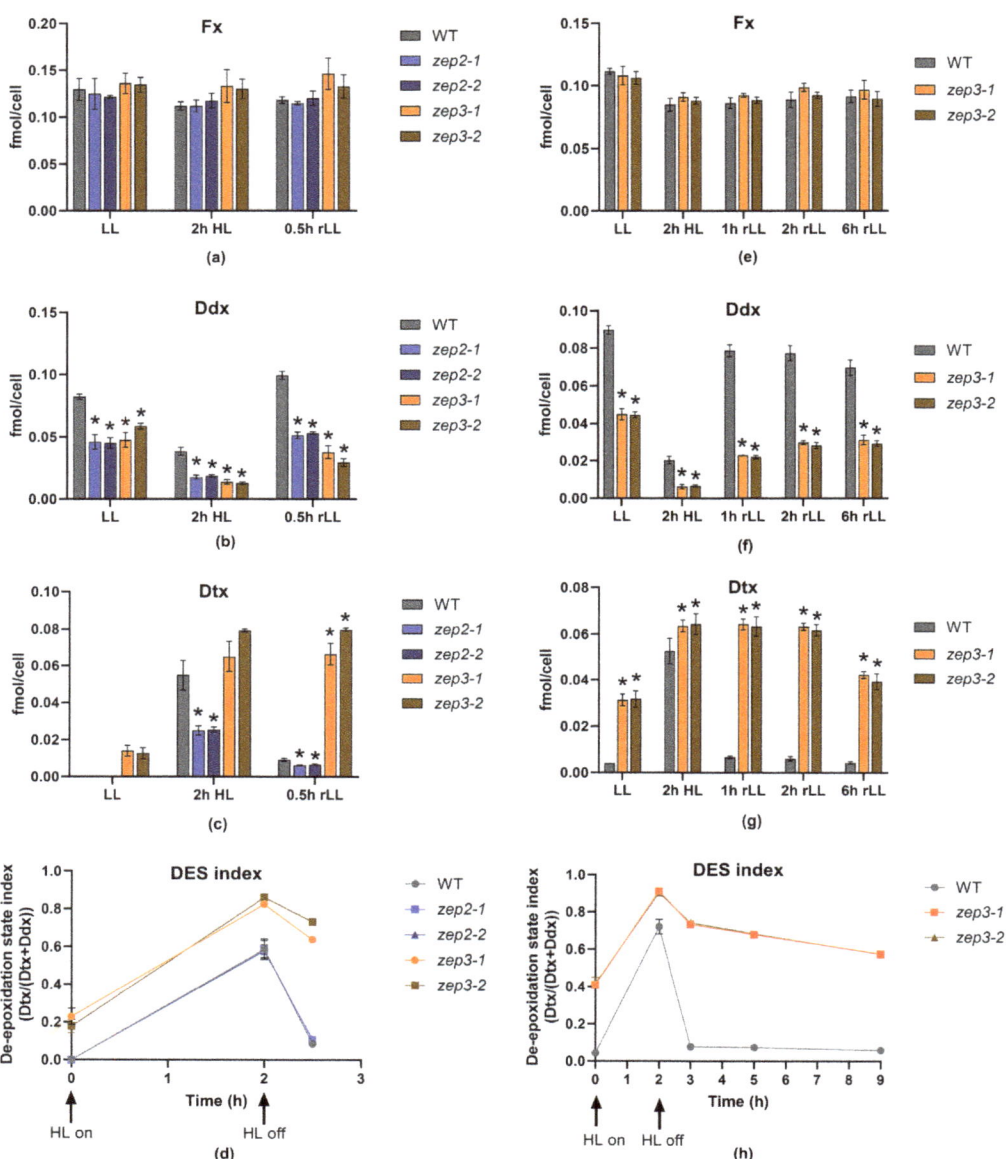

Figure 5. Carotenoid concentration and DES index in WT, *zep2* and *zep3* mutant lines. WT, *zep2* and *zep3* cultures were acclimated to LL and exposed to 2 h of HL before being returned to LL for 0.5 h (rLL). The (**a**) Fx, (**b**) Ddx and (**c**) Dtx cell concentrations are presented as fmol/cell, whereas the (**d**) DES index is calculated as fmol Dtx/fmol (Dtx+Ddx). An additional experiment was performed with only WT and *zep3* lines, where the rLL period was prolonged to 1, 2 and 6 h. The resulting carotenoid concentrations are presented in (**e**) Fx, (**f**) Ddx and (**g**) Dtx. Figure (**h**) describes the DES index pattern resulting from a prolonged recovery time in rLL. All results are presented as the means

of three biological replicates ± SD. Asterisks describe significant differences between carotenoid concentrations in *zep* mutants and WT, as indicated by a two-way ANOVA with Dunnett's multiple comparison tests ($p < 0.05$).

2.4. Loss of ZEP3 Inhibits Relaxation of the Photoprotective Mechanism NPQ

To investigate the effect of loss of ZEP2 and ZEP3 at the physiological level, the growth rate and photosynthetic performance of *zep2* and *zep3* mutants were compared to WT using cultures acclimated to LL or HL. The photophysiological effects were assessed using Chl *a* variable fluorescence for calculations of the photosynthetic (PSII) efficiency (maximum quantum yield, F_v/F_m), the photosynthetic capacity (maximum relative electron transport rate, $rETR_{max}$), the maximum light utilisation coefficient (the slope of the photosynthesis versus irradiance curves, alpha) and the light saturation index ($E_k = rETR_{max}/\text{alpha}$) at the two different light conditions (Figure 6a–d). E_k, alpha and $rETR_{max}$ were derived from rapid light curves. These measurements revealed no or minor differences in photosynthetic performance between *zep2* and *zep3* mutants and WT. The similar photosynthetic performance in all strains is in line with the highly similar cell division rates of mutants and WT in LL and HL (Table 1). Because of the possibility of the *zep3* mutant strains being of interest for commercial cultivation, we also investigated the growth of light fluctuating on a millisecond scale, simulating conditions experienced in a photobioreactor (PBR; Table 1). PBR light conditions did not induce statistically significant growth differences under these conditions either, supporting the possibility of industrial cultivation of *zep3* strains. Also, no statistical differences were found between the maximum NPQ values in *zep* mutants compared to WT—neither when NPQ was induced by a stepwise increase in blue light intensity, nor when NPQ was triggered by exposure to constant high-intensity blue light (Figure 6e,f). In contrast, the relaxation behaviour of NPQ in low-intensity blue light was mutant-specific and clearly deviated from WT (Figure 6f). A lack of ZEP3 strongly inhibited the relaxation of NPQ. After a small but rapid decline within the first minutes in very dim light, the NPQ relaxation curve of *zep3* flattened out, and the NPQ level remained at approximately 70% of the maximum level at the end of the relaxation period. The inhibition of NPQ relaxation correlates with the *zep3* mutants' inability to back-convert Ddx to Dtx when returned to LL and the importance of the presence of Dtx for the performance of NPQ in diatoms [20,21]. Still, the modest relaxation of NPQ despite the stable content of Dtx indicates the additional presence of a short-lived fluorescence quenching mechanism independent of a decline in Dtx [42]. This fast (<1 min) relaxation component has previously been described in the centric diatom *Cyclotella meneghiniana*, and more recently, it has also been observed in *P. tricornutum* (pennate diatom), where it was believed to be absent [42–45]. This fast NPQ mechanism seems to be dependent on the concentration of Dtx and has been interpreted as the relaxation of part of the steady-state Dtx-dependent quenching [42]. However, further studies are needed to clarify the mechanisms behind this and if differences are present between centric and pennate diatoms. The NPQ relaxation pattern of *zep2* was more similar to that of WT but less efficient. NPQ in *zep2* relaxed to approximately 30% of maximum levels, whereas the equivalent number for WT was 15%. The DES index of the *zep2* mutants was close to identical to that of WT and did not correlate with the slower NPQ relaxation behaviour of *zep2*.

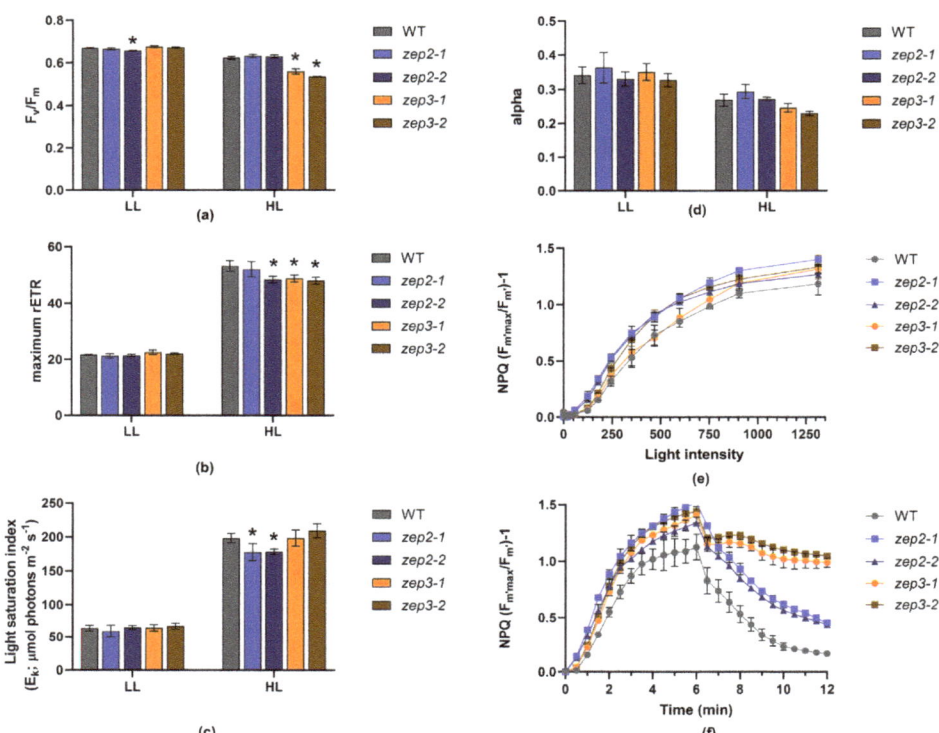

Figure 6. Photophysiological responses of WT, *zep2* and *zep3* mutants. (**a**) The photosynthetic (PSII) efficiency (F_v/F_m), (**b**) the photosynthetic capacity (rETR$_{max}$), (**c**) the light saturation index (E_k) and (**d**) the maximum light utilisation coefficient (alpha) in cells acclimated to either LL or HL. Asterisks describe significant differences between *zep* mutants and WT, as indicated by a two-way ANOVA with Dunnett's multiple comparison tests ($p < 0.05$). NPQ was calculated both as (**e**) a function of increasing blue light intensity (0–1313 µmol photons m^{-2} s^{-1}) and as (**f**) a function of time, where the cells were exposed to 6 min of high-intensity blue light (470 µmol photons m^{-2} s^{-1}), immediately followed by a 6 min recovery period in low-intensity blue light (8 µmol photons m^{-2} s^{-1}). All results are presented as the means of three biological replicates ± SD.

Table 1. Growth rates of WT, *zep2* and *zep3* mutant strains acclimated to LL, HL or PBR conditions. The maximum cell divisions per day during the exponential phase were calculated from three biological replicates of WT, *zep2* and *zep3* mutant lines acclimated to LL (35–40 µmol photons m^{-2} s^{-1}), HL (450–500 µmol photons m^{-2} s^{-1}) or rapidly fluctuating light simulating photobioreactor light conditions (PBR). Values are presented as the mean ± SD. The growth rates in mutant strains did not show statistically significant differences compared to WT in any light condition (one-way ANOVA with Dunnett's multiple comparison tests).

	LL	HL	PBR
WT	1.21 ± 0.17	1.80 ± 0.30	1.65 ± 0.28
zep2-1	1.25 ± 0.14	1.71 ± 0.26	1.34 ± 0.16
zep2-2	1.29 ± 0.12	1.86 ± 0.12	1.52 ± 0.22
zep3-1	1.25 ± 0.06	1.76 ± 0.37	1.45 ± 0.14
zep3-2	1.23 ± 0.05	1.78 ± 0.31	1.28 ± 0.08

3. Materials and Methods

3.1. Structural Comparison and Phylogenetic Analyses of ZEP Proteins

The pdb files of the predicted 3D structures of *P. tricornutum* ZEP1, ZEP2 and ZEP3 were downloaded from the AlphaFold2 server (https://alphafold.ebi.ac.uk/, accessed on 19 February 2024) [46,47]. The Swiss PDB Viewer 4.1 (https://spdbv.unil.ch/) was used to view and analyse the proteins [48]. In the 3D models, the non-conserved regions, including the leader peptides with chloroplast-targeting motifs and transit peptides, were excluded from the models. For the phylogenetic analyses, a protein alignment of 158 full-length ZEP proteins was produced using ClustalW [49] and manually refined using GeneDoc software version 2.7.000 (http://nrbsc.org/gfx/genedoc, accessed on 19 February 2024). The phylogenetic analysis was conducted in MEGA11 software (Version 11, https://www.megasoftware.net/, accessed on 19 February 2024) [50] using the maximum likelihood method and the Le_Gascuel_2008 model [51]. An unrooted radial maximum-likelihood tree was produced, where a group of flavin-binding proteins distantly related to the ZEP proteins served as an outgroup. The percentage of trees in which the associated taxa clustered together is shown by numbers; in total, 100 bootstrap replicates were made. Bootstrap numbers for main clusters with high confidence are shown in the tree. The rate variation model allowed for some sites to be evolutionarily invariable ([+I], 2.15% sites). The tree is drawn to scale, with branch lengths measured in the number of substitutions per site. All positions with less than 80% site coverage were eliminated. There were a total of 436 positions in the final dataset.

3.2. CRISPR/Cas9 Gene Editing of the ZEP2 and ZEP3 Genes

Knockout mutations in the *ZEP2* (Phatr2_5928) and *ZEP3* (Phatr2_10970) genes in *P. tricornutum* were generated using the CRISPR/Cas9 tool adapted for gene editing in diatoms [22,52,53]. The pPtPuc3m diaCas9_sgRNA vector expressing Cas9 and single-guide RNAs (sgRNAs) targeting *ZEP2* or *ZEP3* was delivered to *P. tricornutum* cells by bacterial conjugation, as described by Sharma and coworkers [22]. The cloning of gene-specific adapters into the sgRNA of the pPtPuc3m diaCas9_sgRNA vector was performed as described in the published protocol by Nymark et al. [53]. The *P. tricornutum* cells that were subjected to CRISPR/Cas9 gene editing were derived from clone Pt1 8.6 (CCMP632) from the culture collection of the Provasoli–Guillard National Center for Culture of Marine Phytoplankton, Bigelow Laboratory for Ocean Sciences, East Boothbay, Maine, USA. Screening, identification and isolation of cells containing bi-allelic mutations in *ZEP2* and *ZEP3* were performed as described previously [52,53]. *ZEP2*- and *ZEP3*-specific oligonucleotides used for the creation of the adapters inserted into the sgRNA of the pPtPuc3m diaCas9_sgRNA vector and primers used for screening purposes are presented in Table 2.

Table 2. Adapter sequences, PCR, high-resolution melting (HRM) analyses and sequencing primers.

Oligo or Primer Name	Orientation	Sequence (5'→3')	Purpose
ZEP2-PAM2_F	Forward	TCGAGCGCGTGGAGATACGGAGAG	Adapter for sgRNA
ZEP2-PAM2_R	Reverse	AAACCTCTCCGTATCTCCACGCGC	
ZEP3-PAM2_F	Forward	TCGAAGTACGGTAACATCCATGGT	Adapter for sgRNA
ZEP3-PAM2_R	Reverse	AAACACCATGGATGTTACCGTACT	
ZEP2-PAM12_scrF	Forward	GAATCGATCTGAATTGGCTACG	Screening for zep2 (508 bp amplicon)
ZEP2-PAM12_scrR	Reverse	CGGTGAAAGTGAACTTGTCCAT	
ZEP3-PAM2_scrF	Forward	GCACCACCTTCGAGCAATGT	Screening for zep3 (643 bp amplicon)
ZEP3-PAM2_scrR	Reverse	TCGCCAGCGAAAACCGTGTA	
ZEP2-PAM2_hrmF	Forward	CTCCGGAAGACGTTGCCTTTGA	HRM for zep2 (146 bp amplicon)
ZEP2-PAM2_hrmR	Reverse	TCTCGTACACCGTCACGTCGAA	
ZEP3-PAM2_hrmF	Forward	TGGTCTTTCCTTGGCCAAGGTT	HRM for zep3 (111 bp amplicon)
ZEP3-PAM2_hrmR	Reverse	GTTACTAGCGAGCTGGATGGGT	
M13-rev (−29)	Reverse	CAGGAAACAGCTATGAC	Sequencing primer

3.3. Light Conditions

P. tricornutum WT, *zep2* (*zep2-1*, *zep2-1*) and *zep3* (*zep3-1*, *zep3-2*) mutant strains were grown at 15 °C in f/2 medium [54] made with 0.2 μm sterile filtered and autoclaved seawater from the Trondheim fjord. Experimental light conditions were either continuous white light at 35–40 μmol photons m^{-2} s^{-1} (low light (LL)) or high light (HL) at 450–500 μmol photons m^{-2} s^{-1}. Cultures for estimation of cell division rates and measurements of photosynthetic parameters were cultivated at LL or HL in a growth chamber equipped with neutral white LEDs (4000 K). Because of the potential industrial relevance of the mutant strains, their growth rate was also investigated in light conditions mimicking the light perception of one cell in a PBR. Nanocosm, a LED-based miniature PBR system [55], was programmed to mimic PBR conditions by fluctuating from darkness to 200 μmol photons m^{-2} s^{-1} in a time scale of milliseconds based on the findings of Luo and coworkers [56]. The light intensity was measured with a ULM-500 (Walz, Effeltrich, Germany) light meter equipped with a spherical sensor. Cultivation of algae cells for pigment analyses was performed in a growth room where LL was provided by fluorescent cool daylight tubes (colour code 865/6500 K), whereas a full-spectrum LED lamp (5500 K) was used to achieve HL conditions. The light intensity in the growth room was measured using a LI-250A light meter (LI-COR Biosciences, Lincoln, NE, USA).

3.4. Growth Rates

Cell division rates were estimated in WT, *zep2* and *zep3* mutant lines (three biological replicates for each line) acclimated to either LL, HL or PBR conditions. The cells were grown in 24-well plates (2 mL of culture in each well) at a starting concentration of 30,000 cells mL^{-1}. Growth was measured indirectly by recording the daily increase in in vivo Chl *a* fluorescence (IVF; Ex: 460 nm, Em: 680 nm) for nine days. IVF was measured using a Tecan Spark plate reader at five different points in each well. The averaged IVF values were used to plot growth curves, and the cell division rates were calculated from the exponential part of the curves.

3.5. Measurements of Photosynthetic Parameters

The photosynthetic parameters F_v ($F_m - F_0$)/F_m (photosynthetic efficiency), the maximum relative electron transport rate ($rETR_{max}$; photosynthetic capacity), the maximum light utilisation coefficient (alpha) and the light saturation index ($E_k = rETR_{max}/alpha$) were calculated based on measurements of variable in vivo Chl *a* fluorescence using a Multi-

Color-PAM fluorometer (Walz, Germany). The instrument was equipped with a Peltier cell (US-T/S, Walz) to keep the temperature constant at 15 °C (±0.2 °C) during measurements. Rapid light curves (RLCs) were obtained by exposing the samples to 14 stepwise increasing irradiances of 0–1313 µmol photons m^{-2} s^{-1} (blue (440 nm) measuring and actinic light) after a 5 min incubation period in darkness. Each light step in the RLCs lasted 30 s. The cardinal points (alpha, ETR$_{max}$ and E$_k$) of the light curves were determined by the build-in fitting routine of the PamWin-3 software package (ver. 3.20). NPQ was calculated as a function of the stepwise increasing light intensity from F$_m$ and F$_{m'}$ values generated during measurements of the rapid light curves as (F$_m$/F$_{m'}$) − 1. Additionally, NPQ induction and relaxation were investigated by exposure of LL-acclimated cells to 470 µmol photons m^{-2} s^{-1} of blue light for 6 min, immediately followed by a 6 min incubation period at 8 µmol photons m^{-2} s^{-1} of blue light. The initial F$_m$ value was measured after 5 min of dark incubation, and F$_{m'}$ was measured every 30 s during the light treatments. Cells for measurements of photosynthetic parameters were grown in sterile cell culture flasks with a volume of 30 mL.

3.6. Diatoxanthin in Vivo Stability Experiment (Pigment Analyses)

LL-acclimated WT, *zep2* and *zep3* mutant strains were exposed to 2 h of HL before being returned to LL (rLL) conditions for 0.5 h. The experiment was repeated with WT and *zep3* mutants, where the rLL treatment was prolonged to 1, 2 and 6 h. Three biological replicates were included for each line in both experiments. For each biological replicate, samples for pigment analyses were taken successively from the same culture. Cell concentrations at the time of harvesting were 0.6–1.5 × 10^6 cells mL^{-1}. Cell numbers were determined by flow cytometry using a NovoCyteTM flow cytometer (Agilent, Santa Clara, CA, USA) as described previously [52] or a Multisizer 4e Coulter Counter (Beckmann Coulter, Indianapolis, IN, USA). Pigment analyses were performed by HPLC using a Hewlett-Packard HPLC 1100 Series system (Agilent, Santa Clara, CA, USA) as described previously [38,57]. Cells for pigment analyses were grown in sterile cell culture flasks in a volume of 100 mL.

3.7. Statistics

A two-way ANOVA with Dunnett's multiple comparison tests was carried out using GraphPad Prism software (version 10.1.0, GraphPad, Boston, MA, USA) to determine if there were significant differences ($p < 0.05$) between the pigment concentrations and NPQ values in *zep2* and *zep3* mutants compared to the WT. A one-way ANOVA with Dunnett's multiple comparison tests was used to determine if there were significant differences ($p < 0.05$) between the growth rates in *zep2* and *zep3* mutants compared to the WT using the same software.

4. Conclusions

In this study, we aimed to genetically engineer the marine diatom *P. tricornutum* to enable industrial production of the bioactive pigment diatoxanthin. We used the CRISPR/Cas9 technology for targeted disruption of the ZEP2 and ZEP3 genes. ZEP2 and/or ZEP3 had previously been suggested to be responsible for the enzymatic conversion of Dtx to Ddx in LL conditions. Based on the combined results, we conclude that the presence of ZEP3 is essential for the conversion of Dtx to Ddx in *P. tricornutum*. ZEP2 is unable to compensate for a lack of ZEP3, meaning that ZEP2 and ZEP3 do not have overlapping functions in the Ddx–Dtx cycle. The role of ZEP2 in the carotenoid synthetic pathway of diatoms was not revealed by our study, and a *zep2*–*zep3* double knockout mutant needs to be investigated to determine its function in catalysing the transformation of Zx to Vx. The stability of HL-accumulated Dtx for hours after the removal of *zep3* mutants from the HL source and the WT-like photosynthetic performance and growth rates at all tested light conditions indicate that such strains might function as a commercial-scale production line for the bioactive carotenoid Dtx from diatoms. The feasibility of large-scale cultivation and production of Dtx using the *zep3* strains created in this study will be further investigated together with microalgae companies in an ongoing research project funded by the Research Council of Norway.

Supplementary Materials: The following supporting information can be downloaded at https://www.mdpi.com/article/10.3390/md22040185/s1, Figure S1: Chlorophyll (Chl) a and Chl $c_1 + c_2$ concentration in WT, $zep2$ and $zep3$ mutant lines; Supplementary File S1: Distribution of ZEP proteins in various marine phyla.

Author Contributions: Conceptualisation, M.N.; methodology, C.G., T.B., C.V., Z.B., M.S., P.W. and M.N.; software, C.V.; formal analysis, C.G., T.B., Z.B., P.W. and M.N.; resources, M.N.; data curation, C.G., Z.B., P.W. and M.N.; writing—original draft preparation, C.V., P.W. and M.N.; writing—review and editing, C.G., T.B., C.V., M.S., P.W. and M.N.; visualisation, C.V., P.W. and M.N.; supervision, T.B., P.W. and M.N.; project administration, M.N.; funding acquisition, M.N. All authors have read and agreed to the published version of the manuscript.

Funding: This research was funded by the Research Council of Norway, grant number 344103.

Institutional Review Board Statement: Not applicable.

Data Availability Statement: The ZEP2 and ZEP3 genes have Draft ID Phatr2_5928 and Phatr2_10970, respectively. AlphaFold2 accession numbers are ZEP1: B7FYW4, ZEP2: B7FQV6 and ZEP3: B7FUR7. $Zep2$ and $zep3$ mutant strains can be shared for research purposes. Raw data generated in the present study used for the calculation of pigment concentrations, photophysiological parameters and cell division rates are available on request.

Acknowledgments: The authors thank Ralph Kissen for careful reading and correction of the manuscript.

Conflicts of Interest: The authors declare no conflicts of interest.

References

1. Sandmann, G. Diversity and Origin of Carotenoid Biosynthesis: Its History of Coevolution towards Plant Photosynthesis. *New Phytol.* **2021**, *232*, 479–493. [CrossRef]
2. Meléndez-Martínez, A.J. An Overview of Carotenoids, Apocarotenoids, and Vitamin A in Agro-Food, Nutrition, Health, and Disease. *Mol. Nutr. Food Res.* **2019**, *63*, 1801045. [CrossRef]
3. Ren, Y.; Sun, H.; Deng, J.; Huang, J.; Chen, F. Carotenoid Production from Microalgae: Biosynthesis, Salinity Responses and Novel Biotechnologies. *Mar. Drugs* **2021**, *19*, 713. [CrossRef]
4. Kabir, M.T.; Rahman, M.H.; Shah, M.; Jamiruddin, M.R.; Basak, D.; Al-Harrasi, A.; Bhatia, S.; Ashraf, G.M.; Najda, A.; El-kott, A.F.; et al. Therapeutic Promise of Carotenoids as Antioxidants and Anti-Inflammatory Agents in Neurodegenerative Disorders. *Biomed. Pharmacother.* **2022**, *146*, 112610. [CrossRef] [PubMed]
5. Seth, K.; Kumar, A.; Rastogi, R.P.; Meena, M.; Vinayak, V. Harish Bioprospecting of Fucoxanthin from Diatoms—Challenges and Perspectives. *Algal Res.* **2021**, *60*, 102475. [CrossRef]
6. Pocha, C.K.R.; Chia, W.Y.; Chew, K.W.; Munawaroh, H.S.H.; Show, P.L. Current Advances in Recovery and Biorefinery of Fucoxanthin from *Phaeodactylum Tricornutum*. *Algal Res.* **2022**, *65*, 102735. [CrossRef]
7. Sathasivam, R.; Ki, J.-S. A Review of the Biological Activities of Microalgal Carotenoids and Their Potential Use in Healthcare and Cosmetic Industries. *Mar. Drugs* **2018**, *16*, 26. [CrossRef]
8. Singh, T.; Pandey, V.K.; Dash, K.K.; Zanwar, S.; Singh, R. Natural Bio-Colorant and Pigments: Sources and Applications in Food Processing. *J. Agric. Res.* **2023**, *12*, 100628. [CrossRef]
9. Ávila-Román, J.; García-Gil, S.; Rodríguez-Luna, A.; Motilva, V.; Talero, E. Anti-Inflammatory and Anticancer Effects of Microalgal Carotenoids. *Mar. Drugs* **2021**, *19*, 531. [CrossRef] [PubMed]
10. Peng, J.; Yuan, J.-P.; Wu, C.-F.; Wang, J.-H. Fucoxanthin, a Marine Carotenoid Present in Brown Seaweeds and Diatoms: Metabolism and Bioactivities Relevant to Human Health. *Mar. Drugs* **2011**, *9*, 1806–1828. [CrossRef] [PubMed]
11. Galasso, C.; Corinaldesi, C.; Sansone, C. Carotenoids from Marine Organisms: Biological Functions and Industrial Applications. *Antioxidants* **2017**, *6*, 96. [CrossRef] [PubMed]
12. Bae, M.; Kim, M.-B.; Park, Y.-K.; Lee, J.-Y. Health Benefits of Fucoxanthin in the Prevention of Chronic Diseases. *Biochim. Biophys. Acta Mol. Cell Biol. Lipids* **2020**, *1865*, 158618. [CrossRef] [PubMed]
13. Leong, Y.K.; Chen, C.-Y.; Varjani, S.; Chang, J.-S. Producing Fucoxanthin from Algae—Recent Advances in Cultivation Strategies and Downstream Processing. *Bioresour. Technol.* **2022**, *344*, 126170. [CrossRef]
14. Nymark, M.; Valle, K.C.; Brembu, T.; Hancke, K.; Winge, P.; Andresen, K.; Johnsen, G.; Bones, A.M. An Integrated Analysis of Molecular Acclimation to High Light in the Marine Diatom *Phaeodactylum Tricornutum*. *PLoS ONE* **2009**, *4*, e7743. [CrossRef] [PubMed]

15. Brown, J.S. Photosynthetic Pigment Organization in Diatoms (Bacillariophyceae). *J. Phycol.* **1988**, *24*, 96–102. [CrossRef]
16. Konishi, I.; Hosokawa, M.; Sashima, T.; Maoka, T.; Miyashita, K. Suppressive Effects of Alloxanthin and Diatoxanthin from *Halocynthia Roretzi* on LPS-Induced Expression of pro-Inflammatory Genes in RAW264.7 Cells. *J. Oleo Sci.* **2008**, *57*, 181–189. [CrossRef] [PubMed]
17. Pistelli, L.; Sansone, C.; Smerilli, A.; Festa, M.; Noonan, D.M.; Albini, A.; Brunet, C. MMP-9 and IL-1β as Targets for Diatoxanthin and Related Microalgal Pigments: Potential Chemopreventive and Photoprotective Agents. *Mar. Drugs* **2021**, *19*, 354. [CrossRef] [PubMed]
18. Sansone, C.; Pistelli, L.; Del Mondo, A.; Calabrone, L.; Fontana, A.; Noonan, D.M.; Albini, A.; Brunet, C. The Microalgal Diatoxanthin Inflects the Cytokine Storm in SARS-CoV-2 Stimulated ACE2 Overexpressing Lung Cells. *Antioxidants* **2022**, *11*, 1515. [CrossRef] [PubMed]
19. Sansone, C.; Pistelli, L.; Calabrone, L.; Del Mondo, A.; Fontana, A.; Festa, M.; Noonan, D.M.; Albini, A.; Brunet, C. The Carotenoid Diatoxanthin Modulates Inflammatory and Angiogenesis Pathways In Vitro in Prostate Cancer Cells. *Antioxidants* **2023**, *12*, 359. [CrossRef]
20. Goss, R.; Lepetit, B. Biodiversity of NPQ. *J. Plant Physiol.* **2015**, *172*, 13–32. [CrossRef]
21. Lavaud, J.; Goss, R. The Peculiar Features of Non-Photochemical Fluorescence Quenching in Diatoms and Brown Algae. In *Non-photochemical Quenching and Energy Dissipation in Plants, Algae and Cyanobacteria*; Advances in photosynthesis and respiration (Including bioenergy and related, processes); Demmig-Adams, B., Garab, G., Adams, I.W., Govindjee, Eds.; Springer: Dordrecht, The Netherlands, 2014; Volume 40, pp. 421–443.
22. Sharma, A.K.; Nymark, M.; Sparstad, T.; Bones, A.M.; Winge, P. Transgene-Free Genome Editing in Marine Algae by Bacterial Conjugation—Comparison with Biolistic CRISPR/Cas9 Transformation. *Sci. Rep.* **2018**, *8*, 14401. [CrossRef]
23. Serif, M.; Dubois, G.; Finoux, A.L.; Teste, M.A.; Jallet, D.; Daboussi, F. One-Step Generation of Multiple Gene Knock-Outs in the Diatom *Phaeodactylum Tricornutum* by DNA-Free Genome Editing. *Nat. Commun.* **2018**, *9*, 3924. [CrossRef]
24. Araújo, R.; Vázquez Calderón, F.; Sánchez López, J.; Azevedo, I.C.; Bruhn, A.; Fluch, S.; Garcia Tasende, M.; Ghaderiardakani, F.; Ilmjärv, T.; Laurans, M.; et al. Current Status of the Algae Production Industry in Europe: An Emerging Sector of the Blue Bioeconomy. *Front. Mar. Sci.* **2021**, *7*, 626389. [CrossRef]
25. Dautermann, O.; Lyska, D.; Andersen-Ranberg, J.; Becker, M.; Fröhlich-Nowoisky, J.; Gartmann, H.; Krämer, L.C.; Mayr, K.; Pieper, D.; Rij, L.M.; et al. An Algal Enzyme Required for Biosynthesis of the Most Abundant Marine Carotenoids. *Sci. Adv.* **2020**, *6*, eaaw9183. [CrossRef] [PubMed]
26. Bai, Y.; Cao, T.; Dautermann, O.; Buschbeck, P.; Cantrell, M.B.; Chen, Y.; Lein, C.D.; Shi, X.; Ware, M.A.; Yang, F.; et al. Green Diatom Mutants Reveal an Intricate Biosynthetic Pathway of Fucoxanthin. *Proc. Natl. Acad. Sci. USA* **2022**, *119*, e2203708119. [CrossRef] [PubMed]
27. Cao, T.; Bai, Y.; Buschbeck, P.; Tan, Q.; Cantrell, M.B.; Chen, Y.; Jiang, Y.; Liu, R.-Z.; Ries, N.K.; Shi, X.; et al. An Unexpected Hydratase Synthesizes the Green Light-Absorbing Pigment Fucoxanthin. *Plant Cell* **2023**, *35*, 3053–3072. [CrossRef] [PubMed]
28. Bowler, C.; Allen, A.E.; Badger, J.H.; Grimwood, J.; Jabbari, K.; Kuo, A.; Maheswari, U.; Martens, C.; Maumus, F.; Otillar, R.P.; et al. The *Phaeodactylum* Genome Reveals the Evolutionary History of Diatom Genomes. *Nature* **2008**, *456*, 239–244. [CrossRef] [PubMed]
29. Coesel, S.; Obornik, M.; Varela, J.; Falciatore, A.; Bowler, C. Evolutionary Origins and Functions of the Carotenoid Biosynthetic Pathway in Marine Diatoms. *PLoS ONE* **2008**, *3*, e2896. [CrossRef] [PubMed]
30. Eilers, U.; Dietzel, L.; Breitenbach, J.; Büchel, C.; Sandmann, G. Identification of Genes Coding for Functional Zeaxanthin Epoxidases in the Diatom *Phaeodactylum Tricornutum*. *J. Plant Physiol.* **2016**, *192*, 64–70. [CrossRef]
31. Dautermann, O.; Lohr, M. A Functional Zeaxanthin Epoxidase from Red Algae Shedding Light on the Evolution of Light-harvesting Carotenoids and the Xanthophyll Cycle in Photosynthetic Eukaryotes. *Plant J.* **2017**, *92*, 879–891. [CrossRef]
32. Karas, B.J.; Diner, R.E.; Lefebvre, S.C.; McQuaid, J.; Phillips, A.P.R.; Noddings, C.M.; Brunson, J.K.; Valas, R.E.; Deerinck, T.J.; Jablanovic, J.; et al. Designer Diatom Episomes Delivered by Bacterial Conjugation. *Nat. Commun.* **2015**, *6*, 6925. [CrossRef] [PubMed]
33. Dima, O.; Inzé, D. The Role of Scientists in Policy Making for More Sustainable Agriculture. *Curr. Biol.* **2021**, *31*, R218–R220. [CrossRef] [PubMed]
34. Voigt, B. EU Regulation of Gene-Edited Plants—A Reform Proposal. *Front. Genome Ed.* **2023**, *5*, 1119442. [CrossRef] [PubMed]
35. Jia, X.; Zhang, Q.; Jiang, M.; Huang, J.; Yu, L.; Traw, M.B.; Tian, D.; Hurst, L.D.; Yang, S. Mitotic Gene Conversion Can Be as Important as Meiotic Conversion in Driving Genetic Variability in Plants and Other Species without Early Germline Segregation. *PLoS Biol.* **2021**, *19*, e3001164. [CrossRef] [PubMed]
36. Nymark, M.; Finazzi, G.; Volpe, C.; Serif, M.; de Miranda Fonseca, D.; Sharma, A.; Sanchez, N.; Sharma, A.K.; Ashcroft, F.; Kissen, R.; et al. Loss of CpFTSY Reduces Photosynthetic Performance and Affects Insertion of PsaC of PSI in Diatoms. *Plant Cell Physiol.* **2023**, *64*, 583–603. [CrossRef] [PubMed]
37. Nymark, M.; Volpe, C.; Hafskjold, M.C.G.; Kirst, H.; Serif, M.; Vadstein, O.; Bones, A.M.; Melis, A.; Winge, P. Loss of ALBINO3b Insertase Results in Truncated Light-Harvesting Antenna in Diatoms. *Plant Physiol.* **2019**, *181*, 1257–1276. [CrossRef] [PubMed]
38. Sharma, A.K.; Nymark, M.; Flo, S.; Sparstad, T.; Bones, A.M.; Winge, P. Simultaneous Knockout of Multiple LHCF Genes Using Single SgRNAs and Engineering of a High-Fidelity Cas9 for Precise Genome Editing in Marine Algae. *Plant Biotechnol. J.* **2021**, *19*, 1658–1669. [CrossRef]

39. Niyogi, K.K.; Bjorkman, O.; Grossman, A.R. Chlamydomonas Xanthophyll Cycle Mutants Identified by Video Imaging of Chlorophyll Fluorescence Quenching. *Plant Cell* **1997**, *9*, 1369–1380. [CrossRef] [PubMed]
40. Jin, E.; Feth, B.; Melis, A. A Mutant of the Green Alga *Dunaliella Salina* Constitutively Accumulates Zeaxanthin under All Growth Conditions. *Biotech Bioeng.* **2003**, *81*, 115–124. [CrossRef]
41. Manfellotto, F.; Stella, G.R.; Falciatore, A.; Brunet, C.; Ferrante, M.I. Engineering the Unicellular Alga *Phaeodactylum Tricornutum* for Enhancing Carotenoid Production. *Antioxidants* **2020**, *9*, 757. [CrossRef]
42. Grouneva, I.; Jakob, T.; Wilhelm, C.; Goss, R. A New Multicomponent NPQ Mechanism in the Diatom *Cyclotella Meneghiniana*. *Plant Cell Physiol.* **2008**, *49*, 1217–1225. [CrossRef] [PubMed]
43. Lavaud, J.; Materna, A.C.; Sturm, S.; Vugrinec, S.; Kroth, P.G. Silencing of the Violaxanthin De-Epoxidase Gene in the Diatom *Phaeodactylum Tricornutum* Reduces Diatoxanthin Synthesis and Non-Photochemical Quenching. *PLoS ONE* **2012**, *7*, e36806. [CrossRef]
44. Goss, R.; Ann Pinto, E.; Wilhelm, C.; Richter, M. The Importance of a Highly Active and DeltapH-Regulated Diatoxanthin Epoxidase for the Regulation of the PS II Antenna Function in Diadinoxanthin Cycle Containing Algae. *J. Plant Physiol.* **2006**, *163*, 1008–1021. [CrossRef] [PubMed]
45. Lavaud, J.; Kroth, P.G. In Diatoms, the Transthylakoid Proton Gradient Regulates the Photoprotective Non-Photochemical Fluorescence Quenching beyond Its Control on the Xanthophyll Cycle. *Plant Cell Physiol.* **2006**, *47*, 1010–1016. [CrossRef]
46. Jumper, J.; Evans, R.; Pritzel, A.; Green, T.; Figurnov, M.; Ronneberger, O.; Tunyasuvunakool, K.; Bates, R.; Zidek, A.; Potapenko, A.; et al. Applying and Improving AlphaFold at CASP14. *Proteins* **2021**, *89*, 1711–1721. [CrossRef]
47. Varadi, M.; Bertoni, D.; Magana, P.; Paramval, U.; Pidruchna, I.; Radhakrishnan, M.; Tsenkov, M.; Nair, S.; Mirdita, M.; Yeo, J.; et al. AlphaFold Protein Structure Database in 2024: Providing Structure Coverage for over 214 Million Protein Sequences. *Nucleic Acids Res.* **2024**, *52*, D368–D375. [CrossRef] [PubMed]
48. Guex, N.; Peitsch, M.C. SWISS-MODEL and the Swiss-Pdb Viewer: An Environment for Comparative Protein Modeling. *Electrophoresis* **1997**, *18*, 2714–2723. [CrossRef]
49. Larkin, M.A.; Blackshields, G.; Brown, N.P.; Chenna, R.; McGettigan, P.A.; McWilliam, H.; Valentin, F.; Wallace, I.M.; Wilm, A.; Lopez, R.; et al. Clustal W and Clustal X Version 2.0. *Bioinformatics* **2007**, *23*, 2947–2948. [CrossRef]
50. Tamura, K.; Stecher, G.; Kumar, S. MEGA11: Molecular Evolutionary Genetics Analysis Version 11. *Mol. Biol. Evol.* **2021**, *38*, 3022–3027. [CrossRef]
51. Le, S.Q.; Gascuel, O. An Improved General Amino Acid Replacement Matrix. *Mol. Biol. Evol.* **2008**, *25*, 1307–1320. [CrossRef]
52. Nymark, M.; Sharma, A.K.; Sparstad, T.; Bones, A.M.; Winge, P. A CRISPR/Cas9 System Adapted for Gene Editing in Marine Algae. *Sci. Rep.* **2016**, *6*, 24951. [CrossRef] [PubMed]
53. Nymark, M.; Sharma, A.K.; Hafskjold, M.C.; Sparstad, T.; Bones, A.M.; Winge, P. CRISPR/Cas9 Gene Editing in the Marine Diatom *Phaeodactylum Tricornutum*. *Bio-Protocol* **2017**, *7*, e2442. [CrossRef] [PubMed]
54. Guillard, R.R.L. Culture of Phytoplankton for Feeding Marine Invertebrates. In *Culture of Marine Invertebrate Animals: Proceedings—1st Conference on Culture of Marine Invertebrate Animals Greenport*; Smith, W.L., Chanley, M.H., Eds.; Springer: Boston, MA, USA, 1975; pp. 29–60, ISBN 978-1-4615-8714-9.
55. Volpe, C.; Vadstein, O.; Andersen, G.; Andersen, T. Nanocosm: A Well Plate Photobioreactor for Environmental and Biotechnological Studies. *Lab Chip* **2021**, *21*, 2027–2039. [CrossRef] [PubMed]
56. Luo, H.; Al-Dahhan, M.H. Analyzing and Modeling of Photobioreactors by Combining First Principles of Physiology and Hydrodynamics. *Biotech Bioeng.* **2004**, *85*, 382–393. [CrossRef]
57. Rodriguez, F.; Chauton, M.; Johnsen, G.; Andresen, K.; Olsen, L.M.; Zapata, M. Photoacclimation in Phytoplankton: Implications for Biomass Estimates, Pigment Functionality and Chemotaxonomy. *Mar. Biol.* **2006**, *148*, 963–971. [CrossRef]

Disclaimer/Publisher's Note: The statements, opinions and data contained in all publications are solely those of the individual author(s) and contributor(s) and not of MDPI and/or the editor(s). MDPI and/or the editor(s) disclaim responsibility for any injury to people or property resulting from any ideas, methods, instructions or products referred to in the content.

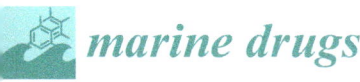

Article

Tisochrysis lutea F&M-M36 Mitigates Risk Factors of Metabolic Syndrome and Promotes Visceral Fat Browning through β3-Adrenergic Receptor/UCP1 Signaling

Mario D'Ambrosio [1,2], Elisabetta Bigagli [1,*], Lorenzo Cinci [1], Manuela Gencarelli [1,†], Sofia Chioccioli [1], Natascia Biondi [3], Liliana Rodolfi [3,4], Alberto Niccolai [3], Francesca Zambelli [1], Annunziatina Laurino [1,‡], Laura Raimondi [1], Mario R. Tredici [3,§] and Cristina Luceri [1]

[1] Department of NEUROFARBA, Section of Pharmacology and Toxicology, University of Florence, Viale Pieraccini 6, 50139 Florence, Italy; cristina.luceri@unifi.it (C.L.)
[2] Enteric Neuroscience Program, Department of Medicine, Section of Gastroenterology and Hepatology, Mayo Clinic, Rochester, MN 55905, USA
[3] Department of Agriculture, Food, Environment and Forestry (DAGRI), University of Florence, Piazzale delle Cascine 18, 50144 Florence, Italy
[4] Fotosintetica & Microbiologica S.r.l., Via di Santo Spirito 14, 50125 Florence, Italy
* Correspondence: elisabetta.bigagli@unifi.it
† Current address: The Leon H. Charney Division of Cardiology, New York University Grossman School of Medicine, New York, NY 55905, USA.
‡ Current address: Department of Molecular and Developmental Medicine, University of Siena, 53100 Siena, Italy.
§ Mario R. Tredici passed away on 17 June 2022.

Abstract: Pre-metabolic syndrome (pre-MetS) may represent the best transition phase to start treatments aimed at reducing cardiometabolic risk factors of MetS. In this study, we investigated the effects of the marine microalga *Tisochrysis lutea* F&M-M36 (*T. lutea*) on cardiometabolic components of pre-MetS and its underlying mechanisms. Rats were fed a standard (5% fat) or a high-fat diet (20% fat) supplemented or not with 5% of *T. lutea* or fenofibrate (100 mg/Kg) for 3 months. Like fenofibrate, *T. lutea* decreased blood triglycerides ($p < 0.01$) and glucose levels ($p < 0.01$), increased fecal lipid excretion ($p < 0.05$) and adiponectin ($p < 0.001$) without affecting weight gain. Unlike fenofibrate, *T. lutea* did not increase liver weight and steatosis, reduced renal fat ($p < 0.05$), diastolic ($p < 0.05$) and mean arterial pressure ($p < 0.05$). In visceral adipose tissue (VAT), *T. lutea*, but not fenofibrate, increased the β3-adrenergic receptor (β3ADR) ($p < 0.05$) and Uncoupling protein 1 (UCP-1) ($p < 0.001$) while both induced glucagon-like peptide-1 receptor (GLP1R) protein expression ($p < 0.001$) and decreased interleukin (IL)-6 and IL-1β gene expression ($p < 0.05$). Pathway analysis on VAT whole-gene expression profiles showed that *T. lutea* up-regulated energy-metabolism-related genes and down-regulated inflammatory and autophagy pathways. The multitarget activity of *T. lutea* suggests that this microalga could be useful in mitigating risk factors of MetS.

Keywords: microalgae; *Tisochrysis lutea*; adipose tissue; lipid metabolism; thermogenesis; β3-adrenergic receptor; UCP-1; inflammation; fenofibrate

1. Introduction

Metabolic syndrome (MetS) is defined as a cluster of metabolic alterations including at least three of the following: abdominal obesity, hypertriglyceridemia, hypertension, low high-density lipoprotein (HDL) cholesterol, and hyperglycemia [1]. Apart from metabolic abnormalities, chronic low-grade inflammation associated with MetS plays a crucial role in increasing cardiovascular diseases and diabetes [2].

The first-line approach in treating MetS relies on improving lifestyle and dietary habits followed by poly-pharmacological strategies able to simultaneously treat individual components of MetS [3]. Another potential approach could be focusing on the pre-disease state, namely pre-metabolic syndrome (pre-MetS), a condition of increased susceptibility to MetS where, however, the diagnostic criteria of MetS are not already met [4]. This pre-disease state could represent the best transition phase to start effective treatments based on dietary interventions.

The marine microalga *Tisochrysis lutea* (*T. lutea*) contains several multitarget bioactive compounds endowed with anti-inflammatory and anti-dyslipidemic properties, such as omega-3 fatty acids, mainly docosahexaenoic acid (DHA), polyphenols, and carotenoids, such as fucoxanthin [5–8]. Unlike other microalgae, *T. lutea* is not approved for human consumption and it is currently mainly used in aquaculture [9]. We were among the first to evaluate the safety of *T. lutea* F&M-M36 in animals, demonstrating that a diet containing a high percentage (20%) of microalgal biomass was well tolerated in the short term with no remarkable systemic toxic effects or organ damage; however, we also highlighted that the relatively high salt and nucleic acids content of the biomass could limit its inclusion in the diet [5]. In the same study, despite rats being fed a well-balanced and iso-caloric diet, we observed an unexpected, positive effect of *T. lutea* F&M-M36 on lipid metabolism [5]. We also recently demonstrated that the *T. lutea* F&M-M36 methanolic extract exerts anti-inflammatory activity in vitro by reducing the Cyclooxygenases-2 (COX-2) and Prostaglandin E2 (PGE2) pathway and NLRP3 inflammasome/microRNA-223 axis, with effects more evident than those of fucoxanthin alone [6]. In rats fed a high-fat and high-fructose diet, dietary supplementation with 12% *T. lutea* exerted anti-inflammatory effects and ameliorated lipid and glucose metabolism probably in virtue of the potential synergy among DHA, fucoxanthin, phytosterols, and fibers [8]. However, the molecular mechanisms involved, including the genes, proteins, and pathways modulated by the microalga and the analysis of its functional and molecular effects compared to existing drugs have been almost unexplored so far.

In this study, the effects of *T. lutea* F&M-M36 on the main components of pre-MetS, blood lipids, glucose, pressure, and inflammation were investigated; furthermore, since *T. lutea* is rich in DHA [8], a natural ligand of the nuclear receptor peroxisome proliferator-activated receptor α (PPARα), its effects were compared to those of fenofibrate, a synthetic ligand of the same receptor currently used in the pharmacotherapy of dyslipidemia [10]. The underlying mechanisms were also explored focusing on adipose tissue, a culprit organ for the regulation of whole-body energy homeostasis and metabolism.

2. Results

2.1. Effects of T. lutea F&M-M36 vs. Fenofibrate on Body and Organs Weight and on Fat Mass

Daily food and calorie intakes were significantly higher in rats fed NF diet compared to the other groups (all, $p < 0.001$), whereas water intake was similar. As a result of the lower calorie intake, the high-fat (HF) diet groups did not show a significantly higher weight gain compared to rats fed normal-fat (NF) diet. However, the HF diet increased epididymal and renal fat weight compared to NF diet ($p < 0.05$ and $p < 0.01$, respectively), but not visceral (mesenteric and retroperitoneal) fat. Fenofibrate did not affect fat depots, while *T. lutea* F&M-M36 significantly decreased renal fat weight compared to the HF diet ($p < 0.05$). Rats fed *T. lutea* F&M-M36 and fenofibrate also showed a significantly higher fecal excretion of lipids compared to HF ($p < 0.05$ and $p < 0.01$, respectively) and NF ($p < 0.05$ and $p < 0.01$, respectively). The increased liver and kidney weight in rats treated with fenofibrate ($p < 0.001$) was not observed in those fed *T. lutea* F&M-M36 (Table 1).

2.2. Effects of T. lutea F&M-M36 and Fenofibrate on Metabolic Profile, Adiponectin, and Blood Pressure

The HF diet significantly increased plasma triglycerides ($p < 0.01$) compared to NF diet but did not impact total cholesterol or high-density lipoprotein (HDL). *T. lutea* and fenofibrate were both able to significantly reduce TG compared to the HF diet ($p < 0.01$ and $p < 0.001$, respectively) (Table 2). The atherogenic index of plasma (AIP) was also reduced by *T. lutea* supplementation ($p < 0.05$) and fenofibrate ($p < 0.01$). Furthermore, both fenofibrate and *T. lutea* significantly counteracted the increase in plasma non-fasting glucose levels induced by the HF diet ($p < 0.001$ and $p < 0.01$, respectively) (Table 2).

Table 1. Effects of *T. lutea* F&M-M36 and fenofibrate on body weight gain, fat weight, food, and water intake.

	NF	HF	HFF	HFT
Weight gain (g)	213.5 ± 7.7	252.5 ± 20.1	208.5 ± 11.6	281.3 ± 11.6
Food intake (g)	51.66 ± 0.3	27.51 ± 0.5 ^^^	31.55 ± 0.5 ^^^	27.51 ± 0.5 ^^^
Calorie intake (kcal)/24 h	195.8 ± 1.3	146.6 ± 2.64 ^^^	168.2 ± 2.4 ^^^	146.3 ± 2.63 ^^^
Water intake (mL)	52.47 ± 2	50.27 ± 1.8	58.27 ± 1.7	52.80 ± 1.2
Fecal lipids excretion (µg/g 24 h dw)	1.4 ± 0.2	2.0 ± 0.2	5.4 ± 1.2 ^^**	4.2 ± 0.6 ^*
Liver (w/bw × 10^{-3})	38.86 ± 0.80	36.85 ± 1.38	65.44 ± 0.95 ***^^^	32.63 ± 0.29
Kidney (w/bw × 10^{-3})	3.23 ± 0.07	3.18 ± 0.10	4.21 ± 0.13 ***^^^	3.04 ± 0.10
Heart (w/bw × 10^{-3})	3.53 ± 0.12	3.38 ± 0.06	3.41 ± 0.09	3.70 ± 0.09
Visceral fat (w/bw × 10^{-3})	1.38 ± 0.14	2.30 ± 0.24	2.04 ± 0.39	1.83 ± 0.22
Epididymal fat (w/bw × 10^{-3})	7.64 ± 0.73	12.37 ± 0.67 ^	10.24 ± 1.61	10.93 ± 1.20
Renal fat (w/bw × 10^{-3})	8.56 ± 1.40	15.89 ± 1.49 ^^	12.46 ± 1.40	10.26 ± 0.55 *

Normal diet (NF), high-fat diet (HF), high-fat diet + fenofibrate (HFF), high-fat diet + *T. lutea* F&M-M36 (HFT), dry weight (dw), ratio of organ weights to body weight (w/bw). Water and food intakes and fecal lipids excretion were evaluated during the third month of treatment, placing rats in metabolic cages for one day. Data are expressed as means ± SE; *n* = 8 rats/group. ^ $p < 0.05$, ^^ $p < 0.01$ and ^^^ $p < 0.001$ vs. NF; * $p < 0.05$, ** $p < 0.01$ and *** $p < 0.001$ vs. HF, by one-way ANOVA and Dunnett's multiple comparisons test.

Table 2. Effects of *T. lutea* F&M-M36 and fenofibrate on plasma lipids, glucose, adiponectin, atherogenic index, uric acid, and blood pressure.

	NF	HF	HFF	HFT
TG (mg/dL)	183.7 ± 15.1	254.0 ± 21.6 ^^	90.5 ± 3.2 ***^^^	141.0 ± 7.9 **
TC (mg/dL)	128 ± 5.1	134 ± 7.0	130 ± 8.3	139 ± 22.2
HDL (mg/dL)	89 ± 5.64	68 ± 7.8	78 ± 6.5	80 ± 10.2
AIP	2.2 ± 0.36	3.5 ± 0.5	1.2 ± 0.1 **	2.0 ± 0.36 *
Glucose (mg/dL)	168.2 ± 9.1	212.1 ± 11.1 ^	137.5 ± 9.4 ***	150.9 ± 9.1 **
Adiponectin (ng/mL)	37.9 ± 3.5	28.9 ± 1.8	80.5 ± 5.9 ***^^^	57.9 ± 3.4 ***^^^
Urinary uric acid (mg/dL)	21.07 ± 4.6	25.05 ± 7.5	14.80 ± 6.1	13 ± 3.9
SBP (mm Hg)	156.2 ± 5.2	159.7 ± 3.6	164.6 ± 2.8	147.9 ± 1.9
DBP (mm Hg)	94.9 ± 6.4	111.7 ± 4.4	105.9 ± 8.1	80.56 ± 4.4 **
MAP (mm Hg)	115.3 ± 5.6	127.7 ± 4.1	125.4 ± 5.5	107.1 ± 4.9 *
RPP (mm Hg bpm)	61,342 ± 2650	68,703 ± 3012	67,409 ± 3093	58,338 ± 1555 *

Normal diet (NF), high-fat diet (HF), high-fat diet + fenofibrate (HFF), and high-fat diet + *T. lutea* F&M-M36 (HFT). Triglycerides (TG), total cholesterol (TC), high density lipoprotein (HDL), atherogenic index of plasma (AIP), SBP (systolic blood pressure), DBP (diastolic blood pressure), MAP (mean arterial pressure), and RPP (rate pressure product). Data are expressed as means ± SE; *n* = 8 rats/group. ^ $p < 0.05$, ^^ $p < 0.01$ and ^^^ $p < 0.001$ vs. NF; * $p < 0.05$, ** $p < 0.01$ and *** $p < 0.001$ vs. HF by one-way ANOVA and Dunnett's multiple comparisons test.

Adiponectin plasma levels were increased by fenofibrate and *T. lutea* compared to the HF diet (both $p < 0.001$); the urinary excretion of uric acid was similar among the groups. Systolic, diastolic, and mean arterial pressures, as well as the rate pressure product were not affected by the HF diet, except for SBP; *T. lutea* F&M-M36 significantly reduced all these parameters ($p < 0.01$, $p < 0.05$ and $p < 0.05$) compared to the HF diet (Table 2).

2.3. Effects of T. lutea F&M-M36 and Fenofibrate on Hepatic Steatosis

Hematoxylin and eosin staining of the liver revealed that the HF diet induced a significant increase in the steatosis score (Figure 1A–E) compared to the NF diet ($p < 0.001$); the score of rats fed *T. lutea* was similar to that of the HF diet (Figure 1D,E); on the contrary, fenofibrate increased the steatosis score compared to the HF diet ($p < 0.001$, Figure 1C,E) and induced hepatocellular ballooning, characterized by hepatocytic diameter enlargement and the presence of lipid droplets (Figure 1C), features of steatotic damage.

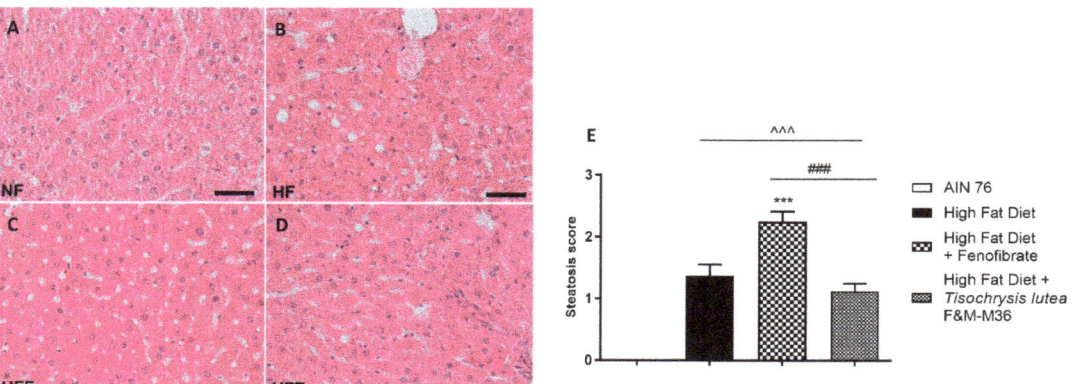

Figure 1. Hematoxylin and eosin staining for histopathological analysis of rat hepatic tissues: (**A**) NF group; (**B**) HF group; (**C**) HFF group; (**D**) HFT group, scale bar 400× magnification; (**E**) steatosis score. Normal diet (NF), high-fat diet (HF), high-fat diet + fenofibrate (HFF), and high-fat diet + *T. lutea* F&M-M36 (HFF). Data are expressed as means ± SE; n = 8 rats/group. ^^^ $p < 0.001$ vs. NF; *** $p < 0.001$ vs. HF; ### $p < 0.001$ vs. HFF, by one-way ANOVA and Dunnett's multiple comparisons test.

2.4. Effects of T. lutea F&M-M36 and Fenofibrate on Glycogen Storage in the Liver

As shown in Figure 2, the HF diet did not modify glycogen storage determined by periodic acid–Schiff (PAS) glycogen staining, compared to the NF diet. Fenofibrate but not *T. lutea* significantly decreased hepatic glycogen levels, compared to the HF diet ($p < 0.01$).

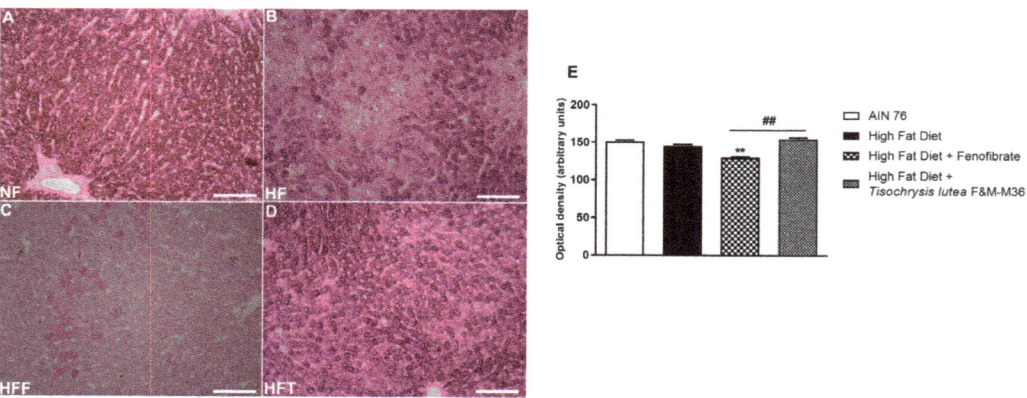

Figure 2. Periodic acid–Schiff (PAS) staining of rat hepatic tissues in the different groups; (**A**) NF group; (**B**) HF group; (**C**) HFF group; (**D**) HFT group. Scale bar 400× magnification. (**E**) glycogen storage. Data are expressed as mean ± SE; n = 8 rats/group. ** $p < 0.01$ vs. HF and ## $p < 0.01$ vs. HFF, by one-way ANOVA and Dunnett's multiple comparisons test.

2.5. Effects of T. lutea F&M-M36 and Fenofibrate on β3ADr, Ucp1, and Glp1r Protein Expression in Visceral Adipose Tissue

Western blot analysis on visceral adipose tissue revealed that the HF diet did not affect type 3 beta adrenergic receptor (β3ADr), Uncoupling Protein 1 (Ucp1), and Glucagon-like peptide-1 receptor (Glp1r) protein expression (Figure 3A–C). However, *T. lutea* but not fenofibrate, significantly increased the expression of β3ADr (Panel A, $p < 0.05$) and Ucp1 (Panel B, $p < 0.001$) compared to the HF diet. At a similar extent to fenofibrate, *T. lutea* also significantly induced Glp1r protein expression compared to the HF diet (Panel C, both $p < 0.001$). On the contrary, in brown adipose tissue, the mRNA expression of β3ADr and Ucp1 was similar among groups (data not shown).

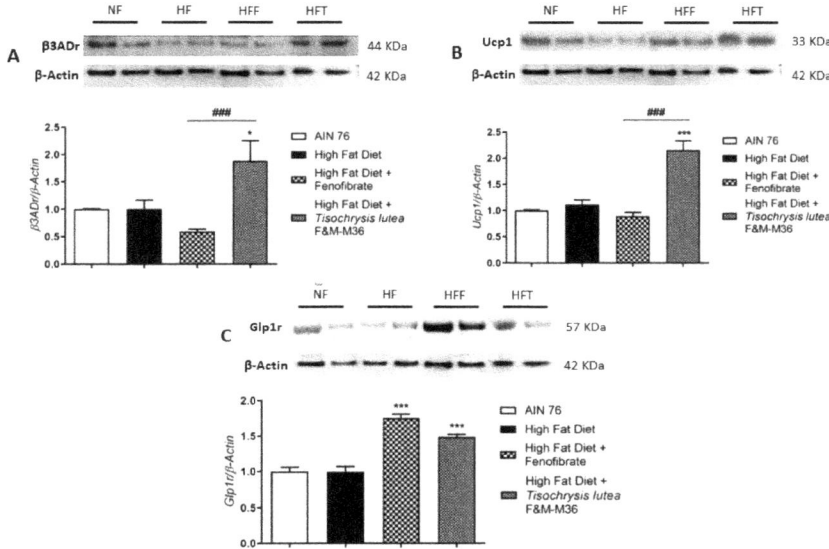

Figure 3. Effect of fenofibrate and *T. lutea* F&M-M36 on type 3 beta adrenergic receptors (β3ADr, (**A**)), Uncoupling Protein 1 (Ucp1, (**B**)) and Glucagon-like peptide-1 receptor (Glp1r, (**C**)) protein expression in visceral adipose tissue by Western-blot analysis. Representative gel images loaded with proteins obtained from two different samples for each experimental group. Normal diet (NF), high-fat diet (HF), high-fat diet + fenofibrate (HFF), and high-fat diet + *T. lutea* F&M-M36 (HFF). Densitometric analysis is expressed as mean ± SE; $n = 8$ rats/group. * $p < 0.05$ and *** $p < 0.001$ vs. HF; ### $p < 0.001$ vs. HFF by one-way ANOVA and Dunnett's multiple comparisons test.

2.6. Effects of T. lutea F&M-M36 and Fenofibrate on Pro-Inflammatory Cytokines mRNA Expression in Visceral Adipose Tissue

As shown in Figure 4, the HF diet slightly induced the mRNA expression of interleukin 1 beta (IL-1β, Figure 4A) interleukin-6 (IL-6, Figure 4B) while not affecting tumor necrosis factor alpha (TNFα, Panel C) compared to the NF diet. Fenofibrate and *T. lutea* F&M-M36 significantly reduced Il-1β ($p < 0.001$ and $p < 0.05$, respectively) and IL-6 ($p < 0.05$ for both) compared to the HF (Figure 4A,B).

2.7. Effect of T. lutea F&M-M36 on Whole-Gene Expression Profiles in Visceral Adipose Tissue

Transcriptomic analysis of whole-gene expression in visceral fat identified 2159 differentially expressed genes between HF diet and *T. lutea*-fed rats ($p < 0.01$), out of which 992 were up-regulated and 1167 were down-regulated. Pathway analysis identified 15 KEGG pathways differentially modulated by *T. lutea* compared to the HF diet, 13 up-regulated, and 2 down-regulated (Table 3). Among up-regulated pathways, it is of interest to mention PPAR signaling and Huntington's, Parkinson's, and Alzheimer's disease pathways since they include several electron transport chain and oxidative phosphorylation genes (several ATP synthases (ATPs, cytochrome c oxidases (COXs), and NADH ubiquinone oxidoreductases (Ndufs)) and peroxisome proliferator-activated receptor gamma (PPARγ). Conversely, down-regulated pathways included cytokine–cytokine receptor interaction and regulation of autophagy (Table 3).

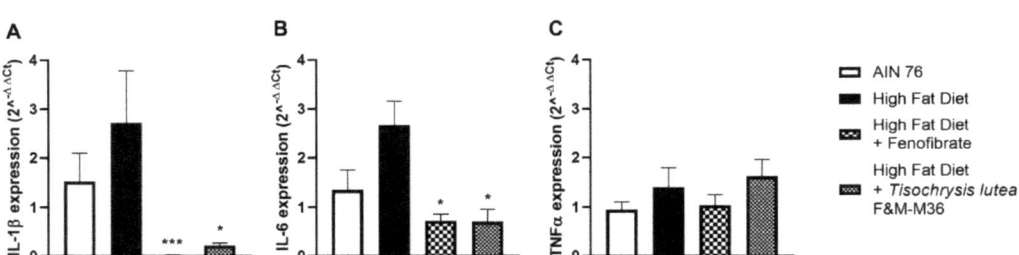

Figure 4. Effect of *T. lutea* F&M-M36 and fenofibrate on interleukin 1β (IL-1β, (**A**)), interleukin 6 (IL-6, (**B**)) and tumor necrosis factor alfa (TNFα, (**C**)) mRNA expression in visceral adipose tissue by real-time PCR. Data are expressed as mean ± SE; n = 8 rats/group. * $p < 0.05$ and *** $p < 0.001$ vs. HF by one-way ANOVA and Dunnett's multiple comparisons test.

Table 3. List of KEGG gene sets differentially modulated by comparing visceral adipose tissue from high-fat diet and high-fat diet + *T. lutea* F&M-M36, divided into 13 up-regulated and 2 down-regulated.

Gene-Set Name	Percent Changed	PermuteP	Gene Symbols
Up-Regulated			
Notch signaling pathway:KEGG-rno04330	50.0	0.002	Dll3 | Dtx1 | Jag2 | Ncstn | Notch3 | Notch4 | Ptcra | Rbpj
Protein export:KEGG-rno03060	44.4	0.04	LOC100361694 | Oxa1l | Sec11c | Spcs2
Mismatch repair:KEGG-rno03430	44.4	0.05	Exo1 | Lig1 | Mlh1 | Pold3
Galactose metabolism:KEGG-rno00052	41.7	0.03	Gaa | Galk1 | Hk2 | Hk3 | Pfkl
Endocrine and other factor-regulated calcium reabsorption:KEGG-rno04961	33.3	0.02	Ap2b1 | Ap2m1 | Clta | Cltb | Cltc | Dnm2 | Plcb3 | Plcb4 | Prkcg
PPAR signaling pathway:KEGG-rno03320	33.3	0.01	Acox1 | Acsbg1 | Dbi | Fabp4 | Fabp5 | LOC681458 | Mmp1 | Nr1h3 | Pparg | Scd1 | Slc27a1 | Ubc
Huntington's disease:KEGG-rno05016	31.9	0.00	Ap2b1 | Ap2m1 | Atp5g1 | Atp5g2 | Atp5g3 | Atp5hl1 | Atp5o | Clta | Cltb | Cltc | Cox4i2 | Cox5b | Dnali1 | Grm5 | LOC688963 | Mt-co1 | Ndufa10 | Ndufa6 | Ndufb10 | Ndufb11 | Ndufb2 | Ndufs7 | Ndufv1 | Plcb3 | Plcb4 | Pparg | Sod1 | Tp53 | Uqcrh | Vdac3
Gap junction:KEGG-rno04540	31.3	0.02	Adcy5 | Gnai2 | Grm5 | Htr2a | Plcb3 | Plcb4 | Prkcg | Tuba3a | Tubb4b | Tubb5
Bacterial invasion of epithelial cells:KEGG-rno05100	31.3	0.02	Arpc1a | Cdc42 | Clta | Cltb | Cltc | Ctnnb1 | Cttn | Dnm2 | Pik3r2 | Pxn
Pancreatic secretion:KEGG-rno04972	30.8	0.03	Adcy5 | Atp2a3 | Cela2a | Clca1 | Cpa1 | Ctrb1 | Pla2g1b | Plcb3 | Plcb4 | Prkcg | Rap1b | Slc4a2
Antigen processing and presentation:KEGG-rno04612	28.9	0.04	Calr | Ctsb | Hsp90aa1 | LOC680121 | LOC688090 | Psme2 | RT1-CE3 | RT1-Da | RT1-M1-4 | RT1-M6-2 | RT1-T18

Table 3. Cont.

Gene-Set Name	Up-Regulated		
	Percent Changed	PermuteP	Gene Symbols
Parkinson's disease:KEGG-rno05012	28.4	0.004	Atp5g1 | Atp5g2 | Atp5g3 | Atp5hl1 | Atp5o | Cox4i2 | Cox5b | Gp1bb | LOC688963 | Mt-co1 | Ndufa10 | Ndufa6 | Ndufb10 | Ndufb11 | Ndufb2 | Ndufs7 | Ndufv1 | Th | Uba1 | Ubc | Ube2l3 | Uqcrh | Vdac3
Alzheimer's disease:KEGG-rno05010	25.0	0.03	Atp2a3 | Atp5g1 | Atp5g2 | Atp5g3 | Atp5hl1 | Atp5o | Calm1 | Cox4i2 | Cox5b | Grin2c | LOC688963 | Mt-co1 | Ncstn | Ndufa10 | Ndufa6 | Ndufb10 | Ndufb11 | Ndufb2 | Ndufs7 | Ndufv1 | Plcb3 | Plcb4 | Uqcrh
Down-regulated			
Gene-Set Name	*Percent Changed*	*PermuteP*	*gene symbols*
Cytokine-cytokine receptor interaction:KEGG-rno04060	26.0	0.0085	Ccl12 | Ccr6 | Cd40 | Csf2rb | Cxcl11 | Cxcl13 | Cxcr4 | Egf | Ifna2 | Ifnar2 | Il11ra1 | Il12b | Il22 | LOC100910178 | Lta | Osmr | Pdgfrb | RGD1561246 | Tnfrsf12a | Tnfrsf21 | Tnfrsf8
Regulation of autophagy:KEGG-rno04140	40	0.049	Becn1 | Ifna2 | Prkaa2 | RGD1561246

3. Discussion

High-fat diet is a critical risk factor for the development of obesity and related metabolic disorders [11]. In this study, a high-fat diet (30%) administered to Sprague Dawley rats for 3 months did not induce a frank MetS, but rather a pre-MetS, the initial stage of the disease. There is no consensus on the criteria for defining pre-MetS in humans [12,13], but Gesteiro et al. recently proposed to consider the cardiometabolic risk and the closeness to the cut-off criteria for the diagnosis of MetS [14]. In our model, because of the lower food and calorie intakes, rats fed the HF diet showed a similar weight gain compared to rats fed the normal-fat diet; however, the HF diet had a negative impact on blood lipids and fat depots. Indeed, the HF diet increased renal and epididymal fat deposits, blood triglycerides, and glucose but did not induce obesity or hypertension or a significant increase in visceral adipose tissue, therefore better recapitulating the features of pre-MetS. This stage of the disease can be the ideal timepoint to start dietary interventions aimed at reducing risk factors by acting on the same cardiometabolic routes of overt MetS.

In our previous study on the safety of a diet containing 20% of *T. lutea*, we reported that the relatively high salt and nucleic acid content of the biomass represented a safety concern limiting its inclusion in the diet [5]. Notably, by decreasing the dose to 5%, which is more achievable than dietary consumption, in the present study, we did not observe signs of adverse effects, including histopathological alterations in any organ or abnormalities in water consumption, diuresis or uric acid excretion, indicating that the sub-chronic administration of *T. lutea* is safe in rats, at this dose. On the contrary, Mayer et al. reported a marked increase in water intake in rats fed 12% Tiso with no other relevant abnormalities [8].

This is the first study comparing the effects of a dietary intervention with those of fenofibrate, a widely employed anti-dyslipidemic drug. Its effects, such as those of DHA, are mediated through the activation of PPAR-α, leading to expression of genes involved in lipid metabolism and through reducing lipoprotein lipase [15]. Despite being less effective than fenofibrate, dietary treatment with *T. lutea* reduced plasma triglycerides by nearly 50% without increasing lipid accumulation in the liver; at variance, rats treated with fenofibrate showed enhanced hepatic lipid accumulation, an adverse effect previously reported in ob/ob mice [16]. Non-fasting glucose levels were also decreased by *T. lutea* to the same extent as fenofibrate. These positive effects on lipid and glucose metabolisms agree with the results of Meyer et al., who also reported a significant reduction in body weight, but their animals were fed a high-fat and high-fructose diet, and the dose of *T. lutea* was 12% [8]. Like fenofibrate, *T. lutea* reduced the atherogenic index of plasma, a metabolic syndrome and atherogenicity biomarker [17,18]; *T. lutea* also enhanced adiponectin, an adipocyte-secreted anti-inflammatory protein associated with lower inflammation and with increased antioxidant defenses [19,20].

Interestingly, renal fat accumulation was significantly reduced by *T. lutea* but not by fenofibrate; this result is of relevance since perirenal fat correlates with metabolic risk factors in obese subjects and in patients with chronic kidney disease and type 2 diabetes [21–23]. Other than being suggested as an independent predictor of MetS, para-and perirenal fat are also positively correlated with diastolic blood pressure in overweight and obese healthy subjects [24]. Consistently, we observed reduced diastolic blood pressure and renal fat in rats treated with *T. lutea* but not with fenofibrate; mechanistically, the reduction in perirenal fat may limit the compression of renal lymphatics and veins, the renal hydrostatic pressure, and the activation of the renin–angiotensin–aldosterone system [24]. Collectively, these data indicate that *T. lutea* may exert a protective effect against cardiometabolic risk factors of MetS.

Our study is the first to report the molecular mechanisms involved in these effects, focusing on adipose tissue, a key player in energy metabolism. In addition to the well-known role of white adipose tissue (WAT) in storing energy in the form of triglycerides, mammals, including adult humans, are also equipped with brown adipose tissue (BAT) that uses fatty acids and glucose at a high rate and dissipates energy as heat for non-shivering thermogenesis [25]. Adaptive thermogenesis in BAT is principally dependent on the activation of UCP1, a mitochondrial protein specific to brown adipocytes, which uncouples electron transport from ATP production, thereby generating heat [25]. β3-adrenergic receptors are among the predominant regulators of this process and most of the strategies to enhance lipolysis and thermogenesis converge into the stimulation of these receptors [26]. Cold exposure, β3 receptors agonists, but also dietary factors can induce the so-called "WAT browning" process characterized by the presence of UCP1-expressing beige or brown-like adipocytes displaying the same thermogenic function of brown adipocytes [26]. By increasing energy expenditure and regulating glucose and lipid metabolism, "WAT browning" seems a promising approach for MetS and obesity [27].

Our results demonstrate that *T. lutea* increases the expression of the β3-adrenergic receptor and UCP1 in visceral but not in brown fat, suggesting that this microalga stimulates visceral WAT browning and thermogenesis without affecting the metabolic activity of BAT. Various bioactive compounds of *T. lutea* biomass can exert a positive effect on WAT browning; among them, the literature extensively reported that PUFAs, especially ω-3 PUFAs, increase WAT browning and energy expenditure through UCP1-dependent mechanisms. The DHA content in *T. lutea* F&M-M36 is 1.01% of dry matter [5,7], equivalent to an average DHA intake of 13.89 mg/day/rat, and for a 70 kg human, it corresponds to a daily intake of about 2 g, the minimal effective dose to lower plasma triglycerides [28]. *T. lutea* F&M-M36 biomass also contains 0.6% (dry weight) of the carotenoid fucoxanthin [5,7]; fucoxanthin showed anti-obesity and anti-diabetic effects in mice by promoting the expression of the UCP1 and β3-adrenergic receptors in WAT [29–31]. In addition, the methanolic extract of *T. lutea* F&M-M36 contains 6.22 mg of gallic acid equivalents of phenols per gram, and in particular, phenolic acid derivatives of hydroxybenzoic and gallic acids [6]. The ability of phenolic compounds to induce WAT browning is largely demonstrated and may involve the activation of β3 signaling pathways [32,33].

Increased fecal lipid excretion was also observed in rats fed *T. lutea* or treated with fenofibrate. Data in mice indicate that fenofibrate decreases cholesterol absorption by reducing the expression of the intestinal cholesterol transporter Niemann-Pick C1-Like 1 (NPC1L1), thereby increasing fecal neutral sterol excretion [34]. Orlistat, another well-known drug able to increase fecal lipid excretion, selectively inhibits gastrointestinal lipase activity, thereby preventing the absorption of dietary fat [35]. The increased lipid excretion observed in *T-lutea*-fed rats may be due to ω-3 and fucoxanthin; indeed, eicosapentaenoic acid (EPA) and DHA limit cholesterol uptake and are transported by down-regulating

NPC1L1 [36], while fucoxanthin inhibits gastrointestinal lipase activity and suppresses triglyceride absorption, thereby increasing the fecal excretions of lipids [37,38].

Pathway analysis on adipose tissue whole-gene expression profiles suggested that *T.lutea* increased the adipose tissue metabolic activity. Indeed, among the genes belonging to the most significantly up-regulated pathways, we found multiple energy metabolism-related genes, electron transport chain genes, and those relevant for the control of oxidative phosphorylation and mitochondrial functions, such as *ATP5g*, *Cox4i2*, and *Cox5b* [39,40]. Genes such as *Acox-1*, *FABP4* and *FABP5PPAR*, and *PPARg*, belonging to PPAR signaling, are implicated in thermogenesis, lipolysis promotion, and adipocytes differentiation [40–45]. In particular, the overexpression of the mitochondrial *Cox4i2* gene and the β-oxidation *Acox-1* gene was associated with β3-adrenergic receptor activation in adipose tissue [40]. The down-regulation of autophagy is also consistent with the maintenance of fat browning through β-adrenergic stimulation [46].

The inflammation of visceral adipose tissue is also a trigger for the induction and spreading of low-grade systemic inflammation; the down-regulation of the cytokine–cytokine receptor pathway, including several chemokines and interleukins, suggests that *T. lutea* also exerts anti-inflammatory actions in the adipose tissue, thus contributing to the mitigation of chronic low-grade inflammation. It is also intriguing that both fenofibrate and *T. lutea* F&M-M36 induced the expression of GLP1R, down-regulated that of pro-inflammatory cytokines IL-6 and IL-1β in adipose tissue, and increased adiponectin plasma levels, thus suggesting that some of the metabolic effects observed may in part be due to the amplification of incretin action and its known anti-inflammatory effects [47,48].

Collectively, our data suggest that the a role of *T. lutea* F&M-M36 on visceral fat browning is at least in part mediated by the activation of β3ADR/UCP1 signaling in visceral fat, but further studies using appropriate knock-out models are needed to validate this mechanistic pathway.

The ability of *T. lutea* F&M-M36 to target multiple components of pre-MetS suggests that this microalga is a promising candidate for mitigating risk factors associated with metabolic syndrome.

4. Materials and Methods

4.1. Microalgae Cultivation and Production

T. lutea F&M-M36 biomass belongs to the Fotosintetica & Microbiologica (F&M) S.r.l. Culture Collection (Florence, Italy), and was produced at Archimede Ricerche S.r.l. (Camporosso, Imperia, Italy) in GWP®-II photobioreactors [49] in a semi-batch mode in F medium [50]. The biomass was harvested by centrifugation, frozen, lyophilized, and powdered. The powdered biomass was stored at $-20\ °C$ until use.

4.2. Animals and Treatment Design

All procedures were carried out in agreement with the European Union Regulations on the Care and Use of Laboratory Animals (OJ of ECL 358/1, 18 December 1986) and according to Italian regulations on the protection of animals used for experimental and other scientific purposes (DM 116/1992), after approval from the Italian Ministry for Scientific Research (ID 1137/2015; date of approval 28 October 2015).

After 1 week of acclimatization in plastic cages equipped with soft wood bedding, a water bottle, and basic equipment, male Sprague Dawley rats (Nossan S.r.l., Milan, Italy), aged 6–8 weeks, were divided into 4 experimental groups; rats fed AIN-76 diet (NF—5% of fat; $n = 8$), rats fed high-fat diet (HF—30% of fat; $n = 8$), rats fed a HF diet, supplemented with 5% *T. lutea* F&M-M36 biomass (HFT—30% of fat; $n = 8$), and rats fed a HF diet, supplemented with 100 mg/Kg Fenofibrate for 2 months, after the first month of feeding (HFF—30% of fat; $n = 8$).

Water and food were available ad libitum; the lighting regime was a standard 12 h light and 12 h dark regime, the temperature was maintained constant at $21 \pm 2\ °C$. At the end of the study, the rats were euthanized by inhalation of CO_2, and blood samples were collected in tubes containing an anticoagulant (EDTA) to separate plasma. Following the sacrifice, kidney, hearth, liver, visceral, epididymal, and renal adipose tissue were weighed and stored either at −20 °C or −80 °C for further analyses. The experimental diets were prepared using components purchased from Piccioni Laboratories (Gessate, Milan, Italy). All the diets were prepared in accordance with the standard AIN76 diet. In the HF and HFT diets, the amount of proteins, lipids, carbohydrates, and fibers were adjusted in accordance with the contents of these components in the microalgal biomass (Table 4). The AIN76 diet provided 3.79 kcal/g, while HF and HFT diets provided 5.33 and 5.32 kcal/g, respectively.

Table 4. Composition of the experimental diets (g/100 g of diet).

	AIN-76 Diet (NF)	High-Fat Diet (HF)	T. lutea F&M-M36 Enriched Diet (HFT)
Lyophilized algal biomass			5
Corn oil	5	3	**2**
Lard	-	30	30
Sucrose	50	34	**33.4**
Starch	15		
Casein	20	24.6	**22.5**
Cellulose	5	2	**1.1**
Mineral Mix AIN 76	3.5	4.1	4.1
Vitamin Mix AIN 76	1	1.3	1
Coline	0.2	0.26	0.26
DL Methionine	0.3	0.4	0.4

Values in bold indicate constituents of the diets that were adjusted to compensate for components deriving from algal biomass.

4.3. Blood Pressure Measurement

Systolic and diastolic blood pressures, mean arterial pressure (MAP), and heart rate (HR) were measured in conscious rats by the noninvasive computerized tail-cuff method (Visitech BP-2000 Series II Blood Pressure Analysis System, Apex, NC, USA). Before the recording, 2 days of training were performed for each animal. The same researcher performed all measurements, repeated 10 times, in a quiet environment; the highest and lowest values were discarded. The values recorded in the rats of each experimental group were reported as mean ± SEM. The rate pressure product (RPP), which is an indirect index of myocardial oxygen consumption, was calculated in accordance with [51].

4.4. Food and Water Consumption

During the third month of treatment, the animals were placed in metabolic cages for one day to accurately measure water and food daily consumption and the 24 h urine and feces production. Daily calorie intake was calculated by multiplying the daily food intake (g) by the total energy of the diet (kcal/g).

4.5. Macroscopic Examinations and Histological Analyses

A complete necropsy, including the examination of the external surface of all orifices and of the cranial, thoracic, abdominal, and pelvic cavities and viscera, was conducted on all rats. The main organs (heart, kidneys, liver, and fat) were weighed. For histological analyses, tissue samples were stored in neutral formaldehyde and embedded in paraffin wax. Sections (5 μm) were stained with a standard hematoxylin and eosin procedure.

Microscopic analysis was performed using the ACT-2U software (Nikon, Instruments Europe, Badhoevedorp, The Netherlands) connected via a camera to the microscope (Optiphot-2; Nikon). Hepatic fat content was evaluated by quantifying the extent of fat droplets in each liver section using the ImageJ software (ImageJ 1.33 image analysis software (https://rsb.info.nih.gov/ij, accessed on 1 May 2023) and expressed as the mean number of lipid droplets for microscopic field. The steatosis score was graded based on the percentage of lipid droplets within the hepatocytes: Grade 0 (healthy, <5%), Grade 1 (mild, 5–33%), Grade 2 (moderate, 34–66%), and Grade 3 (severe, >66%) [52].

4.6. Blood Biochemistry

Plasma levels of TC, HDL, Triglycerides, and Glucose were measured with the Reflotron® Plus system (Roche Diagnostics GmbH, Mannheim, Germany) using specific test strips. The atherogenic risk was evaluated by calculating the atherogenic index plasma (AIP) as the log (TAG/HDL-C) [53].

4.7. Fecal Lipid Content

Fecal lipid content was measured from dried fecal samples (about 30 mg) in accordance with [54]. Briefly, dried fecal samples (about 30 mg) were re-suspended in 500 µL of normal saline. Then, 500 µL of chloroform–methanol (2:1, v/v) were added to extract the lipids.

4.8. Periodic Acid–Schiff (PAS) Staining

The detection of glycogen in liver tissue was performed on histological slices (4 µm tick). Briefly, tissues were oxidized in 0.5% periodic acid solution (0.5 g of periodic acid in 100 mL distilled water) for 5 min. Washed in distilled water; placed in Schiff reagent (bis-N-aminosulfonic acid) for 15 min; washed in lukewarm tap water for 5 min; counterstained in Mayer's hematoxylin for 1 min; washed in tap water for 5 min. Microscopic images were evaluated using the ACT-2U software program (Nikon, Instruments Europe, Badhoevedorp, The Netherlands) connected via a camera to the microscope (Optiphot-2; Nikon).

4.9. Western Blot

For Western Blot analysis, protein extraction was performed on 50 mg of visceral adipose tissue in accordance with [55]. The total protein content was estimated by using the Bio-Rad DC protein assay kit (Bio-Rad, Segrate, Milan, Italy), using a bovine serum albumin (BSA) standard solution (ranging from 0.2 to 2 mg/mL) for the calibration curve.

Twenty micrograms of proteins were separated on 4–20% SDS-PAGE (Thermo Fisher scientific, Waltham, MA, USA) and transferred into PVDF membranes (60 min at 398 mA) using standard procedures. Blots were incubated overnight at 4 °C with a specific primary antibody (Table 5) diluted in phosphate-buffered saline (PBS) containing 5% BSA or 5% non-fat dry milk and 0.05% Tween 20. The antigen–antibody complexes were visualized using appropriate secondary antibodies (1:10,000, diluted in PBS containing 5% albumin or 5% non-fat dry milk and 0.05% Tween 20), and left for 1 h at room temperature. Blots were then extensively washed with PBS containing 0.1% Tween 20 and developed using an enhanced chemiluminescence detection system (Pierce, Rodano, Italy). Exposition and developing time were standardized for all blots. Densitometric analysis was performed using the public domain NIH Image program (Image J software Version 1.50i, National Institute of Health, Bethesda, MD, USA). Each gel was loaded with all the experimental groups to standardize the image acquisition and densitometric analysis. Data are presented as mean ± SEM of four different gel preparations and were reported as arbitrary units (AU), consisting of the ratio between the level of the target protein expression and that of the β-Actin.

Table 5. Primary antibodies used for Western blot analysis (WB).

Antibody	Dilution	Supplier
β3ADr	1:500	Santa Cruz Biotechnology Inc. Dallas, TX, USA (SC-515763)
UCP-1	1:500	Santa Cruz Biotechnology Inc. Dallas, TX, USA (SC-2934184)
GLP1r	1:200	Santa Cruz Biotechnology Inc. Dallas, TX, USA (sc-390774)
β-Actin	1:1000	Bioss Antibodies Woburn, MS, USA (bs-0061R)

4.10. Total RNA Extraction and Real-Time PCR

Total RNA was extracted by using TRIzol extraction reagent (Invitrogen, Carlsbad, CA, USA). First-strand cDNA synthesis was performed using the Revert Aid RT Kit, in accordance with manufacturer's instruction (Thermo Scientific, Waltham, USA. qRT-PCR assays were carried out in Rotor-Gene® qPCR System (Qiagen, Hilden, Germany), using SsoAdvanced Universal SYBR Green Supermix (Biorad, Hercules, CA, USA). Briefly, each reaction was performed in a final volume of 10 µL containing 1 µL of the cDNA, 1 µL of forward and 1 µL of reverse primers, 5 µL of SsoAdvanced universal SYBR Green supermix and 1 µL of nuclease-free water. Primers were designed based on the mouse GenBank sequences for IL-6, IL-1β, and TNFa, and are reported in Table 6. The amplification protocol was based on an initial heat activation at 95 °C for 30 s, followed by 35 cycles of denaturation at 95 °C for 15 s and combined annealing/extension at 60 °C for 30 s. The relative expression of mRNA was normalized by β-Actin and calculated by the $2^{-\Delta\Delta Ct}$ method.

Table 6. Primer sequences used for real-time PCR.

Gene	Primer Forward	Primer Reverse
β-Actin	TACAGCTTCACCACCACAGC	TGGCCATCTCTTGCTCGAAG
IL-1β	GACTTCACCATGGAACCCGT	GGAGACTGCCCATTCTCGAC
IL-6	GTGGCTAAGGACCAAGACCA	TAGCACACTAGGTTTGCCGAG
TNFα	AACACACGAGACGCTGAAGT	TCCAGTGAGTTCCGAAAGCC
ADRB3	ACTCACCGCTCAACAGGTTT	TTCTGGAGAGTTGCGGTTCC
UCP1	CCGAAACTGTACAGCGGTCT	CAGGAGTGTGGTGCAAAACC

4.11. Gene Expression Profiling

Total RNA was extracted from visceral fat by using the RNeasy Mini kit Plus (Macherey-Nagel), in accordance with the manufacturer's protocol. RNA concentration and purity was determined by using a NanoPhotometer spectrophotometer (IMPLEN, München, Germany).

Transcriptomic analyses were performed using a two-color microarray protocol, in which a pool of RNA (50 ng) extracted from the HFT group ($n = 6$) was contrasted with a reference RNA (50 ng) obtained by pooling an equal amount of RNA samples extracted from HF rats ($n = 6$).

RNA samples were labeled using the Agilent Quick Amp Labeling Kit (Agilent Technologies, Santa Clara, CA, USA), following the manufacturer's protocol (Two-Color Microarray-Based Gene Expression Analysis Low Input Quick Amp Labeling Version 6.9.1). The RNA Spike-In kit (Agilent Technologies) was also used to monitor and calibrate the linearity, sensitivity, and accuracy of the microarray workflow. Yields of cRNA and the dye incorporation rate were measured with the NanoPhotometer spectrophotometer (IMPLEN). Sample mixture was loaded into the Agilent Rat GE 8 × 60 K v2 Oligo 60-mer microarrays, in Agilent microarray chambers (G2534A) at 65° for 18 h. Fluorescent signal intensities were detected using the Agilent Scan Control 7.0 Software on an Agilent DNA Microarray Scanner, at a resolution of 2 µm. Data were acquired using the Agilent Feature Extraction 9.5.3.1 software. Image analysis and initial quality control were performed using the same software. The genes of interest were those that exhibited a PValueLogRatio (statistical significance on the LogRatio per each gene between red and green channels) of <0.01.

Pathway analysis was performed by means of GO-Elite software, version 1.2.5, an open source, freely available (http://www.genmapp.org/go_elite accessed on 17 January 2023), using the list of the differentially expressed genes with a statistical significance of less than 0.01 and a fold change (FC) of ≥ 2 or ≤ 2 as input data.

4.12. Statistics

Statistical analyses were conducted using the GraphPad Prism 8.02 software (GraphPad, San Diego, CA, USA) program. The D'Agostino and Pearson omnibus normality test was applied to verify the Gaussian distribution of each variable. Differences among groups were analyzed by using one-way ANOVA and Dunnett's multiple comparisons test or by Kruskal–Wallis and Dunn's multiple comparisons tests, when appropriate. Results are presented as means ± SEM. Significance was assigned at $p < 0.05$.

Author Contributions: Conceptualization, C.L. and E.B.; methodology, C.L., E.B., L.C., L.R. (Laura Raimondi), M.R.T., N.B. and L.R. (Liliana Rodolfi); validation, C.L., E.B. and L.R. (Laura Raimondi); formal analysis, C.L. and M.D.; investigation, M.D., L.C., A.L., F.Z., M.G., S.C. and C.L.; resources, C.L., A.N., N.B., L.R. (Liliana Rodolfi), L.R. (Laura Raimondi) and M.R.T.; writing—original draft preparation, E.B.; writing—review and editing, all authors; supervision, C.L. and E.B.; funding acquisition, C.L. and M.R.T. All authors have read and agreed to the published version of the manuscript.

Funding: This research was co-funded by Ente Cassa di Risparmio Firenze grant numbers: 2015.0919 and 2018.1002 and Regione Toscana (Italy) under Par-FAS 2007–2013 Projects (Centro di Competenza VALORE).

Institutional Review Board Statement: The animal study protocol was approved by the Italian Ministry of Health-Direzione generale della sanità animale e dei farmaci veterinari (n° 1137/2017/PR, 28 October 2015).

Data Availability Statement: The data that support the findings of this study are available on request from the corresponding author E.B. (elisabetta.bigagli@unifi.it).

Conflicts of Interest: *T. lutea* F&M-M36 belongs to F&M S.r.l. Culture Collection, where M.R.T. had and L.R. has a financial interest. The other authors have no conflict of interest.

References

1. Huang, P.L. A comprehensive definition for metabolic syndrome. *Dis. Model Mech.* **2009**, *2*, 231–237. [CrossRef] [PubMed]
2. Hotamisligil, G. Inflammation and metabolic disorders. *Nature* **2006**, *444*, 860–867. [CrossRef] [PubMed]
3. Grundy, S.M. Drug therapy of the metabolic syndrome: Minimizing the emerging crisis in polypharmacy. *Nat. Rev. Drug Discov.* **2006**, *5*, 295–309. [CrossRef] [PubMed]
4. Koizumi, K.; Oku, M.; Hayashi, S.; Inujima, A.; Shibahara, N.; Chen, L.; Igarashi, Y.; Tobe, K.; Saito, S.; Kadowaki, M.; et al. Identifying pre-disease signals before metabolic syndrome in mice by dynamical network biomarkers. *Sci. Rep.* **2019**, *9*, 8767. [CrossRef] [PubMed]
5. Bigagli, E.; Cinci, L.; Niccolai, A.; Biondi, N.; Rodolfi, L.; D'Ottavio, M.; D'Ambrosio, M.; Lodovici, M.; Tredici, M.R.; Luceri, C. Preliminary data on the dietary safety, tolerability and effects on lipid metabolism of the marine microalga *Tisochrysis lutea*. *Algal. Res.* **2018**, *34*, 244–249. [CrossRef]
6. Bigagli, E.; D'Ambrosio, M.; Cinci, L.; Niccolai, A.; Biondi, N.; Rodolfi, L.; Dos Santos Nascimiento, L.B.; Tredici, M.R.; Luceri, C. A Comparative In Vitro Evaluation of the Anti-Inflammatory Effects of a *Tisochrysis lutea* Extract and Fucoxanthin. *Mar. Drugs* **2021**, *19*, 334. [CrossRef]
7. Niccolai, A.; Chini Zittelli, G.; Rodolfi, L.; Biondi, N.; Tredici, M.R. Microalgae of interest as food source: Biochemical composition and digestibility. *Algal Res.* **2019**, *42*, 101617. [CrossRef]
8. Mayer, C.; Richard, L.; Côme, M.; Ulmann, L.; Nazih, H.; Chénais, B.; Ouguerram, K.; Mimouni, V. The Marine Microalga, *Tisochrysis lutea*, Protects against Metabolic Disorders Associated with Metabolic Syndrome and Obesity. *Nutrients* **2021**, *13*, 430. [CrossRef]
9. Custódio, L.; Soares, F.; Pereira, H.; Barreira, L.; Vizetto-Duarte, C.; Rodrigues, M.J.; Rauter, A.P.; Albericío, F.; Varela, J. Fatty acid composition and biological activities of Isochrysis galbana T-ISO, *Tetraselmis* sp. and *Scenedesmus* sp.: Possible application in the pharmaceutical and functional food industries. *J. Appl. Phycol.* **2014**, *26*, 151–161. [CrossRef]
10. Tenenbaum, A.; Fisman, E.Z. Fibrates are an essential part of modern anti-dyslipidemic arsenal: Spotlight on atherogenic dyslipidemia and residual risk reduction. *Cardiovasc. Diabetol.* **2012**, *11*, 125. [CrossRef]
11. Duan, Y.; Zeng, L.; Zheng, C.; Song, B.; Li, F.; Kong, X.; Xu, K. Inflammatory Links Between High Fat Diets and Diseases. *Front. Immunol.* **2018**, *9*, 2649. [CrossRef] [PubMed]
12. Vidigal Fde, C.; Ribeiro, A.Q.; Babio, N.; Salas-Salvadó, J.; Bressan, J. Prevalence of metabolic syndrome and pre-metabolic syndrome in health professionals: Latinmets brazil study. *Diabetol. Metab. Syndr.* **2015**, *7*, 6. [CrossRef] [PubMed]
13. de las Fuentes, L.; Brown, A.L.; Mathews, S.J.; Waggoner, A.D.; Soto, P.F.; Gropler, R.J.; Dávila-Román, V.G. Metabolic syndrome is associated with abnormal left ventricular diastolic function independent of left ventricular mass. *Eur. Heart J.* **2007**, *28*, 553–559. [CrossRef] [PubMed]
14. Gesteiro, E.; Megía, A.; Guadalupe-Grau, A.; Fernandez-Veledo, S.; Vendrell, J.; González-Gross, M. Early identification of metabolic syndrome risk: A review of reviews and proposal for defining pre-metabolic syndrome status. *Nutr. Metab. Cardiovasc. Dis.* **2021**, *31*, 2557–2574. [CrossRef]
15. Ferreira, A.V.; Parreira, G.G.; Green, A.; Botion, L.M. Effects of fenofibrate on lipid metabolism in adipose tissue of rats. *Metabolism* **2006**, *55*, 731–735. [CrossRef]
16. Zhang, Y.; Jia, X.B.; Liu, Y.C.; Yu, W.Q.; Si, Y.H.; Guo, S.D. Fenofibrate enhances lipid deposition via modulating PPARγ, SREBP-1c, and gut microbiota in ob/ob mice fed a high-fat diet. *Front. Nutr.* **2022**, *9*, 971581. [CrossRef]
17. Zhang, X.; Zhang, X.; Li, X.; Feng, J.; Chen, X. Association of metabolic syndrome with atherogenic index of plasma in an urban Chinese population: A 15-year prospective study. *Nutr. Metab. Cardiovasc. Dis.* **2019**, *29*, 1214–1219. [CrossRef]

18. Wu, J.; Zhou, Q.; Wei, Z.; Wei, J.; Cui, M. Atherogenic Index of Plasma and Coronary Artery Disease in the Adult Population: A Meta-Analysis. *Front. Cardiovasc. Med.* **2021**, *8*, 817441. [CrossRef]
19. Rosenson, R.S. Effect of fenofibrate on adiponectin and inflammatory biomarkers in metabolic syndrome patients. *Obes. Silver Spring* **2009**, *17*, 504–509. [CrossRef]
20. Lodovici, M.; Bigagli, E.; Tarantini, F.; Di Serio, C.; Raimondi, L. Losartan reduces oxidative damage to renal DNA and conserves plasma antioxidant capacity in diabetic rats. *Exp. Biol. Med.* **2015**, *240*, 1500–1504. [CrossRef]
21. Manno, C.; Campobasso, N.; Nardecchia, A.; Triggiani, V.; Zupo, R.; Gesualdo, L.; Silvestris, F.; De Pergola, G. Relationship of para- and perirenal fat and epicardial fat with metabolic parameters in overweight and obese subjects. *Eat Weight Disord.* **2019**, *24*, 67–72. [CrossRef] [PubMed]
22. D'Marco, L.; Salazar, J.; Cortez, M.; Salazar, M.; Wettel, M.; Lima-Martínez, M.; Rojas, E.; Roque, W.; Bermúdez, V. Perirenal fat thickness is associated with metabolic risk factors in patients with chronic kidney disease. *Kidney Res. Clin. Pract.* **2019**, *38*, 365–372. [CrossRef] [PubMed]
23. Guo, X.L.; Tu, M.; Chen, Y.; Wang, W. Perirenal Fat Thickness: A Surrogate Marker for Metabolic Syndrome in Chinese Newly Diagnosed Type 2 Diabetes. *Front. Endocrinol.* **2022**, *13*, 850334. [CrossRef] [PubMed]
24. De Pergola, G.; Campobasso, N.; Nardecchia, A.; Triggiani, V.; Caccavo, D.; Gesualdo, L.; Silvestris, F.; Manno, C. Para- and perirenal ultrasonographic fat thickness is associated with 24-h mean diastolic blood pressure levels in overweight and obese subjects. *BMC Cardiovasc. Disord.* **2015**, *15*, 108. [CrossRef] [PubMed]
25. El Hadi, H.; Di Vincenzo, A.; Vettor, R.; Rossato, M. Food Ingredients Involved in White-to-Brown Adipose Tissue Conversion and in Calorie Burning. *Front. Physiol.* **2019**, *9*, 1954. [CrossRef] [PubMed]
26. Tabuchi, C.; Sul, H.S. Signaling Pathways Regulating Thermogenesis. *Front. Endocrinol.* **2021**, *12*, 595020. [CrossRef]
27. Ricquier, D. Uncoupling protein 1 of brown adipocytes, the only uncoupler: A historical perspective. *Front. Endocrinol.* **2011**, *2*, 85. [CrossRef]
28. Park, Y.; Harris, W.S. Dose-dependent effects of n-3 polyunsaturated fatty acids on platelet activation in mildly hypertriglyceridemic subjects. *J. Med. Food* **2009**, *12*, 809–813. [CrossRef]
29. Maeda, H.; Hosokawa, M.; Sashima, T.; Murakami-Funayama, K.; Miyashita, K. Anti-obesity and anti-diabetic effects of fucoxanthin on diet-induced obesity conditions in a murine model. *Mol. Med. Rep.* **2009**, *2*, 897–902. [CrossRef]
30. Maeda, H.; Hosokawa, M.; Sashima, T.; Funayama, K.; Miyashita, K. Fucoxanthin from edible seaweed, Undaria pinnatifida, shows antiobesity effect through UCP1 expression in white adipose tissues. *Biochem. Biophys. Res. Commun.* **2005**, *332*, 392–397. [CrossRef]
31. Wu, M.T.; Chou, H.N.; Huang, C.J. Dietary fucoxanthin increases metabolic rate and upregulated mRNA expressions of the PGC-1alpha network, mitochondrial biogenesis and fusion genes in white adipose tissues of mice. *Mar. Drugs* **2014**, *12*, 964–982. [CrossRef] [PubMed]
32. Hu, J.; Wang, Z.; Tan, B.K.; Christian, M. Dietary polyphenols turn fat "brown": A narrative review of the possible mechanisms. *Trends Food Sci. Technol.* **2020**, *97*, 221–232. [CrossRef]
33. Kang, N.H.; Mukherjee, S.; Yun, J.W. Trans-Cinnamic Acid Stimulates White Fat Browning and Activates Brown Adipocytes. *Nutrients* **2019**, *11*, 577. [CrossRef]
34. Valasek, M.A.; Clarke, S.L.; Repa, J.J. Fenofibrate reduces intestinal cholesterol absorption via PPARalpha-dependent modulation of NPC1L1 expression in mouse. *J. Lipid Res.* **2007**, *48*, 2725–2735. [CrossRef] [PubMed]
35. Johnson, R.; Schwartz, S.M. Pharmacologic and Pharmacodynamic Equivalence of 2 Formulations of Orlistat. *Clin. Pharmacol. Drug Dev.* **2018**, *7*, 773–780. [CrossRef] [PubMed]
36. Yang, F.; Chen, G.; Ma, M.; Qiu, N.; Zhu, L.; Li, J. Fatty acids modulate the expression levels of key proteins for cholesterol absorption in Caco-2 monolayer. *Lipids Health Dis.* **2018**, *17*, 32. [CrossRef] [PubMed]
37. Matsumoto, M.; Hosokawa, M.; Matsukawa, N.; Hagio, M.; Shinoki, A.; Nishimukai, M.; Miyashita, K.; Yajima, T.; Hara, H. Suppressive effects of the marine carotenoids, fucoxanthin and fucoxanthinol on triglyceride absorption in lymph duct-cannulated rats. *Eur. J. Nutr.* **2010**, *49*, 243–249. [CrossRef]
38. Ha, A.W.; Kim, W.K. The effect of fucoxanthin rich power on the lipid metabolism in rats with a high fat diet. *Nutr. Res. Pract.* **2013**, *7*, 287–293. [CrossRef]
39. Wei, X.H.; Guo, X.; Pan, C.S.; Li, H.; Cui, Y.C.; Yan, L.; Fan, J.Y.; Deng, J.N.; Hu, B.H.; Chang, X.; et al. Quantitative Proteomics Reveal That Metabolic Improvement Contributes to the Cardioprotective Effect of T89 on Isoproterenol-Induced Cardiac Injury. *Front. Physiol.* **2021**, *12*, 653349. [CrossRef]
40. Suárez, J.; Rivera, P.; Arrabal, S.; Crespillo, A.; Serrano, A.; Baixeras, E.; Pavón, F.J.; Cifuentes, M.; Nogueiras, R.; Ballesteros, J.; et al. Oleoylethanolamide enhances β-adrenergic-mediated thermogenesis and white-to-brown adipocyte phenotype in epididymal white adipose tissue in rat. *Dis. Model Mech.* **2014**, *7*, 129–141. [CrossRef]
41. Dou, H.X.; Wang, T.; Su, H.X.; Gao, D.D.; Xu, Y.C.; Li, Y.X.; Wang, H.Y. Exogenous FABP4 interferes with differentiation, promotes lipolysis and inflammation in adipocytes. *Endocrine* **2020**, *67*, 587–596. [CrossRef] [PubMed]
42. Mita, T.; Furuhashi, M.; Hiramitsu, S.; Ishii, J.; Hoshina, K.; Ishimura, S.; Fuseya, T.; Watanabe, Y.; Tanaka, M.; Ohno, K.; et al. FABP4 is secreted from adipocytes by adenyl cyclase-PKA- and guanylyl cyclase-PKG-dependent lipolytic mechanisms. *Obes. Silver Spring* **2015**, *23*, 359–367. [CrossRef] [PubMed]

43. Senga, S.; Kobayashi, N.; Kawaguchi, K.; Ando, A.; Fujii, H. Fatty acid-binding protein 5 (FABP5) promotes lipolysis of lipid droplets, de novo fatty acid (FA) synthesis and activation of nuclear factor-kappa B (NF-κB) signaling in cancer cells. *Biochim. Biophys. Acta Mol. Cell Biol. Lipids.* **2018**, *1863*, 1057–1067. [CrossRef] [PubMed]
44. Jeong, Y.S.; Hong, J.H.; Cho, K.H.; Jung, H.K. Grape skin extract reduces adipogenesis- and lipogenesis-related gene expression in 3T3-L1 adipocytes through the peroxisome proliferator-activated receptor-γ signaling pathway. *Nutr. Res.* **2012**, *32*, 514–521. [CrossRef] [PubMed]
45. Chen, K.; Wang, L.; Yang, W.; Wang, C.; Hu, G.; Mo, Z. Profiling of differentially expressed genes in adipose tissues of multiple symmetric lipomatosis. *Mol. Med. Rep.* **2017**, *16*, 6570–6579. [CrossRef]
46. Ferhat, M.; Funai, K.; Boudina, S. Autophagy in Adipose Tissue Physiology and Pathophysiology. *Antioxid. Redox Signal.* **2019**, *3*, 487–501. [CrossRef]
47. Lee, Y.S.; Park, M.S.; Choung, J.S.; Kim, S.S.; Oh, H.H.; Choi, C.S.; Ha, S.Y.; Kang, Y.; Kim, Y.; Jun, H.S. Glucagon-like peptide-1 inhibits adipose tissue macrophage infiltration and inflammation in an obese mouse model of diabetes. *Diabetologia* **2012**, *55*, 2456–2468. [CrossRef]
48. Izaguirre, M.; Gómez-Ambrosi, J.; Rodríguez, A.; Ramírez, B.; Becerril, S.; Valentí, V.; Moncada, R.; Unamuno, X.; Silva, C.; de la Higuera, M.; et al. GLP-1 Limits Adipocyte Inflammation and Its Low Circulating Pre-Operative Concentrations Predict Worse Type 2 Diabetes Remission after Bariatric Surgery in Obese Patients. *J. Clin. Med.* **2019**, *8*, 479. [CrossRef]
49. Tredici, M.R.; Rodolfi, L.; Biondi, N.; Bassi, N.; Sampietro, G. Techno-economic analysis of microalgal biomass production in a 1-ha Green Wall Panel (GWP®) plant. *Algal Res.* **2016**, *19*, 253–263. [CrossRef]
50. Guillard, R.R.L.; Ryther, J.H. Studies of marine planktonic diatoms. I. Cyclotella nana Hustedt and Detonula confervacea Cleve. *Can. J. Microbiol.* **1962**, *8*, 229–239. [CrossRef]
51. Whitman, M.; Jenkins, C. Rate pressure product, age predicted maximum heart rate or heart rate reserve. Which one better predicts cardiovascular events following exercise stress echocardiography? *Am. J. Cardiovasc. Dis.* **2021**, *11*, 450–457. [PubMed]
52. Takahashi, Y.; Fukusato, T. Histopathology of nonalcoholic fatty liver disease/nonalcoholic steatohepatitis. *World J. Gastroenterol.* **2014**, *20*, 15539–15548. [CrossRef] [PubMed]
53. Shen, S.W.; Lu, Y.; Li, F.; Yang, C.J.; Feng, Y.B.; Li, H.W.; Yao, W.F.; Shen, Z.H. Atherogenic index of plasma is an effective index for estimating abdominal obesity. *Lipids Health Dis.* **2018**, *17*, 11. [CrossRef]
54. Kraus, D.; Yang, Q.; Kahn, B.B. Lipid Extraction from Mouse Feces. *Bio-Protoc.* **2015**, *5*, e1375. [CrossRef] [PubMed]
55. Diaz Marin, R.; Crespo-Garcia, S.; Wilson, A.M.; Sapieha, P. RELi protocol: Optimization for protein extraction from white, brown and beige adipose tissues. *MethodsX* **2019**, *6*, 918–928. [CrossRef] [PubMed]

Disclaimer/Publisher's Note: The statements, opinions and data contained in all publications are solely those of the individual author(s) and contributor(s) and not of MDPI and/or the editor(s). MDPI and/or the editor(s) disclaim responsibility for any injury to people or property resulting from any ideas, methods, instructions or products referred to in the content.

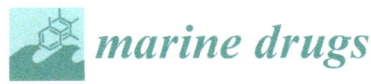 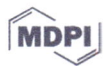

Article

Extraction and Purification of Highly Active Astaxanthin from *Corynebacterium glutamicum* Fermentation Broth

Jan Seeger, Volker F. Wendisch and Nadja A. Henke *

Genetics of Prokaryotes, CeBiTec, Bielefeld University, 33615 Bielefeld, Germany
* Correspondence: n.henke@uni-bielefeld.de

Abstract: The marine carotenoid astaxanthin is one of the strongest natural antioxidants and therefore is used in a broad range of applications such as cosmetics or nutraceuticals. To meet the growing market demand, the natural carotenoid producer *Corynebacterium glutamicum* has been engineered to produce astaxanthin by heterologous expression of genes from the marine bacterium *Fulvimarina pelagi*. To exploit this promising source of fermentative and natural astaxanthin, an efficient extraction process using ethanol was established in this study. Appropriate parameters for ethanol extraction were identified by screening ethanol concentration (62.5–97.5% v/v), temperature (30–70 °C) and biomass-to-solvent ratio (3.8–19.0 $mg_{CDW}/mL_{solvent}$). The results demonstrated that the optimal extraction conditions were: 90% ethanol, 60 °C, and a biomass-to-solvent ratio of 5.6 $mg_{CDW}/mL_{solvent}$. In total, 94% of the cellular astaxanthin was recovered and the oleoresin obtained contained 9.4 mg/g astaxanthin. With respect to other carotenoids, further purification of the oleoresin by column chromatography resulted in pure astaxanthin (100%, HPLC). In addition, a 2,2-diphenyl-1-picrylhydrazyl (DPPH) radical scavenging assay showed similar activities compared to esterified astaxanthin from microalgae and a nine-fold higher antioxidative activity than synthetic astaxanthin.

Keywords: astaxanthin; *Corynebacterium glutamicum*; extraction; antioxidant; DPPH

Citation: Seeger, J.; Wendisch, V.F.; Henke, N.A. Extraction and Purification of Highly Active Astaxanthin from *Corynebacterium glutamicum* Fermentation Broth. *Mar. Drugs* **2023**, *21*, 530. https://doi.org/10.3390/md21100530

Academic Editors: Donatella Degl'Innocenti and Marzia Vasarri

Received: 23 September 2023
Revised: 6 October 2023
Accepted: 9 October 2023
Published: 11 October 2023

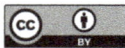

Copyright: © 2023 by the authors. Licensee MDPI, Basel, Switzerland. This article is an open access article distributed under the terms and conditions of the Creative Commons Attribution (CC BY) license (https://creativecommons.org/licenses/by/4.0/).

1. Introduction

Initially used as a feed additive for fish and crustaceans [1,2], the red-colored marine carotenoid astaxanthin has gained much attention for human consumption due to its various health-promoting effects. Based on its molecular structure, consisting of a hydrocarbon backbone with conjugated C-C double bonds (nonpolar) and terminal oxy-functionalized ionone rings (polar) at both sides [3], astaxanthin exhibits anti-inflammatory [4,5], anti-cancer [6] as well as cardioprotective activities [7,8]. As its antioxidative activity is 100 times stronger than α-tocopherol [9], astaxanthin is also used for UV protection and anti-aging applications in the cosmetics industry [10,11]. While still being dominated by astaxanthin obtained by chemical synthesis [12,13], the astaxanthin market is predicted to grow with a CAGR of 17.2%, reaching USD 6.9 billion in 2030 [14]. However, synthetic astaxanthin is not considered for human consumption [15] resulting in an increasing demand for natural astaxanthin. Common hosts for the production of natural astaxanthin are the microalgae *Haematococcus lacustris* (formerly *Haematococcus pluvialis*) (Chlorophyta), the yeast *Xanthophyllomyces dendrorhous* and the Gram-negative bacterium *Paracoccus carotinifaciens* [9,12,16]. Another source of astaxanthin that has been exploited are shells of crustaceans that occur as byproducts in food processing [17–19].

The costs of downstream processing contribute significantly to the overall production costs. Here, the capital investment and operational costs for each unit operation as well as the overall efficacy to recover the product from the cultivation broth need to be considered [20,21]. Due to its polar-nonpolar-polar structure, astaxanthin is incorporated into the cell membrane [22] or stored intracellularly within lipid droplets [23], depending on the organism. For both, microalgae and yeast, classical preprocessing methods such as (freeze-)drying [16,24,25], ball-milling [13], and high-pressure homogenization [26] have been used prior to extraction. Other processes to disrupt or permeabilize the cell envelope involved enzymatic treatment [27], pulsed electric fields [23], microwaves [28] or ultrasound [27,29]. The extraction itself can be carried out by organic solvents [13,24,25], supercritical fluids [26,30], vegetable oils [31] or eutectic solvents [32].

The natural producer of the C50 carotenoid decaprenoxanthin *C. glutamicum* [33], known for amino acid production in million-ton scale [34], has been engineered to produce astaxanthin. Therefore, the β-carotene hydroxylase (CrtZ) and β-carotene ketolase (CrtW) from *Fulvimarina pelagi*, a Mn(II) oxidizing marine bacterium [35], were introduced into the strain [36]. The production was further improved by constructing a fusion protein of CrtZ and CrtW (CrtZ~W), resulting in a promising host for large-scale astaxanthin production (see Supplementary Figure S1) [37]. Compared to algae-derived astaxanthin, which occurs mainly as mono- and diesters, bacterial astaxanthin is synthesized in an unesterified form [9,12].

As previous studies concerning astaxanthin extraction have shown, several opportunities exist how astaxanthin can be extracted, depending on the used organisms and chemicals. In this study, a fast and simple extraction process using organic solvents should be established, resulting in an astaxanthin oleoresin, which is to be treated further to obtain a purified product. For the choice of extraction solvent, solubility of the product, toxicity and ecological impact are important points to be considered [38]. The solvents, namely ethanol, acetone and ethyl acetate, were chosen from the intersecting set of preferrable solvents for green chemistry [39] and the European guidelines for solvents approved for the production of foodstuffs and food ingredients [40]. Subsequently, the solvent polarity, the extraction temperature and the biomass-to-solvent ratio were optimized, as theses parameters critically effect the extraction efficiency [41]. Finally, the antioxidant activity of the corynebacterial astaxanthin was determined.

2. Results
2.1. Optimization of Astaxanthin Extraction Parameters

In the first instance, ethanol, acetone and ethyl acetate were tested for their suitability for the extraction of astaxanthin from *C. glutamicum* cells. Extraction with ethanol yielded 1.4 ± 0.1 mg/g_{CDW} astaxanthin, which was significantly more than the 0.88 ± 0.1 mg/g_{CDW} and 1.1 ± 0.03 mg/g_{CDW} that were extracted by acetone and ethyl acetate, respectively (Figure 1A). Although ethanol seemed to be most promising, the extracted astaxanthin amount corresponded to only 64.7 ± 0.1% of the initial cellular astaxanthin content. Apart from astaxanthin, the precursor carotenoids β-carotene and lycopene were extracted to a non-proportional lesser extent, namely 32.6 ± 0.1% and 27.1 ± 0.1%, resulting in partial depletion of non-targeted carotenoids. To improve the extraction efficiency, the polarity of the solvent was changed by altering the ratio of ethanol and water within the extraction mixture. As shown in Figure 1B, the addition of water improved the extraction efficiency compared to pure ethanol. At 90% ethanol, the extraction efficiency reached its maximum with 98.9 ± 2.3% and remained stable up to 80% ethanol. A further reduction below 80% ethanol resulted in a clearly decreased extraction efficiency. To verify that the extraction temperature of 60 °C from the extraction protocol for corynebacterial carotenoids [42] still applies or could potentially be reduced, temperatures ranging from 30 to 70 °C were tested (Figure 1C). The results showed a clear optimum at 60 °C with lower extraction efficiencies below and above this value. So far, a biomass-to-solvent ration of 3.8 mg_{CDW}/$mL_{solvent}$ was used. To reduce the amount of used solvent, the biomass-to-solvent ratio was altered in a range of 3.8–19.0 mg_{CDW}/$mL_{solvent}$ (Figure 1D). The cut-off in extraction efficiency was set to 90%, which was reached at a ratio of 5.6 mg_{CDW}/$mL_{solvent}$.

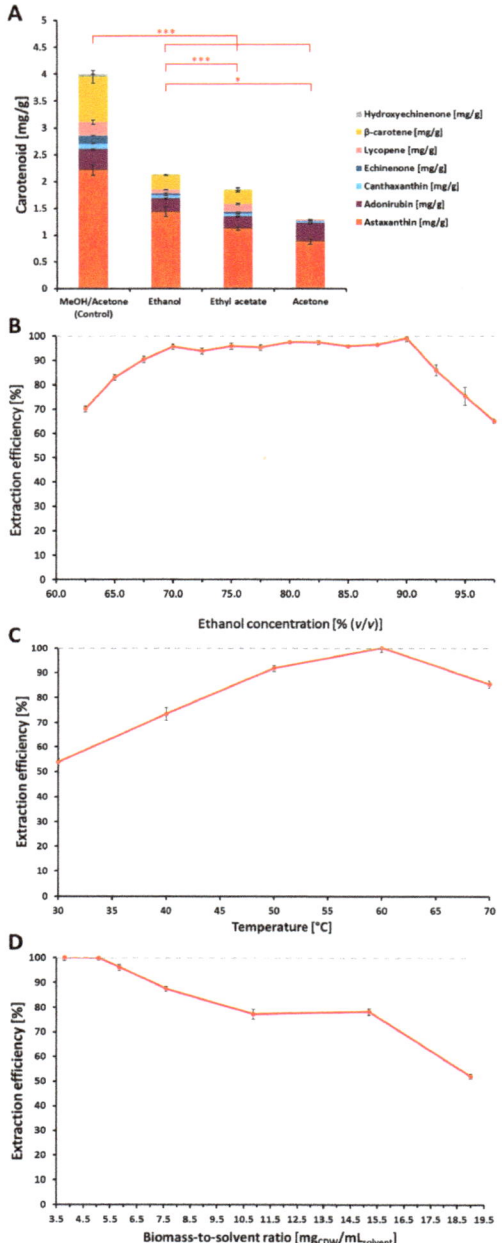

Figure 1. Optimization of astaxanthin extraction parameters. (**A**) Solvent screening. Extraction yield is given in mg/g for methanol:acetone (7:3) as control, ethanol, acetone and ethyl acetate. Statistical differences are given for astaxanthin (* for $p < 0.05$, *** for $p < 0.001$). (**B**) Ethanol concentration. Extraction efficiency [%] of astaxanthin is given in relation to methanol:acetone (7:3) as control. (**C**) Extraction temperature. Extraction efficiency [%] of astaxanthin is given in relation to the extraction at 90% ethanol at 60 °C. (**D**) Biomass-to-solvent ratio. Extraction efficiency [%] of astaxanthin is given in relation to the extraction at 90% ethanol at 60 °C and 3.8 $mg_{CDW}/mL_{solvent}$.

2.2. Preparation of Astaxanthin Oleoresin

In order to obtain quantitative amounts of astaxanthin, the optimized extraction parameters were used to scale up the extraction process from a small-scale shaking system (reaction tubes; volume = 1 mL) into a technical scale with a stirred vessel (volume = 1 L). As the agitation of the milliliter system, which was used for the optimization of extraction parameters, could not directly be transferred into the stirred system, the influence of the agitation rate was investigated by a volumetric mass transfer model. The linear correlation between the volumetric mass transfer coefficient of astaxanthin from the biomass into the solvent is shown in Figure 2, where the k_La increased from 0.39 min^{-1} at 200 rpm to 0.56 min^{-1} at 500 rpm. Subsequently, 500 rpm was chosen for further extractions.

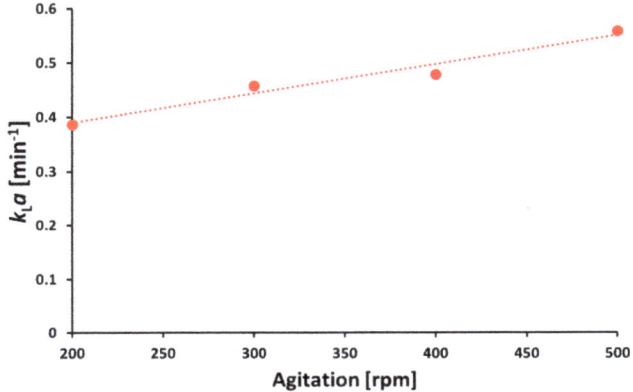

Figure 2. Volumetric mass transfer coefficient of astaxanthin. k_La values in stirred extraction vessel at 60 °C with varying agitation rates calculated using mass transfer kinetic model. R^2 = 0.96.

Applying the agitation of 500 rpm determined in the k_La experiment, 2.07 mg/g astaxanthin was extracted into the liquid phase, which can be considered as the complete cellular content (Table 1). As already observed during the solvent screening, some carotenoids, such as β-carotene, lycopene and echinenone were not completely extracted, which contributed to astaxanthin purity. During the removal of the solvent by vacuum rotary evaporation, the solvent was recovered and could potentially be used for further extractions. Overall, the resulting oleoresin contained 9.4 mg/g astaxanthin and 14.7 mg/g total carotenoids (Table 2), corresponding to a recovery of 94% of the initial cellular astaxanthin content.

Table 1. Astaxanthin extraction in stirred vessel. Extraction yield of the respective carotenoid is given in mg/g$_{CDW}$. Extraction efficiency [%] is given in relation to the initial cellular carotenoid content determined by the control extraction.

Carotenoid	Extraction Yield [mg/g$_{CDW}$]	Extraction Efficiency [%]
Astaxanthin	2.07	108
Adonirubin	0.30	101
Canthaxanthin	0.10	94
Echinenone	0.02	20
Hydroxyechinenone	0.03	106
Lycopene	0.07	11
β-carotene	0.41	67
Total carotenoids	3.00	91

Table 2. Carotenoid content in astaxanthin oleoresin. Content is given in mg/$g_{oleoresin}$. Recovery [%] is given in relation to the initial cellular carotenoid content determined by the control extraction.

Carotenoid	Oleoresin [mg/$g_{oleoresin}$]	Recovery [%]
Astaxanthin	9.41	94
Adonirubin	1.75	112
Canthaxanthin	0.48	87
Echinenone	0.11	18
Hydroxyechinenone	0.13	94
Lycopene	0.48	14
β-carotene	2.37	70
Total carotenoids	14.7	75

2.3. Astaxanthin Purification by Column Chromatography

The astaxanthin containing oleoresin, obtained by rotary vacuum evaporation, was loaded onto a C18 column for purification and the collected fractions were analyzed to identify the astaxanthin fraction. HPLC analysis showed that all precursor carotenoids that were present in the oleoresin (Figure 3A) were separated and a high purity astaxanthin fraction was obtained (Figure 3B). In total, 80% of the loaded astaxanthin was collected as pure astaxanthin. Both the astaxanthin oleoresin and the purified astaxanthin were used for subsequent testing of antioxidant activities.

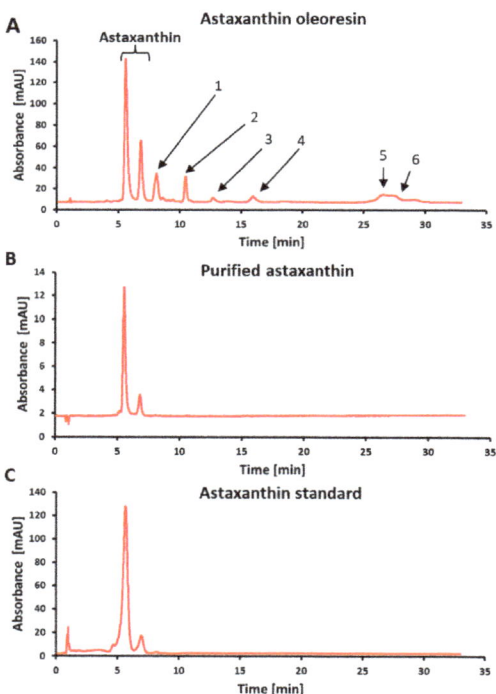

Figure 3. Purification of astaxanthin by column chromatography. (**A**) Astaxanthin oleoresin from *C. glutamicum*. 1: Adonirubin, 2: Canthaxanthin, 3: Hydroxyechinenone, 4: Echinenone, 5: Lycopene, 6: β-carotene. (**B**) Purified astaxanthin from oleoresin. (**C**) Astaxanthin standard.

2.4. Antioxidant Properties of Corynebacterial Astaxanthin

A DPPH radical scavenging assay [43] was used to assess the antioxidant properties of the corynebacterial astaxanthin both in the oleoresin and in the column-purified astaxanthin. The astaxanthin purified by column chromatography possessed an EC_{50} value of 4.5 ± 0.2 µg/mL, thus, showing about five-fold higher antioxidant activity as compared to BHT and ascorbic acid and about nine-fold higher antioxidant activity than synthetic astaxanthin (EC_{50} of 41.9 ± 0.7 µg/mL; Table 3). The EC_{50} value of the corynebacterial astaxanthin oleoresin was found to be 3.7 ± 0.6 µg/mL, while the astaxanthin esters from *H. lacustris* had a value of 3.2 ± 0.2 µg/mL.

Table 3. Antioxidant properties of corynebacterial astaxanthin. Antioxidant activities are given as EC_{50} [µg/mL] in comparison to other antioxidants.

Antioxidant	EC_{50} [µg/mL]
BHT	22.4 ± 0.5 [a]
Ascorbic acid	22.9 ± 0.1 [a]
Synthetic astaxanthin	41.9 ± 0.7
Astaxanthin esters from *H. lacustris*	3.2 ± 0.2 [b]
Astaxanthin oleoresin from *C. glutamicum*	3.7 ± 0.6 [b]
Purified astaxanthin from *C. glutamicum*	4.5 ± 0.2 [b]

[a,b] Mean values followed by the same letter are not significantly different to each other.

3. Discussion

In order to meet the growing market demand as well as consumer requirements for natural astaxanthin, the industrial workhorse *C. glutamicum* has been engineered to produce astaxanthin [36,37]. To be economically competitive, not only must the bacterial cultivation be optimized, but also the downstream process for product recovery [20,21]. The recovery of astaxanthin is particularly challenging as the molecule is incorporated within the biomass [22,23], as well as being susceptible to heat, light and oxygen [44]. Since dehydration of the biomass is costly [9], this step should be avoided. Instead, the fermentation broth was centrifuged and the cell pellet was directly used for extraction (Figure 4). Among the three organic solvents ethanol, acetone and ethyl acetate tested for the extraction of astaxanthin, ethanol showed the most promising results. Ethanol has also been used for the extraction of astaxanthin from *X. dendrorhous* [23,45], shrimp [18] and *H. lacustris* [13,25]. To improve the extraction, the polarity of the solvent was varied and showed an optimum with 98.9% extraction efficiency at a solvent-water ratio of 90%. Ahmad and colleagues also found that 90% ethanol worked best for the extraction of astaxanthin from microalgae [46]. The optimum extraction temperature was determined to be at 60 °C. The decrease in extraction efficiency at higher temperatures could be explained by the breakdown of astaxanthin as it was shown that astaxanthin already degrades at 70 °C [47]. In the next optimization step, the biomass-to-solvent ratio was almost doubled, compared to the initial ratio, reaching 5.60 $mg_{CDW}/mL_{solvent}$. However, this ratio is still low in relation to other studies, where biomass-to-solvent ratios of 16.7, 181.8, 250 $mg_{CDW}/mL_{solvent}$ were applied for *X. dendrorhous* [45], *H. lacustris* [25] and *Jaagichlorella luteoviridis* (formerly *Chlorella luteoviridis*) (Chlorophyta) [46], respectively. The optimized extraction conditions were successfully scaled up into a liter scale to obtain quantitative amounts of corynebacterial astaxanthin. After solvent removal by vacuum rotary evaporation, the astaxanthin oleoresin contained 9.4 mg/g astaxanthin, which is in the same range as oleoresins obtained by ethanol extraction from shrimp (3.4 mg/g [48], 15.6 mg/g [18]). By contrast, the extraction of *H. lacustris* with supercritical carbon dioxide ($scCO_2$) yielded oleoresins that contained 96.2 mg/g [49] and 125 mg/g [50] astaxanthin which is about one magnitude higher. A total astaxanthin recovery of 94% was achieved which is higher than the recoveries obtained by Molino et al. [13] using ethanol (67% recovery) and acetone (86% recovery) in an accelerated solvent extraction process. For the extraction using $scCO_2$, 80.6% of the cellular astaxanthin content could be recovered [50]. With respect to other carotenoids, column chromatography purification of the corynebacterial astaxanthin oleoresin yielded 100% (HPLC) pure astaxanthin. A purity of 85.1% was achieved by Hu and colleagues [48], who used a silica gel column in comparison to the C18 column used in this study.

To investigate the antioxidant properties of the corynebacterial astaxanthin, the DPPH radical scavenging assay was used. Initially introduced by Marsden Blois in 1958 [43], this assay has been applied in various studies to determine the antioxidant activities of natural compounds and extracts [51–54]. The assay is based on the neutralization of the DPPH radical by donated electrons from the antioxidants, which results in an absorption shift of DPPH [43]. EC_{50} values of the positive controls ascorbic acid (22.9 µg/mL) and BHT (22.4 µg/mL) were in line with the published data obtained by Chintong et al. [18]. The astaxanthin containing oleoresin of *C. glutamicum* showed a higher antioxidant activity (EC_{50} = 3.7 µg/mL) compared with different extracts from shrimp (17.5 µg/mL; 6.3 µg/mL) [18,55], crab (50.93 µg/mL) [19], *Chromochloris zofingiensis* (formerly *Chlorella zofingiensis*) (Chlorophyta) (1040 µg/mL) [56] and the common astaxanthin production host *X. dendrorhous* (31.79 µg/mL) [45]. We also measured the activity of esterified astaxanthin from *H. lacustris* (3.2 µg/mL), which was comparable to our corynebacterial extract. Recently, another study measured EC_{50} values ranging from 15.39 to 56.25 µg/mL for *H. lacustris* extracts [57]. The purified corynebacterial astaxanthin had an EC_{50} value of 4.5 µg/mL which is more than nine times higher than the activity of the pure synthetic astaxanthin (41.9 µg/mL). Column chromatography purified astaxanthin from *Rhodotorula toruloides* (formerly *Rhodosporidium toruloides*) (Fungi, Basidiomycota) showed an even higher activity with an EC_{50} value of 0.97 µg/mL [24]. The superior activity of the astaxanthin produced by *C. glutamicum* compared to the synthetic astaxanthin might be explained by the molecule's different stereoisomers. In bacteria and algae, the (3S,3'S) isomer is predominantly produced, while the synthetic version consists of a 1:2:1 mixture of the three isomers (3S,3'S, 3R,3'S and 3R,3'R) [47]. The strain used in this study expresses the β-carotene hydroxylase and β-carotene ketolase from the marine bacterium *Fulvimarina pelagi* [36,37], synthesizing the (3S,3'S) isomer. Using superoxide anion radical as well as hydroxyl radical assays, it was shown that the antioxidant activity of synthetic astaxanthin was inferior compared to natural astaxanthin comprised of the (3S,3'S) isomer [58]. This is in line with the results from Liu and colleagues, who also found that the (3S,3'S) isomer had a higher antioxidant activity in the ABTS radical scavenging assay and a superior oxygen radical absorbance capacity (ORAC) than the other isomers [59]. Interestingly, the latter study found no differences among the three isomers using the DPPH radical scavenging assay. Discrepancies in the DPPH assay parameters influence the experimental outcome [60] and therefore, a direct comparison of the antioxidant activities to our results is difficult. In general, the reason for the higher antioxidant activity of the (3S,3'S) isomer remains to be solved. Compared to the oleoresin, the activity of the purified astaxanthin was slightly lower. This might be due to the additional presence of other carotenoids such as β-carotene and canthaxanthin in the oleoresin, contributing to the antioxidant activity [61,62]. Similar synergistic effects were also observed by Sindhu and Sherief who referred the high antioxidant activity of their shrimp extract to the combination of astaxanthin and poly unsaturated fatty acids measured by different in vitro antioxidant activity assays [63].

Compared to other astaxanthin downstream processes from algae or yeast [64], this study provides a fast and simple workflow, without the need for extensive equipment or expensive chemicals (Figure 4). In the end, 94% product recovery within the astaxanthin oleoresin was achieved. Both the oleoresin and the purified astaxanthin showed high antioxidative activity in an in vitro DPPH assay. However, further studies are necessary to test the suitability of this corynebacterial astaxanthin for application as a cosmetic ingredient. Therefore, the antioxidant activity could be investigated by cell-based in vitro assays, e.g., with keratinocytes [65] or with stem-cell-based complex skin models [66,67]. Another aspect to be considered is, that astaxanthin, as all carotenoids, is poorly soluble in water and possesses a low bioavailability [11]. Furthermore, free astaxanthin shows a reduced stability compared to the esterified version [68]. These limitations could be overcome by different delivery systems, e.g., liposomes, emulsions and nanoparticles [11,44].

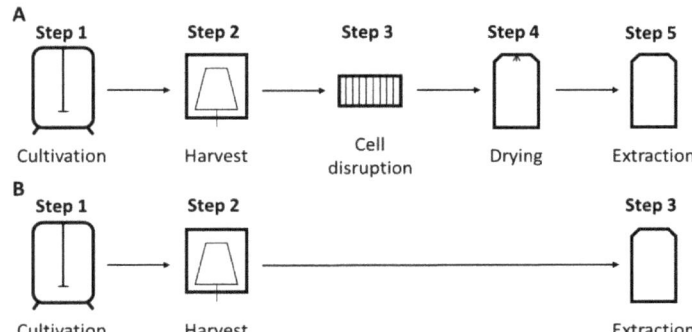

Figure 4. Comparison of astaxanthin downstream processes. Unit operations of each process are shown schematically. Options for further purification or treatment of the extract, e.g., column chromatography, are not shown. (**A**) Common downstream process for algae and yeast derived astaxanthin [64,65]. (**B**) Downstream process of astaxanthin derived from *C. glutamicum* established in this study.

4. Materials and Methods

4.1. Chemicals and Biomass

If not stated differently, chemicals were purchased by Carl Roth (Karlsruhe, Germany) or Sigma-Aldrich (St. Louis, MA, USA). Solvents for extraction and analysis were HPLC grade. The astaxanthin producing *C. glutamicum* strain (Pathway: Supplementary Figure S1) was cultivated in CGXII minimal medium, supplemented with 4% (w/v) glucose in baffled shake flasks on a rotary shaker (120 rpm) at 30 °C [37]. For the optimization of the extraction parameters, 0.5 mL culture was harvested after 48 h of cultivation at 20,000× g for 10 min. For the extraction in the stirred bottle reactor, culture was harvested accordingly after 48 h of cultivation at 10,000× g for 20 min. Water content of the cell pellet was determined by drying it completely.

4.2. Optimization of Extraction Parameters

4.2.1. Solvent Screening

In order to find an appropriate solvent for the extraction of astaxanthin, ethanol, acetone and ethyl acetate were tested. The cell pellet was extracted with 1 mL solvent at 1000 rpm for 30 min (Thermomixer comfort, Eppendorf, Hamburg, Germany). The biomass-to-solvent ratio and temperature were kept constant at 3.8 mg$_{CDW}$/mL$_{solvent}$ and at 60 °C, respectively. After centrifugation at 20,000× g for 10 min, the supernatant was analyzed via HPLC. The extraction efficiency was determined by comparison with the extraction protocol for corynebacterial carotenoids used for analytical purposes (7:3 mixture of methanol:acetone), which assumes that all carotenoids are extracted from the cell [42]. The extraction was performed in triplicates.

4.2.2. Ethanol Concentration

To determine the optimal ethanol concentration, the water content and the dry mass of harvested cultures were determined. Based on the water content of the biomass, absolute ethanol and ddH$_2$O were added accordingly, to reach the desired ethanol concentration (v/v). As the cell pellet already contained a certain amount of water, ethanol concentrations ranging from 62.5 to 97.5% (v/v) were tested. The cell pellet was extracted with 1 mL total solvent at 1000 rpm for 30 min (Thermomixer comfort, Eppendorf, Hamburg, Germany). The biomass-to-solvent ratio and temperature were kept constant at 3.8 mg$_{CDW}$/mL$_{solvent}$ and at 60 °C, respectively. The extraction efficiency was determined by comparison with the extraction protocol for corynebacterial carotenoids (7:3 mixture of methanol:acetone) [42]. The extraction was performed at least in duplicates.

4.2.3. Temperature

To determine the optimal extraction temperature, samples were extracted with 1 mL 90% (v/v) ethanol at temperatures ranging from 30 to 70 °C, following the same procedure as in Section 4.2.1. The extraction efficiency was determined by comparison with the extraction using 90% (v/v) ethanol at 60 °C (optimum from Section 4.2.2). The extraction was performed in triplicates.

4.2.4. Biomass-to-Solvent Ratio

Under previous conditions, 3.8 mg$_{CDW}$/mL$_{solvent}$ was used for extraction. To determine the optimal biomass-to-solvent ratio, the already optimized parameters were used and biomass-to-solvent ratios ranging from 3.8 to 19.0 mg$_{CDW}$/mL$_{solvent}$ were tested. The extraction efficiency was determined by comparison with the biomass-to-solvent ratio of 3.8 mg$_{CDW}$/mL$_{solvent}$ (optimum from Section 4.2.3). The extraction was performed in triplicates.

4.3. Astaxanthin Extraction

Astaxanthin extraction was performed in a 1 L stirred bottle reactor equipped with an anchor stirrer (DWK Life Sciences, Mainz, Germany). Temperature and agitation were controlled by a magnetic stirrer with heating plate and temperature probe (IDL GmbH, Nidderau, Germany). Centrifuged biomass from cultivation with a water content of 80–85% (w/w) was used. Based on the amount of dry substance, respective amounts of absolute ethanol and ddH$_2$O were added to reach 5.6 mg$_{CDW}$/mL$_{solvent}$ with an ethanol concentration of 90% (v/v). Extraction was performed at 60 °C and 500 rpm for 20 min. Liquid crude extract was analyzed by HPLC and was used for preparation of the astaxanthin oleoresin. The extraction efficiency was determined by comparison with the extraction protocol for corynebacterial carotenoids (7:3 mixture of methanol:acetone) [42].

Kinetic Model

To describe the extraction kinetic and to evaluate the influence of different agitation rates on the extraction, the mass transfer kinetic model proposed by Handayani et al. [69] was applied. This model assumes that the limiting step of the extraction is the mass transfer of astaxanthin from the biomass into the solvent. The rate of mass transfer can be written as:

$$dN_A/dt = k_L * A * [C_{Ae} - C_A] \tag{1}$$

with dN_A/dt as the rate of astaxanthin mass transfer [mg/min], C_A and C_{AE} are the concentrations of astaxanthin in liquid and at equilibrium [mg/L], respectively. k_L is the mass transfer coefficient and A the surface area. As the process was carried out in batch mode, the volume (V) was kept constant.

$$dN_A = V dC_A \tag{2}$$

Substitution of (2) into (1) results in

$$V dC_A/dt = k_L * A * [C_{Ae} - C_A] \tag{3}$$

$$dC_A/dt = k_L * A/V * [C_{Ae} - C_A] \tag{4}$$

$$dC_A/dt = k_L * a * [C_{Ae} - C_A] \tag{5}$$

With $k_L * a$ being the volumetric mass transfer coefficient. Considering that at the beginning of the process ($t = 0$), the astaxanthin concentration in the liquid is zero ($C_A = 0$) and the concentration of astaxanthin at any time is $C_A = C_A$, integration of (3) yields

$$C_A = C_{AE} * [1 - \exp(-k_L * a * t)] \tag{6}$$

For this model, the parameters C_A, k_L and a were estimated by nonlinear least squares fit of the experimental data. The agitation rate was varied as indicated and samples were drawn at 2, 5, 10, 15, 20, 25, 30, 35, 40 min.

4.4. Preparation of Astaxanthin Oleoresin

Liquid crude extract (Section 4.3) was concentrated to one-twentieth of the initial volume by vacuum rotary evaporation (VV2000, Heidolph Instruments, Schwabach, Germany). Absolute ethanol was added in a relation of 7:1 to the concentrated crude extract and the mixture was vigorously shaken for 3 min. Supernatant was separated from solid precipitate and the liquid phase was removed by vacuum rotary evaporation. The oleoresin obtained was stored at −20 °C until further usage. The carotenoid recovery was calculated by comparison with the cellular carotenoid content determined with the extraction protocol for corynebacterial carotenoids (7:3 mixture of methanol:acetone) [42].

4.5. Purification by Column Chromatography

For further purification, astaxanthin oleoresin was resolubilized in methanol and injected into a flash chromatography system (Reveleris X2, Büchi Labortechnik, Flawil, Switzerland) equipped with a 12 g FlashPure EcoFlex C18 column (Büchi Labortechnik, Flawil, Switzerland). Methanol:water (9:1) (A) and methanol (B) were used as mobile phases. The injection volume was 1 mL and a gradient flow at a rate of 30 mL min^{-1} was used as per the following: 0 min B: 0%, 8 min B: 100%, 25.7 min B: 100%. Collected fractions were analyzed by HPLC.

4.6. Quantification of Carotenoids

The quantification of carotenoids (Structure: Supplementary Figure S2) was performed as previously described [42]. Standards were used for standard calibration curves using lycopene (ExtraSynthese, Genay, France), β-carotene (Sigma-Aldrich, St. Louis, MA, USA), canthaxanthin (VWR, Darmstadt, Germany), echinenone (Sigma-Aldrich, St. Louis, MA, USA), adonirubin (CaroteNature, Münsingen, Switzerland), 3-hydroxyechinenone (CaroteNature, Münsingen, Switzerland) and astaxanthin (Sigma-Aldrich, St. Louis, MA, USA).

4.7. DPPH Assay

The radical scavenging activity test was carried out as described [18] with slight modifications. Serial dilutions of the respective antioxidant (3.125–100 µg/mL; for column chromatography purified astaxanthin: 0.64–20.5 µg/mL) were prepared in methanol. In case of the oleoresin from *C. glutamicum* and the esterified astaxanthin from *H. lacustris*, the antioxidant concentration refers to the amount of free astaxanthin. In total, 0.4 mL of each dilution was mixed with 0.4 mL of the DPPH solution (0.18 mM in methanol) and incubated at room temperature for 30 min in the dark. The absorbance at 517 nm was determined photometrically (UV-VIS Spectrophotometer UV-1650PC, Shimadzu, Kyoto, Japan). The radical scavenging activity was calculated as follows:

$$\text{DPPH scavenging activity (\%)} = (A_{control} - (A_{sample} - A_{sample\ blank}))/A_{control} \tag{7}$$

with $A_{control}$, A_{sample} and $A_{sample\ blank}$ being the absorbances of the DPPH solution without antioxidant, antioxidant solution with DPPH and the antioxidant solution without DPPH, respectively. EC$_{50}$ value (efficient concentration when 50% of the radial is reduced) was expressed in µg/mL (related to the respective antioxidant) and was calculated by plotting the antioxidant concentration against the scavenging activity. The measurements were performed in triplicates. Butylated hydroxytoluene (Merck KGaA, Darmstadt, Germany), ascorbic acid (Karlsruhe, Germany), astaxanthin esters from *Haematococcus pluvialis* (Sigma-Aldrich, St. Louis, MA, USA) and synthetic astaxanthin (Sigma-Aldrich, St. Louis, MA, USA) were used for comparison.

Supplementary Materials: The following supporting information can be downloaded at: https://www.mdpi.com/article/10.3390/md21100530/s1, Figure S1: Astaxanthin biosynthesis pathway in *C. glutamicum*. Scheme of the astaxanthin biosynthesis pathway based on the central carbon metabolism, including respective precursor carotenoids. Heterologous expression of CrtY, CrtW, CrtZ. Enzymes are given in abbreviated form next to the reaction. GAP: Glyceraldehyde 3-phosphate; DXS: 1-deoxy-D-xylulose-5-phosphate synthase; MEP: 2-C-methyl-D-erythritol 4-phosphate pathway; IPP: Isopentenyl diphosphate; DMAPP: Dimethylallyl pyrophosphate; Idi: Isopentenyl pyrophosphate isomerase; GGPPS: Geranylgeranyl pyrophosphate synthase; GGPP: Geranylgeranyl pyrophosphate; CrtB: Phytoene synthase; CrtI: Phytoene desaturase; CrtY: Lycopene cyclase; CrtW: β-carotene ketolase; CrtZ: β-carotene hydroxylase. Figure S2: Structure of carotenoids detected by HPLC in this study. Oxy-functionalization is highlighted in red.

Author Contributions: Conceptualization, N.A.H. and V.F.W.; methodology, J.S. and N.A.H.; experimental performance J.S.; writing—original draft preparation, J.S.; writing—review and editing, V.F.W. and N.A.H.; visualization, J.S.; funding acquisition, V.F.W. and N.A.H. All authors have read and agreed to the published version of the manuscript.

Funding: This research was funded by BMBF project KaroTec, grant number 03VP09460, and support for the Open Access Publication Fund of Bielefeld University.

Data Availability Statement: Not applicable.

Acknowledgments: The authors thank Kai Schülke from Organic Chemistry and Biocatalysis at Bielefeld University and Fabian Schmitfranz from Genetics of Prokaryotes at Bielefeld University for supporting the laboratory work.

Conflicts of Interest: The authors declare no conflict of interest. The funders had no role in the design of the study; in the collection, analyses, or interpretation of data; in the writing of the manuscript; or in the decision to publish the results.

References

1. Lim, K.C.; Yusoff, F.M.; Shariff, M.; Kamarudin, M.S. Astaxanthin as feed supplement in aquatic animals. *Rev. Aquac.* **2018**, *10*, 738–773. [CrossRef]
2. Pereira da Costa, D.; Campos Miranda-Filho, K. The use of carotenoid pigments as food additives for aquatic organisms and their functional roles. *Rev. Aquac.* **2020**, *12*, 1567–1578. [CrossRef]
3. Higuera-Ciapara, I.; Félix-Valenzuela, L.; Goycoolea, F.M. Astaxanthin: A Review of its Chemistry and Applications. *Crit. Rev. Food Sci. Nutr.* **2007**, *46*, 185–196. [CrossRef]
4. Chang, M.X.; Xiong, F. Astaxanthin and its Effects in Inflammatory Responses and Inflammation-Associated Diseases: Recent Advances and Future Directions. *Molecules* **2020**, *25*, 5342. [CrossRef] [PubMed]
5. Kohandel, Z.; Farkhondeh, T.; Aschner, M.; Pourbagher-Shahri, A.M.; Samarghandian, S. Anti-inflammatory action of astaxanthin and its use in the treatment of various diseases. *Biomed. Pharmacother.* **2022**, *145*, 112179. [CrossRef] [PubMed]
6. Faraone, I.; Sinisgalli, C.; Ostuni, A.; Armentano, M.F.; Carmosino, M.; Milella, L.; Russo, D.; Labanca, F.; Khan, H. Astaxanthin anticancer effects are mediated through multiple molecular mechanisms: A systematic review. *Pharmacol. Res.* **2020**, *155*, 104689. [CrossRef] [PubMed]
7. Kishimoto, Y.; Yoshida, H.; Kondo, K. Potential Anti-Atherosclerotic Properties of Astaxanthin. *Mar. Drugs* **2016**, *14*, 35. [CrossRef] [PubMed]
8. Pashkow, F.J.; Watumull, D.G.; Campbell, C.L. Astaxanthin: A Novel Potential Treatment for Oxidative Stress and Inflammation in Cardiovascular Disease. *Am. J. Cardiol.* **2008**, *101*, S58–S68. [CrossRef] [PubMed]
9. Shah, M.M.R.; Liang, Y.; Cheng, J.J.; Daroch, M. Astaxanthin-producing green microalga *Haematococcus pluvialis*: From single cell to high value commercial products. *Front. Plant Sci.* **2016**, *7*, 172296. [CrossRef]
10. Saraiva, S.M.; Miguel, S.P.; Araujo, A.R.T.S.; Rodrigues, M.; Ribeiro, M.P.; Coutinho, P. Cosmetic industry: Natural secondary metabolites for beauty and aging. In *Natural Secondary Metabolites*; Springer: Cham, Switzerland, 2023; pp. 853–891.
11. Lima, S.G.M.; Freire, M.C.L.C.; Oliveira, V.S.; Solisio, C.; Converti, A.; Lima, A.A.N. Astaxanthin Delivery Systems for Skin Application: A Review. *Mar. Drugs* **2021**, *19*, 511. [CrossRef]

12. Kumar, S.; Kumar, R.; Kumari, A.; Panwar, A. Astaxanthin: A super antioxidant from microalgae and its therapeutic potential. *J. Basic Microbiol.* **2022**, *62*, 1064–1082. [CrossRef]
13. Molino, A.; Rimauro, J.; Casella, P.; Cerbone, A.; Larocca, V.; Chianese, S.; Karatza, D.; Mehariya, S.; Ferraro, A.; Hristoforou, E.; et al. Extraction of astaxanthin from microalga *Haematococcus pluvialis* in red phase by using generally recognized as safe solvents and accelerated extraction. *J. Biotechnol.* **2018**, *283*, 51–61. [CrossRef] [PubMed]
14. Astaxanthin Market Size, Share, Growth & Trends Report 2030. Market Analysis Report, Grand View Research, San Francisco, CA. Available online: https://www.grandviewresearch.com/industry-analysis/global-astaxanthin-market (accessed on 24 August 2023).
15. Li, J.; Zhu, D.; Niu, J.; Shen, S.; Wang, G. An economic assessment of astaxanthin production by large scale cultivation of *Haematococcus pluvialis*. *Biotechnol. Adv.* **2011**, *29*, 568–574. [CrossRef] [PubMed]
16. Hayashi, M.; Ishibashi, T.; Kuwahara, D.; Hirasawa, K. Commercial Production of Astaxanthin with *Paracoccus carotinifaciens*. *Adv. Exp. Med. Biol.* **2021**, *1261*, 11–20.
17. Sharayei, P.; Azarpazhooh, E.; Zomorodi, S.; Einafshar, S.; Ramaswamy, H.S. Optimization of ultrasonic-assisted extraction of astaxanthin from green tiger (*Penaeus semisulcatus*) shrimp shell. *Ultrason. Sonochem.* **2021**, *76*, 105666. [CrossRef]
18. Chintong, S.; Phatvej, W.; Rerk-Am, U.; Waiprib, Y.; Klaypradit, W. In Vitro Antioxidant, Antityrosinase, and Cytotoxic Activities of Astaxanthin from Shrimp Waste. *Antioxidants* **2019**, *8*, 128. [CrossRef]
19. Abd El-Ghany, M.N.; Hamdi, S.A.; Elbaz, R.M.; Aloufi, A.S.; Sayed, R.R.E.; Ghonaim, G.M.; Farahat, M.G. Development of a Microbial-Assisted Process for Enhanced Astaxanthin Recovery from Crab Exoskeleton Waste. *Fermentation* **2023**, *9*, 505. [CrossRef]
20. Kumar, R.; Ghosh, A.K.; Dhurandhar, R.; Chakrabortty, S. Downstream process: Toward cost/energy effectiveness. In *Handbook of Biofuels*; Elsevier: Amsterdam, The Netherlands, 2022; pp. 249–260.
21. Straathof, A.J.J. The Proportion of Downstream Costs in Fermentative Production Processes. In *Comprehensive Biotechnology*, 2nd ed.; Elsevier: Amsterdam, The Netherlands, 2011; pp. 811–814.
22. McNulty, H.P.; Byun, J.; Lockwood, S.F.; Jacob, R.F.; Mason, R.P. Differential effects of carotenoids on lipid peroxidation due to membrane interactions: X-ray diffraction analysis. *Biochim. Biophys. Acta—Biomembr.* **2007**, *1768*, 167–174. [CrossRef]
23. Aguilar-Machado, D.; Delso, C.; Martinez, J.M.; Morales-Oyervides, L.; Montanez, M.; Raso, J. Enzymatic Processes Triggered by PEF for Astaxanthin Extraction from *Xanthophyllomyces dendrorhous*. *Front. Bioeng. Biotechnol.* **2020**, *8*, 552006. [CrossRef] [PubMed]
24. Tran, T.N.; Tran, N.-T.; Tran, T.-A.; Pham, D.-C.; Su, C.-H.; Nguyen, H.C.; Barrow, C.J.; Ngo, D.-N. Highly Active Astaxanthin Production from Waste Molasses by Mutated *Rhodosporidium toruloides* G17. *Fermentation* **2023**, *9*, 148. [CrossRef]
25. Jaime, L.; Rodriguez-Meizoso, I.; Cifuentes, A.; Santoyo, S.; Suarez, S.; Ibanez, E.; Senorans, F.J. Pressurized liquids as an alternative process to antioxidant carotenoids' extraction from *Haematococcus pluvialis* microalgae. *LWT Food Sci. Technol.* **2010**, *43*, 105–112. [CrossRef]
26. Hasan, M.; Azhar, M.; Nangia, H.; Bhatt, P.C.; Panda, B.P. Influence of high-pressure homogenization, ultrasonication, and supercritical fluid on free astaxanthin extraction from β-glucanase-treated *Phaffia rhodozyma* cells. *Prep. Biochem. Biotechnol.* **2016**, *46*, 116–122. [CrossRef] [PubMed]
27. Michelon, M.; de Matos de Borba, T.; da Silva Rafael, R.; Burkert, C.A.V.; de Medeiros Burkert, J.F. Extraction of carotenoids from *Phaffia rhodozyma*: A comparison between different techniques of cell disruption. *Food Sci. Biotechnol.* **2012**, *21*, 1–8. [CrossRef]
28. Choi, S.K.; Kim, J.H.; Park, Y.S.; Kim, Y.J.; Chang, H.I. An efficient method for the extraction of astaxanthin from the red yeast *Xanthophyllomyces dendrorhous*. *J. Microbiol. Biotechnol.* **2007**, *17*, 847–852. [PubMed]
29. Zou, T.-B.; Jia, Q.; Li, H.W.; Wang, C.X.; Wu, H.F. Response Surface Methodology for Ultrasound-Assisted Extraction of Astaxanthin from *Haematococcus pluvialis*. *Mar. Drugs* **2013**, *11*, 1644–1655. [CrossRef]
30. Molino, A.; Mehariya, S.; Iovine, A.; Larocca, V.; Di Sanzo, G.; Martino, M.; Casella, P.; Chianese, S.; Musmarra, D. Extraction of Astaxanthin and Lutein from Microalga *Haematococcus pluvialis* in the Red Phase Using CO_2 Supercritical Fluid Extraction Technology with Ethanol as Co-Solvent. *Mar. Drugs* **2018**, *16*, 432. [CrossRef]
31. Kang, C.D.; Sim, S.J. Direct extraction of astaxanthin from *Haematococcus* culture using vegetable oils. *Biotechnol. Lett.* **2008**, *30*, 441–444. [CrossRef] [PubMed]
32. Pitacco, W.; Samori, C.; Pezzolesi, L.; Gori, V.; Grillo, A.; Tiecco, M.; Vagnoni, M.; Galletti, P. Extraction of astaxanthin from *Haematococcus pluvialis* with hydrophobic deep eutectic solvents based on oleic acid. *Food Chem.* **2022**, *379*, 132156. [CrossRef]
33. Heider, S.A.E.; Peters-Wendisch, P.; Wendisch, V.F. Carotenoid biosynthesis and overproduction in *Corynebacterium glutamicum*. *BMC Microbiol.* **2012**, *12*, 198. [CrossRef] [PubMed]
34. Wendisch, V.F. Metabolic engineering advances and prospects for amino acid production. *Metab. Eng.* **2020**, *58*, 17–34. [CrossRef]
35. Kang, I.; Oh, H.-M.; Lim, S.-I.; Ferriera, S.; Giovannonni, S.J.; Cho, J.-C. Genome sequence of *Fulvimarina pelagi* HTCC2506T, a Mn(II)-oxidizing alphaproteobacterium possessing an aerobic anoxygenic photosynthetic gene cluster and Xanthorhodopsin. *J. Bacteriol.* **2010**, *192*, 4798–4799. [CrossRef] [PubMed]
36. Henke, N.A.; Heider, S.A.E.; Peters-Wendisch, P.; Wendisch, V.F. Production of the marine carotenoid astaxanthin by metabolically engineered *Corynebacterium glutamicum*. *Mar. Drugs* **2016**, *14*, 124. [CrossRef]
37. Henke, N.A.; Wendisch, V.F. Improved astaxanthin production with *Corynebacterium glutamicum* by application of a membrane fusion protein. *Mar. Drugs* **2019**, *17*, 621. [CrossRef] [PubMed]

38. Pagels, F.; Pereira, R.N.; Vicente, A.A.; Guedes, A.C. Extraction of Pigments from Microalgae and Cyanobacteria—A Review on Current Methodologies. *Appl. Sci.* **2021**, *11*, 5187. [CrossRef]
39. Alfonsi, K.; Colberg, J.; Dunn, P.J.; Fevig, T.; Jennings, S.; Johnson, T.A.; Kleine, H.P.; Knight, C.; Nagy, M.A.; Perry, D.A.; et al. Green chemistry tools to influence a medicinal chemistry and research chemistry based organisation. *Green Chem.* **2008**, *10*, 31–36. [CrossRef]
40. Directive 2009/32/EC of the European Parliament and of the Council on the Approximation of the Laws of the Member States on Extraction Solvents Used in the Production of Foodstuffs and Food Ingredients. 2009. Available online: https://eur-lex.europa.eu/legal-content/EN/TXT/?uri=CELEX:02009L0032-20100916#E0008 (accessed on 23 August 2023).
41. Zhang, Q.W.; Lin, L.G.; Ye, W.C. Techniques for extraction and isolation of natural products: A comprehensive review. *Chin. Med.* **2018**, *13*, 20. [CrossRef]
42. Göttl, V.L.; Pucker, B.; Wendisch, V.F.; Henke, N.A. Screening of Structurally Distinct Lycopene β-Cyclases for Production of the Cyclic C40 Carotenoids β-Carotene and Astaxanthin by *Corynebacterium glutamicum*. *J. Agric. Food Chem.* **2023**, *71*, 7765–7776. [CrossRef] [PubMed]
43. Blois, M.S. Antioxidant Determinations by the Use of a Stable Free Radical. *Nature* **1958**, *181*, 1199–1200. [CrossRef]
44. Chen, S.; Wang, J.; Feng, J.; Xuan, R. Research progress of Astaxanthin nano-based drug delivery system: Applications, prospects and challenges? *Front. Pharmacol.* **2023**, *14*, 1102888. [CrossRef] [PubMed]
45. Cheng, X.Y.; Xiong, Y.J.; Yang, M.M.; Zhu, M.J. Preparation of astaxanthin mask from *Phaffia rhodozyma* and its evaluation. *Process Biochem.* **2019**, *79*, 195–202. [CrossRef]
46. Ahmad, N.; Mounsef, J.R.; Lteif, R. A simple and fast experimental protocol for the extraction of xanthophylls from microalga *Chlorella luteoviridis*. *Prep. Biochem. Biotechnol.* **2021**, *51*, 1071–1075. [CrossRef] [PubMed]
47. Li, Y.; Fengping, M.; Yahong, G.; Dayan, L.; Chengwu, Z.; Mingtao, Z. Accurate quantification of astaxanthin from *Haematococcus* crude extract spectrophotometrically. *Chin. J. Oceanol. Limnol.* **2012**, *30*, 627–637. [CrossRef]
48. Hu, J.; Lu, W.; Lv, M.; Wang, Y.; Ding, R.; Wang, L. Extraction and purification of astaxanthin from shrimp shells and the effects of different treatments on its content. *Rev. Bras. Farmacogn.* **2019**, *29*, 24–29. [CrossRef]
49. Ruiz-Domínguez, M.C.; Espinosa, C.; Paredes, A.; Palma, J.; Jaime, C.; Vilchez, C.; Cerezal, P. Determining the Potential of *Haematococcus pluvialis* Oleoresin as a Rich Source of Antioxidants. *Molecules* **2019**, *24*, 4073. [CrossRef] [PubMed]
50. Machmudah, S.; Shotipruk, A.; Goto, M.; Sasaki, M.; Hirose, T. Extraction of astaxanthin from *Haematococcus pluvialis* using supercritical CO_2 and ethanol as entrainer. *Ind. Eng. Chem. Res.* **2006**, *45*, 3652–3657. [CrossRef]
51. Parry, J.; Su, L.; Luther, M.; Zhou, K.; Yurawecz, M.P.; Whittaker, P.; Yu, L. Fatty acid composition and antioxidant properties of cold-pressed marionberry, boysenberry, red raspberry, and blueberry seed oils. *J. Agric. Food Chem.* **2005**, *53*, 566–573. [CrossRef] [PubMed]
52. Sendra, J.M.; Sentandreu, E.; Navarro, J.L. Reduction kinetics of the free stable radical 2,2-diphenyl-1-picrylhydrazyl (DPPH•) for determination of the antiradical activity of citrus juices. *Eur. Food Res. Technol.* **2006**, *223*, 615–624. [CrossRef]
53. Ramadan, M.F.; Kroh, L.W.; Mörsel, J.T. Radical Scavenging Activity of Black Cumin (*Nigella sativa* L.), Coriander (*Coriandrum sativum* L.), and Niger (*Guizotia abyssinica* Cass.) Crude Seed Oils and Oil Fractions. *J. Agric. Food Chem.* **2003**, *51*, 6961–6969. [CrossRef]
54. Liu, Z.; Li, H.; Qi, Y.; Zhu, Z.; Huang, D.; Zhang, K.; Pan, J.; Wen, L.; Zou, Z. *Cinnamomum camphora* leaves as a source of proanthocyanidins separated using microwave-assisted extraction method and evaluation of their antioxidant activity in vitro. *Arab. J. Chem.* **2021**, *14*, 103328. [CrossRef]
55. Abdelmalek, B.E.; Sila, A.; Ghlissi, Z.; Taktak, M.A.; Ayadi, M.A.; Bougatef, A. The Influence of Natural Astaxanthin on the Formulation and Storage of Marinated Chicken Steaks. *J. Food Biochem.* **2016**, *40*, 393–403. [CrossRef]
56. Sun, Z.; Liu, J.; Zeng, X.; Huangfu, J.; Jiang, Y.; Wang, M.; Chen, F. Astaxanthin is responsible for antiglycoxidative properties of microalga *Chlorella zofingiensis*. *Food Chem.* **2011**, *126*, 1629–1635. [CrossRef]
57. Tan, Y.; Ye, Z.; Wang, M.; Manzoor, M.F.; Aadil, R.M.; Tan, X.; Liu, Z. Comparison of Different Methods for Extracting the Astaxanthin from *Haematococcus pluvialis*: Chemical Composition and Biological Activity. *Molecules* **2021**, *26*, 3569. [CrossRef] [PubMed]
58. Capelli, B.; Bagchi, D.; Cysewski, G.R. Synthetic astaxanthin is significantly inferior to algal-based astaxanthin as an antioxidant and may not be suitable as a human nutraceutical supplement. *Nutrafoods* **2013**, *12*, 145–152. [CrossRef]
59. Liu, X.; Luo, Q.; Rakariyatham, K.; Cao, Y.; Goulette, T.; Liu, X.; Xiao, H. Antioxidation and anti-ageing activities of different stereoisomeric astaxanthin in vitro and in vivo. *J. Funct. Foods* **2016**, *25*, 50–61. [CrossRef]
60. Kedare, S.B.; Singh, R.P. Genesis and development of DPPH method of antioxidant assay. *J. Food Sci. Technol.* **2011**, *48*, 412. [CrossRef] [PubMed]
61. Rohmah, M.; Rahmadi, A.; Raharjo, S. Bioaccessibility and antioxidant activity of β-carotene loaded nanostructured lipid carrier (NLC) from binary mixtures of palm stearin and palm olein. *Heliyon* **2022**, *8*, e08913. [CrossRef]
62. Castangia, I.; Manca, M.L.; Razavi, S.H.; Nacher, A.; Diez-Sales, O.; Peris, J.E.; Allaw, A.; Terencio, M.C.; Usach, I.; Manconi, M. Canthaxanthin Biofabrication, Loading in Green Phospholipid Vesicles and Evaluation of In Vitro Protection of Cells and Promotion of Their Monolayer Regeneration. *Biomedicines* **2022**, *10*, 157. [CrossRef]
63. Sindhu, S.; Sherief, P.M. Extraction, Characterization, Antioxidant and Anti-Inflammatory Properties of Carotenoids from the Shell Waste of Arabian Red Shrimp *Aristeus alcocki*, Ramadan 1938. *Open Conf. Proc. J.* **2011**, *2*, 95–103.

64. Rodríguez-Sifuentes, L.; Marszalek, J.E.; Hernández-Carbajal, G.; Chuck-Hernández, C. Importance of Downstream Processing of Natural Astaxanthin for Pharmaceutical Application. *Front. Chem. Eng.* **2021**, *2*, 601483. [CrossRef]
65. Gironde, C.; Rigal, M.; Dufour, C.; Furger, C. AOP1, a New Live Cell Assay for the Direct and Quantitative Measure of Intracellular Antioxidant Effects. *Antioxidants* **2020**, *9*, 471. [CrossRef]
66. Kim, B.S.; Kwon, Y.W.; Kong, J.-S.; Park, G.T.; Gao, G.; Han, W.; Kim, M.-B.; Lee, H.; Kim, J.H.; Cho, D.-W. 3D cell printing of in vitro stabilized skin model and in vivo pre-vascularized skin patch using tissue-specific extracellular matrix bioink: A step towards advanced skin tissue engineering. *Biomaterials* **2018**, *168*, 38–53. [CrossRef]
67. Lee, J.; Böschke, R.; Tang, P.-C.; Hartmann, B.H.; Heller, S.; Koehler, K.R. Hair Follicle Development in Mouse Pluripotent Stem Cell-Derived Skin Organoids. *Cell Rep.* **2018**, *22*, 242–254. [CrossRef] [PubMed]
68. Snell, T.W.; Carberry, J. Astaxanthin Bioactivity Is Determined by Stereoisomer Composition and Extraction Method. *Nutrients* **2022**, *14*, 1522. [CrossRef]
69. Handayani, A.D.; Sutrisno Indraswati, N.; Ismadji, S. Extraction of astaxanthin from giant tiger (*Panaeus monodon*) shrimp waste using palm oil: Studies of extraction kinetics and thermodynamic. *Bioresour. Technol.* **2008**, *99*, 4414–4419. [CrossRef]

Disclaimer/Publisher's Note: The statements, opinions and data contained in all publications are solely those of the individual author(s) and contributor(s) and not of MDPI and/or the editor(s). MDPI and/or the editor(s) disclaim responsibility for any injury to people or property resulting from any ideas, methods, instructions or products referred to in the content.

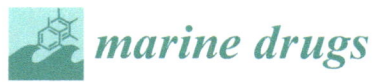 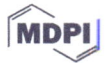

Article

Discovery and Anti-Inflammatory Activity of a Cyanobacterial Fatty Acid Targeting the Keap1/Nrf2 Pathway

Fatma H. Al-Awadhi [1,2], Emily F. Simon [1], Na Liu [1,3], Ranjala Ratnayake [1], Valerie J. Paul [4] and Hendrik Luesch [1,*]

[1] Department of Medicinal Chemistry and Center for Natural Products, Drug Discovery and Development (CNPD3), University of Florida, Gainesville, FL 32610, USA; fatalawadhi@ufl.edu or fatma.h@ku.edu.kw (F.H.A.-A.); simonemily@ufl.edu (E.F.S.); mls_liun@ujn.edu.cn (N.L.); rratnayake@cop.ufl.edu (R.R.)

[2] Department of Pharmaceutical Chemistry, Faculty of Pharmacy, Kuwait University, P.O. Box 24923, Safat 13110, Kuwait

[3] School of Biological Science and Technology, University of Jinan, Jinan 250022, China

[4] Smithsonian Marine Station, Fort Pierce, FL 34949, USA; paul@si.edu

* Correspondence: luesch@cop.ufl.edu

Abstract: The monounsaturated fatty acid 7(*E*)-9-keto-hexadec-7-enoic acid (**1**) and three structurally related analogues with different oxidation states and degrees of unsaturation (**2**–**4**) were discovered from a marine benthic cyanobacterial mat collected from Delta Shoal, Florida Keys. Their structures were elucidated using NMR spectroscopy and mass spectrometry. The structure of **1** contained an α,β-unsaturated carbonyl system, a key motif required for the activation of the Keap1/Nrf2−ARE pathway that is involved in the activation of antioxidant and phase II detoxification enzymes. Compounds **1**–**4** were screened in ARE-luciferase reporter gene assay using stably transfected HEK293 cells, and only **1** significantly induced Nrf2 activity at 32 and 10 μM, whereas **2**–**4** were inactive. As there is crosstalk between inflammation and oxidative stress, subsequent biological studies were focused on **1** to investigate its anti-inflammatory potential. Compound **1** induced *Nqo1*, a well-known target gene of Nrf2, and suppressed *iNos* transcript levels, which translated into reduced levels of nitric oxide in LPS-activated mouse macrophage RAW264.7 cells, a more relevant model for inflammation. RNA sequencing was performed to capture the effects of **1** on a global level and identified additional canonical pathways and upstream regulators involved in inflammation and immune response, particularly those related to multiple sclerosis. A targeted survey of marine cyanobacterial samples from other geographic locations, including Guam, suggested the widespread occurrence of **1**. Furthermore, the previous isolation of **1** from marine diatoms and green algae implied a potentially important ecological role across marine algal eukaryotes and prokaryotes. The previous isolation from sea lettuce raises the possibility of dietary intervention to attenuate inflammation and related disease progression.

Keywords: marine cyanobacteria; fatty acids; inflammation; RNA sequencing; NF-κB; immune function; multiple sclerosis

Citation: Al-Awadhi, F.H.; Simon, E.F.; Liu, N.; Ratnayake, R.; Paul, V.J.; Luesch, H. Discovery and Anti-Inflammatory Activity of a Cyanobacterial Fatty Acid Targeting the Keap1/Nrf2 Pathway. *Mar. Drugs* 2023, 21, 553. https://doi.org/10.3390/md21110553

Academic Editors: Donatella Degl'Innocenti and Marzia Vasarri

Received: 14 September 2023
Revised: 21 October 2023
Accepted: 23 October 2023
Published: 25 October 2023

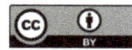

Copyright: © 2023 by the authors. Licensee MDPI, Basel, Switzerland. This article is an open access article distributed under the terms and conditions of the Creative Commons Attribution (CC BY) license (https://creativecommons.org/licenses/by/4.0/).

1. Introduction

Inflammation is a process that involves the activation of immune and non-immune cells as a protective mechanism in response to exposure to toxins, pathogens and infection, as well as tissue injury [1]. Although intermittent or acute inflammation is crucial for tissue repair, recovery and survival, progression to chronic inflammation is undesirable. Chronic inflammation underlies the pathogenesis of several diseases including diabetes, chronic obstructive pulmonary disorder (COPD), chronic kidney disease, cancer, neurodegenerative and cardiovascular diseases. It has been recognized as the most significant cause of death worldwide, with more than 50% of deaths attributed to the aforementioned underlying pathogenesis [1]. One of the causative factors of inflammation is oxidative stress, which results from the overproduction of reactive oxygen species (ROS) in excessive amounts that cannot all be neutralized by the endogenous antioxidant defense mechanisms [2]. A significant body of evidence supports the link between oxidative stress and inflammation [2–4]. High levels of ROS not only damage cellular structures, including lipids, proteins and nucleic acid, but also activate a variety of transcriptional factors, resulting in differential expression of genes involved in inflammatory pathways that ultimately lead to chronic inflammation and can even progress to cancer [3,5,6].

To combat these damaging effects of oxidative stress, cells are equipped with antioxidant defensive mechanisms responsible for the clearance of ROS and maintenance of cellular redox homeostasis. Kelch ECH-associated protein 1 (Keap1)/nuclear factor erythroid 2-related factor 2 (Nrf2)−antioxidant response element (ARE) signaling is a key cytoprotective pathway involved in the induction of phase II detoxification enzymes and therefore protects cells from the accumulation of toxic metabolites [3]. Keap1, a negative regulator of Nrf2 in the cytoplasm, is a cysteine-rich protein (27 cysteine residues) and, upon alkylation of specific Cys residues (usually C151) by electrophiles, induces Nrf2 translocation to the nucleus, where it binds to the ARE and induces the expression of antioxidant genes (*NQO1*, *HO-1*) and suppresses NF-κB-dependent proinflammatory genes (*iNOS*, *COX2*) [3,7–10]. Hence, the Keap1/Nrf2−ARE pathway is considered a promising therapeutic target for the management of several inflammatory and oxidative-stress-mediated diseases. This is further supported by the fact that bardoxolone methyl, which is an Nrf2 activator, has reached phase III clinical trials for the management of diabetic kidney disease (NCT03550443) [11].

Among the well-established Nrf2 activators are molecules bearing an α,β-unsaturated carbonyl moiety [7,8]. They activate Nrf2 via electrophilic modification of cysteine residues on the Keap1 protein through the 1,4-conjugate addition (Michael) reaction [7,8]. Their chemical reactivity and specific molecular architecture dictate the target profile in the cysteome within and beyond Keap1, producing a net effect. Levels of pleiotropic effects at the target level and downstream signaling contribute to both therapeutic efficacy and toxicity, which has to be taken into consideration. The α,β-unsaturated moiety-bearing Nrf2 activator dimethyl fumarate has been approved by the FDA for the management of multiple sclerosis, while several other multi-target drug candidates are in clinical trials for various indications, including curcumin (impaired glucose tolerance and insulin resistance; NCT01052025), licochalcone A (squamous cell carcinoma; NCT03292822) and parthenolide (cancer; NCT00133341) (Figure 1) [7].

Several marine-derived Nrf2 modulators have been reported [12]. In particular, marine algae are known for their cytoprotective effects, and several secondary metabolites have been isolated and characterized as inducers of the Keap1/Nrf2−ARE pathway [13,14]. Marine cyanobacteria are a rich source of structurally diverse secondary metabolites that elicit a wide range of biological activities [15–18]. Several natural products containing an α,β-unsaturated carbonyl system have been isolated from marine benthic cyanobacteria and are reported to induce the activation of Nrf2, including anaenamides C and D (*Hormoscilla* sp.), honaucin A (*Leptolyngbya crossbyana*), and malyngamide F acetate (*Lyngbya majuscula*) (Figure 1) [19–21].

Our efforts to explore field collections of marine cyanobacterial mats from the Florida Keys and Guam have led to the discovery of a monounsaturated fatty acid bearing an α,β-unsaturated carbonyl (**1**) in addition to three related analogues (**2–4**; Figure 2A). Herein, we describe their isolation, structure elucidation and Nrf2−ARE activity. We report the anti-inflammatory effects of the active compound **1** in lipopolysaccharide (LPS)-stimulated mouse macrophages and captured global transcriptional responses to identify pathways modulated by **1**.

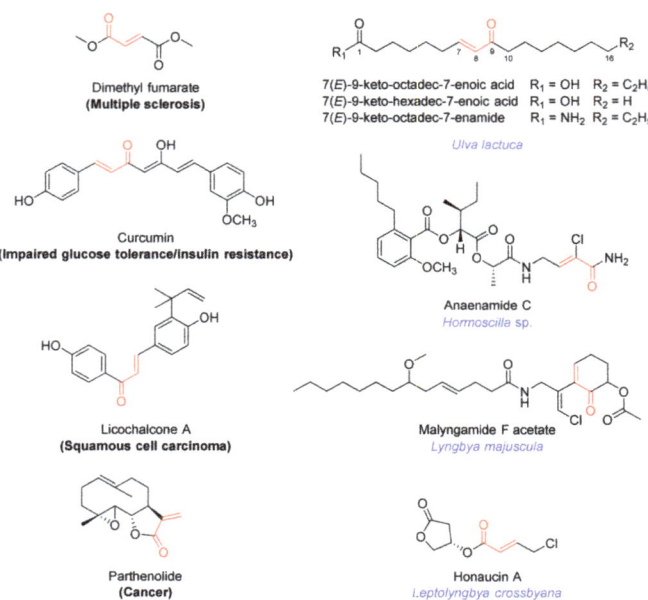

Figure 1. Chemical structures of selected Nrf2 activators bearing an α,β-unsaturated carbonyl motif which are either FDA-approved (dimethyl fumarate) or in clinical trials (curcumin, licochalcone A, pathenolide), isolated from algae (monounsaturated fatty acids) or marine cyanobacteria (anaenamide C, malyngamide F acetate, honaucin A).

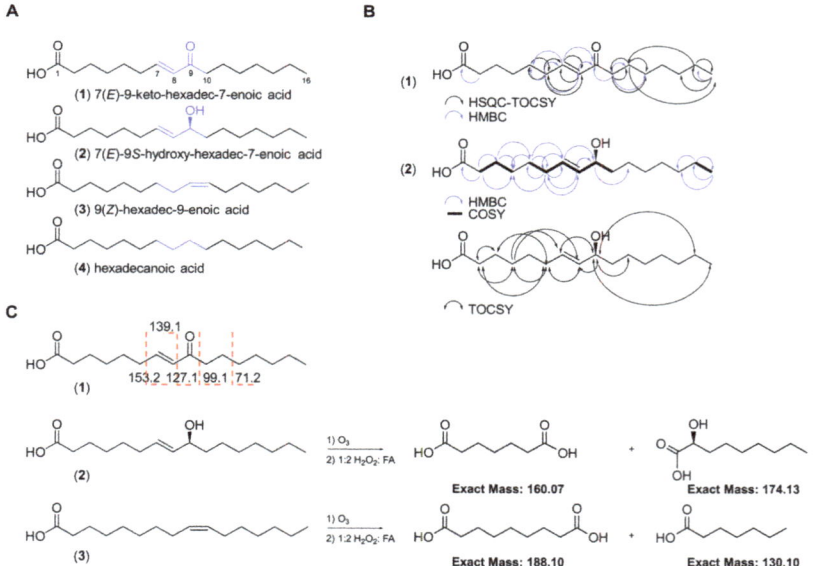

Figure 2. Chemical structures of the four fatty acids (**1**–**4**) isolated from the marine cyanobacterial mat VPFK21-7. (**A**) Key differences in the structures of compounds **1**–**4** are highlighted. (**B**) Key HSQC-TOCSY, HMBC, COSY and TOCSY correlations for compounds **1** and **2**. (**C**) ESI-MS/MS fragmentation and ozonolysis reactions to confirm the position of the double bond in compounds **1**–**3**.

2. Results

2.1. Isolation and Structure Elucidation

The red marine cyanobacterial mat (VPFK21-7) collected off Delta Shoal in the Florida Keys was freeze-dried and extracted with 1:1 EtOAc−MeOH. The non-polar extract was subsequently partitioned between EtOAc and H_2O. The EtOAc soluble fraction was then fractionated with silica gel column chromatography using a gradient system starting with 30% EtOAc−Hex and ending with 1:1 EtOAc−MeOH to afford four fractions. The fractions eluting with 30% EtOAc−Hex and EtOAc were further purified by reversed-phase HPLC, resulting in the isolation of four fatty acid type compounds differing in oxidation status and degree of unsaturation (**1–4**, Figure 2).

The HRESIMS spectrum of **1** in the negative mode showed an ion peak at m/z 267.1964 [M − H]$^-$, suggesting a molecular formula of $C_{16}H_{28}O_3$ which corresponds to 7(E)-9-keto-hexadec-7-enoic acid, a known compound previously isolated from the marine diatom *Skeletonema marinoi* and green alga *Ulva lactuca* [14,22]. Analysis of the ^{1}H NMR spectrum acquired in CDCl$_3$ revealed the characteristic two olefinic protons H-7 (δ_H 6.83, *dt*) and H-8 (δ_H 6.08, *d*) indicative of a Michael acceptor motif present in **1**. Compound **1** possessed the same ^{1}H and ^{13}C NMR chemical shifts, deduced from the ^{1}H NMR and HSQC spectra, to the known compound previously isolated from *Ulva lactuca* (Table 1; Figure 2) [14]. The planar structure was confirmed via HMBC and HSQC-TOCSY and the position of the olefinic double bond was established by selective 1D TOCSY and ESI-MS/MS fragmentation (Figures 1 and S1). The fragmentation of the [M − H]$^-$ ion of **1** showed the same fragmentation pattern as **1** isolated from the diatom *Chaetoceros karianus* [23]. A strong fragment ion peak at m/z 127.1 was evident, which corresponds to the cleavage across C-8/C-9. Compound **1** was also isolated through chemical investigations of four other marine cyanobacteria collected from the Florida Keys and Guam, suggesting a widespread occurrence and potentially important ecological role (see experimental section and Supporting Information).

Table 1. NMR spectral data for the isolated fatty-acid-type compounds (**1–4**) in CDCl$_3$.

C/H No.	1		2		3	4
	δ_H (*J* in Hz)	δ_C [a], mult [b]	δ_H (*J* in Hz)	δ_C [a], mult [b]	δ_H (*J* in Hz)	δ_H (*J* in Hz)
OH	−	−	−	−	−	−
1	−	177.2, qC	−	176.6, qC	−	−
2	2.35, t (7.4)	33.7, CH$_2$	2.37, t (7.4)	33.5, CH$_2$	2.37, t (7.4)	2.37, t (7.4)
3	1.65, m	24.8, CH$_2$	1.67, m	24.5, CH$_2$	1.67, m	1.67, m
4	1.31, m	31.7, CH$_2$	1.37, m	28.7, CH$_2$	1.32, m	1.28, m
5	1.49, m	27.9, CH$_2$	1.40, m	28.7, CH$_2$	1.32, m	1.28, m
6	2.21, dt (7.1, 6.9)	32.3, CH$_2$	2.05, dt (7.1, 6.9)	32.1, CH$_2$	1.32, m	1.28, m
7	6.83, dt (15.3, 6.9)	147.1, CH	5.63, dt (15.3, 6.9)	132.1, CH	1.32, m	1.28, m
8	6.11, dd (15.3, 7.1)	130.3, CH	5.47, dd (15.3, 7.1)	133.2, CH	2.02, dt (6.9, 6.3)	1.28, m
9	−	201.0, qC	4.06, dt (7.1, 6.8)	73.3, CH	5.34, m	1.28, m
9-OH	−	−	−	−	−	−
10	2.54, m	40.2, CH$_2$	1.57, 1.49, m	37.3, CH$_2$	5.34, m	1.28, m
11	1.62, m	24.2, CH$_2$	1.33, m	25.4, CH$_2$	2.02, dt (6.9, 6.3)	1.28, m
12, 13	1.37, m	28.7, CH$_2$	1.30, m	29.1, CH$_2$	1.32, m	1.28, m
14	1.37, m	28.7, CH$_2$	1.30, m	31.9, CH$_2$	1.32, m	1.28, m
15	1.32, m	22.5, CH$_2$	1.31, m	22.5, CH$_2$	1.32, m	1.28, m
16	0.9, t (7.0)	14.1, CH$_3$	0.9, t (7.0)	14.1, CH$_3$	0.9, t (7.0)	0.9, t (7.0)

[a] ^{13}C values were deduced from HSQC and HMBC spectra. [b] Multiplicity derived from the HSQC spectrum.

The HRESIMS spectrum of the optically active compound **2** ([α]$_D^{20}$ + 23 (*c* 0.01, MeOH)) in the negative mode showed an ion peak at m/z 269.2119 [M − H]$^-$, suggesting a molecular formula of $C_{16}H_{30}O_3$ with two degrees of unsaturation. Analysis of the ^{1}H NMR spectrum of **2** and direct comparison with **1** revealed the presence of the two characteristic olefinic proton signals H-7 (δ_H 5.63, *dt*) and H-8 (δ_H 5.47, *dd*), with an *E* configuration based on their coupling constant (J = 15.3 Hz) and allylic proton H-6 (δ_H 2.05, dt), which were all shifted upfield compared to **1**. Additionally, a new methine signal H-9 (δ_H 4.06, dt) was evident in the ^{1}H NMR spectrum of **2**. Taken together, these data suggest that the C-9 keto carbonyl in **1** is replaced by a hydroxy–methine in compound **2**. The proposed structure was further confirmed through analysis of the HMBC data, which showed the presence of only one carbonyl (δ_C 176.6) corresponding to the carboxylic acid as in **1** but missing keto carbonyl (Tables 1 and S1; Figure 2). The position of the double bond was confirmed via an ozonolysis reaction followed by oxidative workup to generate two fragments, which were detected by ESIMS in the negative mode (m/z 159.12 [M − H]$^-$ corresponding to the dicarboxylic acid fragment and 173.08 [M − H]$^-$ corresponding to the alpha hydroxy carboxylic acid fragment), suggesting the cleavage of alkene at C-7/C-8 (Figures 2C and S4). The configuration at C-9 was determined to be S based on a comparison of the optical rotation sign of **2** with the previously reported analogue 8(E)-10(S)-hydroxy-hexadec-8-enoic acid, which had a positive optical rotation sign [24]. Taken together, the structure of **2** corresponds to 7(E)-9S-hydroxy-hexadec-7-enoic acid, a known compound previously isolated from the marine diatom *Thalassiosira rotula* [25].

Analysis of the ^{1}H NMR spectrum of **3** and direct comparison with **2** revealed the presence of two olefinic protons, H-9 and H-10 (δ_H 5.34, 2H), and the absence of the methine H-9 (δ_H 4.06, dt) present in **2** (Figure 2). The proposed structure was confirmed with HRESIMS, which gave the expected ion peak that showed 16 mass units of difference compared to **2**, suggesting the lack of one oxygen. The HRESIMS spectrum of **3** in the negative mode showed an ion peak at m/z 253.2170 [M − H]$^-$, suggesting a molecular formula of $C_{16}H_{30}O_2$ with one degree of unsaturation, which corresponds to palmitoleic acid. The position of the double bond was established via an ozonolysis reaction followed by oxidative workup to cleave the alkene and generate a dicarboxylic acid fragment. The fragment was detected by ESIMS in the negative mode, which showed an ion peak at m/z 187.11 [M − H]$^-$, suggesting the cleavage of the alkene at C-9/C-10 (Figures 2C and S4). The Z configuration of the double bond was established following a selective homonuclear decoupling of the allylic methylenes (δ_H 2.04) followed by subsequent measurement of the coupling constant of the olefinic protons (δ_H 5.34, J = 11.1 Hz) and comparison with the coupling constants of commercially available E/Z isomers of the same compound (Figure S5) [26]. The coupling constants and the ^{1}H NMR signals of olefinic protons following homonuclear decoupling were consistent with the published data of isomeric methyl ester derivatives of **3** [26]. Analysis of other proton signals in **3** further confirmed the structural assignments, including the alpha protons H$_2$-2 (δ_H 2.37, t, 2H); two allylic methylenes, H$_2$-8 and H$_2$-11 (δ_H 2.04, q, 4H); one methylene at the beta carbon of the carboxylic acid, H$_2$-3 (δ_H 1.66, m, 2H); the methylene chains H$_2$-4 to H$_2$-7 and H$_2$-11 to H$_2$-15 (δ_H 1.29–1.33, m, 16H); and one terminal methyl group, H$_3$-16 (δ_H 0.9, t, 3H) (Figure 2; Tables 1 and S1).

Analysis of the ^{1}H NMR spectrum of **4** and direct comparison with **3** revealed the absence of the two olefinic protons, H-7 and H-8 (δ_H 5.37, m, 2H), present in **3**. The proposed structure was confirmed by HRESIMS, which gave the expected ion peak that showed 2 mass units of difference to **3**, suggesting the lack of a double bond (Figure 2). The HRESIMS spectrum of **4** in the negative mode showed an ion peak at m/z 255.2325 [M − H]$^-$, suggesting a molecular formula of $C_{16}H_{32}O_2$ with a lower unsaturation number (1), which corresponds to palmitic acid. The structure was deduced via analysis of the ^{1}H NMR spectrum, indicating a long-chain fatty acid without branching. The ^{1}H NMR spectrum acquired in CDCl$_3$ revealed signals indicative of methylene protons at the alpha carbon H$_2$-2 (δ_H 2.37, t, 2H), one methylene at the beta carbon of the carboxylic acid H$_2$-3 (δ_H 1.66, q, 2H), the methylene chain H$_2$-4 to H$_2$-15 (δ_H 1.32, m, 12H) and one terminal methyl group, H$_3$-16 (δ_H 0.9, t, 3H) (Figure 2; Table 1).

2.2. Biological Activity

2.2.1. ARE-Luciferase Reporter Assay

As compound **1** was reported previously to be the Nrf2/ARE activator in IMR-32 cells [14], we aimed to investigate the Nrf2/ARE activity of the isolated analogues alongside **1**. The four fatty acids were screened in an ARE-luciferase reporter gene assay for 24 h using stably transfected HEK293 cells. Compound **1**, bearing an α,β-unsaturated carbonyl system, induced Nrf2 activity 48- and 11-fold at 32 and 10 µM, respectively, and was slightly active at 3.2 µM. On the other hand, compounds **2–4** were not active in this assay (Figure 3A). A cell viability assay was also carried out in parallel under the same conditions and none of the tested compounds were toxic at 32 µM (Figure 3B). Comparing the chemical structures of the fatty acids **1–4** with their corresponding ARE-luc activity suggests that the electrophilic Michael acceptor motif is essential for activity. As **1** was the only active compound in this assay, we carried out all subsequent biological studies using **1** that was isolated from VPFK 21-7.

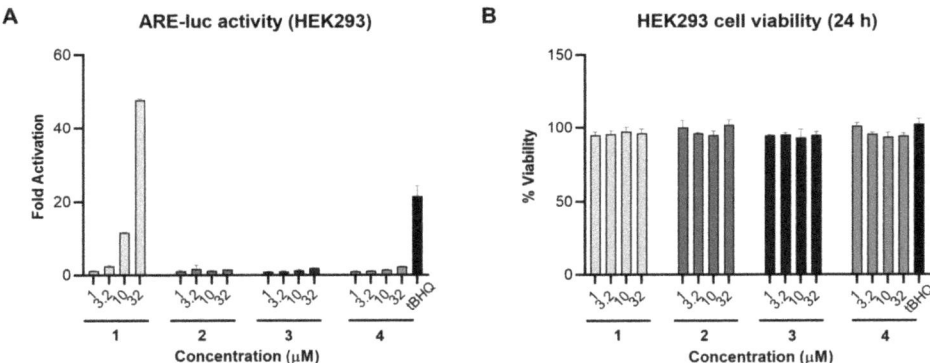

Figure 3. Nrf2/ARE activity for compounds **1–4** in HEK293 cells. (**A**) Compound **1** activated the ARE-luc reporter (24 h) in a dose-dependent manner. tBHQ was used as a positive control. (**B**) Cell viability in HEK293 cells after 24 h treatment with **1–4** measured by MTT. Data represent mean ± SD (n = 3).

2.2.2. NO Production

The anti-inflammatory activity of **1** was subsequently tested by measuring the levels of nitric oxide (NO) in LPS-activated mouse macrophage RAW264.7 cells, a more relevant model for inflammation. In this assay, **1** dose-dependently reduced NO levels up to 3.2 µM (Figure 4A). The cell viability was measured in RAW264.7 cells using MTT, and none of the tested concentrations of **1** were cytotoxic under these conditions (Figure 4B).

2.2.3. Nqo1 and iNos Transcript Levels

To investigate whether the reduction in NO levels caused by **1** was a result of transcriptional regulation, the relative transcript levels of NAD(P)H:quinone oxidoreductase 1 (Nqo1), the mRNA level of a well-known target gene of Nrf2, was measured. Compound **1** dose-dependently induced *Nqo1* transcript levels with pronounced effects observed at 32 and 10 µM (9.8- and 4.6-fold induction, respectively). Concomitantly, **1** suppressed *iNos* transcript levels 5.0- and 2.0-fold at 32 and 10 µM, respectively (Figure 4C,D). *iNos* is an NF-κB target gene which encodes the synthesis of NO. As expected, the suppression of *iNos* transcript levels by **1** translated into reduced levels of nitric oxide in LPS-activated mouse macrophage RAW264.7 cells (Figure 4A).

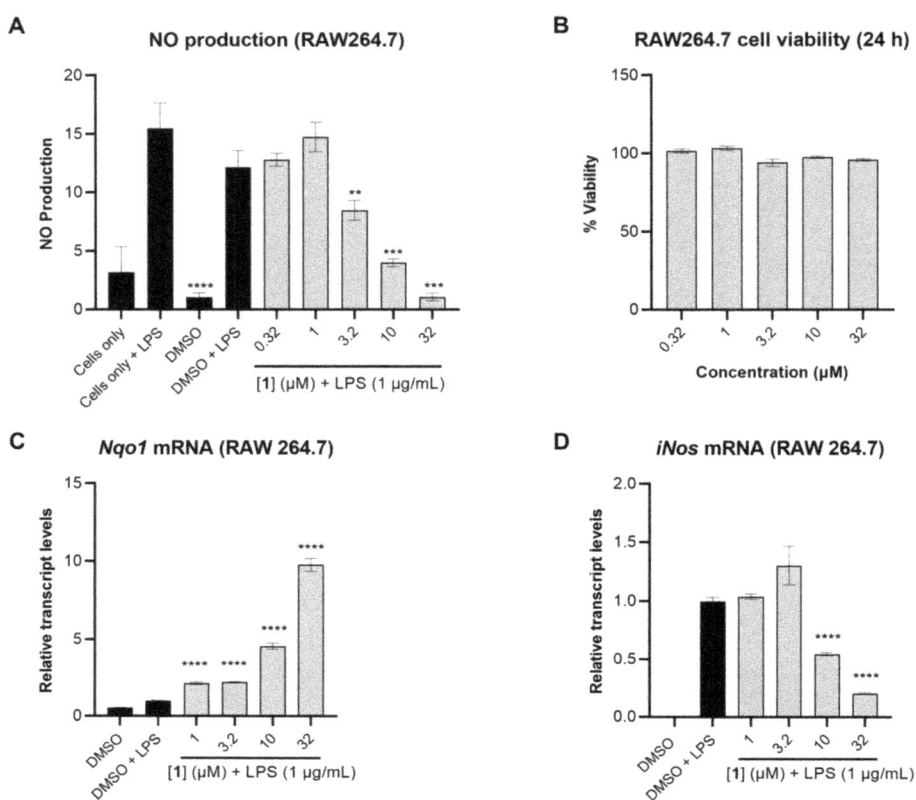

Figure 4. The anti-inflammatory effects of **1** in RAW264.7 cells. (**A**) NO production in RAW264.7 cells measured after 24 h using Griess reagent. The cells were pretreated with **1** at different concentrations for 1 h followed by stimulation with LPS (1 μg/mL). (**B**) Cell viability in RAW264.7 after 24 h treatment with **1** measured using MTT assay. (**C,D**) Relative transcript levels of *Nqo1* and *iNos* measured by TaqMan analysis, using actin as endogenous control. RAW264.7 cells were pretreated with compound **1** at different concentrations for 1 h followed by LPS stimulation (1 μg/mL). RNA was extracted following 12 h incubation. Data represent mean ± SD (n = 3). The asterisks denote significance of $p < 0.05$ relative to DMSO + LPS using two-tailed unpaired t-test (** denotes $p \leq 0.01$, *** denotes $p \leq 0.001$, **** denotes $p \leq 0.0001$).

2.2.4. RNA Sequencing

Given the effect of **1** on *Nqo1* and *iNos* mRNA levels linked to two different transcription factors (Nrf2 vs. NF-κB), we aimed to further capture its effects in mouse macrophage RAW264.7 cells on a global level and explore additional pathways that might be modulated. RNA sequencing was performed using three different concentrations of **1** (32, 10 and 3.2 μM), encompassing the entire activity range (Figure 5). This was followed by Ingenuity Pathway Analysis (IPA) of differentially expressed genes using the cutoff criteria of a 1.5-fold change (exp log ratio 0.586) and p-value of 0.05 to focus on biologically and statistically significant changes. Using these criteria, a total of 671 genes (at 32 μM), 325 genes (at 10 μM) and 130 genes (at 3.2 μM) were identified as differentially expressed (exp log ratio 0.586 and p-value of 0.05).

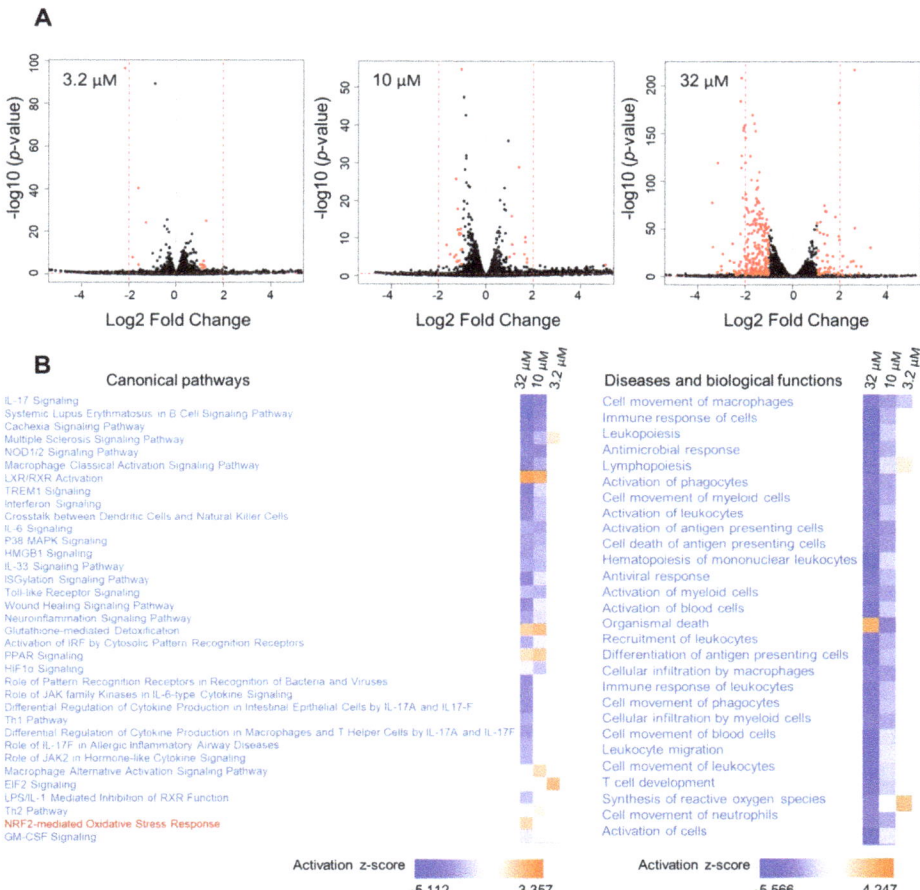

Figure 5. Analysis of RNA sequencing data of **1** at three concentrations. (**A**) Volcano plots of the differentially regulated genes obtained from the RNA sequencing data of **1**, with cutoff values of log2 fold change > 1 and *p*-value < 0.05. (**B**) Heatmap showing selected canonical pathways involved in inflammation and top biological functions of **1** derived from comparison analysis of the three datasets using IPA.

At the concentration where **1** showed the most potent activity (32 µM, Figure 4), the dataset was highly enriched with genes involved in inflammatory pathways, and at 10 µM similar results were noted but with differences in z-scores and *p*-values (Figure 5B). At 3.2 µM, where the compound showed only marginal activity (Figure 4), these pathways were not enriched (Figure 5B).

Analysis of RNA sequencing data of **1** at 32 µM and 10 µM revealed immunological and inflammatory diseases, immune cell trafficking and inflammatory response to be among the top hits in the IPA list of diseases and functions. Additionally, functions related to lipid metabolism and free radical scavenging (synthesis of reactive oxygen species) were also detected. The analysis supports the beneficial functions of **1**, as the activation status of some of the diseases and functions underlying the aforementioned categories were predicted to be decreased based on the activation z-scores. As expected, the Nrf2-mediated oxidative stress response and glutathione-mediated detoxification pathways were evident in the analysis with positive z-scores (Table 2). Additionally, several other canonical pathways with negative z-scores, which strongly correlate with inflammation, were detected (Table 2).

Table 2. Selected immune and inflammatory canonical pathways modulated by **1** at 32 µM based on RNA-seq and IPA.

Canonical Pathway	Activation z-Score	p-Value	No. of Molecules	Selected Genes
Role of hypercytokinemia/hyperchemokinemia in the pathogenesis of Influenza	−5.112	4.85×10^{-27}	30	IL33, CCL2, IFNB1, IL1A, IFIT3
Pathogen-induced cytokine storm signaling pathway	−5.091	4.85×10^{-23}	50	IL33, CCL2, CXCL9, CSF2, NOS2
Role of pattern recognition receptors in recognition of bacteria and viruses	−2.887	1.10×10^{-17}	29	IL33, CSF2, TNFSF10, IFNB1, IL1A
Multiple sclerosis signaling pathway	−3.402	1.03×10^{-12}	28	IL33, CSF2, TNFSF10, IL1A, IL36A
NOD1/2 signaling pathway	−3.138	8.86×10^{-13}	26	IL33, CCL2, CSF2, TNFSF10, NOS2
TREM1 signaling	−3.638	3.42×10^{-12}	17	CCL2, CSF2, CD86, IL6, IL1B
Macrophage classical activation signaling pathway	−3.400	5.92×10^{-12}	25	IL33, CSF2, TNFSF10, NOS2
IL-17 signaling	−4.146	6.02×10^{-09}	21	IL33, CCL2, MMP3, CSF2, NOS2
Interferon signaling	−3.162	9.25×10^{-09}	10	IFIT1 *, IFNB1, IFIT3 *, ISG15
Neuroinflammation signaling pathway	−2.449	1.84×10^{-08}	27	CCL2, MMP3, NOX1, NOS2
Differential regulation of cytokine production in macrophages and T-helper cells	−2.646	1.19×10^{-07}	7	CCL2, CSF2, IL6, IL1B, CCL4
LXR/RXR activation	2.840	3.04×10^{-07}	15	IL33, CCL2, NOS2, IL1A, IL36A
Toll-like receptor signaling	−2.111	3.68×10^{-07}	12	IL33, IL1A, IL36A, IL1B, TLR8
LPS-IL-1-mediated inhibition of RXR function	−2.000	1.81×10^{-05}	19	IL33, IL1A, IL36A, IL1B, FABP4
Glutathione-mediated detoxification *	1.633	2.58×10^{-05}	7	Gsta4, GSTA5 *, GSTA3, MGST2
HMGB1 signaling	−2.646	5.89×10^{-05}	14	IL33, CCL2, CSF2, TNFSF10, IL1A
P38 MAPK signaling	−2.530	1.64×10^{-04}	11	IL33, IL1A, IL36A, IL1B, PLA2G4C
PPAR signaling	1.265	2.75×10^{-05}	10	IL33, IL1A, IL36A, IL1B
NRF2-mediated oxidative stress response *	1.414	2.22×10^{-03}	14	GSTA5, GSTA3, NQO1, PRDX1

* The genes involved in these pathways were upregulated.

Hypercytokinemia/hyperchemokinemia and pathogen-induced cytokine storm were the top two canonical pathways that were downregulated. Next, pattern recognition receptor (PRR) signaling was identified as downregulated; this receptor recognizes specific molecules on the surface of pathogens and induces the innate immune response, which in turn activates downstream signaling pathways that activate transcriptional responses and trigger the expression and release of pro-inflammatory genes to initiate host defense [27]. Also downregulated were NOD-like receptors, members of PRRs which activate the innate immune system in response to cellular stress and injury and therefore are associated with a wide range of inflammatory conditions [28]. In addition to NF-κB and MAPK, NOD1/2 is involved in the activation of interferon (IFN) signaling, which was strongly attenuated based on our analysis [29]. IL-17 signaling, a critical pathway involved in the pathogenesis of several inflammatory and autoimmune diseases, was also downregulated [30]. In these conditions, IL-17 induces the sustained production of inflammatory cytokines and chemokines, including IL-1, IL-6, IL-1β, TNF, CCL2 and CSF, as well as matrix metalloproteinases such as MMP3 and MMP9, all of which were detected and found to be downregulated in response to **1** [31]. Additional players in the pathogenesis of inflammatory and autoimmune diseases that were downregulated were the high-mobility group box 1 (HMGB1) and p38 mitogen-activated protein kinases (MAPK) signaling [32,33]. Interestingly, peroxisome proliferator-activated receptor (PPAR) signaling weas upregulated. PPARs are ligand-activated transcriptional regulators involved in lipid metabolism and therefore implicated in the regulation of several cellular processes [34]. PPARs heterodimerize with retinoic X receptors (RXR)—which were also upregulated—and upon ligand (unsaturated fatty acids) binding they regulate the expression of downstream target genes [34].

The top upstream regulator identified in the analysis was lipopolysaccharide (LPS), which was predicted to be inhibited with activation z-scores of −11.621 and −5.491 at 32 and 10 μM, respectively (Figure S6). Interestingly, the upstream analysis identified dexamethasone, which was predicted to be activated with positive z-scores of 4.210 and 5.299 at 32 and 10 μM, respectively. The analysis identified 116 genes out of 202 (at 32 μM) in the dataset with measurement directions consistent with its activation, suggesting that compound **1** functions similarly to dexamethasone (Figure 6A). Dexamethasone is a steroidal drug known for its anti-inflammatory activity. Several studies supported the effect of dexamethasone in inhibiting *iNos* expression and NO production including LPS-treated macrophages [35–43]. Dexamethasone was also reported to inhibit TNFα secretion and LPS-induced activation of p38 MAPK signaling. Furthermore, a study supported its effects of inhibiting *IL-1β* expression via inhibition of NF-κB/Rel and AP1 in LPS-stimulated RAW264.7 cells [36,44]. The upstream analysis identified 11 genes (downregulated: *CCL2, NOS2, IL-6, IL-1β, MMP9, CCL4, IL-10, CCL3L3, CCND1, BCL2L1*; upregulated: *GCLM*) in the dataset with the same measurement direction as the Nrf2 activator bardoxolone methyl, a natural product-derived triterpenoid (z-score 3.251; *p*-value 5.82×10^{-11}) which has reached phase III clinical trials for the treatment of diabetic kidney disease [11]. Nrf2 (NFE2L2) was detected as an upstream regulator and predicted to be activated (z-score 4.198), with 40 out of 53 genes having a measurement direction consistent with its activation (Figure 6B). The analysis also identified NF-κB as an upstream regulator that is predicted to be inhibited (z-score −4.170) based on 30 out of 52 genes having a measurement direction consistent with its inhibition, including *IL-6, IL-10, IL-1β, NOS, MMP3* and *MMP9*, which were all significantly downregulated (Figure 6B). In line with the reported crosstalk between the Nrf2 and NF-κB pathways [45,46], the mechanistic network of the upstream regulator Nrf2 shows and predicts HMOX1 activation as a key player mediating the crosstalk through the reported inhibition of proinflammatory genes of NF-κB (Figure 6C) [47].

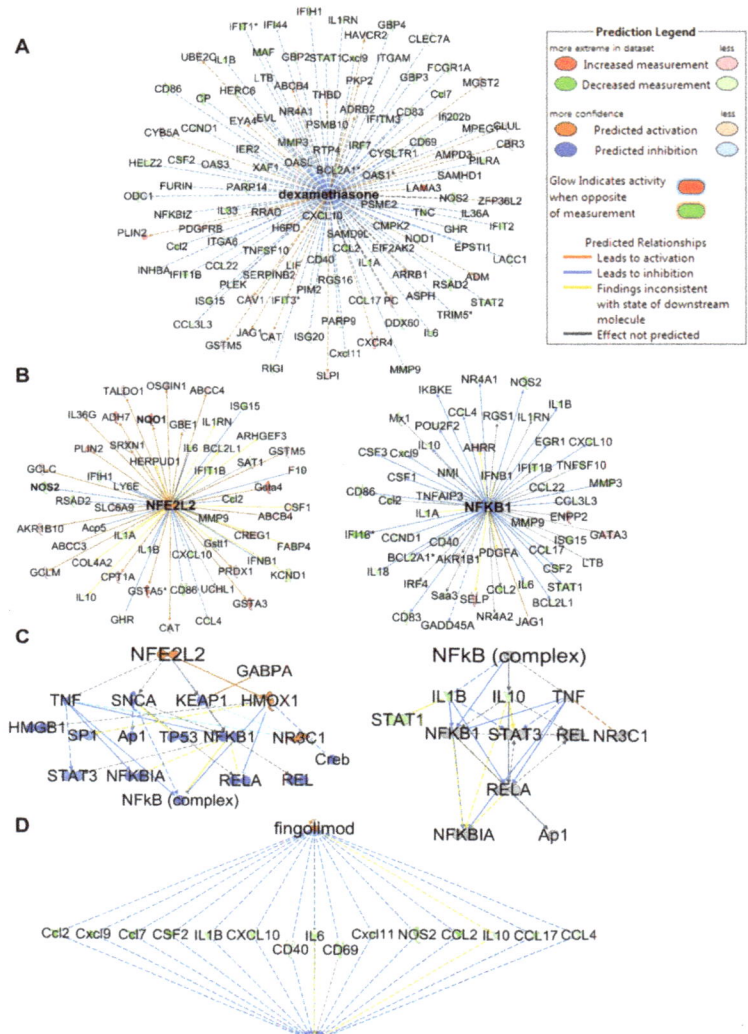

Figure 6. IPA analysis of RNA sequencing data at 32 μM. (**A**) Upstream regulator network of dexamethasone showing all genes with measurement directions consistent with dexamethasone's predicted activation state. (**B**) Upstream regulator networks of Nrf2 (NFE2L2) and NF-κB showing the modulated target genes in response to **1**. (**C**) Mechanistic networks of Nrf2 (NFE2L2) and NF-κB demonstrating the crosstalk between the two pathways via HMOX1 activation. (**D**) Regulator effect network of the Nrf2 activator fingolimod, predicted to be activated as it downregulates the same set of genes that are downregulated in the dataset in response to **1**. The asterisks on some genes indicate that multiple identifiers in the dataset file map to a single gene.

Analysis of regulator effect networks at 32 μM identified the known ARE activators fingolimod, resveratrol and curcumin to have similar effects as **1** [6,48]. These networks connect the upstream regulator through differentially regulated genes in the dataset to a relevant phenotype (Figure 6D). Fingolimod, a natural product-derived drug for the treatment of multiple sclerosis, is known for its immunosuppressive and neuroprotective effects and is currently in phase 2 clinical trials for inflammation (NCT04675762). Studies have supported the neuroprotective effects of fingolimod in multiple sclerosis, which are mediated through downregulation of IL-17 signaling and inhibition of NF-κB translocation and NO production in astrocytes [48–50]. Interestingly, relapsed multiple sclerosis appeared in the analysis list of diseases and was predicted to be decreased based on the activation z-score -2.058 (p-value 2.28×10^{-12}) with 22 genes involved. Also, multiple sclerosis signaling was one of the top canonical pathways identified in the analysis and was predicted to be downregulated. Resveratrol, a plant-derived polyphenolic compound known for its antioxidant and anti-inflammatory activities, also appeared in the analysis, modulating a set of genes with similar measurement direction as **1** (Figure S7). Resveratrol was reported to decrease the production of *IL-6*, *TNF-α* and *IL-17* expression in HTLV-1-infected T cells, as well as reduce NO production and inhibit *iNos* expression in LPS-stimulated RAW264.7 cells [51].

3. Discussion

Marine cyanobacteria are prolific producers of bioactive secondary metabolites with diverse structures, including polyketides, modified peptides and fatty acid derivatives such as fatty acid amides [15–18]. Here, we report for the first time the discovery and isolation of a cyanobacterial C16 monounsaturated fatty acid (**1**) and its hydroxy-containing analogue (**2**), which were previously reported in marine diatoms and a green alga, in addition to two other structurally related analogues (**3–4**), all differing in their oxidation status. Compound **1**, characterized by the presence of a conjugated enone motif, has been previously isolated from the green alga *Ulva lactuca* and was reported to induce Nrf2/ARE activity in IMR-32 cells [14]. Also, it is an isomer of the anti-inflammatory (*E*)-9-oxohexadec-10-enoic acid isolated from the red alga *Gracilaria verrucosa*, which was reported to inhibit the production of NO, IL-6 and TNFα in LPS-stimulated RAW264.7 cells [24]. Furthermore, **1** and its isomer were also co-isolated from the diatom *Chaetoceros karianus*, which both exhibited a dual agonist activity towards human PPARα and PPARγ [23]. The co-existence of both the keto- and hydroxy-monounsaturated fatty acids has been reported previously, as **1** and **2** were isolated from the marine diatom *Skeletonema marinoi* [22]. C18 analogues of **1** and **2**, namely (*E*)-11-oxo-octadeca-12-enoic acid and (*E*)-11-hydroxy-octadeca-12-enoic acid, were isolated from a marine green alga, *Ulva fasciata* [52]. Furthermore, the methyl ester derivatives of **1** and **2** have been reported from the marine diatom *Thalassiosira rotula*, in which the extract was methylated prior to purification of both derivatives [25].

In this study, we also report the discovery of **1** from cyanobacterial samples collected from five distinct geographical locations in Guam and Florida Keys. The widespread distribution of these secondary metabolites across different organisms and geographical locations highlights their evolutionary importance, which prompted us to investigate their bioactivity to better understand their pervasiveness in the marine environment. C16 acid (**1**) and its derivatives 7(*E*)-9-keto-octadec-7-enoic acid (C18 acid) and 7(*E*)-9-keto-octadec-7-enamide (C18 amide) from *Ulva lactuca* demonstrated Nrf2/ARE activity in IMR-32 human neuroblastoma, a widely used cellular model for oxidative stress, with the highest ARE activation induced by the C18 acid derivative of **1** with no observed effects on viability [14]. The C18 acid also induced many ARE-regulated antioxidant genes in vitro, including *Nqo1*, and hence highlighting the potential of these unsaturated fatty acids for chemoprevention to protect from cancer and other oxidative-stress-mediated diseases. Due to the established crosstalk between oxidative stress and inflammation, we investigated the anti-inflammatory potential of **1** in RAW264.7 mouse macrophage cells, a relevant cellular model for inflammation. Compound **1** suppressed the LPS-induced transcript levels of the NF-κB target gene *iNos*, which translated into reduced production of NO. This data inversely correlated with *Nqo1* transcript levels, which showed a strong dose-dependent induction in response to **1**, suggesting that the anti-inflammatory activity of **1** is mediated through ARE activation. Our analysis of LPS-induced global changes in transcript levels following treatment with **1** identified many additional canonical pathways and regulator networks linked to inflammation, immune response and related diseases, particularly multiple sclerosis. Recent evidence highlights the role of Nrf2 as a regulator of innate immune response via direct and indirect interactions with major components and signaling pathways of the immune system, including Toll-like receptor signaling, the NF-κB pathway and the type-1 interferon system [53], all of which were found to be downregulated in our IPA analysis. Furthermore, Nrf2 has been reported to be involved in the regulation of immune cell recruitment, as well as cytokine release and transcriptional activation of proinflammatory cytokines such as IL-6 and IL-1β, which were downregulated in response to **1** in LPS-stimulated macrophages.

Oxidative stress and high levels of ROS have been reported to underlie the pathogenesis of several neurodegenerative disorders, including multiple sclerosis. In multiple sclerosis, macrophages and microglia activation contribute to increased levels of ROS, dysregulated immunity and enhanced inflammatory response, ultimately resulting in mitochondrial dysfunction, neuroinflammation, demyelination and axonal degeneration, key features of the disease [54]. High levels of ROS in multiple sclerosis were reported to activate immune cells to induce kinases and redox-sensitive transcription factors, including MAPKs, AP1 and NF-κB. NF-κB activation in turn upregulates the expression of several genes implicated in the pathogenesis of multiple sclerosis, such as *TNFα*, *iNos* and *IL1α/IL1β* [55]. Increased levels of TNFα, IL-6 and IL-10 were evident in the blood of an LPS-treated animal model of multiple sclerosis [54]. Interestingly, our transcriptomic analysis revealed downregulation of all these markers in response to **1**. An increasing body of evidence supports the involvement of Nrf2 in the pathogenesis of multiple sclerosis in particular, where loss of Nrf2 resulted in a rapid onset and more severe clinical course of the disease [54]. The role of Nrf2 activation as a potential therapeutic target was further supported following the FDA approval of the Nrf2 activator dimethyl fumarate for the treatment of remitting–relapsing multiple sclerosis [54–56]. The drug was shown to induce *Nqo1* expression levels in patients' blood following 4–6 weeks' treatment, with more patients likely to have undetected disease activity a year later [54,57]. In a mouse model of multiple sclerosis, dimethyl fumarate treatment reduced the severity of symptoms and preserved myelination compared to Nrf2$^{-/-}$ mice [55,56]. Interestingly, our transcriptomic analysis identified multiple sclerosis signaling as among the top five canonical pathways that were downregulated, in addition to the predicted inhibition of relapsed multiple sclerosis in the list of diseases. Also, the identification of the multiple sclerosis drug fingolimod in regulator effect networks, in addition to resveratrol and curcumin, which were all preclinically investigated as Nrf2 activators in experimental models of multiple sclerosis, further supports the role of the Nrf2-ARE signaling pathway activation in combating the hallmark features of the disease and highlights the potential beneficial applications of **1** [55].

4. Materials and Methods

4.1. Biological Material

Samples of VPFK21-7, a red cyanobacterial mat, were collected from Delta Shoal in the Florida Keys on 24 September 2021. While the taxonomy of this cyanobacterium has not been confirmed, the fine filaments were only ~5 μm in width and were fairly uniform, suggesting mostly one filament type in the sample. Samples of the cyanobacterium DRTO-73, which correspond microscopically with *Leptolyngbya* sp., were collected from Loggerhead Key, Florida on 21 May 2013 [58]. Samples of the cyanobacterium VPG 18-62 red leathery mat were collected from Tanguisson Reef flat in Guam on 7 April 2018.

Two other cyanobacteria, HL-CN2011-062 (DRTO-46) and HL-CN2015-131 (DRTO-89), were collected from Fort Jefferson on 24 May 2011 and Loggerhead Key on 9 May 2015, respectively. This is a diverse group of benthic filamentous cyanobacteria. Voucher specimens have been retained at the Smithsonian Marine Station for all samples.

4.2. General Experimental Procedures

^{1}H and 2D NMR spectra for **1** (0.4 mg) and **2** (0.3 mg) in CDCl$_3$ were recorded on a Bruker 800-MHz/63 mm Avance III Spectrometer (Bruker Biospin Corporation, Billerica, MA, USA) and Bruker Avance Neo-600-MHz Spectrometer using a 1.7 mm tube, respectively. ^{1}H NMR spectra for **3** (0.2 mg) and **4** (0.8 mg) in CDCl$_3$ were recorded on a Cryo 600-MHz/54 mm Bruker Avance III HD. The spectra were referenced using the residual solvent signal ($\delta_{H/C}$ 7.26/77.0 (CDCl$_3$)). The HRESIMS data were obtained in the negative mode using the high-resolution LC Q-Exactive orbitrap mass spectrometer (ThermoSci, Waltham, MA, USA) equipped with the APCI/ESI multimode ion source detector. The LRESIMS data were acquired in the negative mode using the TSQ Altis plus triple quadrupole mass spectrometer equipped with Vanquish LC system (ThermoSci). The optical rotation was measured using a JASCO P-2000 polarimeter.

4.3. Extraction and Isolation

Samples of the VP FK21-7 red mat cyanobacterium were freeze-dried and subjected to non-polar extraction using EtOAc−MeOH (1:1) and polar extraction using 30% aq EtOH. The non-polar extract (2724 mg) was partitioned between EtOAc and H$_2$O. The EtOAc fraction (80.5 mg) was concentrated and subjected to silica gel chromatography using the following gradient: (30% EtOAc−Hex, 100% EtOAc, 10% MeOH−EtOAc, 1:1 EtOAc−MeOH, and finally 100% MeOH). The fraction that eluted with 100% EtOAc (12 mg) was purified by semipreparative reversed-phase HPLC [Synergi Hydro 4u-RP, 250 × 10.0 mm; flow rate, 2.0 mL/min; PDA detection 200–800 nm] using a linear MeOH−H$_2$O gradient (20–100% MeOH over 15 min, 100% MeOH for 20 min) to afford **1** and **2** in a 1:1 mixture (1.5 mg) eluting at t_R 21.6 min. The mixture was further purified by HPLC using an analytical column [Synergi 4u Hydro-RP 80A, 150 × 4.60 mm, 4 micron; flow rate 0.5 mL/min, PDA detection 200–800 nm] with a linear ACN−H$_2$O gradient (20–100% ACN for 10 min, 100% ACN for 15 min) to afford **1** (0.4 mg), eluting at t_R 12.2 min, and **2** (0.3 mg), eluting at t_R 12.0 min. The Si fraction that eluted with 30% EtOAc−Hex (34.3 mg) was partially purified (11.6 mg) by semipreparative reversed-phase HPLC [Synergi Hydro 4u-RP, 250 × 10.0 mm; flow rate, 2.0 mL/min; PDA detection 200–800 nm] using a linear MeOH−H$_2$O gradient (20–100% MeOH over 15 min, 100% MeOH for 20 min) to afford **3** (0.8 mg), eluting at t_R 26.5 min, and **4** (0.8 mg), eluting at t_R 28.3 min. Compound **3** was repurified by HPLC using analytical column [Synergi 4u Hydro-RP 80A, 150 × 4.60 mm, 4 micron; flow rate 0.5 mL/min, PDA detection 200–800 nm] using a linear ACN−H$_2$O gradient (20–100% ACN for 10 min, 100% ACN for 15 min) to afford **3** (0.2 mg) eluting at t_R 17.3 min.

7(*E*)-9-Keto-hexadec-7-enoic acid (**1**): colorless, amorphous powder; ^{1}H and 2D NMR data (CDCl$_3$), Table 1; HRESIMS *m/z* 267.1964 [M − H]$^-$ (calcd. for C$_{16}$H$_{27}$O$_3$, 268.3970).

7(*E*)-9*S*-Hydroxy-hexadec-7-enoic acid (**2**): colorless, amorphous powder; $[\alpha]_D^{20}$ + 23 (*c* 0.01, MeOH); ^{1}H and 2D NMR data (CDCl$_3$), Tables 1 and S1; HRESIMS *m/z* 269.2119 [M − H]$^-$ (calcd. for C$_{16}$H$_{29}$O$_3$, 270.4130).

9(*Z*)-Hexadec-9-enoic acid (**3**): colorless, amorphous powder; ^{1}H NMR and HSQC data (CDCl$_3$), Tables 1 and S1; HRESIMS *m/z* 253.2170 [M − H]$^-$ (calcd. for C$_{16}$H$_{29}$O$_2$, 254.4140).

Hexadecanoic acid (**4**): colorless, amorphous powder; ^{1}H NMR data (CDCl$_3$), Table 1; HRESIMS *m/z* 255.2325 [M − H]$^-$ (calcd. for C$_{16}$H$_{31}$O$_2$, 256.4300).

Isolation of Compound **1** from Other Cyanobacteria Samples

Samples of the filamentous cyanobacterium DRTO-73 collected from Loggerhead Key, Florida were freeze-dried, extracted and fractionated as described previously [58]. The 20% *i*PrOH/CH$_2$Cl$_2$ was purified by reversed-phase HPLC [Synergi Hydro 4u-RP, 250 × 10.0 mm; flow rate, 2.0 mL/min; PDA detection 200–800 nm] using a linear MeOH−H$_2$O gradient (60–100% MeOH over 10 min, 100% MeOH for 20 min) to afford **1** (0.6 mg) and which was repurified by HPLC [Synergi 4u Hydro-RP 80A, 150 × 4.60 mm, 4 micron; flow rate 0.5 mL/min, PDA detection 200–800 nm] using a linear ACN−H$_2$O gradient (20–100% ACN for 10 min, 100% ACN for 15 min) to afford **1** (0.1 mg) eluting at t_R 12.2 min.

The freeze-dried material of the cyanobacterium VPG18-67 red leathery mat collected in Guam (73.35 g) was subjected to non-polar extraction using EtOAc−MeOH (1:1) and polar extraction using EtOH−H_2O (1:1). The non-polar extract (2.4 g) was partitioned between hexanes and 80% MeOH in H_2O. The methanolic phase was dried and further partitioned between EtOAc and H_2O. The EtOAc layer was concentrated and subjected to silica gel chromatography by using hexane and increasing gradients of EtOAc (10, 20, 40, 60, 80%), 100% EtOAc, MeOH and increasing gradients of EtOAc (20, 40, 60, 80%), and finally with 100% MeOH. The 60% EtOAc/hexane Si fraction was purified by reversed-phase HPLC [Luna C18, 250 × 4.60 mm, 4 micron; flow rate 0.8 mL/min, PDA detection 200–800 nm] using a linear ACN−H_2O gradient (10–95% ACN for 30 min, 95% ACN for 10 min) to afford **1** (0.4 mg) eluting at t_R 28.3 min.

The freeze-dried material (20.56 g) of the cyanobacterium HL-CN2011-062 (DRTO-46) collected from Fort Jefferson was extracted and partitioned as described for the sample VPG18-67. The EtOAc-partitioned fraction (60.47 mg) was subjected to silica gel chromatography by using CH_2Cl_2 and increasing gradients of *i*PrOH (2, 4, 6, 8, 10, 20, 40, 60, 80%), 100% *i*PrOH, and finally with 100% MeOH. The fraction that was eluted with 2 and 4% *i*PrOH/CH_2Cl_2 contained compound **1** based on the characteristic downfield signals in the ^{1}H NMR spectrum characteristic of the Michael acceptor motif. A total of 4 mg was then purified by reversed-phase HPLC [Synergi 4u Hydro-RP 80A, 150 × 4.60 mm, 4 micron; flow rate 1 mL/min, PDA detection 200–800 nm] using a linear ACN−H_2O gradient (15–100% ACN for 25 min, 100% ACN for 10 min) to afford **1** (0.4 mg) eluting at t_R 20.1 min.

The freeze-dried material (2.88 g) of the cyanobacterium HL-CN2015-131 (DRTO-89) collected from Loggerhead Key was extracted, partitioned and fractionated as described for HL-CN2011-062. The fraction that was eluted with 6 and 8% *i*PrOH/CH_2Cl_2 contained compound **1** based on the characteristic downfield signals in the ^{1}H NMR spectrum characteristic of the Michael acceptor motif. A total of 4.63 mg was then purified by reversed-phase HPLC using the same column and method described for HL-CN2011-062 to afford 0.2 mg of **1**.

4.4. Ozonolysis and Oxidative Workup

Compounds **2** and **3** (50 µg each) were dissolved in 3 mL of CH_2Cl_2 followed by bubbling of ozone into the solution at −78 °C for 20 min. The solution was then dried, and the residues were resuspended in H_2O_2−HCOOH (1:2) for 20 min at 70 °C. The resulting mixture was subsequently evaporated and subjected to ESIMS analysis in the negative mode to detect the generated dicarboxylic acid fragments.

4.5. Cell Culture

HEK293 ARE-luc cells (SL-0042-NP; Signosis) (human embryonic kidney cells stably transfected with firefly luciferase reporter gene) and RAW264.7 cells (ATCC) (mouse macrophagic cells) were cultured using Dulbecco's Modified Eagle's Medium (DMEM; Invitrogen) supplemented with 10% fetal bovine serum (FBS; Sigma, St. Louis, MO, USA), 1% antibiotic–antimycotic (Invitrogen, Waltham, MA, USA) and maintained at 37 °C humidified air and 5% CO_2.

4.6. ARE-Luciferase Reporter Assay

HEK293 ARE-luc cells (10,000 cells/well) were seeded in 96-well plates (Costar 96-well white solid plates; COS3917) and incubated overnight to attach. The cells were then treated with different concentrations of compounds, positive control (tBHQ, 10 µM) and solvent control (DMSO; 0.5% *v/v*). Following 24 h incubation, luciferase activity was detected using BriteLite detection reagent (PerkinElmer, Waltham, MA, USA) following the manufacturer's instructions. The luminescence was read using the Envision plate reader (PerkinElmer). Cell viability assay was performed in parallel under the same conditions and time points.

4.7. NO Assay

RAW264.7 cells (20,000 cells/well) were seeded in 96-well plates and allowed to attach overnight. The cells were then pretreated for 1 h with different concentrations of compounds **1** and **2**, and solvent control (DMSO; 0.5% v/v) followed by stimulation with 1 µg/mL LPS. Non-stimulated cells (no LPS) were also tested simultaneously. Following 24 h incubation, the production of NO in the cell supernatant was assessed by measuring the concentration of nitrile, which is an oxidative product of NO. Briefly, 50 µL of culture supernatant was mixed with 50 µL of Griess reagent (Promega) according to the manufacturer's instructions. The absorbance was measured at 540 nm using a SpectraMax M5 plate reader (Molecular Devices, SAN Jose, CA, USA). NO production was calculated based on a standard reference curve generated for fresh nitrite standard solution. Cell viability assay was performed in parallel under the same conditions and time points.

4.8. Cell Viability Assay

HEK293 ARE-luc cells (10,000 cells/well) and RAW264.7 cells (20,000 cells/well) were seeded in 96-well plates and allowed to attach overnight. The cells were then treated with different concentrations of compounds, positive control (tBHQ, 10 µM) and solvent control (DMSO; 0.5% v/v). Following 24 h incubation, cell viability was measured using 3-(4,5-dimethylthiazol-2-yl)-2,5-diphenyltetrazoliumbromide according to the manufacturer's instructions (Promega, Madison, WI, USA).

4.9. RNA Extraction and RT-qPCR Analysis of Nqo1 and iNos Transcript Levels in RAW264.7 Cells

RAW264.7 cells (250,000 cells/well) were seeded in 6-well plates and allowed to attach overnight. After overnight incubation, the media in each well were replaced with fresh media prior to treatment with **1** at 32, 10, 3.2 and 1 µM and solvent control (0.5% DMSO) for 1 h. After 1 h, the cells were stimulated with1 µg/mL LPS. Non-stimulated cells (no LPS) were also tested simultaneously. After 12 h incubation, RNA was isolated using an RNeasy mini kit (Qiagen, Hilden, Germany) according to the manufacturer's protocol. cDNA synthesis was carried out using SuperScript II reverse transcriptase and oligo (dT) (Invitrogen). qPCR was carried out after reverse transcription on a reaction solution (25 µL) prepared using a 1 µL aliquot of cDNA, 12.5 µL of TaqMan gene expression assay mix, 1.25 µL of 20× TaqMan gene expression assay mix and 10.25 µL of RNase-free water. The qPCR experiment was performed using an ABI 7300 sequence detection system. The thermocycler program used was 2 min at 50 °C, 10 min at 95 °C, 15 s at 95 °C (40 cycles) and 1 min at 60 °C. iNos (Mm00440502_m1) and NQO1 (Mm01253561_m1) were used as target genes and mouse ACTB (#4352933, Applied Biosystems, Waltham, MA, USA) was used as endogenous control.

4.10. Illumina Sequencing Library Construction

RNA samples were measured by the QUBIT fluorescent method (Invitrogen) and Agilent Bioanalyzer. A total of 500 ng high-quality total RNA with a RIN of 10 was used for library construction using the reagents provided in the NEBNext Poly(A) mRNA Magnetic Isolation Module (New England Biolabs, Ipswich, MA, USA, catalog # E7490) and the NEBNext Ultra II Directional RNA Library Prep Kit (New England Biolabs, catalog # E7760) according to the manufacturer's user guide. Briefly, 500 ng of total RNA was used for mRNA isolated using the NEBNext Poly(A) mRNA Magnetic Isolation Module (New England Biolabs, catalog # E7490). Then, the poly A-enriched RNA was fragmented in a NEBNext First Strand Synthesis Buffer via incubation at 94 °C for the desired time. This step was followed by first-strand cDNA synthesis using reverse transcriptase and random hexamer primer. Synthesis of ds cDNA was conducted using the 2nd strand master mix provided in the kit, followed by end repair and dA tailing. At this point, Illumina adaptors were ligated to the sample. Finally, the library was amplified, followed by purification with AMPure beads (Beckman Coulter, Brea, CA, USA, catalog # A63881). The library size and mass were assessed by analysis in the Agilent TapeStation using a High Sensitivity DNA1000 Screen Tape. Typically, a 250–900 library peak was observed, with the highest peak at ~420 bp. Barcoded libraries were pooled equimolarly for sequencing simultaneously for NavaSeq 6000 S4 2 × 150 cycles run as described below. RNA-seq library performed at UF ICBR Gene Expression Core (https://biotech.ufl.edu/gene-expression-genotyping/, accessed on 26 May 2023, RRID:SCR_019145).

4.11. Illumina NovaSeq6000 Sequencing

Normalized libraries were submitted to the "Free Adapter Blocking Reagent" protocol (FAB, Cat# 20024145) to minimize the presence of adaptor dimers and index hopping rates. The library pool was diluted to 0.8 nM and sequenced on one S4 flow cell lane (2 × 150 cycles) of the Illumina NovaSeq6000. The instrument's computer utilized the NovaSeq Control Software v1.6. Cluster and SBS consumables were v1.5. The final loading concentration of the library was 120 pM with 1% PhiX spike-in control. One lane generated 2.5–3 billion paired-end reads (~950 Gb) with an average Q30% $\geq$ 92.5% and Cluster PF = 85.4%. FastQ files were generated using the BCL2fastQ function in the Illumina BaseSpace portal. The Illumina NovaSeq 6000 was used to sequence the libraries for 2 × 150 cycles. Sequencing was performed with ICBR NextGen Sequencing (https://biotech.ufl.edu/next-gen-dna/, RRID:SCR_019152, accessed on 26 May 2023). The data were deposited with the GEO accession number GSE240402.

5. Conclusions

In conclusion, we report the discovery of a C16 monounsaturated fatty acid containing an α,β-unsaturated carbonyl (**1**) for the first time from a benthic marine cyanobacterial mat, in addition to three structurally related analogues (**2–4**). These compounds were previously known from diatoms and algae and may play an important ecological role. The α,β-unsaturated carbonyl motif appeared to be critical for their Nrf2−ARE activity. The relationship of **1** and **2** suggests that oxidation reduction or vice versa can serve as an on/off switch for antioxidant and anti-inflammatory activity. Given the established crosstalk between the Nrf2 and NF-κB pathways, we evaluated the anti-inflammatory potential of **1** in LPS-stimulated mouse macrophages, reducing NO production through a transcriptional mechanism by lowering *iNos* transcript levels. We also demonstrated the effect of **1** on global transcript changes induced by LPS via RNA sequencing and identified additional inflammatory pathways besides the Keap1/Nrf2−ARE pathway modulated by **1**. Transcriptomic analysis identified many additional canonical pathways and regulatory networks linked to inflammation and immune function and related diseases, particularly multiple sclerosis, for which a Nrf2 activator (dimethyl fumarate) is FDA-approved. Our study raises the question of whether therapeutic or preventive effects can be achieved with such oxidized fatty acids. The diversity of organisms producing the compounds allows us to target those that are easiest to grow. While we studied the effects of **1** from a marine cyanobacterium, a previous isolation from the dietary seaweed *Ulva lactuca*, which is easily amenable to culturing, suggests that therapeutic properties could be retrieved through diet or supplementation. This class of α,β-unsaturated carbonyl-containing fatty acids could also serve as chemical probes to aid in understanding the molecular basis underlying several inflammatory and oxidative-stress mediated diseases, where the cytoprotective Keap1/Nrf2−ARE pathway serves as a target.

Supplementary Materials: The following supporting information can be downloaded at: https://www.mdpi.com/article/10.3390/md21110553/s1, ^{1}H NMR, HSQC, HSQC-TOCSY, HMBC, 1D TOCSY for 7(*E*)-9-keto-hexadec-7-enoic acid (**1**) in CDCl$_3$; ^{1}H NMR, HSQC, COSY, HMBC, TOCSY for 7(*E*)-9*S*-hydroxy-hexadec-7-enoic acid (**2**) in CDCl$_3$; ^{1}H NMR, HSQC, band-selective HSQC for 9(*Z*)-hexadec-9-enoic acid (**3**) in CDCl$_3$; ^{1}H NMR spectrum for hexadecanoic acid (**4**) in CDCl$_3$; Table S1: NMR spectral data for 7(*E*)-9*S*-hydroxy-hexadec-7-enoic acid (**2**) and 9(*Z*)-hexadec-9-enoic acid (**3**); Figure S1: ESI-MS/MS spectra for **1**; Figures S2 and S3: HRMS data for (**1–4**); Figure S4: LRMS data for ozonolysis products of **2** and **3**; Figure S5: homonuclear decoupling of **1** and *E*/*Z* commercially available standards; Figure S6: upstream regulator network for LPS; Figure S7: regulator effect networks of the Nrf2 activators.

Author Contributions: Conceptualization: H.L. Sample collection: F.H.A.-A., V.J.P. and H.L. Design of experiments: F.H.A.-A., R.R. and H.L. Performing experiments (chemistry): F.H.A.-A., E.F.S. and N.L. Performing experiments (biology): F.H.A.-A. Writing—original draft preparation: F.H.A.-A. Writing—review and editing: H.L. Project supervision—R.R. and H.L. All authors have read and agreed to the published version of the manuscript.

Funding: This research was supported by the National Institutes of Health (grant R01CA172310) and the Debbie and Sylvia DeSantis Chair professorship (H.L.). F.H.A. is the recipient of the L'Oréal-UNESCO for Women in Science Middle East Regional Young Talents Grant.

Institutional Review Board Statement: Not applicable.

Informed Consent Statement: Not applicable.

Data Availability Statement: Data presented in this study are available within this article and Supplementary Materials.

Acknowledgments: We thank Yanping Zhang from the Gene Expression and Genotyping Core and Fahong Yu from the Bioinformatics Core of the Interdisciplinary Center for Biotechnology Research for RNA sequencing and assistance with data analysis. We acknowledge the Florida Institute of Oceanography for supporting the use of R/V Bellows and the National Park Service for their permission to collect within Dry Tortugas National Park (permit # DRTO-2015-SCI-0008). We thank the Guam Department of Agriculture Division of Aquatic and Wildlife Resources for collection permits.

Conflicts of Interest: H.L. is the co-founder of Algevity Extracts LLC that negotiates licenses for technology related to fatty acid seaweed constituents and their activities.

Sample Availability: Data are included in the article or Supporting Information. Raw data will be made available upon request.

References

1. Furman, D.; Campisi, J.; Verdin, E.; Carrera-Bastos, P.; Targ, S.; Franceschi, C.; Ferrucci, L.; Gilroy, D.W.; Fasano, A.; Miller, G.W.; et al. Chronic Inflammation in the Etiology of Disease across the Life Span. *Nat. Med.* **2019**, *25*, 1822–1832. [CrossRef] [PubMed]
2. Lugrin, J.; Rosenblatt-Velin, N.; Parapanov, R.; Liaudet, L. The Role of Oxidative Stress during Inflammatory Processes. *Biol. Chem.* **2014**, *395*, 203–230. [CrossRef] [PubMed]
3. Hussain, T.; Tan, B.; Yin, Y.; Blachier, F.; Tossou, M.C.B.; Rahu, N. Oxidative Stress and Inflammation: What Polyphenols Can Do for Us? *Oxid. Med. Cell. Longev.* **2016**, *2016*, 7432797. [CrossRef]
4. Wardyn, J.D.; Ponsford, A.H.; Sanderson, C.M. Dissecting Molecular Cross-Talk between Nrf2 and NF-κB Response Pathways. *Biochem. Soc. Trans.* **2015**, *43*, 621–626. [CrossRef]
5. Singh, A.; Kukreti, R.; Saso, L.; Kukreti, S. Oxidative Stress: A Key Modulator in Neurodegenerative Diseases. *Molecules* **2019**, *24*, 1583. [CrossRef] [PubMed]
6. Magesh, S.; Chen, Y.; Hu, L. Small Molecule Modulators of Keap1-Nrf2-ARE Pathway as Potential Preventive and Therapeutic Agents. *Med. Res. Rev.* **2012**, *23*, 687–726. [CrossRef]
7. Egbujor, M.C.; Buttari, B.; Profumo, E.; Telkoparan-Akillilar, P.; Saso, L. An Overview of NRF2-Activating Compounds Bearing α,β-Unsaturated Moiety and Their Antioxidant Effects. *Int. J. Mol. Sci.* **2022**, *23*, 8466. [CrossRef]
8. Liang, S.T.; Chen, C.; Chen, R.X.; Li, R.; Chen, W.L.; Jiang, G.H.; Du, L.L. Michael Acceptor Molecules in Natural Products and Their Mechanism of Action. *Front. Pharmacol.* **2022**, *13*, 1033003. [CrossRef]
9. Hur, W.; Sun, Z.; Jiang, T.; Mason, D.E.; Peters, E.C.; Zhang, D.D.; Luesch, H.; Schultz, P.G.; Gray, N.S. A Small-Molecule Inducer of the Antioxidant Response Element. *Chem. Biol.* **2010**, *17*, 537–547. [CrossRef]
10. Wang, R.; Mason, D.E.; Choe, K.P.; Lewin, A.S.; Peters, E.C.; Luesch, H. In Vitro and in Vivo Characterization of a Tunable Dual-Reactivity Probe of the Nrf2-ARE Pathway. *ACS Chem. Biol.* **2013**, *8*, 1764–1774. [CrossRef] [PubMed]
11. Kanda, H.; Yamawaki, K. Bardoxolone Methyl: Drug Development for Diabetic Kidney Disease. *Clin. Exp. Nephrol.* **2020**, *24*, 857–864. [CrossRef]
12. Boo, Y.C. Natural Nrf2 Modulators for Skin Protection. *Antioxidants* **2020**, *9*, 812. [CrossRef] [PubMed]
13. Bousquet, M.S.; Ratnayake, R.; Pope, J.L.; Chen, Q.Y.; Zhu, F.; Chen, S.; Carney, T.J.; Gharaibeh, R.Z.; Jobin, C.; Paul, V.J.; et al. Seaweed Natural Products Modify the Host Inflammatory Response via Nrf2 Signaling and Alter Colon Microbiota Composition and Gene Expression. *Free Radic. Biol. Med.* **2020**, *146*, 306–323. [CrossRef]

14. Wang, R.; Paul, V.J.; Luesch, H. Seaweed Extracts and Unsaturated Fatty Acid Constituents from the Green Alga *Ulva lactuca* as Activators of the Cytoprotective Nrf2-ARE Pathway. *Free Radic. Biol. Med.* **2013**, *57*, 141–153. [CrossRef] [PubMed]
15. Yadav, P.; Singh, R.P.; Kumar, A.; Singh, P.K.; Gupta, R.K. Therapeutic Potential of Cyanobacteria as a Producer of Novel Bioactive Compounds. In *Cyanobacterial Biotechnology in the 21st Century*; Springer Nature: Singapore, 2023; pp. 237–252.
16. Leão, P.N.; Martins, T.P.; Abt, K.; Reis, J.P.A.; Figueiredo, S.; Castelo-Branco, R.; Freitas, S. Incorporation and Modification of Fatty Acids in Cyanobacterial Natural Products Biosynthesis. *Chem. Commun.* **2023**, *59*, 4436–4446. [CrossRef] [PubMed]
17. Shiels, K.; Tsoupras, A.; Lordan, R.; Zabetakis, I.; Murray, P.; Kumar Saha, S. Anti-Inflammatory and Antithrombotic Properties of Polar Lipid Extracts, Rich in Unsaturated Fatty Acids, from the Irish Marine Cyanobacterium *Spirulina subsalsa*. *J. Funct. Foods* **2022**, *94*, 105124. [CrossRef]
18. Demay, J.; Bernard, C.; Reinhardt, A.; Marie, B. Natural Products from Cyanobacteria: Focus on Beneficial Activities. *Mar. Drugs* **2019**, *17*, 320. [CrossRef]
19. Brumley, D.A.; Gunasekera, S.P.; Sauvage, T.; Dos Santos, L.A.H.; Chen, Q.Y.; Paul, V.J.; Luesch, H. Discovery, Synthesis, and Biological Evaluation of Anaenamides C and D from a New Marine Cyanobacterium, *Hormoscilla* sp. *J. Nat. Prod.* **2022**, *85*, 581–589. [CrossRef]
20. Mascuch, S.J.; Boudreau, P.D.; Carland, T.M.; Pierce, N.T.; Olson, J.; Hensler, M.E.; Choi, H.; Campanale, J.; Hamdoun, A.; Nizet, V.; et al. Marine Natural Product Honaucin A Attenuates Inflammation by Activating the Nrf2-ARE Pathway. *J. Nat. Prod.* **2018**, *81*, 506–514. [CrossRef]
21. Villa, F.A.; Lieske, K.; Gerwick, L. Selective MyD88-Dependent Pathway Inhibition by the Cyanobacterial Natural Product Malyngamide F Acetate. *Eur. J. Pharmacol.* **2010**, *629*, 140–146. [CrossRef]
22. Fontana, A.; D'Ippolito, G.; Cutignano, A.; Romano, G.; Lamari, N.; Gallucci, A.M.; Cimino, G.; Miralto, A.; Ianora, A. LOX-Induced Lipid Peroxidation Mechanism Responsible for the Detrimental Effect of Marine Diatoms on Zooplankton Grazers. *ChemBioChem* **2007**, *8*, 1810–1818. [CrossRef] [PubMed]
23. Moldes-Anaya, A.; Sæther, T.; Uhlig, S.; Nebb, H.I.; Larsen, T.; Eilertsen, H.C.; Paulsen, S.M. Two Isomeric C16 Oxo-Fatty Acids from the Diatom *Chaetoceros karianus* Show Dual Agonist Activity towards Human Peroxisome Proliferator-Activated Receptors (PPARs) α/γ. *Mar. Drugs* **2017**, *15*, 148. [CrossRef] [PubMed]
24. Hung, T.D.; Hye, J.L.; Eun, S.Y.; Shinde, P.B.; Yoon, M.L.; Hong, J.; Dong, K.K.; Jung, J.H. Anti-Inflammatory Constituents of the Red Alga *Gracilaria verrucosa* and Their Synthetic Analogues. *J. Nat. Prod.* **2008**, *71*, 232–240.
25. D'Ippolito, G.; Cutignano, A.; Briante, R.; Febbraio, F.; Cimino, G.; Fontana, A. New C16 Fatty-Acid-Based Oxylipin Pathway in the Marine Diatom *Thalassiosira rotula*. *Org. Biomol. Chem.* **2005**, *3*, 4065–4070. [CrossRef] [PubMed]
26. Santalova, E.A.; Denisenko, V.A. Analysis of the Configuration of an Isolated Double Bond in Some Lipids by Selective Homonuclear Decoupling. *Nat. Prod. Commun.* **2017**, *12*, 1913–1916. [CrossRef]
27. Li, D.; Wu, M. Pattern Recognition Receptors in Health and Diseases. *Signal Transduct. Target. Ther.* **2021**, *6*, 291. [CrossRef]
28. Moreira, L.O.; Zamboni, D.S. NOD1 and NOD2 Signaling in Infection and Inflammation. *Front. Immunol.* **2012**, *3*, 328. [CrossRef]
29. Mukherjee, T.; Hovingh, E.S.; Foerster, E.G.; Abdel-Nour, M.; Philpott, D.J.; Girardin, S.E. NOD1 and NOD2 in Inflammation, Immunity and Disease. *Arch. Biochem. Biophys.* **2019**, *670*, 69–81. [CrossRef] [PubMed]
30. Qian, Y.; Kang, Z.; Liu, C.; Li, X. IL-17 Signaling in Host Defense and Inflammatory Diseases. *Cell. Mol. Immunol.* **2010**, *7*, 328–333. [CrossRef]
31. Ruiz de Morales, J.M.G.; Puig, L.; Daudén, E.; Cañete, J.D.; Pablos, J.L.; Martín, A.O.; Juanatey, C.G.; Adán, A.; Montalbán, X.; Borruel, N.; et al. Critical Role of Interleukin (IL)-17 in Inflammatory and Immune Disorders: An Updated Review of the Evidence Focusing in Controversies. *Autoimmun. Rev.* **2020**, *19*, 102429. [CrossRef]
32. Yi, Y.S.; Son, Y.J.; Ryou, C.; Sung, G.H.; Kim, J.H.; Cho, J.Y. Functional Roles of P38 Mitogen-Activated Protein Kinase in Macrophage-Mediated Inflammatory Responses. *Mediators Inflamm.* **2014**, *2014*, 352371. [CrossRef]
33. Magna, M.; Pisetsky, D.S. The Role of HMGB1 in the Pathogenesis of Inflammatory and Autoimmune Diseases. *Mol. Med.* **2014**, *20*, 138–146. [CrossRef]
34. Tyagi, S.; Gupta, P.; Saini, A.; Kaushal, C.; Sharma, S. The Peroxisome Proliferator-Activated Receptor: A Family of Nuclear Receptors Role in Various Diseases. *J. Adv. Pharm. Technol. Res.* **2011**, *2*, 236. [CrossRef] [PubMed]
35. Crinelli, R.; Antonelli, A.; Bianchi, M.; Gentilini, L.; Scaramucci, S.; Magnani, M. Selective Inhibition of NF-κB Activation and TNF-α Production in Macrophages by Red Blood Cell-Mediated Delivery of Dexamethasone. *Blood Cells Mol. Dis.* **2000**, *26*, 211–222. [CrossRef] [PubMed]
36. Jeon, Y.J.; Han, S.H.; Lee, Y.W.; Lee, M.; Yang, K.H.; Kim, H.M. Dexamethasone Inhibits IL-1β Gene Expression in LPS-Stimulated RAW 264.7 Cells by Blocking NF-κB/Rel and AP-1 Activation. *Immunopharmacology* **2000**, *48*, 173–183. [CrossRef]
37. Kent, L.M.; Smyth, L.J.C.; Plumb, J.; Clayton, C.L.; Fox, S.M.; Ray, D.W.; Farrow, S.N.; Singh, D. Inhibition of Lipopolysaccharide-Stimulated Chronic Obstructive Pulmonary Disease Macrophage Inflammatory Gene Expression by Dexamethasone and the P38 Mitogen-Activated Protein Kinase Inhibitor N-Cyano-N'-(2-{[8-(2,6- Difluorophenyl)-4-(4-Fluoro-2-Methylphenyl)-7-oxo-7,8-dihydropyrido[2,3-d] pyrimidin-2-yl]amino}ethyl)guanidine (SB706504). *J. Pharmacol. Exp. Ther.* **2009**, *328*, 458–468. [PubMed]
38. Zhao, Y.; Shen, X.F.; Cao, K.; Ding, J.; Kang, X.; Guan, W.X.; Ding, Y.T.; Liu, B.R.; Du, J.F. Dexamethasone-Induced Myeloid-Derived Suppressor Cells Prolong Allo Cardiac Graft Survival through INOS- and Glucocorticoid Receptor-Dependent Mechanism. *Front. Immunol.* **2018**, *9*, 282. [CrossRef] [PubMed]

39. Qureshi, A.A.; Tan, X.; Reis, J.C.; Badr, M.Z.; Papasian, C.J.; Morrison, D.C.; Qureshi, N. Inhibition of Nitric Oxide in LPS-Stimulated Macrophages of Young and Senescent Mice by δ-Tocotrienol and Quercetin. *Lipids Health Dis.* **2011**, *10*, 239. [CrossRef]
40. Golde, S.; Coles, A.; Lindquist, J.A.; Compston, A. Decreased INOS Synthesis Mediates Dexamethasone-Induced Protection of Neurons from Inflammatory Injury in Vitro. *Eur. J. Neurosci.* **2003**, *18*, 2527–2537. [CrossRef] [PubMed]
41. Walker, G.; Pfeilschifter, J.; Kunz, D. Mechanisms of Suppression of Inducible Nitric-Oxide Synthase (INOS) Expression in Interferon (IFN)-γ-Stimulated RAW 264.7 Cells by Dexamethasone. Evidence for Glucocorticoid-Induced Degradation of INOS Protein by Calpain as a Key Step in Post-Transcriptional Regulation. *J. Biol. Chem.* **1997**, *272*, 16679–16687.
42. Kunz, D.; Walker, G.; Eberhardt, W.; Pfeilschifter, J. Molecular Mechanisms of Dexamethasone Inhibition of Nitric Oxide Synthase Expression in Interleukin 1β-Stimulated Mesangial Cells: Evidence for the Involvement of Transcriptional and Posttranscriptional Regulation. *Proc. Natl. Acad. Sci. USA* **1996**, *93*, 255–259. [CrossRef] [PubMed]
43. Korhonen, R.; Lahti, A.; Hämäläinen, M.; Kankaanranta, H.; Moilanen, E. Dexamethasone Inhibits Inducible Nitric-Oxide Synthase Expression and Nitric Oxide Production by Destabilizing MRNA in Lipopolysaccharide-Treated Macrophages. *Mol. Pharmacol.* **2002**, *62*, 698–704. [CrossRef]
44. Jeon, Y.J.; Han, S.H.; Lee, Y.W.; Yea, S.S.; Yang, K.H. Inhibition of NF-Kappa B/Rel Nuclear Translocation by Dexamethasone: Mechanism for the Inhibition of INOS Gene Expression. *Biochem. Mol. Biol. Int.* **1998**, *45*, 435–441. [PubMed]
45. Nair, S.; Doh, S.T.; Chan, J.Y.; Kong, A.N.; Cai, L. Regulatory Potential for Concerted Modulation of Nrf2- and Nfkb1-Mediated Gene Expression in Inflammation and Carcinogenesis. *Br. J. Cancer* **2008**, *99*, 2070–2082. [CrossRef] [PubMed]
46. Lee, D.F.; Kuo, H.P.; Liu, M.; Chou, C.K.; Xia, W.; Du, Y.; Shen, J.; Chen, C.T.; Huo, L.; Hsu, M.C.; et al. KEAP1 E3 Ligase-Mediated Downregulation of NF-κB Signaling by Targeting IKKβ. *Mol. Cell* **2009**, *36*, 131–140. [CrossRef]
47. Alcaraz, M.J.; Vicente, A.M.; Araico, A.; Dominguez, J.N.; Terencio, M.C.; Ferrándiz, M.L. Role of Nuclear Factor-κB and Heme Oxygenase-1 in the Mechanism of Action of an Anti-Inflammatory Chalcone Derivative in RAW 264.7 Cells. *Br. J. Pharmacol.* **2004**, *142*, 1191–1199. [CrossRef]
48. Jiménez-Villegas, J.; Ferraiuolo, L.; Mead, R.J.; Shaw, P.J.; Cuadrado, A.; Rojo, A.I. NRF2 as a Therapeutic Opportunity to Impact in the Molecular Roadmap of ALS. *Free Radic. Biol. Med.* **2021**, *173*, 125–141. [CrossRef]
49. Pournajaf, S.; Dargahi, L.; Javan, M.; Pourgholami, M.H. Molecular Pharmacology and Novel Potential Therapeutic Applications of Fingolimod. *Front. Pharmacol.* **2022**, *13*, 352371. [CrossRef]
50. Colombo, E.; Di Dario, M.; Capitolo, E.; Chaabane, L.; Newcombe, J.; Martino, G.; Farina, C. Fingolimod May Support Neuroprotection via Blockade of Astrocyte Nitric Oxide. *Ann. Neurol.* **2014**, *76*, 325–337. [CrossRef]
51. Meng, T.; Xiao, D.; Muhammed, A.; Deng, J.; Chen, L.; He, J. Anti-Inflammatory Action and Mechanisms of Resveratrol. *Molecules* **2021**, *26*, 229. [CrossRef]
52. Abou-ElWafa, G.S.E.; Shaaban, M.; Shaaban, K.A.; El-Naggar, M.E.E.; Laatsch, H. Three New Unsaturated Fatty Acids from the Marine Green Alga *Ulva fasciata* Delile. *Z. Naturforschung B* **2009**, *64*, 1199–1207. [CrossRef]
53. Van der Horst, D.; Carter-Timofte, M.E.; van Grevenynghe, J.; Laguette, N.; Dinkova-Kostova, A.T.; Olagnier, D. Regulation of Innate Immunity by Nrf2. *Curr. Opin. Immunol.* **2022**, *78*, 102247. [CrossRef] [PubMed]
54. Brandes, M.S.; Gray, N.E. NRF2 as a Therapeutic Target in Neurodegenerative Diseases. *ASN Neuro* **2020**, *12*, 1–23. [CrossRef] [PubMed]
55. Michaličková, D.; Hrnčíř, T.; Canová, N.K.; Slanař, O. Targeting Keap1/Nrf2/ARE Signaling Pathway in Multiple Sclerosis. *Eur. J. Pharmacol.* **2020**, *873*, 172973. [CrossRef]
56. Maldonado, P.P.; Guevara, C.; Olesen, M.A.; Orellana, J.A.; Quintanilla, R.A.; Ortiz, F.C. Neurodegeneration in Multiple Sclerosis: The Role of Nrf2-Dependent Pathways. *Antioxidants* **2022**, *11*, 1146. [CrossRef]
57. Hammer, A.; Waschbisch, A.; Kuhbandner, K.; Bayas, A.; Lee, D.H.; Duscha, A.; Haghikia, A.; Gold, R.; Linker, R.A. The NRF2 Pathway as Potential Biomarker for Dimethyl Fumarate Treatment in Multiple Sclerosis. *Ann. Clin. Transl. Neurol.* **2018**, *5*, 668–676. [CrossRef]
58. Al-Awadhi, F.H.; Paul, V.J.; Luesch, H. Structural Diversity and Anticancer Activity of Marine-Derived Elastase Inhibitors: Key Features and Mechanisms Mediating the Antimetastatic Effects in Invasive Breast Cancer. *ChemBioChem* **2018**, *19*, 815. [CrossRef]

Disclaimer/Publisher's Note: The statements, opinions and data contained in all publications are solely those of the individual author(s) and contributor(s) and not of MDPI and/or the editor(s). MDPI and/or the editor(s) disclaim responsibility for any injury to people or property resulting from any ideas, methods, instructions or products referred to in the content.

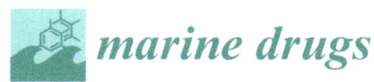

Review

Anti-Inflammatory Effects of Bioactive Compounds from Seaweeds, Bryozoans, Jellyfish, Shellfish and Peanut Worms

Md Khursheed [†], Hardik Ghelani [†], Reem K. Jan and Thomas E. Adrian *

College of Medicine, Mohammed Bin Rashid University of Medicine, and Health Sciences, Dubai P.O. Box 505055, United Arab Emirates; md.khursheed@mbru.ac.ae (M.K.); hardik.ghelani@mbru.ac.ae (H.G.); reem.jan@mbru.ac.ae (R.K.J.)
* Correspondence: thomas.adrian@mbru.ac.ae; Tel.: +971-504472604
† These authors contributed equally to this work.

Abstract: Inflammation is a defense mechanism of the body in response to harmful stimuli such as pathogens, damaged cells, toxic compounds or radiation. However, chronic inflammation plays an important role in the pathogenesis of a variety of diseases. Multiple anti-inflammatory drugs are currently available for the treatment of inflammation, but all exhibit less efficacy. This drives the search for new anti-inflammatory compounds focusing on natural resources. Marine organisms produce a broad spectrum of bioactive compounds with anti-inflammatory activities. Several are considered as lead compounds for development into drugs. Anti-inflammatory compounds have been extracted from algae, corals, seaweeds and other marine organisms. We previously reviewed anti-inflammatory compounds, as well as crude extracts isolated from echinoderms such as sea cucumbers, sea urchins and starfish. In the present review, we evaluate the anti-inflammatory effects of compounds from other marine organisms, including macroalgae (seaweeds), marine angiosperms (seagrasses), medusozoa (jellyfish), bryozoans (moss animals), mollusks (shellfish) and peanut worms. We also present a review of the molecular mechanisms of the anti-inflammatory activity of these compounds. Our objective in this review is to provide an overview of the current state of research on anti-inflammatory compounds from marine sources and the prospects for their translation into novel anti-inflammatory drugs.

Keywords: anti-inflammatory activity; inflammatory pathways; marine drugs; macroalgae; marine seaweeds; bryozoans; medusozoa; mollusks

Citation: Khursheed, M.; Ghelani, H.; Jan, R.K.; Adrian, T.E. Anti-Inflammatory Effects of Bioactive Compounds from Seaweeds, Bryozoans, Jellyfish, Shellfish and Peanut Worms. *Mar. Drugs* 2023, 21, 524. https://doi.org/10.3390/md21100524

Academic Editors: Donatella Degl'Innocenti, Marzia Vasarri and Marc Diederich

Received: 1 September 2023
Revised: 22 September 2023
Accepted: 27 September 2023
Published: 30 September 2023

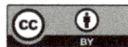

Copyright: © 2023 by the authors. Licensee MDPI, Basel, Switzerland. This article is an open access article distributed under the terms and conditions of the Creative Commons Attribution (CC BY) license (https://creativecommons.org/licenses/by/4.0/).

1. Introduction

The vast diversity of the marine ecosystem ensures the availability of a wide range of bioactive compounds with biological effects in various disease conditions. There is a diverse range of species found in the marine ecosystem. Indeed, 14 out of 35 animal phyla are exclusively found in the marine environment [1]. This variation creates different marine habitats that are hotspots of biodiversity. Moreover, this biodiversity is not constant but is dynamic in nature [2]. Several efforts have been made to make a census of marine biodiversity in different regions of the world so that we can obtain the benefits of region-specific marine biodiversity. These efforts and challenges have previously been reviewed [3].

Marine biodiversity has motivated researchers across the world to investigate novel compounds that may be valuable for the treatment of various disease conditions. Bioactive compounds have been identified and extracted from various marine organisms and shown to be useful in various pathological conditions as described in a recent review [4]. Interestingly, many of these compounds with valuable pharmaceutical properties are in different phases of preclinical and clinical investigation [5]. Bioactive compounds from marine sources have shown immunomodulatory effects [6], activity against diseases such as type 2 diabetes mellitus [7] or anti-cancer properties [8,9]. Many bioactive compounds show anti-inflammatory activity [10,11]. For example, Frondanol is a sea-cucumber-derived intestinal extract that exhibits anti-inflammatory properties in a dextran sodium sulfate (DSS)-induced colitis mouse model [12]. Notably, several marine-derived compounds appear valuable in inflammatory bowel disease (IBD) [13].

Bioactive compounds have distinct chemical and functional properties [14]. In a previous review, we summarized the chemical and anti-inflammatory properties of major bioactive compounds from echinoderms (sea cucumbers, sea urchins, and starfish) [15]. However, there are other major marine species that produce bioactive compounds and few of these are approved for clinical use. The current review summarizes the anti-inflammatory properties of compounds derived from species other than echinoderms.

2. Methods

For this proposed review article preparation, we searched the keywords "Seaweed" + "Anti-inflammatory", "Bryozoans" + "Anti-inflammatory", "Jellyfish" + "Anti-inflammatory", "Shellfish" + "Anti-inflammatory" and "Peanut worm" + "Anti-inflammatory" in PubMed, Scopus, Web of Science, American Chemical Society, Elsevier, MDPI and Springer database from 2010 to 2023. The inclusion criteria encompassed only original research articles published in English between 2010 and 2023 that are thoroughly aligned with the theme of this review article. Updated articles related to the anti-inflammatory activity of bioactive compounds from various marine organisms (seaweed, bryozoan, jellyfish, shellfish and peanut worms) species are summarized and subdivided into subsections similar to those used in our review on anti-inflammatory compounds from echinoderms for the convenience of the reader [15].

3. Seaweed as a Marine Source for Anti-Inflammatory Activity

Seaweed is a popular food source rich in bioactive compounds, polysaccharides, fatty acids, peptides, proteins and vitamins. Seaweeds have several potential therapeutic activities, including anti-bacterial, anti-viral, anti-cancer, antioxidant and anti-inflammatory [16,17]. Seaweeds are classified into three groups based on pigment content; for example, Ochrophyta and Phaeophyceae (brown), Chlorophyta (green) and Rhodophyta (red) seaweeds containing fucoxanthin, chlorophyll A, chlorophyll B, phycocyanin and phycoerythrin [18–20]. The most diverse are the red seaweeds, with more than 7000 species, followed by the brown and green seaweeds, with approximately 2030 and 600 species, respectively [21]. Researchers have been isolating, purifying and screening the secondary metabolites from these organism for bioactivity in recent decades. Here, we summarize the anti-inflammatory activity of compounds isolated from various seaweed species (Figure 1 and Table 1).

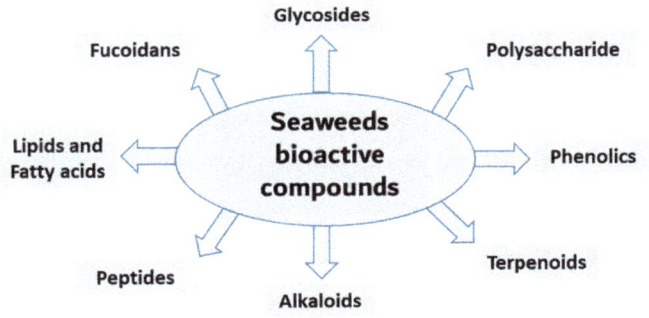

Figure 1. Main classes of seaweed bioactive compounds.

Table 1. Anti-inflammatory bioactive substances derived from seaweed.

Species	Bioactive Compounds/ Extracts/ Purified Compounds	Model	Anti-Inflammatory Activity	Ref.
Eisenia bicyclis	Phlorofucofuroeckol A (compound purified by HPLC and characterized by NMR).	Lipopolysaccharide (LPS)-stimulated RAW 264.7 macrophages.	Suppresses LPS-induced nitric oxide (NO) production at 10 µg/mL. In this study, 10 µM AMT 2-amino-5,6-dihydro-6-methyl-4H-1,3-thiazine was used as a positive control.	[22]
Ecklonia stolonifera	Phlorofucofuroeckol B (compound purified by HPLC and characterized by NMR).	LPS-stimulated microglial cells.	Inhibits secretion of tumor necrosis factor (TNF)-α, interleukin (IL)-1β and IL-6, downregulates the transcription of cycloxygenase (COX)-2 and iNOS synthase, inhibits IκB-α/NF-κB and Akt/ERK/JNK pathways at concentrations of 10 µM–40 µM.	[23]
Ecklonia cava	Dieckol (compound purified by HPLC and characterized by NMR).	LPS-stimulated microglial cells.	Suppresses LPS-induced mRNA expression of inflammatory mediators COX-2 and iNOS and NO production at concentrations 50 µg/mL to 300 µg/mL. Inhibits IL-1β and TNFα production. Reduces mRNA expression of NF-κB and p38 MAPK.	[24]
Ecklonia cava	Dieckol (commercial dieckol is used in this study).	Carrageenan-triggered inflammation in mice.	Dieckol inhibits carrageenan-triggered inflammation, leukocyte infiltration and formation of pro-inflammatory regulators such as TNFα, IL1β, IL6, etc. at dosages from 5 mg/kg–20 mg/kg bodyweight.	[25]
Ishige okamurae	Diphloretho-hydroxycarmalol purified from aqueous methanol extract through HPLC and characterized by NMR.	LPS-induced RAW 264.7 cells and TNF-α-stimulated C2C12 myotubes.	Downregulates mRNA expression of pro-inflammatory cytokines, reduces NO production and reduces protein expression of NF-κB and p38 MAPK at concentration ranges from 6 to 200 µg/mL.	[26]
Ishige okamurae	Diphloretho-hydroxycarmalol purified from aqueous methanol extract through HPLC and characterized by NMR.	LPS-stimulated RAW 264.7 macrophages.	Downregulates IκB-α and NF-κB protein expression and inhibits IL-6 production by downregulating STAT5 activation and SOCS1 augmentation at concentration ranges from 12.5 to 100 µM.	[27]
Ishige foliacea	Octaphlorethol A purified from aqueous ethanolic extract and characterized by LC/MS and NMR.	CpG- stimulated C57BL/6 mice bone-marrow-derived macrophages and bone-marrow-derived dendritic cells.	Exhibits anti-inflammatory activity by octaphlorethol A by transcriptional regulation of NF-κB through MAPK at concentration ranges from 1.5 to 50 µM.	[28]
Saccharina japonica	Fucoidan purified from ethanolic extract by dialysis and HPLC.	LPS-stimulated RAW 264.7 macrophages and LPS-induced zebrafish embryonic cells.	Reduces the production of NO and downregulates the expression of MAPK (including p38, ENK and JNK) and NF-κB (including p65 and IκBα/ IκBβ) signaling pathways at concentration ranges from 12.5 to 50 µg/mL.	[29]

Table 1. Cont.

Species	Bioactive Compounds/ Extracts/ Purified Compounds	Model	Anti-Inflammatory Activity	Ref.
Colpomenia sinuosa	Fucoidan purified from ethanol:formaldehyde:water solvent system through acid extraction and purification.	In vitro NO scavenging assay and RBC hemolysis and PCM-induced hepatic injury in rat.	Prevents paracetamol-induced hepatic oxidative stress and decreases NO, iNOS, TNFα, IL-1β and IL-6 in liver tissue at a concentration of 10 to 50 µg/mL.	[30]
Fucus vesiculosus	Fucoidan from *Fucus vesiculosus* purchased from Sigma.	LPS-stimulated RAW 264.7 macrophages and LPS-induced zebrafish embryonic cells.	Decreases secretion of NO, prostaglandin (PG) E2, TNFα and IL-1β at concentration ranges from 0.5 to 10 µg/mL.	[31]
Fucus vesiculosus	Fucoidan crude hot water extract.	UV-induced inflammation in HaCaT cells.	Decreases production of NO, PGE2, IL-1β and TNFα, and inhibits NF-κB, Akt, ERK, p38 MAPK and JNK pathways regulated by nc886-PKR.	[32]
Sargassum fulvellum	Sulfated polysaccharides purified from ethanolic extract by HPLC.	LPS-stimulated RAW 264.7 macrophages and LPS-induced zebrafish embryonic cells.	Suppresses production of NO, TNFα, IL-1β and IL-6, downregulates expression of iNOS and COX-2 in LPS-stimulated RAW 264.7 cells, improves survival rate and reduces cell death, reactive oxygen species (ROS) and NO in LPS-stimulated zebrafish at concentration ranges from 25 to 100 µg/mL.	[33]
Sargassum horneri	Alginic acid purified from ethanolic extract by HPLC and GC/MS.	LPS-stimulated RAW 264.7 and human haCaT cells and particulate-matter-stimulated inflammation in keratinocytes and fibroblasts	Suppresses PGE2 production via COX-2 inhibition, decreases pro-inflammatory cytokines and abates NF-κB and MAPK pathways in the model system at concentration ranges from 50 to 125 µg/mL.	[34]
Grifola frondosa	Laminarin purified from water extract by dialysis.	LPS-stimulated RAW 264.7 macrophages.	Inhibits NO and PGE2 production, suppresses pro-inflammatory cytokine (TNF-α and IL-6) secretion and inactivates NF-κB pathway at concentration ranges from 50 to 200 µg/mL.	[35]
Padina boryana	Fucosterol purified from ethanolic extract by HPLC.	Particulate matter and LPS-stimulated RAW 264.7 macrophages.	Inactivates NF-kB and MPAK pathways and suppresses iNOS, COX-2, pro-inflammatory cytokines and PGE2 mRNA expression at concentration ranges from 12.5 to 50 µg/mL.	[36]
Stypopodium flabelliforme	Epitaondiol purified from marine metabolite.	In vitro sPLA2 activity, 12-O-tetradecanoylphorbol-13-acetate (TPA)-induced mouse ear edema model.	Inhibits phospholipase A2 production, suppresses eicosanoid (LTB4 and TXB2) release and reduces TPA-induced mouse ear inflammation at approximately 3.8 µM.	[37]

Table 1. Cont.

Species	Bioactive Compounds/ Extracts/ Purified Compounds	Model	Anti-Inflammatory Activity	Ref.
Laurencia glandulifera	Neorogioltriol purified from many solvent fractions by HPLC.	LPS-stimulated RAW 264.7 macrophages, DSS-induced colitis in mice.	Suppresses macrophage activation, promotes M2-like anti-inflammatory phenotype and suppresses DSS-induced colitis by reducing tissue damage and pro-inflammatory cytokine production.	[38]
Dunaliella tertiolecta	Ergosterol purified from lipid extract by HPLC and analyzed by GC/MS.	LPS- and ConA-stimulated sheep peripheral blood mononuclear cells.	Inhibits pro-inflammatory cytokines (TNF-α, IL-6, IL-1β and IL-10) production at concentration of 0.2 to 0.8 mg/mL.	[39]
Sargassum muticum	Apo-9′-fucoxanthinone.	LPS-stimulated RAW 264.7 macrophages and LPS-induced zebrafish embryonic cells.	Suppresses mRNA expression of inflammatory mediators such as iNOS, COX-2 and pro inflammatory cytokines, and modulates NF-κB and MPAK signaling pathways	[40]
Amansia multifida	Lectin purified by sodium salt extraction and HPLC.	Carrageenan-triggered inflammation models in rat.	Reduces parameters of the inflammatory process such as edema formation and leukocyte migration, and modulates levels of proinflammatory cytokines, IL-1β and TNF-α.	[41]
Bryothamnion triquetrum	Lectin.	Carrageenan-triggered inflammation in rat.	Inhibits vascular and cellular events of an acute inflammatory response, and inhibits neutrophil migration to inflammation sites via suppression of TNF-α and IL-1β production at different concentrations in different models.	[42]
Ulva spp.	Peptide fractions purified from enzyme hydrolysate and characterized by FPLC.	LPS and ConA-stimulated rat spleen mononuclear cells.	Modulates TLR4 and the NFκB/p38/JNK pathway at 0.01 g/L to 0.1g/L.	[43]
Caulerpa peltata, Caulerpa racemosa	Caulerpin purified from ethanolic extract and crystalized from liquid portioning.	DSS-induced colitis in mice.	Reduces inflammatory infiltrates and the levels of the proinflammatory cytokines, increases the levels of the anti-inflammatory cytokine IL-10 and suppresses NF-κB p65 expression.	[44]
Gracilaria opuntia	Azocinyl morpholinone alkaloid purified from ethanol:methanol extract by HPLC.	Carrageenan-triggered inflammation in rat. In vitro anti-inflammatory model using 5-LOX inhibition assay.	Reduces edema formation by 6 h and exhibits a selective inhibitory effect on COX-2 and 5-LOX activity at a concentration of approximately 0.08 mg/mL.	[45]
Ulva pertusa	3-Hydroxy-4,7-megastigmadien-9-one purified from aqueous ethanol extract by MPLC.	CpG-stimulated C57BL/6 mice bone-marrow-derived dendritic cells.	Inhibits IL-12 p40, IL-6 and TNF-α production and blocks MAPKs and NF-κB pathways at concentration ranges from 0.1 to 50 μM.	[46]

Table 1. Cont.

Species	Bioactive Compounds/ Extracts/ Purified Compounds	Model	Anti-Inflammatory Activity	Ref.
Laelia undulata	Floridoside purified from methanolic extract by thin-layer chromatography.	LPS-stimulated BV-2 microglia cells.	Inhibits the production of NO and ROS and downregulates the protein and gene expression levels of iNOS and COX-2 by significantly blocking the phosphorylation of p38 and ERK in LPS-stimulated BV-2 cells at concentration ranges from 10 to 50 µM.	[47]
Cymopolia barbata	Cymopol and cyclocymopol purified from various non-polar extract through HPLC.	DSS-induced colitis in mice, zebrafish tail wound model and RAW 264.7 macrophages.	Attenuates neutrophil migration and reduces the colon inflammation at the in vitro concentration of 1 to 3 µM and 0.1 to 0.4 g/kg body weight.	[48]
Sargassum siliquastrum	Sargachromanol G isolated from aqueous methanol and other solvent and then purified from HPLC.	LPS- and RANKL-stimulated RAW 264.7 macrophages	Reduces the expression of pro-inflammatory cytokines, suppresses NO and PGE2 production via inhibition of iNOS and COX-2 and inhibits RANKL-induced activation of NF-κB by suppressing RANKL-mediated IκB-α degradation at concentration ranges from 10 to 40 µM.	[49,50]

3.1. Anti-Inflammatory Phenolic Compounds from Seaweed

Phenolic compounds are secondary metabolites that are found in many natural extracts and are known for their antioxidant potential. Seaweed is also a rich source of various phenolic compounds, such as flavonoids and tannins, obtained by different extraction methods [49–51]. As shown in Figure 2, many categories of phenolic compounds are obtained from seaweeds [51]. The best-studied phenolic compounds are phlorotannins, which exhibit anti-inflammatory effects in addition to other biological activities [52]. A methanol extract of the brown seaweed *Eisenia bicyclis* and its CH_2Cl_2 sub-fraction have potent anti-inflammatory effects in LPS-stimulated RAW 264.7 macrophages by inhibiting NO production [22]. Fucosterol, purified through column chromatography from the CH_2Cl_2 sub-fraction also decreases NO production via the suppression of iNOS expression [22]. Furthermore, the ethyl acetate sub-fraction of the methanolic extract and chromatographic sub-fractions 1-6 yielded phlorofucofuroeckol A (Figure 2A), eckol, dieckol, phlorofucofuroeckol-A, dioxinodehydroeckol and 7-phloroeckol, which also inhibit NO production in a dose-dependent manner in LPS-stimulated macrophages [22]. Interestingly, similar sub-fractions were extracted from an ethanolic extract and its ethyl acetate sub-fraction from another seaweed, *Ecklonia cava* [53]. These also resulted in significant decreases in the expression of IL1β, IFNγ and interferon stimulatory gene (SGI15) in the olive flounder animal model [53]. The related phlorotannin, phlorofucofuroeckol B (PFFB) (Figure 2B), was isolated and chromatographically purified using NMR from an ethanol extract of the brown algae *Ecklonia stolonifera* [23]. PFFB suppressed the inflammatory response in LPS-stimulated BV2 microglial cells by downregulating the PGE_2, TNF-α, IL-1β and IL-6 [23]. Furthermore, this study demonstrated that the inhibition of inflammation is via the downregulation of IκB-α/NF-κB mediated by Akt/ERK/JNK pathways [23]. Dieckol (Figure 2C) was isolated from a methanol extract of *Ecklonia cava* powder, with diethyl sub-fractionation, chromatographic purification and NMR characterization [24]. Dieckol decreased NO production via the suppression of iNOS and COX-2 and also inhibited the generation of proinflammatory cytokines IL-1β and TNF-α through suppressing the activation of NF-κB and p38 MAPK in LPS-induced microglial cells [24]. Furthermore, a study using commercially available dieckol revealed the inhibition of carrageenan-triggered inflammation and leukocyte infiltration and reduced pro-inflammatory cytokines (TNF-α, IL-1β, and IL-6) in a mouse model [25]. A recent study demonstrated an increased production of NO and ROS in LPS-treated zebrafish embryos following treatment of an ethyl acetate fraction from *Ecklonia maxima*, which included dieckol [54]. Another compound, diphlorethohydroxycarmalol (DPHC) (Figure 2D), was isolated and purified from the edible brown seaweed *Ishige okamurae*. DPHC suppressed the production of IL-6 via the inhibition of phosphorylation and translocation of NF-κB in LPS-stimulated RAW 264.7 macrophages [27]. Cytokine signaling 1 (SOCS1) suppression functions as a negative feedback regulator of Janus kinase (Jak)-signal transducer and activator of transcription (STAT) signaling [27]. DPHC downregulated STAT5 and upregulated SOCS1 in macrophages [27]. DPHC attenuated several inflammatory symptoms (ear edema, lymph node size, serum IgE level and mast cell infiltration) in an experimental atopic dermatitis-induced inflammatory mouse model [27]. In another study, DPHC purified from the same seaweed also reduced the expression of pro-inflammatory cytokines and suppressed muscle RING-finger protein (MuRF)-1 and muscle atrophy F-box (MAFbx)/atrgoin-1 in LPS-induced RAW 264.7 macrophages [26]. These protein complexes are well known in muscle atrophy via NF-κB and MAPK signaling pathways in TNF-α-stimulated C2C12 myotubes [26]. This study also showed DPHC docking in the TNFα inhibitory site in a simulation [26]. Another interesting compound, octaphlorethol A (Figure 2E), is a phenolic compound isolated from the ethanolic extract, purified from chromatography and further characterized by LC/MS and NMR, belonging to *Ishige foliacea*, which inhibits pro-inflammatory cytokines, MAPK and NF-κB pathways in CpG oligodeoxynucleotides (CpG)-stimulated primary murine bone-marrow-derived macrophages and dendritic cells [28].

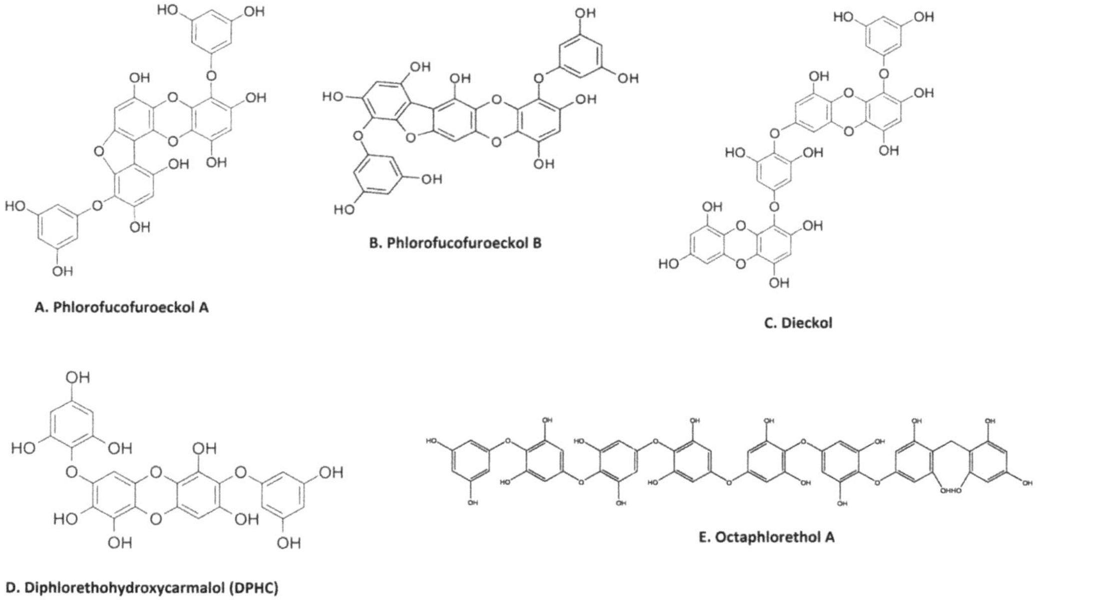

Figure 2. Major anti-inflammatory phenolic compounds isolated from seaweeds (**A**). Phlorofucofuroeckol A from *Eisenia bicyclis*; [22] (**B**). phlorofucofuroeckol B from *Ecklonia stolonifera* [23]; (**C**). dieckol from *Ecklonia cava* [24]; (**D**). diphlorethohydroxycarmalol (DPHC) from *Ishige okamurae* [27]; (**E**) octaphlorethol A from *Ishige foliacea* [55] (structures reproduced with permission from the publisher).

3.2. Anti-Inflammatory Polysaccharides from Seaweed

Polysaccharides are major components of seaweed that have attracted much attention because of various health benefits [11,56]. Sulfated seaweed polysaccharides show significant anti-inflammatory activity in several inflammatory models [57]. The major compounds are alginic acid and fucoidans, which have various biological effects reflecting their chemical diversity [58] as shown in Figure 3. These compounds are major anti-inflammatory components of seaweed polysaccharides. For example, brown seaweed *Sachharina japonica*-derived fucoidan galactofucan (Figure 3A) demonstrated anti-inflammatory activity by reducing the production of NO and the expression of MAPK (including p38, ENK and JNK) and NF-κB (including p65 and IKKα/IKKβ) signaling pathways in endotoxin-stimulated RAW 264.7 macrophages [29]. Similarly, sulfated fucoidan (Figure 3B) isolated from *Colpomenia sinuosa* prevented oxidative stress and inflammation in the paracetamol-induced hepatic injury and inflammation rat model, as evidenced by suppressing the hepatic levels of thiobarbituric acid reactive substances, NO, iNOS, TNF-α, IL-1β and IL-6 while increasing glutathione and glutathione peroxidase enzyme activity [30]. Fucoidan, extracted from *Fucus vesiculosus*, inhibited LPS-induced inflammatory responses in RAW 264.7 macrophages and zebrafish larvae by suppressing NO and PGE2 secretion via iNOS and COX-2 inhibition as well as reducing the expression and secretion of TNF-α and IL-1β [31]. An ethanol fraction of the hot water extract from the edible seaweed *Laminaria japonica* (which contains abundant fucoidan) suppressed the production of PGE_2 and expression of MMP-9, COX-2 and pro-inflammatory cytokines in the UV-induced inflammation model of the human keratinocyte (HaCaT) cell line [32]. Interestingly, Nagahwatta et al. purified sulfated fucoidan from the leaves of *Ecklonia maxima* and demonstrated a reduction in proinflammatory cytokines such as PGE2, NO, TNFα IL6 and IL1β in RAW 264.7 macrophages [59]. Furthermore, a recent study revealed that fucoidan had a curative effect mediated by the downregulation of the aryl hydrocarbon receptor and phosphodiesterase 4 in an ulcerative colitis rat model [60]. More recently, sulfated polysaccharides (Figure 3C) isolated from the edible brown seaweed *Sargassum fulvellum* significantly and concentration-dependently decreased the production of the inflammatory mediators NO, PGE2, TNF-α, IL-1β and IL-6, and suppressed the expression of COX-2 and iNOS in LPS-stimulated RAW 264.7 macrophages [33]. Furthermore, these sulfated polysaccharides improve survival and decrease cell death, ROS production and NO levels in LPS-stimulated zebrafish [33]. Another recent study showed the anti-inflammatory effect of a sulfated polysaccharide extracted from *Codium fragile*. This study demonstrated the reduction in PGE2, NO, IL1β, IL6 and TNFα in LPS-induced RAW 264.7 macrophages [61]. The sulfation of seaweed-derived low-molecular-weight fucoidans increases the potency of their anti-inflammatory properties [62]. In contrast, the non-sulfated polysaccharide, alginic acid (Figure 3D), from *Padina boryana*, showed marked anti-inflammatory activity in particulate-matter-stimulated inflammation in human HaCaT immortalized keratinocytes and dermal fibroblasts (HDF) [63]. Alginic acid reduced PGE_2 and COX-2 and inflammatory cytokines (IL-1β and IL-6) via the suppression of the NF-κB and MAPK pathways [63]. Alginic acid, purified from *Sargassum wightii*, demonstrated anti-inflammatory potential in adjuvant-induced arthritic rats by reducing paw edema and COX, lipoxygenase (LOX) and myeloperoxidase levels [64]. Furthermore, it also reduced the levels of COX-2, IL-6 and TNF-α and inhibited certain key molecular mediators (such as p-p38 MAPK, P-Erk1/2 and P-JNK) of the NF-κB and MAPK pathways in Chinese fine dust (CFD)-treated HaCaT cells [34]. β-Linked polysaccharides, including β-glucans, are known to possess immunomodulatory and anti-proliferative activities. Laminarin, a water-soluble β-glucan isolated from *Grifola frondose*, reduced NO and PGE2 production and suppressed the secretion of pro-inflammatory cytokines via the downregulation of NF-κB in endotoxin-stimulated macrophages [35].

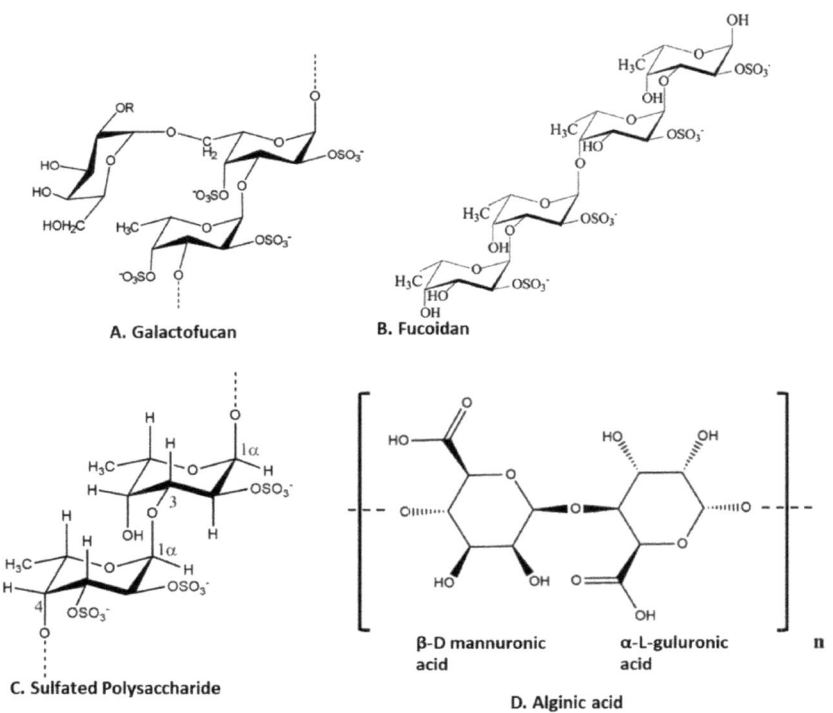

Figure 3. Structure of anti-inflammatory polysaccharides isolated from seaweeds. (**A**). Galactofucans or G-Fucoidan [65]; (**B**). fucoidan found in brown algae [66]; (**C**): sulfated polysaccharides in brown algae [67]; (**D**). alginic acid from brown algae [63] (structures reproduced with permission from the publisher).

3.3. Anti-Inflammatory Terpenoids from Seaweed

Terpenoids are the largest group of natural products with specialized secondary metabolites [68]. These naturally occurring chemical compounds are highly diverse in chemical structure [68]. Although many biological activities of plant-derived terpenoids have been reported, there are several marine-source-based terpenoids that have been isolated and screened for their biological activity in the last few decades [69]. Fucosterol, epitaondiol, neorogioltriol, pacifenol, ergosterol and 7-dehydroporiferasterol, pheophytin A and apo-9′-fucoxanthinone are a few potent anti-inflammatory terpenoids isolated from various species of seaweed [69]. For example, fucosterol (Figure 4A), isolated from *Padina boryana*, reduced particulate matter (PM)-induced inflammation in macrophages by modulating the NF-κB and MAPK pathways [36]. It significantly suppressed the expression of inflammatory mediators such as iNOS, COX-2, pro-inflammatory cytokines and PGE2 [36]. Epitaondiol isolated from various seaweeds, inhibited COX pathway activity. For example, epitaondiol (Figure 4B), isolated from *Stypopodium flabelliforme*, inhibited the production of phospholipase A2 and eicosanoids (LTB4 and TXB2) and modulated the COX pathway in the in vitro isolated human neutrophils and the 12-O-Tetradecanoylphorbol-13-acetate (TPA)-induced mouse ear oedema model [37]. Neorogioltriol (Figure 4C), and two related diterpene neorogioldiol and O11,15-cyclo-14-bromo-14,15-dihydrorogiol-3,11-diol, were isolated from a red algae *Laurencia glandulifera* [38]. These compounds exhibit anti-inflammatory effects in M2-type macrophages via an increased expression of arginase1, MRC1, IRAK-M and the transcription factor C/EBPβ [38]. The anti-inflammatory activity of neorogioldiol and O11,15-cyclo-14-bromo-14,15-dihydrorogiol-3,11-diol was also demonstrated in a DSS-induced colitis mice model where they reduced tissue damage and pro-inflammatory cytokine production in vivo. Ergosterol (Figure 4D) and 7-dehydroporiferasterol (Figure 4E) derivatives, isolated from *Dunaliella tertiolecta*, suppressed pro-inflammatory cytokines in sheep peripheral blood mononuclear cells stimulated with LPS [39]. Apo-9-fucoxanthinone (AF), isolated from *Sargassum muticum*, showed potent anti-inflammatory activity in LPS-stimulated macrophages by suppressing the mRNA expression of several inflammatory mediators, such as iNOS, COX-2 and pro-inflammatory cytokines [40]. These effects of AF are mainly due to the modulation of NF-κB and MPAK signaling pathways [40].

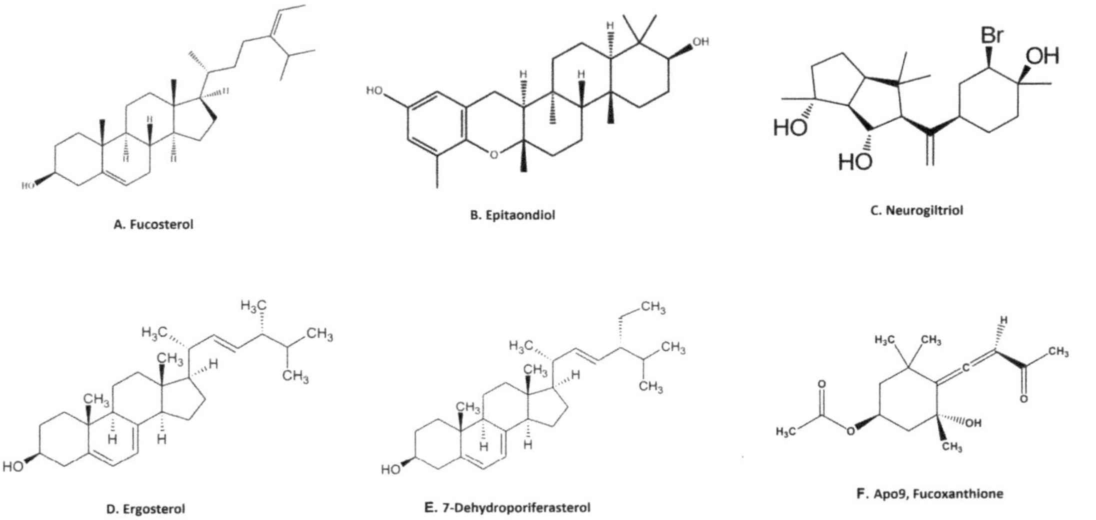

Figure 4. Structure of anti-inflammatory terpenoid extracted from seaweed. (**A**). Fucosterol [36]; (**B**). epitaondiol [37]; (**C**). neurogiltriol [38]; (**D**). ergosterol [39]; (**E**). 7-dehydroporiferasterol [39]; (**F**). Apo9, fucoxanthione [40] (structures reproduced with permission from the publisher).

3.4. Anti-Inflammatory Proteins and Peptides from Seaweed

Lectins, isolated from seaweed, are glycoproteins involved in cellular adhesion. Some of these lectins have anti-inflammatory activity. A 30 kDa lectin derived from *Amansia multifida* has anti-inflammatory effects, reducing edema formation in a paw edema model, leukocyte migration and oxidative stress in a carrageenan-induced peritonitis model and proinflammatory cytokine (IL-1β and TNF-α) expression in a carrageenan-induced rat paw edema model [41]. Another study demonstrated the anti-inflammatory effects of a 9kDa lectin isolated from *Bryothamnion triquetrum* [42]. This lectin inhibited the production of proinflammatory cytokines involved in the migration of neutrophils in a carrageenan-induced peritonitis mice model [42]. These findings suggest that the anti-inflammatory effects of this lectin are mediated by the inhibition of leukocyte recruitment [42]. In another study, a mucin-binding hololectin isolated from red marine algae demonstrated anti-nociceptive and anti-inflammatory responses, reducing abdominal writhing and the paw-licking time in carrageenan-induced peritonitis and paw edema models [70]. Hololectin caused a similar inhibition of neutrophil migration in a peritonitis model and also suppressed paw edema, which was induced by carrageenan, dextran or serotonin [70]. A big anti-inflammatory effect (23–44 kDa) from the green seaweed *Caulerpa cupressoides* revealed a decrease in carrageenan-induced rat paw edema and neutrophil infiltration via a reduction in the expression of IL-1, IL-6, TNF-α and COX-2 [71]. Lectins from red algae and their other potential biomedical applications have been previously summarized in the review [72]. Only a limited number of papers reporting the anti-inflammatory activity of lectins from green seaweeds have been published. However, lectins from red and green algae have distinct structures [73]. A recent review documented the structural diversity among various algal species [73]. The authors classified the lectins from red and brown algae as *Oscillatoria agardhii* agglutinin homolog (OAAH) and the green seaweed as *Galanthus nivalis* agglutinin (GNA) [73]. A study on the structural features of N-glycans of seaweed glycoproteins was performed on 15 economically important seaweeds (12 red and brown seaweeds, 2 green seaweeds and 1 sea grass) [74]. Interestingly, this study revealed the absence of typical plant-based lectins with a complex structure of N-glycans (β1-2 xylosyl and α 1-3 fucosyl) in algae and seagrass [74]. Moreover, the study showed the absence of high manose-type N-glycan (M5–M9) in the green seaweed *Ulva pertusa* [74]. A study on peptide fractions of approximately 2160 kDa from green seaweed *Ulva* spp. showed it exerting immunomodulatory actions in vitro, consistent with an anti-inflammatory effect depending on Toll-like receptor 4 (TLR4) and the NFκB/p38/JNK pathway [43].

3.5. Anti-Inflammatory Alkaloids from Seaweed

Anti-inflammatory alkaloids are commonly found in plants, but there are limited studies identifying and characterizing the activity of such compounds from seaweeds [75]. Only limited studies have investigated the anti-inflammatory effects of seaweed alkaloids [75]. Caulerpin (Figure 5A) is an indole alkaloid with anti-inflammatory activity isolated from several different species of seaweed [76]. This compound is one of the main products in a study of the anti-inflammatory effect of methanolic extracts from *Caulerpa racemosa* [76]. Caulerpin reduced inflammation in DSS-induced ulcerative colitis, where it suppressed inflammatory infiltration and reduced the levels of colonic proinflammatory cytokines (IL-6, IL-17, TNF-α and IFN-γ) while increasing the expression of the anti-inflammatory cytokine IL-10 [44]. These effects of caulerpin were accompanied by a reduction in the expression of NF-κB p65, suggesting that the anti-inflammatory effects are mediated by blocking the activation of NF-κB [44]. Anti-inflammatory alkaloids forming red algae of the genus *Gracilaria* have been identified [77]. An aqueous extract containing polyphenols, flavonoids and ascorbic acid from *Gracilaria tenuistipitata* had anti-inflammatory activity in a hepatitis C virus model [78]. Treatment with this extract inhibited COX-2 activity, the synthesis of PGE$_2$, nuclear translocation of NF-κB p65 and expression of TNF-α, IL-1β and iNOS in HCV-infected cells [78]. Fractions of a methanol extract, analyzed by mass spectroscopy, from *Gracilaria changii* reduced the expression of TNF-α and IL-6 in phorbol 12-myristate 13-acetate (PMA)-stimulated U937 cells [79]. An anti-inflammatory alkaloid, azocinyl morpholinone (Figure 5B), isolated from *Gracilaria opuntia* selectively inhibited COX-2 and 5-LOX activity and thereby reduced inflammation in a murine carrageenan-induced paw edema model [45].

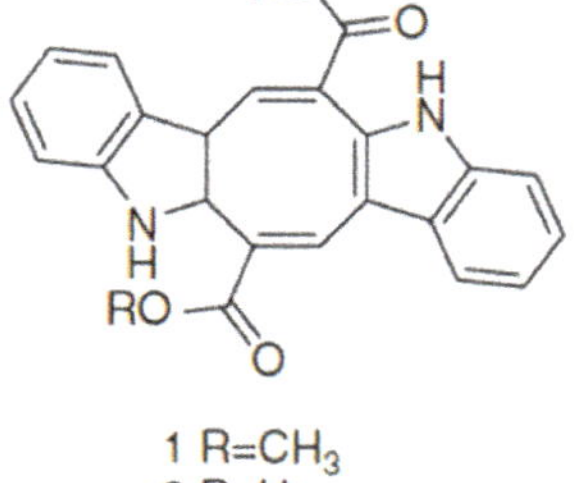

A. Caulerpin

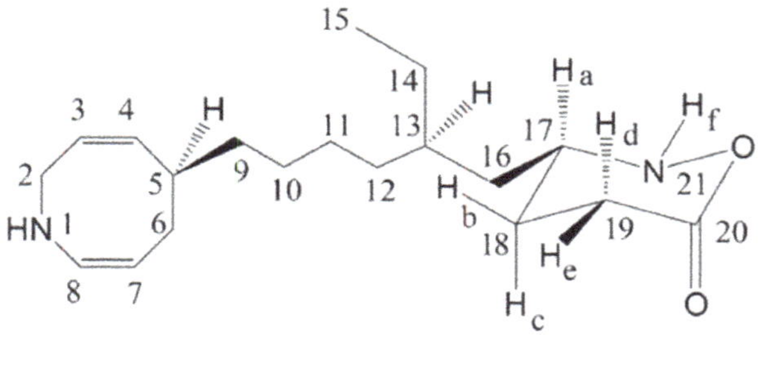

1 R=CH$_3$
2 R=H

B. Azocinyl morpholinone

Figure 5. Structure of anti-inflammatory alkaloids: (**A**). caulerpin [80]; (**B**). azocinyl morpholinone [45] (structures reproduced with permission from the publisher).

3.6. Other Anti-Inflammatory Compounds from Seaweed

3-Hydroxy-4,7-megastigmadien-9-one isolated from *Ulva pertusa* markedly inhibits interleukin (IL)-12 p40, IL-6 and TNF-α cytokine production [46]. The compound exhibits anti-inflammatory activity through the inhibition of MAPK by the dephosphorylation of ERK1/2, JNK12 and p38, as well as inhibition of the NF-κB pathway by the dephosphorylation of IκBα in CpG-stimulated bone-marrow-derived dendritic cells [46]. This study also demonstrated that the compound downregulates the TLR9 promoter activity through AP1 and NF-κB [46]. Floridoside (Figure 6A) is another anti-inflammatory compound derived from Laelia undulata, and inhibits the production of NO and ROS in LPS-stimulated BV2 microglial cells [47]. This study demonstrated the floridoside-mediated downregulation of iNOS and COX-2 by blocking the phosphorylation of p38 and ERK in LPS-stimulated BV-2 cells [47]. A non-polar extract from *Cymopolia barbata* and its primary active component cymopol (Figure 6B) were analyzed for their anti-inflammatory properties [48]. Purified cymopol upregulates the Nrf2 transcription activity and reduces the expression of proinflammatory genes such as iNOS, COX2, PGE2 and Nqo1 with an expected reduction of NO in macrophages and mouse embryonic fibroblasts in an Nrf2-dependent manner [48]. Cymopol-containing extracts also attenuate neutrophil migration in a zebrafish tail wound model [48] and reduce DSS-induced colitis, as measured by fecal lipocalin concentration [48]. Further analysis of DSS-induced mice treated with a cymopol fraction and the non-polar extract through RNA-seq revealed the enrichment of mucosal-associated microbiome genera [48]. Another compound sargachromanol G (Figure 6C), isolated by chromatography from *Sargassum siliquastrum*, reduces the expression of pro-inflammatory cytokines (TNF-α, IL-1β and IL-6) and also suppresses inflammatory markers such as NO and PGE2 production via the inhibition of iNOS and COX-2 in RAW 264.7 cells [81]. A study of sargachromanol G on osteoclast differentiation revealed the inhibition of the receptor activator of the NF-κB ligand (RANKL)-induced activation of NF-κB by suppressing RANKL-mediated IκB-α degradation [82]. The study further explored the mechanism of action of sargachromanol G and demonstrated the inhibition of mitogen-activated protein kinases (p38, JNK and ERK) in RANKL-stimulated RAW 264.7 macrophages [82]. A recent study showed anti-inflammatory activity of an ethanol extract of *Sargassum siliquastrum* in RAW 264.7 cells by the inhibition of NO and proinflammatory cytokines such as TNFα and IL-6 [83]. Further studies are needed to explore these anti-inflammatory active agents responsible.

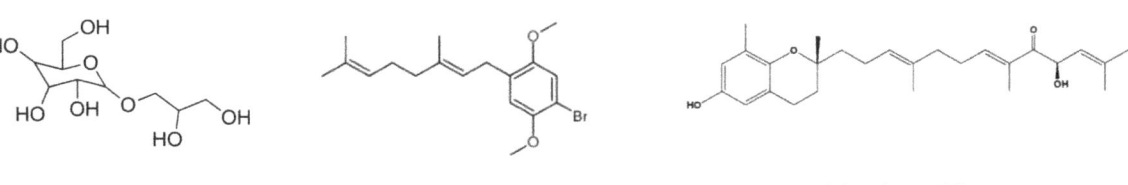

Figure 6. Structure of few important anti-inflammatory compounds from seaweed: (**A**). floridoside from *Laelia undulata* [84]; (**B**). cymopol from *Cymopolia barbata* [48]; (**C**). sargachromanol G from *Sargassum siliquastrum* [81] (structures reproduced with permission from the publisher).

4. Bryozoans as Marine Source for Anti-Inflammatory Activity

Marine bryozoans are a diverse group of invertebrates, inhabiting everywhere from intertidal waters to deep seas in both tropical and polar regions [85]. Diverse species of bryozoans are found in the North Sea, the United Kingdom, the northern Mediterranean and Adriatic, North Pacific around Japan, New Zealand and Antarctica [86]. Bryozoans produce bioactive compounds that are an important source of bioactive compounds important for their development as drugs [87]. They have attracted attention due to the discovery of the remarkable anti-neoplastic activity of bryostatins [88]. A host of secondary metabolites, including alkaloids, sphingolipids, sterols, macrocyclic lactones, other tetracyclic terpenoid lactones and sulfur-containing aromatic compounds, have been isolated from bryozoans [87]. However, in our search for the anti-inflammatory activity of bioactive compounds isolated from marine bryozoans for this review, we found only five papers (Table 2). Two major chemical classes, macrocyclic lactones (bryostatin-1) and alkaloids (convolutamydine A and bromotryptamine) isolated from various species of bryozoan, have been evaluated for anti-inflammatory activity [88]. Bryostatins are macrocyclic lactones first isolated and characterized from Bugula neritina [88]. In a study, around 21 bryostatins were isolated and studied; however, bryostatin (bryos-1) (Figure 7A) has received the most attention from the scientific community as a therapeutic option in several inflammatory diseases [89]. For example, bryos1 has been extensively evaluated as a drug of choice for multiple sclerosis (MS) [90]. The characteristic etiology of MS involves inflammation and myelin damage, which involves multiple steps, including the overexpression of pro-inflammatory cytokines, induction of oxidative stress, overexpression and high levels of activity of matrix metalloproteases (MMPs) and loss of the blood–brain barrier (BBB), which ultimately lead to the immune-mediated destruction of neuronal myelin damage and neuronal degeneration [90]. Bryos-1 was reviewed as a target of multiple MMPs, including MMP 1, 3, 9, 10 and 11, in various models [91]. Moreover, the downregulation of MMP-9 expression and its activation by Bryos-1 reduced hemorrhagic transformation followed by ischemia–reperfusion injuries in an aged female rats model [92]. Bryos-1 also demonstrated an increase in the IL-4-induced expression of the anti-inflammatory marker arginase-1, as well as tissue repair promoting the M2 macrophage phenotype in murine peritoneal macrophages [93]. Similar to its effect on dendritic cells, bryos-1 suppresses the production of pro-inflammatory cytokines (IL-12 and IL-6) while increasing the production of the anti-inflammatory cytokine (IL-10) [94]. A recent study demonstrated the anti-neuroinflammatory effects of the bryos-1 analogue, bryologs, both in vitro and in vivo [95]. In contrast to anti-inflammatory activity, bryos-1 enhances proinflammatory effects by increasing CCL2, IL-10, TNFα, etc., in the context of the analysis of bryos-1 as a latency-reversing agent in HIV pathophysiology [96].

Similarly, bryos-1 also demonstrated to be effectively anti-inflammatory during carcinogenesis. For example, bryos-1 downregulated COX-2 mRNA expression in the mucosa of 1,2-dimethylhydrazine (DMH)-induced colorectal carcinogenesis in rats [93]. Furthermore, it induces the anti-inflammatory phenotype of macrophages and antigen-presenting cells (APCs) [93]. It upregulates the CD86 protein, which is required for the activation of T cells upon their binding to APCs in bone-marrow-derived dendritic cells (BMDCs) [93]. Moreover, recently, the Food and Drug Administration (FDA) approved bryos-1 as an orphan drug in combination therapy with paclitaxel for the treatment of esophageal carcinoma [97].

Convolutamydine A (Figure 7B), an oxindole alkaloid isolated from marine bryozoan species *Amathia convoluta*, was evaluated for anti-inflammatory activity. Convolutamydine A and its two analogues (ISA003 and ISA147) inhibit the formalin-induced licking response at doses as low as 10 μg/kg. These compounds also inhibit leukocyte migration and the production of NO, PGE2 and inflammatory cytokines (IL-6 and TNF-α) in the subcutaneous air pouch (SAP) model of carrageenan-induced inflammation. Furthermore, convolutamydine A and the two analogues reduce NO and PGE2 production by the downregulation of COX-2 and iNOS in cultured macrophages [98]. Recently, Di et.al isolated 13 new bromotryptamines (Figure 7C) and two new imidazole alkaloids (Figure 7D) from the bryozoan Flustra foliacea and evaluated their in vitro anti-inflammatory activity [99]. Several of these newly isolated alkaloids, flustramine Q, flustramine S, flustramine U, Nα-methyldeformylflustrabromine, 6-bromo-N, N-dimethyltryptamine, 6-bromoindole-3-carbaldehyde and deformylflustrabromine B, decreased the dendritic cell secretion of the pro-inflammatory cytokine IL-12 p40 while flustrimidazole A and flustramine T increased the secretion of the anti-inflammatory cytokine IL-10 in monocyte-derived dendritic cells [99].

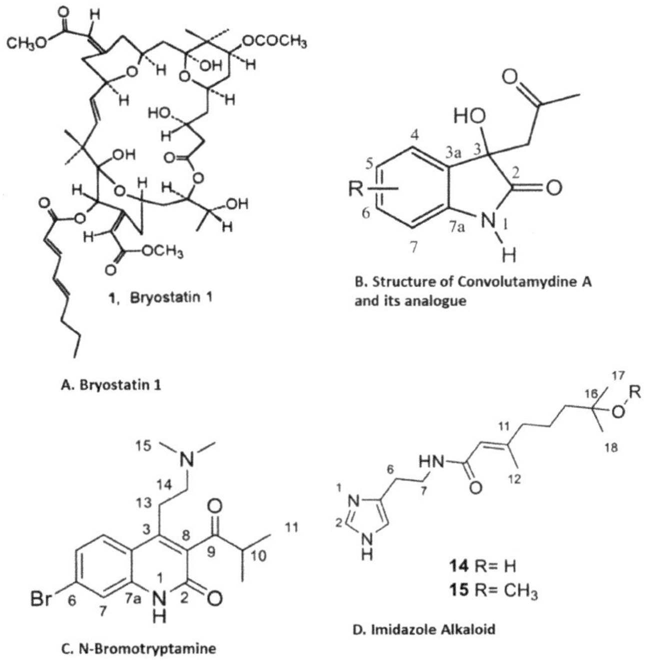

Figure 7. Structure of anti-inflammatory compounds extracted from bryzoans: (**A**). bryostatin 1 [88]; (**B**). convolutamydine A [98]; (**C**). N-bromotryptamine [99]; (**D**). imidazol alkaloids [99] (structures reproduced with permission from the publisher).

Table 2. Anti-inflammatory substances derived from bryozoans.

Species	Bioactive Compounds/ Extracts/ Purified Compound	Model Controls	Anti-inflammatory Activity	Ref.
Bugula neritina	Bryostatin-1 purified and procured from Sigma.	DMH-induced colorectal carcinogenesis in rat as positive control and infection with *Syphacia muris*.	Downregulates COX-2 mRNA expression in colorectal mucosa at 5 µg/kg body weight for 4 weeks.	[93]
	Purified bryostatin-1 procured from Tocris.	Stimulated macrophages, antigen-presenting cells and bone-marrow-derived dendritic cells.	Activates T cell via upregulation of CD86. Increases IL-4-induced expression of arginase-1 and increases M2 macrophages. Suppresses production of pro-inflammatory cytokines (IL-12 and IL-6) while increasing the production of anti-inflammatory cytokine (IL-10) at concentration ranges from 20 to 200 nM.	[94]
	Purified bryostatin-1.	Acute cerebral ischemia in aged rat model. R-tPA is used as a positive control.	Suppresses MMP-9 by upregulating PKCε at 2.5 mg/kg body weight.	[92]

Table 2. *Cont.*

Species	Bioactive Compounds/ Extracts/ Purified Compound	Model Controls	Anti-inflammatory Activity	Ref.
Amathia convolute	Isatin converted by acetome and dienthlamine at room temperature to convolutamydine A.	Carrageenan-induced inflammation model. LPS-stimulated macrophages.	Suppresses leucocyte migration, reduces the production of NO and PGE2 by downregulating iNOS and COX-2 and decreases IL-6 and TNF-α production at 0.1 to 10 mg/kg body weight.	[98]
Flustra foliacea	Bromotryptamine and imidazole alkaloids purified through chromatography and characterized by NMR.	Monocyte-derived dendritic cells.	Decreases pro-inflammatory cytokine IL-12p40 and increases secretion of the anti-inflammatory cytokine IL-10 at 10 µg/mL.	[99]

5. Anti-Inflammatory Compounds from Jellyfish

In the past, jellyfish have elicited unpleasant sentiments in European culture, while they are regarded as a valuable source of bioactive substances and are utilized in traditional food and medicine on the Asian continent [100]. In addition to their nutritional and medicinal benefits in the Chinese pharmacopeia, jellyfish have recently been designated as a novel food in Western countries due to their unexploited source of important nutrients, novel bioactive metabolites and lead compounds [100]. In the last decade, extracts derived from different species of jellyfish have been evaluated for pharmacological properties. Despite this, our literature search for anti-inflammatory activities of bioactive compounds isolated from jellyfish produced only limited results (Table 3). Polysaccharides isolated from the jellyfish *Rhopilema esculentum* modulate oxidative stress and inflammation in the DSS-induced colitis model in mice [101]. These polysaccharides reduced myeloperoxidase (MPO) activity, levels of pro-inflammatory cytokines and NO levels in mice with colitis [101]. The polysaccharides also downregulate the NF-κB signaling pathway in colonic tissue, as evident by reducing the phosphorylation of p65 and IKB [101]. Bile salt (Figure 8A) derivatives isolated from a fungus (*Penicillium chrysogenum* J08NF-4), which specifically grows on the jellyfish *Nemopilema nomurai*, demonstrated a suppression of the NO level in LPS-stimulated RAW 264.7 macrophages [102]. Interestingly, the study also shows the downregulation of many proinflammatory molecules, including iNOS and TNF-α [102]. Molecular docking studies revealed that one these bile salt derivates, a bile salt trifluoroacetate, has a ligand-binding domain for the PPARγ receptor that activates PPARγ and suppresses the phosphorylation of the NF-κB p65 subunit, leading to the downregulation of pro-inflammatory mediators [102]. Monoterpene derivatives (Figure 8B) isolated from the same fungus also exhibit PPARγ receptor agonistic activity in molecular docking studies and also suppress PPARγ-mediated inflammatory markers in Ac2F liver cells [103]. A recent study showed anti-inflammatory properties of collagen hydrolysate from jellyfish in a high-fat diet mice model. This study demonstrated the reduction in proinflammatory cytokines such as TNFβ, IL1β and IL6 [104].

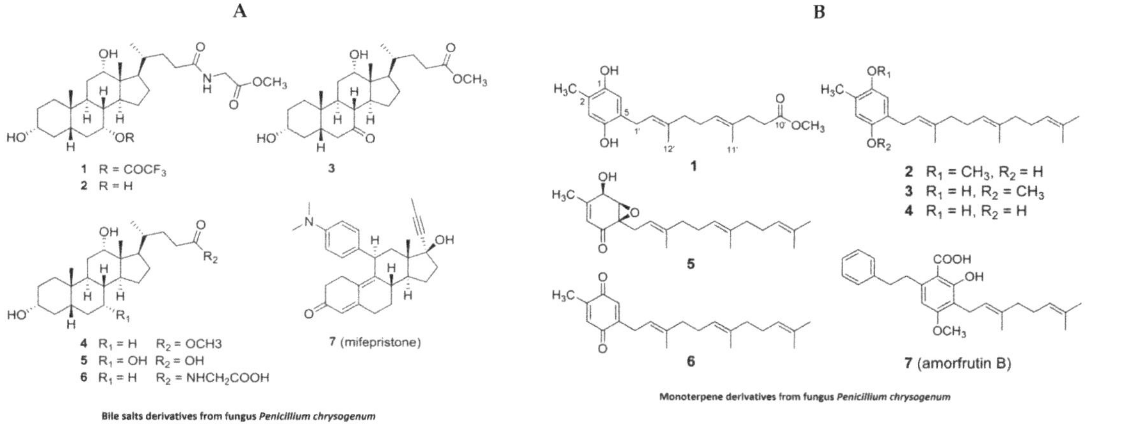

Figure 8. Structure of anti-inflammatory bile salts and monoterpenes derivative from jellyfish: (**A**). bile salts derivatives [102]; (**B**). monoterpene derivatives from jellyfish fungus penicillium chrysogenum [103] (structures reproduced with permission from the publisher).

6. Anti-Inflammatory Compounds from Shellfish

Shellfish constitute a major seafood component [105]. Common subgroups of shellfish are crustaceans, bivalves (mollusks), gastropods (univalves) and cephalopods [105]. Important crustaceans are prawns, shrimp, lobster, crab and krill. Bivalves (two shells) include clam, mussel, oyster and scallops [105]. Univalves (single shell) include cockle, whelk, limpet, abalone and snail. While cephalopods lack an external shell, they are also considered to be shellfish, and this group includes octopus, cuttlefish and squid [105]. Shellfish foods have a high nutrition value, as shown by a high protein digestibility and corrected amino acid score [105]. They are also rich in Omega 3 fatty acids, carotenoids and vitamins [105]. In addition to their high nutritive value, shellfish are also considered as a valuable source of nutraceutical compounds [105]. Here, we summarize the anti-inflammatory activities of bioactive compounds isolated from shellfish, including mussels, clams and other mollusks [106] (Table 3). A novel peptide (EGLLGDVF) isolated and characterized from the green mussel *Perna viridis* has potent anti-inflammatory activity, inhibiting the production of pro-inflammatory cytokines, reducing the activation of NO and COX-2 and downregulating iNOS and COX-2 expression in LPS-stimulated RAW 264.7 macrophages [107]. Similarly, high-molecular-weight peptides isolated from the blue mussel *Mytilus edulis* exhibited marked anti-inflammatory activity, modulating NF-κB and MAPK pathways in LPS-stimulated RAW 264.7 macrophages [108]. *Mytilus coruscus* is a Korean hard-shelled mussel that is heavily exploited for food. Various bioactive compounds (peptides and lipids) from this mussel have been isolated and tested for their anti-inflammatory potential. A novel peptide consisting of 10 amino acid residues (GVSLLQQFFL) was isolated, which effectively blocks NO production in LPS-stimulated RAW 264.7 macrophages [109]. A high-molecular-weight α-d-Glucan named MP-A, also isolated from this hard-shelled mussel, exerts anti-inflammatory activity in LPS-stimulated THP1 cells by inhibiting cytokine production and suppressing iNOS and COX-2 expression via TLR4/NF-κB/MAPK pathway inhibition [110]. A lipid extract from this hard-shelled mussel increases the production of the anti-inflammatory cytokine (IL-10) and suppresses pro-inflammatory cytokines via the downregulation of toll-like receptor (TLR-4) signaling in a lipopolysaccharide (LPS)-challenged mouse model [111]. The lipid extract of this hard-shelled mussel also showed anti-inflammatory activity in adjuvant-induced (AIA) and collagen-induced arthritis (CIA) in rat models, suppressing markers of inflammation such as leukotriene B4 (LTB4), prostaglandin E2 (PGE2) and thromboxane B2 (TXB2) in the ankle joint synovial fluid of treated rats [112]. Green-lipped mussels (*Perna canaliculus*) are heavily cultivated in New Zealand. The oil fractions Lyprinol and Cadalmin from green-lipped mussels are promoted as functional foods with numerous health benefits [113]. These lipid fractions markedly suppressed iNOS and COX-2 and downregulated inflammatory cytokine genes via the inhibition of the NF-κB/MAPK pathways in LPS-stimulated RAW 264.7 murine macrophages [113]. A clinical trial of Lyprinol (PSCOl524) showed a beneficial effect on the bronchoconstriction of 24 asthma patients [114]. Recently, an interesting research article isolated a peptide from the Asiatic hard clam *Meretrix meretrix* and tested its anti-inflammatory potential [115]. The isolated 6 amino acid peptide (HKGQCC) significantly inhibited NO, COX-2, TNF-α and IL-1β in LPS-stimulated RAW 264.7 cells [115]. The in vitro digestion of this peptide resulted in the generation of a tetrapeptide (GQCC) that further downregulates inflammatory gene expression in an LPS-stimulated zebrafish model [115]. The abalone (*Haliotis discus hannai*) is a large marine gastropod mollusk that is a valuable seafood product [116]. An 11-amino-acid peptide (EMDEAQDPSEW) isolated from abalone has potent anti-inflammatory activity by inhibiting MAPK and NF-κB signaling pathways in human fibrosarcoma (HT1080) cells [116]. Phenoloxidase (PO), purified from the hemolymph of the dietary shellfish *Haliotis discus hannai*, has anti-inflammatory effects on LPS-induced HT 29, reducing levels of pro-inflammatory cytokines, including IL4, IL5 and IFNγ and PGE$_2$ [117]. In a recent study, three lipid fractions (neutral lipids, glycolipids and phospholipids) from the eggs of a common dietary shellfish *Ammodytes personates* downregulated proinflammatory cytokines in an LPS-induced RAW 264.7 macrophage model. The downregulation of NFkB signaling through MAPK signaling pathways was also seen [118].

Table 3. Anti-inflammatory substances derived from jellyfish and shellfish.

Marine Source	Species	Bioactive Compounds/ Extracts/Purified	Model	Anti-Inflammatory Activity	Ref.
Jellyfish	*Rhopilema esculentum*	Skin polysaccharide and monosaccharide composition analysis.	DDS-induced colitis mice model.	Reduces MPO activity, pro-inflammatory cytokines and NO levels. Downregulates NF-κB at 50 and 100 mg/kg bodyweight.	[101]
	Nemopilema nomurai Penicillium chrysogenum J08NF-4	Bile acid derivates and monoterpene purified from fungal strain through HPLC.	LPS-stimulated RAW 264.7 cells.	Suppresses production of cytokines. Activates PPARγ-mediated NF-κB inhibition at 10 to 50 μM.	[102,103]
Shellfish	*Perna viridis* (Green mussel)	Peptide (EGLLGDVF) purified of about 850 Da.	LPS-stimulated RAW 264.7 cells.	Suppresses pro-inflammatory cytokines. Downregulates iNOS and COX-2.	[107]
	Mytilus edulis (Blue mussel)	Peptide fraction obtained from enzyme hydrolysate.	LPS-stimulated RAW 264.7 macrophages.	Inhibits the NF-κB/MPAK signaling pathway at concentration ranges from 50 to 200 μg/mL.	[108]
	Mytilus coruscus (Korean hard-shelled mussel)	Peptide (GVSLLGGPPL) purified and characterized from enzyme hydrolysate.	LPS-stimulated RAW 264.7 cells.	Reduces NO production.	[109]
	Mytilus coruscus (Korean hard-shelled mussel)	Lipid extract (HMLE).	Adjuvant-induced and collagen-induced arthritis.	Suppresses markers of inflammation such as LTB4, PGE2 and TXB2 in ankle joint synovial fluid.	[112]

Table 3. Cont.

Marine Source	Species	Bioactive Compounds/ Extracts/Purified	Model	Anti-Inflammatory Activity	Ref.
Jellyfish	*Mytilus coruscus* (Korean hard-shelled mussel)	Lipid extract (HMLE) and analyzed by gas chromatography.	LPS-challenged MS Dowley rats model using adjuvant-induced arthritis as positive control.	Increases the production of IL-10 and suppresses IL-1, IL-6 and TNF-α via downregulation of TLR-4 signaling pathways at 100mg/kg body weight.	[111]
	Mytilus coruscus (Korean hard-shelled mussel)	α-d-Glucan (MP-A) purified by chromatography obtained.	THP1 differentiated by PMA and then stimulated by LPS.	Inhibits cytokine production, downregulates iNOS and COX-2 and inhibits TLR4/NF-κB/MAPK pathway at 10 to 200 μg/mL.	[110]
	Perna canaliculus (Green-lipped mussel)	Oil fraction (GLMO) purified form obtained.	LPS-stimulated RAW 264.7 cells.	Inhibits iNOS and COX-2. Downregulates cytokine gene expression via NF-κB/MAPK pathway at 50 to 300 μg/mL.	[113]
	Meretrix meretrix (Clam)	Peptide (HK and GQCC) purified from enzyme hydrolysate through HPLC.	Human blood in vitro assays, LPS-stimulated RAW 264.7 cells and zebrafish.	Inhibits NO, NO, TNF-α, IL-1β and COX-2 at 50 to 250 μg/mL.	[115]
	Haliotis discus hannai (Mollusk)	Peptide purified and characterized of approximately 1234.41 Da.	PMA-challenged human fibrosarcoma (HT1080) cells.	Inhibits MMPs expression via modulation of MAPK and NF-κB pathway at 50 and 100 μM.	[116]

7. Anti-Inflammatory Compounds Derived from Peanut Worms

Peanut worms are a class of unsegmented marine annelids commonly found in marine benthic ecosystems and used as a functional food in many places, including South China and the Philippines [119]. Many compounds with anti-inflammatory activity have been identified in peanut worm species [119] (Table 4). For example, a study reported the anti-inflammatory activity of an aqueous extract from the body wall of *Sipunculus nudus* in different rat and mouse models such as a carrageenan-induced rat paw oedema model, Dextran-induced rat paw oedema model, cotton-pellet-induced chronic inflammation granuloma rat model, carrageenan-induced peritonitis mouse model, xylene-induced ear oedema model and acetic-acid-induced vascular permeability mice model [120]. In another study, the researchers established the presence of hydrophobic amino-acid-rich peptides within the collagen fraction of the peanut worm *Sipunculus nudus* [121]. They demonstrated the anti-inflammatory function of a novel peptide mediated through a reduction of nitric oxide (NO) in LPS-stimulated RAW 264.7 macrophages [121]. Furthermore, the authors confirmed the inhibitory effect of peptides on the mRNA expression of iNOS, TNFα, IL6 and COX-2 [121]. Another research group from China identified a similar peptide fraction of peanut worm powder [122]. They demonstrated the peptide-mediated induction of skin wound healing function in mice within four days of a wound and complete healing within 28 days [122]. Furthermore, they established that the wound-healing property of these peptides is mediated by a reduction in the expression of proinflammatory cytokines such as TNFα and IL1β [122]. The peptides also had anti-scar activity due to the reduction in TGFβ1 mRNA [122]. Another important species of peanut worm is *Phascolosoma esculenta*, commonly used as a functional food in China [123]. An oligosaccharide fraction extracted from this species by enzymatic hydrolysis has anti-inflammatory effects in an *Escherichia coli*-induced sepsis mouse model via a reduction in the expression of the proinflammatory cytokines TNFα and IL1β and an enhanced expression of IL10 [123].

Table 4. Anti-inflammatory compounds derived from peanut worms.

Marine Source	Species	Bioactive Compounds/Extracts/ Purified	Model	Anti-Inflammatory Activity and Dose	Ref.
Peanut worms	Sipunculus nudus	Hot water extract.	Carragenan-induced rat paw oedema model, DSS-induced rat paw oedema model, etc.	Paw edema is reduced by 50–60% within 4h in the test models at concentration of 200 mg/kg body weight.	[120]
	Phascolosoma esculenta	Oligosaccharide was purified from body wall by enzymatic hydrolysis Sephadex column chromatography. Characterized by mass spec.	Anti-inflammatory mice sepsis model used through intraperitoneal injection of E. coli.	Reduces IL1β and TNFα and enhanced anti-oxidant enzyme activity at a dose of 10 to 50 mg/kg body weight	[123]
	Sipunculus nudus	Anti-inflammatory peptides were purified from peanut worm powder through enzymatic as well as HPLC and sequenced by Q-TOF-ESI-MS/MS. Same peptides were synthesized in the laboratory.	LPS-induced RAW 264.7 macrophages.	Reduces IL1β and TNFα, and also decreases the expression of iNOS. Decreases the level of NO production at dose ranges from 30 to 120 mM.	[121]
	Sipunculus nudus	Collagen peptides were purified from coelomic wall by enzyme hydrolysis and then characterized through SDS and FTIR. Amino acid composition and molecular weight distribution were also determined.	In vitro and in vivo wound healing models were tested.	Enhances wound healing by reducing excessive inflammation in skin of mice through decreasing IL1β and TNFα by using SNCP ointment (2 g/mL).	[122]

8. Conclusions and Future Perspective

Marine biodiversity provides a promising resource for pharmacology. Seaweeds are a major source of bioactive compounds with potent anti-inflammatory effects. Major categories of seaweed-derived bioactive compounds include phenolic compounds, polysaccharides, glycoproteins, polypeptides, terpenoids and alkaloids. These compounds strongly inhibit lipoxygenases and cyclooxygenases and decrease the ROS and NOS levels. Moreover, these compounds also downregulate proinflammatory cytokines such as IL6 and TNFα through the inhibition of NF-κB pathways. Bryozoans provide another rich source of marine pharmaceutical compounds. Compounds from these organisms include bryostatin-1, which exhibits strong anti-inflammatory activity. Jellyfish and shellfish provide a major marine resource widely used for food and as nutraceuticals. However, some of them have been investigated and this has revealed multiple bioactive compounds, including bile acids, monoterpenes, lipids and peptides, with anti-inflammatory activity. This review covers the anti-inflammatory activity of bioactive compounds from seaweed, bryozoans, jellyfish and shellfish. It complements our previous review of anti-inflammatory compounds from echinoderms. These reviews can serve as a source of summarized information for standardizing marine sources and developing analytical methods to quantify anti-inflammatory compounds. By integrating these approaches, we can develop safer and more effective anti-inflammatory agents from marine sources. New technologies and close collaborations between institutional and industrial investigators are crucial for the development of marine-derived bioactive compounds to be successful as novel therapeutics in treating or preventing chronic diseases.

Funding: Supported in part by funding from Mohammed Bin Rashid University of Medicine and Health Sciences and from the Jalila Foundation.

Acknowledgments: This work was supported in part by Mohammed Bin Rashid University of Medicine and Health Sciences (MBRU) and the Al Jalila Foundation for Post-Doctoral Research Fellowship awards to H.G. and M.K.

Conflicts of Interest: The authors have no conflict of interest.

References

1. Sala, E.; Knowlton, N. Global Marine Biodiversity Trends. *Annu. Rev. Environ. Resour.* **2006**, *31*, 93–122. [CrossRef]
2. Renema, W.; Bellwood, D.R.; Braga, J.C.; Bromfield, K.; Hall, R.; Johnson, K.G.; Lunt, P.; Meyer, C.P.; McMonagle, L.B.; Morley, R.J.; et al. Hopping hotspots: Global shifts in marine biodiversity. *Science* **2008**, *321*, 654–657. [CrossRef]
3. Costello, M.J.; Coll, M.; Danovaro, R.; Halpin, P.; Ojaveer, H.; Miloslavich, P. A Census of Marine Biodiversity Knowledge, Resources, and Future Challenges. *PLoS ONE* **2010**, *5*, e12110. [CrossRef]
4. Mayer, A.M.S.; Guerrero, A.J.; Rodríguez, A.D.; Taglialatela-Scafati, O.; Nakamura, F.; Fusetani, N. Marine Pharmacology in 2016–2017: Marine Compounds with Antibacterial, Antidiabetic, Antifungal, Anti-Inflammatory, Antiprotozoal, Antituberculosis and Antiviral Activities; Affecting the Immune and Nervous Systems, and Other Miscellaneous Mechanisms of Action. *Mar. Drugs* **2021**, *19*, 49. [PubMed]
5. Papon, N.; Copp, B.R.; Courdavault, V. Marine drugs: Biology, pipelines, current and future prospects for production. *Biotechnol. Adv.* **2022**, *54*, 107871. [CrossRef]
6. Montuori, E.; de Pascale, D.; Lauritano, C. Recent Discoveries on Marine Organism Immunomodulatory Activities. *Mar. Drugs* **2022**, *20*, 422. [CrossRef] [PubMed]
7. Egbuna, C.; Awuchi, C.G.; Kushwaha, G.; Rudrapal, M.; Patrick-Iwuanyanwu, K.C.; Singh, O.; Odoh, U.E.; Khan, J.; Jeevanandam, J.; Kumarasamy, S.; et al. Bioactive Compounds Effective Against Type 2 Diabetes Mellitus: A Systematic Review. *Curr. Top. Med. Chem.* **2021**, *21*, 1067–1095. [CrossRef]
8. Alves, C.; Diederich, M. Marine Natural Products as Anticancer Agents. *Mar. Drugs* **2021**, *19*, 447. [CrossRef] [PubMed]
9. Khalifa, S.A.M.; Elias, N.; Farag, M.A.; Chen, L.; Saeed, A.; Hegazy, M.-E.F.; Moustafa, M.S.; Abd El-Wahed, A.; Al-Mousawi, S.M.; Musharraf, S.G.; et al. Marine Natural Products: A Source of Novel Anticancer Drugs. *Mar. Drugs* **2019**, *17*, 491. [CrossRef]
10. Suleria, H.A.R.; Gobe, G.; Masci, P.; Osborne, S.A. Marine bioactive compounds and health promoting perspectives; innovation pathways for drug discovery. *Trends Food Sci. Technol.* **2016**, *50*, 44–55. [CrossRef]
11. Li, C.-Q.; Ma, Q.-Y.; Gao, X.-Z.; Wang, X.; Zhang, B.-L. Research Progress in Anti-Inflammatory Bioactive Substances Derived from Marine Microorganisms, Sponges, Algae, and Corals. *Mar. Drugs* **2021**, *19*, 572. [CrossRef] [PubMed]
12. Subramanya, S.B.; Chandran, S.; Almarzooqi, S.; Raj, V.; Al Zahmi, A.S.; Al Katheeri, R.A.; Al Zadjali, S.A.; Collin, P.D.; Adrian, T.E. Frondanol, a Nutraceutical Extract from Cucumaria frondosa, Attenuates Colonic Inflammation in a DSS-Induced Colitis Model in Mice. *Mar. Drugs* **2018**, *16*, 148. [CrossRef] [PubMed]
13. Bilal, M.; Nunes, L.V.; Duarte, M.T.S.; Ferreira, L.F.R.; Soriano, R.N.; Iqbal, H.M.N. Exploitation of Marine-Derived Robust Biological Molecules to Manage Inflammatory Bowel Disease. *Mar. Drugs* **2021**, *19*, 196. [CrossRef] [PubMed]
14. Karthikeyan, A.; Joseph, A.; Nair, B.G. Promising bioactive compounds from the marine environment and their potential effects on various diseases. *J. Genet. Eng. Biotechnol.* **2022**, *20*, 14. [CrossRef] [PubMed]
15. Ghelani, H.; Khursheed, M.; Adrian, T.E.; Jan, R.K. Anti-Inflammatory Effects of Compounds from Echinoderms. *Mar. Drugs* **2022**, *20*, 693. [CrossRef]
16. El-Beltagi, H.S.; Mohamed, A.A.; Mohamed, H.I.; Ramadan, K.M.A.; Barqawi, A.A.; Mansour, A.T. Phytochemical and Potential Properties of Seaweeds and Their Recent Applications: A Review. *Mar. Drugs* **2022**, *20*, 342. [CrossRef]
17. Lomartire, S.; Gonçalves, A.M.M. An Overview of Potential Seaweed-Derived Bioactive Compounds for Pharmaceutical Applications. *Mar. Drugs* **2022**, *20*, 141. [CrossRef]
18. Chye, F.Y.; Ooi, P.W.; Ng, S.Y.; Sulaiman, M.R. Fermentation-Derived Bioactive Components from Seaweeds: Functional Properties and Potential Applications. *J. Aquat. Food Prod. Technol.* **2018**, *27*, 144–164. [CrossRef]
19. Ghosh, R.; Banerjee, K.; Mitra, A. Eco-Biochemical Studies of Common Seaweeds in the Lower Gangetic Delta. In *Handbook of Marine Macroalgae, Biotechnology and Applied Phycology*; John Wiley & Sons, Ltd.: New York, NY, USA, 2011; pp. 45–57.
20. Mišurcová, L. Chemical composition of seaweeds. In *Handbook of Marine Macroalgae: Biotechnology and Applied Phycology*; John Wiley & Sons, Ltd.: New York, NY, USA, 2011; pp. 171–192.
21. Kumar, Y.; Tarafdar, A.; Badgujar, P.C. Seaweed as a Source of Natural Antioxidants: Therapeutic Activity and Food Applications. *J. Food Qual.* **2021**, *2021*, 5753391. [CrossRef]
22. Jung, H.A.; Jin, S.E.; Ahn, B.R.; Lee, C.M.; Choi, J.S. Anti-inflammatory activity of edible brown alga Eisenia bicyclis and its constituents fucosterol and phlorotannins in LPS-stimulated RAW264.7 macrophages. *Food Chem. Toxicol.* **2013**, *59*, 199–206. [CrossRef]
23. Yu, D.K.; Lee, B.; Kwon, M.; Yoon, N.; Shin, T.; Kim, N.G.; Choi, J.S.; Kim, H.R. Phlorofucofuroeckol B suppresses inflammatory responses by down-regulating nuclear factor κB activation via Akt, ERK, and JNK in LPS-stimulated microglial cells. *Int. Immunopharmacol.* **2015**, *28*, 1068–1075. [CrossRef]

24. Jung, W.K.; Heo, S.J.; Jeon, Y.J.; Lee, C.M.; Park, Y.M.; Byun, H.G.; Choi, Y.H.; Park, S.G.; Choi, I.W. Inhibitory Effects and Molecular Mechanism of Dieckol Isolated from Marine Brown Alga on COX-2 and iNOS in Microglial Cells. *J. Agric. Food Chem.* **2009**, *57*, 4439–4446. [CrossRef]
25. Li, Z.; Wang, Y.; Zhao, J.; Zhang, H. Dieckol attenuates the nociception and inflammatory responses in different nociceptive and inflammatory induced mice model. *Saudi J. Biol. Sci.* **2021**, *28*, 4891–4899. [CrossRef]
26. Kim, S.Y.; Ahn, G.; Kim, H.S.; Je, J.G.; Kim, K.N.; Jeon, Y.J. Diphlorethohydroxycarmalol (DPHC) Isolated from the Brown Alga Ishige okamurae Acts on Inflammatory Myopathy as an Inhibitory Agent of TNF-α. *Mar. Drugs* **2020**, *18*, 529. [CrossRef] [PubMed]
27. Kang, N.J.; Han, S.C.; Kang, G.J.; Koo, D.H.; Koh, Y.S.; Hyun, J.W.; Lee, N.H.; Ko, M.H.; Kang, H.K.; Yoo, E.S. Diphlorethohydroxycarmalol inhibits interleukin-6 production by regulating NF-κB, STAT5 and SOCS1 in lipopolysaccharide-stimulated RAW264.7 cells. *Mar. Drugs* **2015**, *13*, 2141–2157. [CrossRef] [PubMed]
28. Manzoor, Z.; Mathema, V.B.; Chae, D.; Kang, H.K.; Yoo, E.S.; Jeon, Y.J.; Koh, Y.S. Octaphlorethol A Inhibits the CpG-Induced Inflammatory Response by Attenuating the Mitogen-Activated Protein Kinase and NF-κB Pathways. *Biosci. Biotechnol. Biochem.* **2013**, *77*, 1970–1972. [CrossRef] [PubMed]
29. Chen, X.; Ni, L.; Fu, X.; Wang, L.; Duan, D.; Huang, L.; Xu, J.; Gao, X. Molecular Mechanism of Anti-Inflammatory Activities of a Novel Sulfated Galactofucan from Saccharina japonica. *Mar. Drugs* **2021**, *19*, 430. [CrossRef] [PubMed]
30. Atya, M.E.; El-Hawiet, A.; Alyeldeen, M.A.; Ghareeb, D.A.; Abdel-Daim, M.M.; El-Sadek, M.M. In vitro biological activities and in vivo hepatoprotective role of brown algae-isolated fucoidans. *Environ. Sci. Pollut. Res.* **2021**, *28*, 19664–19676. [CrossRef]
31. Jeong, J.-W.; Hwang, S.J.; Han, M.H.; Lee, D.-S.; Yoo, J.S.; Choi, I.-W.; Cha, H.-J.; Kim, S.; Kim, H.-S.; Kim, G.-Y.; et al. Fucoidan inhibits lipopolysaccharide-induced inflammatory responses in RAW 264.7 macrophages and zebrafish larvae. *Mol. Cell. Toxicol.* **2017**, *13*, 405–417. [CrossRef]
32. Lee, K.S.; Cho, E.; Weon, J.B.; Park, D.; Fréchet, M.; Chajra, H.; Jung, E. Inhibition of UVB-Induced Inflammation by Laminaria japonica Extract via Regulation of nc886-PKR Pathway. *Nutrients* **2020**, *12*, 1958. [CrossRef]
33. Wang, L.; Yang, H.-W.; Ahn, G.; Fu, X.; Xu, J.; Gao, X.; Jeon, Y.-J. In Vitro and In Vivo Anti-Inflammatory Effects of Sulfated Polysaccharides Isolated from the Edible Brown Seaweed, Sargassum fulvellum. *Mar. Drugs* **2021**, *19*, 277. [CrossRef]
34. Fernando, I.P.S.; Jayawardena, T.U.; Sanjeewa, K.K.A.; Wang, L.; Jeon, Y.-J.; Lee, W.W. Anti-inflammatory potential of alginic acid from Sargassum horneri against urban aerosol-induced inflammatory responses in keratinocytes and macrophages. *Ecotoxicol. Environ. Saf.* **2018**, *160*, 24–31. [CrossRef] [PubMed]
35. Su, C.-H.; Tseng, Y.-T.; Lo, K.-Y.; Lai, M.-N.; Ng, L.-T. Differences in anti-inflammatory properties of water soluble and insoluble bioactive polysaccharides in lipopolysaccharide-stimulated RAW264.7 macrophages. *Glycoconj. J.* **2020**, *37*, 565–576. [CrossRef] [PubMed]
36. Jayawardena, T.U.; Sanjeewa, K.K.A.; Lee, H.G.; Nagahawatta, D.P.; Yang, H.W.; Kang, M.C.; Jeon, Y.J. Particulate Matter-Induced Inflammation/Oxidative Stress in Macrophages: Fucosterol from Padina boryana as a Potent Protector, Activated via NF-κB/MAPK Pathways and Nrf2/HO-1 Involvement. *Mar. Drugs* **2020**, *18*, 628. [CrossRef] [PubMed]
37. Gil, B.; Ferrándiz, M.L.; Sanz, M.J.; Terencio, M.C.; Ubeda, A.; Rovirosa, J.; San-Martin, A.; Alcaraz, M.J.; Payá, M. Inhibition of inflammatory responses by epitaondiol and other marine natural products. *Life Sci.* **1995**, *57*, PL25–PL30. [CrossRef] [PubMed]
38. Daskalaki, M.G.; Vyrla, D.; Harizani, M.; Doxaki, C.; Eliopoulos, A.G.; Roussis, V.; Ioannou, E.; Tsatsanis, C.; Kampranis, S.C. Neorogioltriol and Related Diterpenes from the Red Alga Laurencia Inhibit Inflammatory Bowel Disease in Mice by Suppressing M1 and Promoting M2-Like Macrophage Responses. *Mar. Drugs* **2019**, *17*, 97. [CrossRef]
39. Caroprese, M.; Albenzio, M.; Ciliberti, M.G.; Francavilla, M.; Sevi, A. A mixture of phytosterols from Dunaliella tertiolecta affects proliferation of peripheral blood mononuclear cells and cytokine production in sheep. *Veter.-Immunol. Immunopathol.* **2012**, *150*, 27–35. [CrossRef]
40. Kim, E.A.; Kim, S.Y.; Ye, B.R.; Kim, J.; Ko, S.C.; Lee, W.W.; Kim, K.N.; Choi, I.W.; Jung, W.K.; Heo, S.J. Anti-inflammatory effect of Apo-9′-fucoxanthone via inhibition of MAPKs and NF-kB signaling pathway in LPS-stimulated RAW 264.7 macrophages and zebrafish model. *Int. Immunopharmacol.* **2018**, *59*, 339–346. [CrossRef]
41. Mesquita, J.X.; de Brito, T.V.; Fontenelle, T.P.C.; Damasceno, R.O.S.; de Souza, M.H.L.P.; de Souza Lopes, J.L.; Beltramin, L.M.; Barbosa, A.L.d.R.; Freitas, A.L.P. Lectin from red algae Amansia multifida Lamouroux: Extraction, characterization and anti-inflammatory activity. *Int. J. Biol. Macromol.* **2021**, *170*, 532–539. [CrossRef]
42. Fontenelle, T.P.C.; Lima, G.C.; Mesquita, J.X.; Lopes, J.L.d.S.; de Brito, T.V.; Vieira Júnior, F.d.C.; Sales, A.B.; Aragão, K.S.; Souza, M.H.L.P.; Barbosa, A.L.d.R.; et al. Lectin obtained from the red seaweed Bryothamnion triquetrum: Secondary structure and anti-inflammatory activity in mice. *Int. J. Biol. Macromol.* **2018**, *112*, 1122–1130. [CrossRef]
43. Cian, R.E.; Hernández-Chirlaque, C.; Gámez-Belmonte, R.; Drago, S.R.; Sánchez de Medina, F.; Martínez-Augustin, O. Green Alga Ulva spp. Hydrolysates and Their Peptide Fractions Regulate Cytokine Production in Splenic Macrophages and Lymphocytes Involving the TLR4-NFκB/MAPK Pathways. *Mar. Drugs* **2018**, *16*, 235. [CrossRef]
44. Lucena, A.M.M.; Souza, C.R.M.; Jales, J.T.; Guedes, P.M.M.; de Miranda, G.E.C.; de Moura, A.M.A.; Araújo-Júnior, J.X.; Nascimento, G.J.; Scortecci, K.C.; Santos, B.V.O.; et al. The Bisindole Alkaloid Caulerpin, from Seaweeds of the Genus Caulerpa, Attenuated Colon Damage in Murine Colitis Model. *Mar. Drugs* **2018**, *16*, 318. [CrossRef] [PubMed]
45. Makkar, F.; Chakraborty, K. Previously undescribed antioxidative azocinyl morpholinone alkaloid from red seaweed Gracilaria opuntia with anti-cyclooxygenase and lipoxygenase properties. *Nat. Prod. Res.* **2018**, *32*, 1150–1160. [CrossRef] [PubMed]

46. Ali, I.; Manzoor, Z.; Koo, J.E.; Kim, J.E.; Byeon, S.H.; Yoo, E.S.; Kang, H.K.; Hyun, J.W.; Lee, N.H.; Koh, Y.S. 3-Hydroxy-4,7-megastigmadien-9-one, isolated from Ulva pertusa, attenuates TLR9-mediated inflammatory response by down-regulating mitogen-activated protein kinase and NF-κB pathways. *Pharm. Biol.* **2017**, *55*, 435–440. [CrossRef] [PubMed]
47. Kim, M.; Li, Y.X.; Dewapriya, P.; Ryu, B.; Kim, S.K. Floridoside suppresses pro-inflammatory responses by blocking MAPK signaling in activated microglia. *BMB Rep.* **2013**, *46*, 398–403. [CrossRef]
48. Bousquet, M.S.; Ratnayake, R.; Pope, J.L.; Chen, Q.Y.; Zhu, F.; Chen, S.; Carney, T.J.; Gharaibeh, R.Z.; Jobin, C.; Paul, V.J.; et al. Seaweed natural products modify the host inflammatory response via Nrf2 signaling and alter colon microbiota composition and gene expression. *Free Radic. Biol. Med.* **2020**, *146*, 306–323. [CrossRef]
49. Monteiro, P.; Lomartire, S.; Cotas, J.; Marques, J.C.; Pereira, L.; Gonçalves, A.M.M. Call the Eckols: Present and Future Potential Cancer Therapies. *Mar. Drugs* **2022**, *20*, 387. [CrossRef]
50. Jimenez-Lopez, C.; Pereira, A.G.; Lourenço-Lopes, C.; Garcia-Oliveira, P.; Cassani, L.; Fraga-Corral, M.; Prieto, M.A.; Simal-Gandara, J. Main bioactive phenolic compounds in marine algae and their mechanisms of action supporting potential health benefits. *Food Chem.* **2021**, *341*, 128262. [CrossRef]
51. Cotas, J.; Leandro, A.; Monteiro, P.; Pacheco, D.; Figueirinha, A.; Gonçalves, A.M.M.; da Silva, G.J.; Pereira, L. Seaweed Phenolics: From Extraction to Applications. *Mar. Drugs* **2020**, *18*, 384. [CrossRef]
52. Khan, F.; Jeong, G.J.; Khan, M.S.A.; Tabassum, N.; Kim, Y.M. Seaweed-Derived Phlorotannins: A Review of Multiple Biological Roles and Action Mechanisms. *Mar. Drugs* **2022**, *20*, 384. [CrossRef]
53. Yang, H.K.; Jung, M.H.; Avunje, S.; Nikapitiya, C.; Kang, S.Y.; Ryu, Y.B.; Lee, W.S.; Jung, S.J. Efficacy of algal Ecklonia cava extract against viral hemorrhagic septicemia virus (VHSV). *Fish Shellfish. Immunol.* **2018**, *72*, 273–281. [CrossRef]
54. Kim, H.S.; Je, J.G.; An, H.; Baek, K.; Lee, J.M.; Yim, M.J.; Ko, S.C.; Kim, J.Y.; Oh, G.W.; Kang, M.C.; et al. Isolation and Characterization of Efficient Active Compounds Using High-Performance Centrifugal Partition Chromatography (CPC) from Anti-Inflammatory Activity Fraction of Ecklonia maxima in South Africa. *Mar. Drugs* **2022**, *20*, 471. [CrossRef] [PubMed]
55. Lee, S.H.; Kang, S.M.; Ko, S.C.; Lee, D.H.; Jeon, Y.J. Octaphlorethol A, a novel phenolic compound isolated from a brown alga, Ishige foliacea, increases glucose transporter 4-mediated glucose uptake in skeletal muscle cells. *Biochem. Biophys. Res. Commun.* **2012**, *420*, 576–581. [CrossRef]
56. Hentati, F.; Tounsi, L.; Djomdi, D.; Pierre, G.; Delattre, C.; Ursu, A.V.; Fendri, I.; Abdelkafi, S.; Michaud, P. Bioactive Polysaccharides from Seaweeds. *Molecules* **2020**, *25*, 3152. [CrossRef]
57. Zaitseva, O.O.; Sergushkina, M.I.; Khudyakov, A.N.; Polezhaeva, T.V.; Solomina, O.N. Seaweed sulfated polysaccharides and their medicinal properties. *Algal Res.* **2022**, *68*, 102885. [CrossRef]
58. Apostolova, E.; Lukova, P.; Baldzhieva, A.; Katsarov, P.; Nikolova, M.; Iliev, I.; Peychev, L.; Trica, B.; Oancea, F.; Delattre, C.; et al. Immunomodulatory and Anti-Inflammatory Effects of Fucoidan: A Review. *Polymers* **2020**, *12*, 2338. [CrossRef] [PubMed]
59. Nagahawatta, D.P.; Liyanage, N.M.; Jayawardhana, H.; Lee, H.G.; Jayawardena, T.U.; Jeon, Y.J. Anti-Fine Dust Effect of Fucoidan Extracted from Ecklonia maxima Laves in Macrophages via Inhibiting Inflammatory Signaling Pathways. *Mar. Drugs* **2022**, *20*, 413. [CrossRef] [PubMed]
60. Bagalagel, A.; Diri, R.; Noor, A.; Almasri, D.; Bakhsh, H.T.; Kutbi, H.I.; Al-Gayyar, M.M.H. Curative effects of fucoidan on acetic acid induced ulcerative colitis in rats via modulating aryl hydrocarbon receptor and phosphodiesterase-4. *BMC Complement. Med. Ther.* **2022**, *22*, 196. [CrossRef]
61. Wang, L.; Je, J.G.; Huang, C.; Oh, J.Y.; Fu, X.; Wang, K.; Ahn, G.; Xu, J.; Gao, X.; Jeon, Y.J. Anti-Inflammatory Effect of Sulfated Polysaccharides Isolated from Codium fragile In Vitro in RAW 264.7 Macrophages and In Vivo in Zebrafish. *Mar. Drugs* **2022**, *20*, 391. [CrossRef]
62. Chen, C.Y.; Wang, S.H.; Huang, C.Y.; Dong, C.D.; Huang, C.Y.; Chang, C.C.; Chang, J.S. Effect of molecular mass and sulfate content of fucoidan from Sargassum siliquosum on antioxidant, anti-lipogenesis, and anti-inflammatory activity. *J. Biosci. Bioeng.* **2021**, *132*, 359–364. [CrossRef]
63. Jayawardena, T.U.; Sanjeewa, K.K.A.; Wang, L.; Kim, W.S.; Lee, T.K.; Kim, Y.T.; Jeon, Y.J. Alginic Acid from Padina boryana Abate Particulate Matter-Induced Inflammatory Responses in Keratinocytes and Dermal Fibroblasts. *Molecules* **2020**, *25*, 5746. [CrossRef]
64. Sarithakumari, C.H.; Renju, G.L.; Kurup, G.M. Anti-inflammatory and antioxidant potential of alginic acid isolated from the marine algae, Sargassum wightii on adjuvant-induced arthritic rats. *Inflammopharmacol.* **2013**, *21*, 261–268. [CrossRef] [PubMed]
65. Zayed, A.; Avila-Peltroche, J.; El-Aasr, M.; Ulber, R. Sulfated Galactofucans: An Outstanding Class of Fucoidans with Promising Bioactivities. *Mar. Drugs* **2022**, *20*, 412. [CrossRef] [PubMed]
66. Menshova, R.V.; Shevchenko, N.M.; Imbs, T.I.; Zvyagintseva, T.N.; Malyarenko, O.S.; Zaporoshets, T.S.; Besednova, N.N.; Ermakova, S.P. Fucoidans from Brown Alga Fucus evanescens: Structure and Biological Activity. *Front. Mar. Sci.* **2016**, *3*, 129. [CrossRef]
67. Martins, A.; Alves, C.; Silva, J.; Pinteus, S.; Gaspar, H.; Pedrosa, R. Sulfated Polysaccharides from Macroalgae-A Simple Roadmap for Chemical Characterization. *Polymers* **2023**, *15*, 399. [CrossRef]
68. Shagufta, P. Introductory Chapter: Terpenes and Terpenoids. In *Terpenes and Terpenoids*; Shagufta, P., Areej, A.-T., Eds.; IntechOpen: Rijeka, Croatia, 2018; p. Ch. 1.
69. Gross, H.; König, G.M. Terpenoids from marine organisms: Unique structures and their pharmacological potential. *Phytochem. Rev.* **2006**, *5*, 115–141. [CrossRef]

70. Abreu, T.M.; Ribeiro, N.A.; Chaves, H.V.; Jorge, R.J.; Bezerra, M.M.; Monteiro, H.S.; Vasconcelos, I.M.; Mota É, F.; Benevides, N.M. Antinociceptive and Anti-inflammatory Activities of the Lectin from Marine Red Alga Solieria filiformis. *Planta Med.* **2016**, *82*, 596–605. [CrossRef] [PubMed]
71. de Queiroz, I.N.; Quinderé, A.L.; Rodrigues, J.A.; de Sousa Oliveira Vanderlei, E.; Ribeiro, N.A.; da Conceição Rivanor, R.L.; Ribeiro, K.A.; Coura, C.O.; Pereira, K.M.; Chaves, H.V.; et al. Dual effects of a lectin from the green seaweed Caulerpa cupressoides var. lycopodium on inflammatory mediators in classical models of inflammation. *Inflamm. Res.* **2015**, *64*, 971–982. [CrossRef]
72. Singh, R.S.; Walia, A.K. Lectins from red algae and their biomedical potential. *J. Appl. Phycol.* **2018**, *30*, 1833–1858. [CrossRef]
73. Barre, A.; Simplicien, M.; Benoist, H.; Van Damme, E.J.M.; Rougé, P. Mannose-Specific Lectins from Marine Algae: Diverse Structural Scaffolds Associated to Common Virucidal and Anti-Cancer Properties. *Mar. Drugs* **2019**, *17*, 440. [CrossRef]
74. Yoshiie, T.; Maeda, M.; Kimura, M.; Hama, Y.; Uchida, M.; Kimura, Y. Structural features of N-glycans of seaweed glycoproteins: Predominant occurrence of high-mannose type N-glycans in marine plants. *Biosci. Biotechnol. Biochem.* **2012**, *76*, 1996–1998. [CrossRef] [PubMed]
75. Souza, C.R.M.; Bezerra, W.P.; Souto, J.T. Marine Alkaloids with Anti-Inflammatory Activity: Current Knowledge and Future Perspectives. *Mar. Drugs* **2020**, *18*, 147. [CrossRef] [PubMed]
76. Movahhedin, N.; Barar, J.; Fathi Azad, F.; Barzegari, A.; Nazemiyeh, H. Phytochemistry and biologic activities of caulerpa peltata native to oman sea. *Iran. J. Pharm. Res. IJPR* **2014**, *13*, 515–521.
77. de Almeida, C.L.; Falcão Hde, S.; Lima, G.R.; Montenegro Cde, A.; Lira, N.S.; de Athayde-Filho, P.F.; Rodrigues, L.C.; de Souza Mde, F.; Barbosa-Filho, J.M.; Batista, L.M. Bioactivities from marine algae of the genus Gracilaria. *Int. J. Mol. Sci.* **2011**, *12*, 4550–4573. [CrossRef]
78. Chen, K.J.; Tseng, C.K.; Chang, F.R.; Yang, J.I.; Yeh, C.C.; Chen, W.C.; Wu, S.F.; Chang, H.W.; Lee, J.C. Aqueous extract of the edible Gracilaria tenuistipitata inhibits hepatitis C viral replication via cyclooxygenase-2 suppression and reduces virus-induced inflammation. *PLoS ONE* **2013**, *8*, e57704. [CrossRef] [PubMed]
79. Shu, M.H.; Appleton, D.; Zandi, K.; AbuBakar, S. Anti-inflammatory, gastroprotective and anti-ulcerogenic effects of red algae Gracilaria changii (*Gracilariales, Rhodophyta*) extract. *BMC Complement. Altern. Med.* **2013**, *13*, 61. [CrossRef] [PubMed]
80. Ornano, L.; Donno, Y.; Sanna, C.; Ballero, M.; Serafini, M.; Bianco, A. Phytochemical study of Caulerpa racemosa (Forsk.) J. Agarth, an invading alga in the habitat of La Maddalena Archipelago. *Nat. Prod. Res.* **2014**, *28*, 1795–1799. [CrossRef]
81. Yoon, W.J.; Heo, S.J.; Han, S.C.; Lee, H.J.; Kang, G.J.; Kang, H.K.; Hyun, J.W.; Koh, Y.S.; Yoo, E.S. Anti-inflammatory effect of sargachromanol G isolated from Sargassum siliquastrum in RAW 264.7 cells. *Arch. Pharm. Res.* **2012**, *35*, 1421–1430. [CrossRef]
82. Yoon, W.J.; Kim, K.N.; Heo, S.J.; Han, S.C.; Kim, J.; Ko, Y.J.; Kang, H.K.; Yoo, E.S. Sargachromanol G inhibits osteoclastogenesis by suppressing the activation NF-κB and MAPKs in RANKL-induced RAW 264.7 cells. *Biochem. Biophys. Res. Commun.* **2013**, *434*, 892–897. [CrossRef]
83. Min, H.Y.; Kim, H.; Lee, H.J.; Yoon, N.Y.; Kim, Y.K.; Lee, H.Y. Ethanol Extract of Sargassum siliquastrum Inhibits Lipopolysaccharide-Induced Nitric Oxide Generation by Downregulating the Nuclear Factor-Kappa B Signaling Pathway. *Evid. Based Complement. Altern. Med.* **2022**, *2022*, 6160010. [CrossRef]
84. Niu, T.; Fu, G.; Zhou, J.; Han, H.; Chen, J.; Wu, W.; Chen, H. Floridoside Exhibits Antioxidant Properties by Activating HO-1 Expression via p38/ERK MAPK Pathway. *Mar. Drugs* **2020**, *18*, 105. [CrossRef] [PubMed]
85. Taylor, P.D.; Waeschenbach, A. Phylogeny and diversification of bryozoans. *Palaeontology* **2015**, *58*, 585–599. [CrossRef]
86. Wood, A.C.L.; Probert, P.K.; Rowden, A.A.; Smith, A.M. Complex habitat generated by marine bryozoans: A review of its distribution, structure, diversity, threats and conservation. *Aquat. Conserv. Mar. Freshw. Ecosyst.* **2012**, *22*, 547–563. [CrossRef]
87. Tian, X.R.; Tang, H.F.; Tian, X.L.; Hu, J.J.; Huang, L.L.; Gustafson, K.R. Review of bioactive secondary metabolites from marine bryozoans in the progress of new drugs discovery. *Future Med. Chem.* **2018**, *10*, 1497–1514. [CrossRef]
88. Pettit, G.R.; Herald, C.L.; Doubek, D.L.; Herald, D.L.; Arnold, E.; Clardy, J. Isolation and structure of bryostatin 1. *J. Am. Chem. Soc.* **1982**, *104*, 6846–6848. [CrossRef]
89. Raghuvanshi, R.; Bharate, S.B. Preclinical and Clinical Studies on Bryostatins, A Class of Marine-Derived Protein Kinase C Modulators: A Mini-Review. *Curr. Top. Med. Chem.* **2020**, *20*, 1124–1135. [CrossRef] [PubMed]
90. Safaeinejad, F.; Bahrami, S.; Redl, H.; Niknejad, H. Inhibition of Inflammation, Suppression of Matrix Metalloproteinases Induction of Neurogenesis, and Antioxidant Property Make Bryostatin-1 a Therapeutic Choice for Multiple Sclerosis. *Front Pharmacol.* **2018**, *9*, 625. [CrossRef]
91. Ruiz-Torres, V.; Encinar, J.A.; Herranz-López, M.; Pérez-Sánchez, A.; Galiano, V.; Barrajón-Catalán, E.; Micol, V. An Updated Review on Marine Anticancer Compounds: The Use of Virtual Screening for the Discovery of Small-Molecule Cancer Drugs. *Molecules* **2017**, *22*, 1037. [CrossRef] [PubMed]
92. Tan, Z.; Lucke-Wold, B.P.; Logsdon, A.F.; Turner, R.C.; Tan, C.; Li, X.; Hongpaison, J.; Alkon, D.L.; Simpkins, J.W.; Rosen, C.L.; et al. Bryostatin extends tPA time window to 6 h following middle cerebral artery occlusion in aged female rats. *Eur. J. Pharmacol.* **2015**, *764*, 404–412. [CrossRef]
93. Salim, E.I.; Harras, S.F.; Abdalla, A.G.; Mona, M.H. Syphacia muris infection in rats attenuates colorectal carcinogenesis through oxidative stress and gene expression alterations. Implications for modulatory effects by Bryostatin-1. *Acta Parasitol.* **2018**, *63*, 198–209. [CrossRef]
94. Kornberg, M.D.; Smith, M.D.; Shirazi, H.A.; Calabresi, P.A.; Snyder, S.H.; Kim, P.M. Bryostatin-1 alleviates experimental multiple sclerosis. *Proc. Natl. Acad. Sci. USA* **2018**, *115*, 2186–2191. [CrossRef] [PubMed]

95. Abramson, E.; Hardman, C.; Shimizu, A.J.; Hwang, S.; Hester, L.D.; Snyder, S.H.; Wender, P.A.; Kim, P.M.; Kornberg, M.D. Designed PKC-targeting bryostatin analogs modulate innate immunity and neuroinflammation. *Cell Chem. Biol.* **2021**, *28*, 537–545.e4. [CrossRef] [PubMed]
96. Hany, L.; Turmel, M.O.; Barat, C.; Ouellet, M.; Tremblay, M.J. Impact of latency-reversing agents on human macrophage physiology. *Immun. Inflamm. Dis.* **2023**, *11*, e590. [CrossRef] [PubMed]
97. Matias, D.; Bessa, C.; Fátima Simões, M.; Reis, C.P.; Saraiva, L.; Rijo, P. Chapter 2—Natural Products as Lead Protein Kinase C Modulators for Cancer Therapy. In *Studies in Natural Products Chemistry*; Atta ur, R., Ed.; Elsevier: Amsterdam, Netherlands, 2016; Volume 50, pp. 45–79.
98. Fernandes, P.D.; Zardo, R.S.; Figueiredo, G.S.M.; Silva, B.V.; Pinto, A.C. Anti-inflammatory properties of convolutamydine A and two structural analogues. *Life Sci.* **2014**, *116*, 16–24. [CrossRef]
99. Di, X.; Wang, S.; Oskarsson, J.T.; Rouger, C.; Tasdemir, D.; Hardardottir, I.; Freysdottir, J.; Wang, X.; Molinski, T.F.; Omarsdottir, S. Bromotryptamine and Imidazole Alkaloids with Anti-inflammatory Activity from the Bryozoan Flustra foliacea. *J. Nat. Prod.* **2020**, *83*, 2854–2866. [CrossRef] [PubMed]
100. De Domenico, S.; De Rinaldis, G.; Paulmery, M.; Piraino, S.; Leone, A. Barrel Jellyfish (Rhizostoma pulmo) as Source of Antioxidant Peptides. *Mar. Drugs* **2019**, *17*, 134. [CrossRef]
101. Cao, Y.; Gao, J.; Zhang, L.; Qin, N.; Zhu, B.; Xia, X. Jellyfish skin polysaccharides enhance intestinal barrier function and modulate the gut microbiota in mice with DSS-induced colitis. *Food Funct.* **2021**, *12*, 10121–10135. [CrossRef]
102. Liu, S.; Wang, Y.; Su, M.; Song, S.J.; Hong, J.; Kim, S.; Im, D.S.; Jung, J.H. A bile acid derivative with PPARγ-mediated anti-inflammatory activity. *Steroids* **2018**, *137*, 40–46. [CrossRef]
103. Liu, S.; Su, M.; Song, S.J.; Hong, J.; Chung, H.Y.; Jung, J.H. An Anti-Inflammatory PPAR-γ Agonist from the Jellyfish-Derived Fungus Penicillium chrysogenum J08NF-4. *J. Nat. Prod.* **2018**, *81*, 356–363. [CrossRef]
104. Lv, Z.; Zhang, C.; Song, W.; Chen, Q.; Wang, Y. Jellyfish Collagen Hydrolysate Alleviates Inflammation and Oxidative Stress and Improves Gut Microbe Composition in High-Fat Diet-Fed Mice. *Mediat. Inflamm.* **2022**, *2022*, 5628702. [CrossRef]
105. Venugopal, V.; Gopakumar, K. Shellfish: Nutritive Value, Health Benefits, and Consumer Safety. *Compr. Rev. Food Sci. Food Saf.* **2017**, *16*, 1219–1242. [CrossRef] [PubMed]
106. Grienke, U.; Silke, J.; Tasdemir, D. Bioactive compounds from marine mussels and their effects on human health. *Food Chem.* **2014**, *142*, 48–60. [CrossRef] [PubMed]
107. Joshi, I.; Nazeer, R.A. EGLLGDVF: A Novel Peptide from Green Mussel Perna viridis Foot Exerts Stability and Anti-inflammatory Effects on LPS-Stimulated RAW264.7 Cells. *Protein Pept. Lett.* **2020**, *27*, 851–859. [CrossRef] [PubMed]
108. Kim, Y.S.; Ahn, C.B.; Je, J.Y. Anti-inflammatory action of high molecular weight Mytilus edulis hydrolysates fraction in LPS-induced RAW264.7 macrophage via NF-κB and MAPK pathways. *Food Chem.* **2016**, *202*, 9–14. [CrossRef] [PubMed]
109. Kim, E.K.; Kim, Y.S.; Hwang, J.W.; Kang, S.H.; Choi, D.K.; Lee, K.H.; Lee, J.S.; Moon, S.H.; Jeon, B.T.; Park, P.J. Purification of a novel nitric oxide inhibitory peptide derived from enzymatic hydrolysates of Mytilus coruscus. *Fish Shellfish Immunol.* **2013**, *34*, 1416–1420. [CrossRef]
110. Liu, F.; Zhang, X.; Li, Y.; Chen, Q.; Liu, F.; Zhu, X.; Mei, L.; Song, X.; Liu, X.; Song, Z.; et al. Anti-Inflammatory Effects of a Mytilus coruscus α-d-Glucan (MP-A) in Activated Macrophage Cells via TLR4/NF-κB/MAPK Pathway Inhibition. *Mar. Drugs* **2017**, *15*, 294. [CrossRef]
111. Wan, Y.; Fu, Y.; Wang, F.; Sinclair, A.J.; Li, D. Protective Effects of a Lipid Extract from Hard-Shelled Mussel (Mytilus coruscus) on Intestinal Integrity after Lipopolysaccharide Challenge in Mice. *Nutrients* **2018**, *10*, 860. [CrossRef]
112. Li, G.; Fu, Y.; Zheng, J.; Li, D. Anti-inflammatory activity and mechanism of a lipid extract from hard-shelled mussel (Mytilus coruscus) on chronic arthritis in rats. *Mar. Drugs* **2014**, *12*, 568–588. [CrossRef]
113. Chen, J.; Bao, C.; Cho, S.H.; Lee, H.J. Green lipped mussel oil complex suppresses lipopolysaccharide stimulated inflammation via regulating nuclear factor-κB and mitogen activated protein kinases signaling in RAW264.7 murine macrophages. *Food Sci. Biotechnol.* **2017**, *26*, 815–822. [CrossRef]
114. Mickleborough, T.D.; Vaughn, C.L.; Shei, R.J.; Davis, E.M.; Wilhite, D.P. Marine lipid fraction PCSO-524 (lyprinol/omega XL) of the New Zealand green lipped mussel attenuates hyperpnea-induced bronchoconstriction in asthma. *Respir. Med.* **2013**, *107*, 1152–1163. [CrossRef]
115. Joshi, I.; Mohideen, H.S.; Nazeer, R.A. A Meretrix meretrix visceral mass derived peptide inhibits lipopolysaccharide-stimulated responses in RAW264.7 cells and adult zebrafish model. *Int. Immunopharmacol.* **2021**, *90*, 107140. [CrossRef]
116. Gong, F.; Chen, M.-F.; Chen, J.; Li, C.; Zhou, C.; Hong, P.; Sun, S.; Qian, Z.-J. Boiled Abalone Byproduct Peptide Exhibits Anti-Tumor Activity in HT1080 Cells and HUVECs by Suppressing the Metastasis and Angiogenesis in Vitro. *J. Agric. Food Chem.* **2019**, *67*, 8855–8867. [CrossRef]
117. Song, S.Y.; Park, D.H.; Lee, S.H.; Lim, H.K.; Park, J.W.; Jeong, C.R.; Kim, S.J.; Cho, S.S. Purification of phenoloxidase from Haliotis discus hannai and its anti-inflammatory activity in vitro. *Fish Shellfish Immunol.* **2023**, *137*, 108741. [CrossRef]
118. Choi, G.S.; Lim, J.H.; Rod-In, W.; Jung, S.K.; Park, W.J. Anti-inflammatory properties of neutral lipids, glycolipids, and phospholipids isolated from Ammodytes personatus eggs in LPS-stimulated RAW264.7 cells. *Fish Shellfish Immunol.* **2022**, *131*, 1109–1117. [CrossRef]
119. Qi, Y.; Zhou, J.; Shen, X.; Chalamaiah, M.; Lv, S.; Luo, H.; Chen, L. Bioactive Properties of Peptides and Polysaccharides Derived from Peanut Worms: A Review. *Mar. Drugs* **2021**, *20*, 10. [CrossRef] [PubMed]

120. Zhang, C.X.; Dai, Z.R.; Cai, Q.X. Anti-inflammatory and anti-nociceptive activities of Sipunculus nudus L. extract. *J. Ethnopharmacol.* **2011**, *137*, 1177–1182. [CrossRef] [PubMed]
121. Sangtanoo, P.; Srimongkol, P.; Saisavoey, T.; Reamtong, O.; Karnchanatat, A. Anti-inflammatory action of two novel peptides derived from peanut worms (Sipunculus nudus) in lipopolysaccharide-induced RAW264.7 macrophages. *Food Funct.* **2020**, *11*, 552–560. [CrossRef] [PubMed]
122. Lin, H.; Zheng, Z.; Yuan, J.; Zhang, C.; Cao, W.; Qin, X. Collagen Peptides Derived from Sipunculus nudus Accelerate Wound Healing. *Molecules* **2021**, *26*, 1385. [CrossRef]
123. Yang, Z.; Pan, Y.; Chen, J.; Zhang, H.; Wei, H.; Wu, Z.; Liu, L. Anti-inflammatory, anti-oxidative stress effect of Phascolosoma esculenta oligosaccharides on Escherichia coli-induced sepsis mice. *Food Sci. Biotechnol.* **2019**, *28*, 1871–1879. [CrossRef]

Disclaimer/Publisher's Note: The statements, opinions and data contained in all publications are solely those of the individual author(s) and contributor(s) and not of MDPI and/or the editor(s). MDPI and/or the editor(s) disclaim responsibility for any injury to people or property resulting from any ideas, methods, instructions or products referred to in the content.

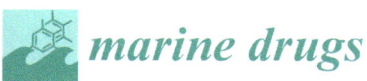

Review

Unlocking the Potential of Octocoral-Derived Secondary Metabolites against Neutrophilic Inflammatory Response

Ngoc Bao An Nguyen [1], Mohamed El-Shazly [2,†], Po-Jen Chen [3,†], Bo-Rong Peng [1,†], Lo-Yun Chen [1], Tsong-Long Hwang [4,5,6,7,8,*] and Kuei-Hung Lai [1,9,10,*]

1. Graduate Institute of Pharmacognosy, College of Pharmacy, Taipei Medical University, Taipei 11031, Taiwan; m303110001@tmu.edu.tw (N.B.A.N.); peng_br@tmu.edu.tw (B.-R.P.); m303110004@tmu.edu.tw (L.-Y.C.)
2. Department of Pharmacognosy, Faculty of Pharmacy, Ain-Shams University, Organization of African Unity Street, Abassia, Cairo 11566, Egypt; mohamed.elshazly@pharma.asu.edu.eg
3. Department of Medical Research, E-Da Hospital, I-Shou University, Kaohsiung 82445, Taiwan; ed113510@edah.org.tw
4. Research Center for Chinese Herbal Medicine, College of Human Ecology, Chang Gung University of Science and Technology, Taoyuan 33303, Taiwan
5. Graduate Institute of Health Industry Technology, College of Human Ecology, Chang Gung University of Science and Technology, Taoyuan 33303, Taiwan
6. Department of Anaesthesiology, Chang Gung Memorial Hospital, Taoyuan 33305, Taiwan
7. Graduate Institute of Natural Products, College of Medicine, Chang Gung University, Taoyuan 33302, Taiwan
8. Department of Chemical Engineering, Ming Chi University of Technology, New Taipei City 24301, Taiwan
9. PhD Program in Clinical Drug Development of Herbal Medicine, College of Pharmacy, Taipei Medical University, Taipei 11031, Taiwan
10. Traditional Herbal Medicine Research Center, Taipei Medical University Hospital, Taipei 11031, Taiwan
* Correspondence: htl@mail.cgu.edu.tw (T.-L.H.); kueihunglai@tmu.edu.tw (K.-H.L.); Tel.: +886-3-211-8800 (ext. 5523) (T.-L.H.); +886-2-2736-1661 (ext. 6157) (K.-H.L.)
† These authors contributed equally to this work.

Abstract: Inflammation is a critical defense mechanism that is utilized by the body to protect itself against pathogens and other noxious invaders. However, if the inflammatory response becomes exaggerated or uncontrollable, its original protective role is not only demolished but it also becomes detrimental to the affected tissues or even to the entire body. Thus, regulating the inflammatory process is crucial to ensure that it is resolved promptly to prevent any subsequent damage. The role of neutrophils in inflammation has been highlighted in recent decades by a plethora of studies focusing on neutrophilic inflammatory diseases as well as the mechanisms to regulate the activity of neutrophils during the overwhelmed inflammatory process. As natural products have demonstrated promising effects in a wide range of pharmacological activities, they have been investigated for the discovery of new anti-inflammatory therapeutics to overcome the drawbacks of current synthetic agents. Octocorals have attracted scientists as a plentiful source of novel and intriguing marine scaffolds that exhibit many pharmacological activities, including anti-inflammatory effects. In this review, we aim to provide a summary of the neutrophilic anti-inflammatory properties of these marine organisms that were demonstrated in 46 studies from 1995 to the present (April 2023). We hope the present work offers a comprehensive overview of the anti-inflammatory potential of octocorals and encourages researchers to identify promising leads among numerous compounds isolated from octocorals over the past few decades to be further developed into anti-inflammatory therapeutic agents.

Keywords: neutrophilic inflammation; octocoral; secondary metabolites; drug leads

Citation: Nguyen, N.B.A.; El-Shazly, M.; Chen, P.-J.; Peng, B.-R.; Chen, L.-Y.; Hwang, T.-L.; Lai, K.-H. Unlocking the Potential of Octocoral-Derived Secondary Metabolites against Neutrophilic Inflammatory Response. *Mar. Drugs* **2023**, *21*, 456. https://doi.org/10.3390/md21080456

Academic Editors: Donatella Degl'Innocenti and Marzia Vasarri

Received: 20 July 2023
Revised: 14 August 2023
Accepted: 16 August 2023
Published: 18 August 2023

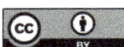

Copyright: © 2023 by the authors. Licensee MDPI, Basel, Switzerland. This article is an open access article distributed under the terms and conditions of the Creative Commons Attribution (CC BY) license (https://creativecommons.org/licenses/by/4.0/).

1. Introduction

Inflammation is an integral response of multicellular organisms that protects the hosts from external harmful factors, such as pathogens and physical and chemical irritants.

It also helps in tissue recovery after injury [1]. It can be classified into acute or chronic inflammatory responses, depending on the duration of the process and cellular activities [2]. Acute inflammation is the first response of the defense system to the invasion of foreign stimuli, which involves a cascade of complicated events. The extravascular migration of immune cells, such as platelets, basophils, neutrophils, eosinophils, mast cells, and macrophages, is one of the characterized features of acute inflammation, which aims to remove inflammatory irritants and facilitate the recovery of tissues [3,4]. The expected result of the acute phase is to eliminate either infectious or non-infectious agents and to restore the tissue to its initial state. If the exogenous stimuli cannot be removed entirely or the reactions of the acute phase are not sufficient to resolve the damage in the inflamed area, the inflammatory state can persist and proceed to the chronic phase [5,6]. Various studies have demonstrated the relationship between chronic inflammation and serious health problems, including type II diabetes, dyslipidemia, chronic kidney diseases, chronic prostatic diseases, cardiovascular diseases, and many types of cancer [7–12].

Neutrophils are the most abundant polymorphonuclear leukocytes, representing 50–70% of all white blood cells. They exhibit a significant role in the acute inflammatory response. Recently, the crucial role of neutrophils in various chronic inflammatory diseases has been investigated by many research groups. This investigation resulted in a wide range of studies focusing on the development of neutrophil-regulating agents as potential anti-inflammatory therapeutics [6,13–18]. Neutrophils act as the first-line defender of the immune system in the battle against noxious stimuli due to their rapid recruitment and various effective mechanisms of defense. The invasion of tissue with either infectious or non-infectious neutrophils triggers alarming signals, resulting in the recruitment and accumulation of neutrophils at the invaded sites. At these sites, neutrophils are activated and deploy their multiple defense mechanisms to protect the area from invaders (Figure 1). The offensive mechanisms of neutrophils include phagocytosis, respiratory burst, degranulation, and the formation of neutrophil extracellular traps [13,19,20].

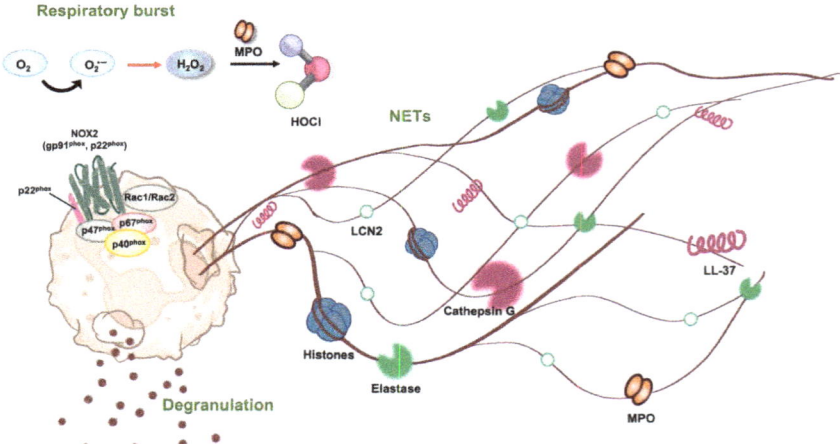

Figure 1. The inflammatory mechanisms employed by neutrophils. When neutrophils are activated they utilize respiratory burst, degranulation, and the formation of neutrophil extracellular traps (NETs) as the primary mechanisms to elicit inflammation.

At the invaded tissue, the activated neutrophils can act as phagocytes that engulf microorganisms, tissue debris, and dead cells in phagosomes similar to macrophages. However, there are some differences in the phagocytosis of neutrophils as compared to that of macrophages, especially in the maturation process of phagosomes. Unlike macrophages, neutrophils contain many types of preformed granules in their cytoplasm used for defense, including primary granules (known as azurophilic granules), secondary granules (referred to as specific granules), tertiary granules (another name for gelatinase granules), and secretory vesicles. For the maturation process, phagosomes require fusions with these granules to perform their degradative function against pathogens and foreign particles. Subsequently, the microorganisms and debris can be degraded and eliminated by granule proteins, and the products of oxygen burst [21].

In addition to phagocytosis, respiratory burst is another defensive method of neutrophils. Reactive oxygen species (ROS) are highly reactive derivatives of oxygen, which are produced by nicotinamide adenine dinucleotide phosphate (NADPH) oxidase complex via respiratory burst in activated neutrophils. Superoxide anions ($O_2^{\bullet-}$) are the initial product of respiratory burst, which are converted into peroxide (H_2O_2) by superoxide dismutase and subsequently into hypochlorous acid (HOCl) by myeloperoxidase (MPO) or hydroxyl radical ($OH^{\bullet}$) through Fenton's reaction in the presence of Fe^{2+}. These ROS can be released into either the phagosome for the disposal of foreign particles or in the extracellular environment in case of too large microorganisms that cannot be phagocytosed. The products of respiratory bursts possess strong oxidizing properties that can oxidize cellular constituents and damage the DNA, resulting in the destruction of pathogens and the removal of foreign particles. Due to their highly reactive and toxic nature, the excessive and prolonged generation of ROS can also cause further damage to the inflamed tissues, resulting in a chronic inflammatory response [22–24].

If the microorganisms are too large to be digested by phagocytosis, degranulation and the formation of neutrophil extracellular traps can be deployed during the response. Azurophilic granules are the primary granules that contain a majority of the pro-inflammatory and antimicrobial proteins such as elastase, myeloperoxidase, cathepsin G, and defensins, which are released to the extracellular environment of the inflammatory site or into the phagosome in a process called degranulation. The remaining defensive mechanism of neutrophils is the extrusion of extracellular traps (NETosis) that are made of decondensed chromatin, elastase, myeloperoxidase, cathepsin G, and histones. The neutrophil extracellular traps (NETs) can prevent the spread of pathogens by capturing and digesting microorganisms. However, NETs can also be injurious to host tissues due to the proteolytic activity of proteases [13].

These offensive mechanisms of neutrophils are double-edged swords that not only protect the host from pathogens and other foreign particles but can also attack the surrounding area in the case of uncontrolled or overwhelmed activation, which results in a subsequent chronic disorder rather than a resolution of inflammation. The overproduction of ROS, especially superoxide anions as well as the activation of elastase enzyme, contribute to the damage of host cells if the activation of neutrophils is out of control. Superoxide anions are the primary reactive oxygen species produced by neutrophils as a defense mechanism of the host in response to contact with foreign stimuli. In addition to the destruction of the invading agents, they can also destroy the surrounding area as well, which may lead to further severe damage to inflamed tissues, especially in the case of imbalanced production [24]. Human neutrophil elastase is one of the proteases that are secreted during degranulation and is a crucial component of the NETs during combat against invading pathogens and sterile agents. The enzyme can degrade not only the foreign proteins in extracellular environments but also the host cell matrix, which can lead to a harmful effect in the case of over-activation. Numerous effects related to tissue damage have been linked to the imbalanced activity of elastase, making it a therapeutic target for various health problems, including chronic obstructive pulmonary disease [25], bronchiectasis [26], colorectal cancer [27], leukemia [28], cystic fibrosis [29], pulmonary arterial hypertension [30], and COVID-19-associated acute respiratory distress syndrome [31]. Due to the pivotal role of superoxide anions and elastase in the pathogenesis of inflammation-induced diseases, their production was selected to evaluate the anti-inflammatory effect of natural products.

Currently, anti-inflammatory drugs are produced from synthetic sources, including nonsteroidal and steroidal drugs. Among them, several neutrophil-targeting anti-inflammatory agents have been used in the clinical stage, such as colchicine, secukinumab, ixekizumab, brodalumab, reparixin, danirixin, sivelestat, and nafamostat. These conventional therapeutic agents exhibit potent effects in the treatment of various inflammation-related diseases, but their adverse effects cannot be ignored. Therefore, there is an increasing number of research studies focusing on the exploration of safer and more effective anti-inflammatory therapeutic agents. Nature was and will be the most valuable and sustainable source for drug discovery. The prolific source of novel lead compounds derived from natural products has been demonstrated via a huge range of studies [32–34]. In recent years, the emergence of marine drug exploration has inspired more research on evaluating different marine organisms, including soft corals, due to their diverse chemical constituents and promising biological effects [35–52]. Soft coral (Figure 2) is the common name of the marine animals classified under the subclass Octocorallia, class Anthozoa of the phylum Cnidaria [53]. They are widely distributed in tropical shallow water or the deep sea [54]. These marine organisms are named "octocorallia" as they possess eight pinnate tentacles on the oral opening of their polyp tubes, which are used as a tool for food capture. Unlike hard corals, more than 60% of the octocoral body is occupied by fleshy parts. Therefore, their defensive mechanism against potential predators mainly relies on the chemical composition contained in the soft tissues [55,56]. The use of soft corals was recorded in ancient literature as a therapeutic ingredient for the treatment of diarrhea, gastrointestinal bleeding, and neurasthenia [57]. In modern times, a great quantity of studies has been conducted in regard to the chemical constituents of soft corals and their pharmacological potentials. Terpenoids and steroids are reported as chemical compositions commonly discovered in these organisms. Secondary metabolites derived from different species of soft corals have shown a diverse range of bioactivities, including cytotoxic, antimicrobial, antimalarial, antifouling, antidiabetic, anxiolytic, antileishmanial, anti-acne, analgesic, antiviral, and anti-inflammatory effects [35–39,45,49–52,58–62]. The promising potential for the pharmacological effects of soft corals has leveraged them to be hot spots in the race for drug discovery.

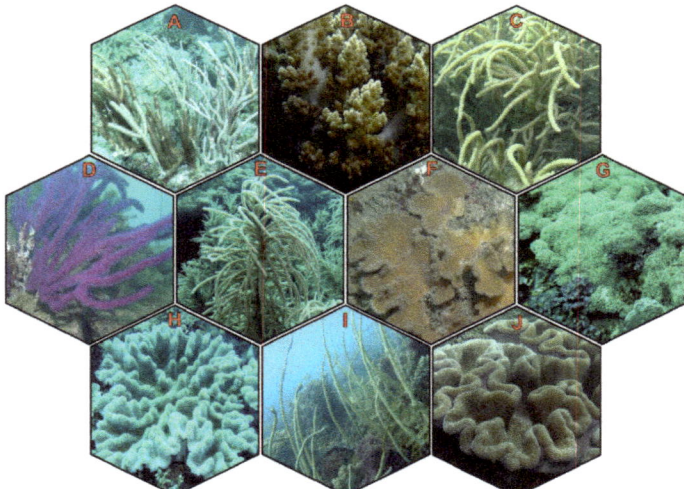

Figure 2. Soft corals that are reported to regulate neutrophilic inflammation. (**A**) *Rumphella* sp.; (**B**) *Litophyton* sp.; (**C**) *Sinularia flexibilis*; (**D**) *Echinomuricea* sp.; (**E**) *Pinnigorgia* sp.; (**F**) *Sinularia brassica*; (**G**) *Briareum* sp.; (**H**) *Lobophytum* sp.; (**I**) *Junceella fragilis*; (**J**) *Sarcophyton* sp.

Aquaculture of soft corals has been conducted since the late 1950s for the purposes of commercialization and preservation. Many techniques, such as coral gardening, microfragmentation, larval enhancement, and direct transplantation, have been developed to meet the demand for the mass production of soft corals [38]. Ex situ and in situ are current approaches to coral cultivation. Whereas in situ practice relies on natural environment for the propagation of soft corals, the ex situ method produces these marine organisms in controlled conditions. Although an ex situ approach is more costly and requires more advanced skills than in situ, it allows the optimization of aquaculture conditions and the elimination of environmental variability so as to facilitate and enhance the biomass and metabolite production of cultivated soft corals. Moreover, there is no interference in the growth of the animals concerning exposure to deleterious factors, such as parasites, competitors, predators, and other hazards [63]. These advantages make ex situ practice a suitable and favorable method of aquaculture to serve the drug discovery journey in marine organisms, particularly soft corals.

Although there are many reviews on these marine organisms, their inhibitory effects targeting neutrophil-mediated inflammation have not been summarized. Therefore, in this review, we aimed to provide a comprehensive summary of marine soft corals' potential as a plentiful resource of neutrophil-targeting anti-inflammatory agents. Superoxide anion generation and elastase release in activated neutrophils were the most common methods used for the evaluation of the anti-inflammatory potential of these marine secondary metabolites.

A total of 299 compounds isolated from different species of the subclass Octocorallia were screened for their anti-inflammatory potential using the aforementioned in vitro tests. Among them, 97 isolates (Table 1) were considered to exhibit significant inhibitory effects on superoxide anion generation and elastase release, with IC_{50} equal to or less than 20 μM. In the current review, the secondary metabolites possessing significant neutrophil-targeting anti-inflammatory effects are classified into sesquiterpenes, diterpenes, biscembranes, steroids, and some miscellaneous compounds. Steroids are the most abundant population with a total of 48 compounds, occupying 49.5% of bioactive agents isolated from octocorals. Ranked in second place, diterpenes comprise 36 derivatives that are classified into 10 subtypes. The remaining 13.4% of 97 potent isolates include 6 sesquiterpenes, 6 biscembranes, 2 α-tocopherol derivatives, a nitrogen-containing compound, and an allenic norterpenoid ketone. The literature investigation was conducted using various scientific databases including PubMed, Google Scholar, ScienceDirect, ResearchGate, and Reaxys. Different keywords, such as "neutrophil", "elastase release", "superoxide anion", "gorgonian", "soft corals", "octocoral", and "secondary metabolites", were used to retrieve original papers studying the target topic.

2. Soft Corals—The Source of Anti-Inflammatory Lead Compounds

2.1. Sesquiterpenes and Derivatives

Sesquiterpenes are a subclass of terpenoids, comprising three units of isoprene in the structure, or having a C15 skeleton with the molecular formula of $C_{15}H_{24}$. They can be acyclic or cyclic with various types of rings making their structures interesting from chemical and biological perspectives [64].

Several chemical studies conducted on *Rumphella antipathies* led to the isolation of bioactive sesquiterpenes, including clovan-2,9-dione (**1**), antipacid B (**2**), and rumphellolide L (**3**) (Figure 3). Clovan-2,9-dione, which was previously described as a synthetic compound, was isolated from a marine natural source as a natural clovane-type sesquiterpenoid for the first time. Antipacid B is a caryophyllane-related sesquiterpenoid possessing a novel bicyclo[5.2.0] carbon core skeleton. Both compounds significantly inhibited superoxide anion generation with IC_{50} values of 11.22 μM and 2.72 μg/mL. They also moderately inhibited elastase release with the IC_{50} values of 23.53 μM and 6.73 μg/mL. Rumphellolide L, a dehydrated product derived from the esterification reaction of the novel sesquiterpene, antipacid A, and a known sesquiterpene, clovane-2β,9α-diol, was also isolated from the same sample of the soft coral *Rumphella antipathies*. It showed a potent elastase release inhibitory effect with an IC_{50} value of 7.63 μM [65,66].

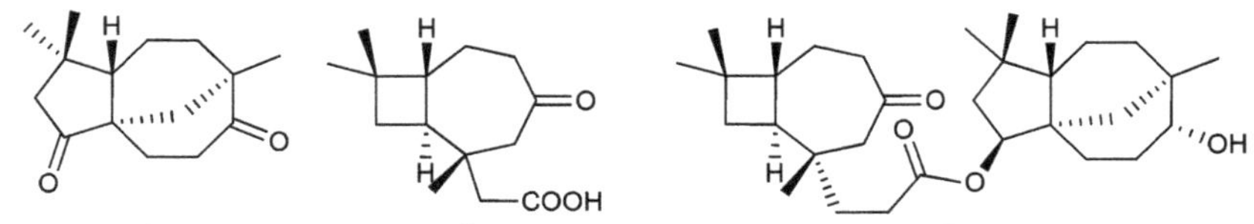

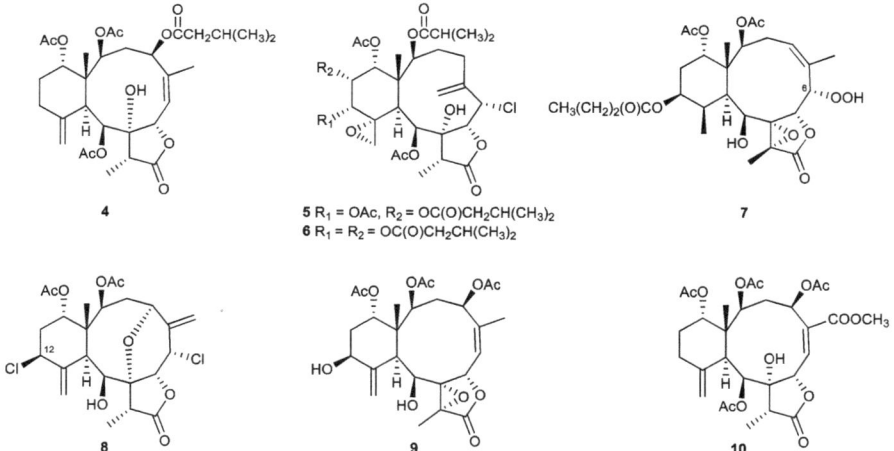

Figure 3. Sesquiterpenes (**1–3**) isolated from *Rumphella antipathies*.

2.2. Diterpenes and Derivatives

Diterpenes are secondary metabolites that comprise four isoprene units possessing the basic molecular formula of $C_{20}H_{32}$. They often exist under highly oxygenated forms with acyclic or cyclic frameworks, which results in a wide range of different carbon skeletons [67]. Within the scope of the current literature-based investigation, four major subtypes of diterpenes, including briarane, cembrane, eunicellin, and xenicane, along with six minor diterpene classes, such as halimane, verticillane, C-2/C-20-cyclized cembranoid skeleton, norcembranoid, capsosane, and lobane, are included in this section.

2.2.1. Briarane-Type Diterpenes

Briaranes are marine metabolites that are featured by a bicyclo[8.4.0]tetradecane skeleton fused with a γ-lactone ring (Figure 4). It was suggested that they are derived from the 3,8-cyclization of cembranes [60].

Figure 4. Briaranes (**4–10**) isolated from the octocorals *Junceella* sp. and *Briareum* sp.

In biological activity assays, three new 8-hydroxybriarane diterpenoids were isolated from the Gorgonian corals *Junceella juncea*, junceols A–C (**4–6**). At 10 µg/mL, they inhibited superoxide anion generation by human neutrophils with 45.64%, 159.60%, and 124.14%, respectively [68].

A new briarane diterpenoid, briarenolide F (**7**), which was isolated from an octocoral *Briareum* sp., was suggested to be the first 6-hydroperoxybriarane derivative. This compound showed a significant inhibitory effect on the generation of superoxide anion by human neutrophils [69].

The chemical investigation of *Briareum* sp. yielded briarenolide J (**8**) which was identified as the first metabolite of a briarane-related natural product. It was found to possess a chlorine atom at C-12. It inhibited the generation of superoxide anions and the release of elastase by human neutrophils with IC_{50} values of 14.98 and 9.96 µM, respectively [70].

In in vitro anti-inflammatory activity assays, it was found that the new polyoxygenated briarane diterpenoid isolated from the octocoral *Briareum excavatum*, briarenol D (**9**), showed a selective inhibitory effect on the release of elastase with an IC$_{50}$ value of 4.65 µM by human neutrophils [71].

In an in vitro anti-inflammatory activity assay, juncin Z (**10**), which was obtained from the gorgonian coral *Junceella fragilis*, showed a 25.56% inhibitory effect on the generation of superoxide anions by human neutrophils at a concentration of 10 µM [72].

2.2.2. Cembrane-Type Diterpenes

Cembrane-type diterpenes (Figure 5) are macrocyclic metabolites that were suggested to be derivatives of geranylgeranyl pyrophosphate. They are structurally diverse with an extended family of subtypes due to the variations in functional groups and patterns of cyclization. Their basic 14-membered ring could be fused to lactones with 5- to 8-atom rings. Several moieties could be attached to the core frameworks, such as epoxide, ester, hydroxyl, peroxide, carboxyl, aldehyde, and ketone groups [58].

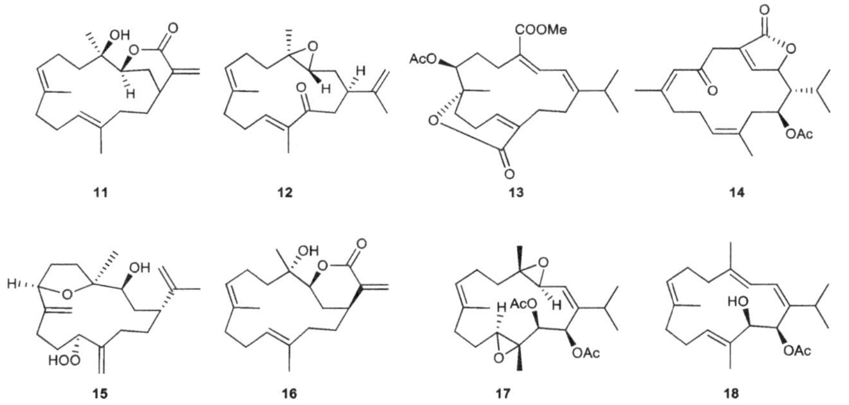

Figure 5. Cembranes (**11–18**) isolated from octocorals.

Lobocrassin B (**11**), which was isolated from the soft coral *Lobophytum crassum*, is a new cembrane metabolite that displayed significant inhibitory effects on the generation of superoxide anion and the release of elastase by human neutrophils, with IC$_{50}$ values of 4.8 and 4.9 µg/mL, respectively. This compound was found to be a stereoisomer of the known cembranes, 14-deoxycrassin [73].

From the ethyl acetate extract of the soft coral *Sinularia arborea*, a new cembrane-type diterpenoid, arbolide C (**12**), was isolated. The new compound significantly inhibited the release of elastase enzyme with an IC$_{50}$ value of 5.13 µg/mL [74].

A known cembrane isolated from the Formosan soft coral *Sarcophyton tortuosum*, emblide (**13**), inhibited elastase release to the extent of 29.2% at 10 µM [75].

A known metabolite, isosarcophytonolide D (**14**), was rediscovered from the cultured soft coral *Sarcophyton glaucum* and showed a 27.12% inhibitory effect on the elastase release at 10 µM [76].

A new cembrane analog, sinulerectol C (**15**), was obtained in the chemical exploration of a Dongsha Atoll soft coral *Sinularia erecta*. At 10 µM, the metabolite inhibited elastase release with an inhibitory rate of 33% [77].

The soft coral *Sinularia flexibilis* afforded a known cembranoid, 14-deoxycrassin (**16**), which inhibited superoxide anion generation and elastase release by human neutrophils with IC$_{50}$ values of 10.8 and 11.0 µM, respectively [59].

A chemical investigation on Formosan soft coral *Klyxum flaccidum* led to the isolation of two potent inhibitors of elastase release. Flaccidodioxide (**17**), a new cembranoid, showed a

17.17% inhibitory effect at 10 μM, whereas the other known analog, 14-O-acetylsarcophytol B (**18**), demonstrated an elastase release inhibitory effect, with an IC$_{50}$ value of 7.22 μM [78].

2.2.3. Eunicellin-Type Diterpenes and Derivatives

Eunicellin-based diterpenes are characterized by a six-carbon ring fused to a ten-carbon ring with an ether bridge that connects C-2 and C-9 or C-4 and C-7 in the latter ring. In some cases, the bond between C-6 and C-7 in the ten-membered ring moiety can be broken to form 6,7-secoeunicellin derivatives [79] (Figure 6).

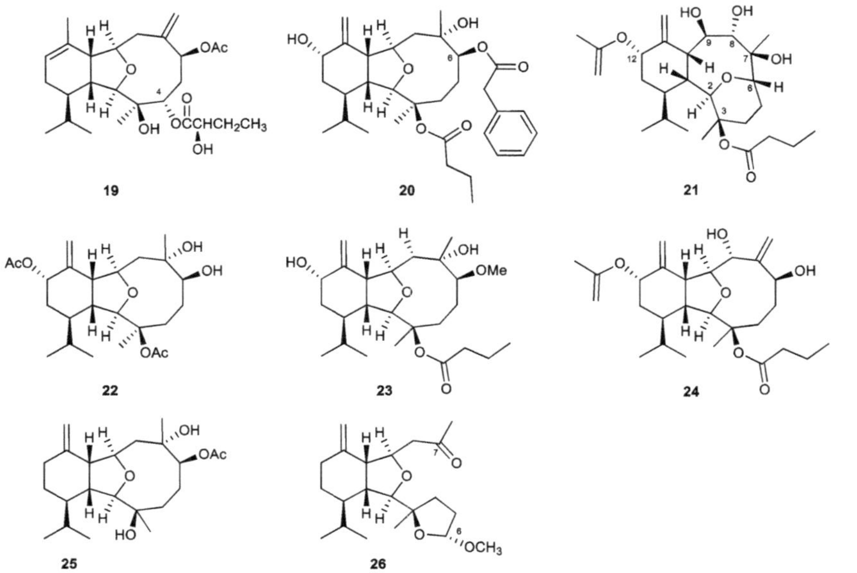

Figure 6. Eunicellines (**19–26**) isolated from *Cladiella* sp. and *Klyxum molle*.

In a chemical exploration of an Indonesian octocoral identified as *Cladiella* sp., a new eunicellin-type diterpenoid that possessed a 2-hydroxybutyroxy group at C-4 was discovered and designated as cladielloide B (**19**). The metabolite showed a significant inhibitory effect on superoxide anion generation and elastase release with IC$_{50}$ values of 5.9 and 6.5 μg/mL, respectively [80].

A chemical examination of the Formosan soft coral *Klyxum molle* resulted in the isolation of the first eunicellin-based metabolite with a phenylacetate moiety at C-6, klymollin M (**20**). The distinct substituent might contribute to the most potent anti-inflammatory activities of **20** toward the generation of superoxide anions (IC$_{50}$ = 3.13 ± 0.39 μM) and elastase release (IC$_{50}$ = 2.92 ± 0.27 μM) when compared to the eunicellines that were derived from the same organic extract of the soft coral [81].

A series of new eunicellin-type diterpenes was discovered in the soft coral *Cladiella krempfi*. Several of them were found to be effective anti-inflammatory agents. Krempfielin K (**21**), which possesses a rare eunicellin skeleton with a highly oxygenated pattern at C-2, C-3, C-6, C-7, C-8, C-9, and C-12, showed a 45.51% inhibitory effect on the release of elastase at a concentration of 10 μM. At the same concentration, krempfielin M (**22**) also significantly inhibited the elastase release (27.30 ± 5.42% inhibition). Krempfielin N (**23**) showed the most potent activity among the isolates, displaying an up to 73.86% inhibitory effect on elastase release at 10 μM, with an IC$_{50}$ value of 4.94 μM. The remaining active eunicelline in this series was krempfielin P (**24**), which inhibited not only elastase release but also the generation of superoxide anion with 35.54% and 23.32% inhibition at 10 μM, respectively [82,83].

A formerly reported eunicellin metabolite, sclerophytin B (**25**), was rediscovered in the chemical exploration of an octocoral of *Cladiella* sp. The compound showed 28.12% inhibitory effects on human neutrophils in terms of the generation of superoxide anions at a concentration of 10 µM [84].

An NMR-guided chemical examination of the octocoral *Cladiella* sp. afforded the first secoeunicellin possessing two tetrahydrofuran moieties, which was named cladieunicellin X (**26**). In comparison with the other novel metabolite that was isolated from the same sample of soft coral (cladieunicellin W), the novel 6,7-secoeunicellin was found to display a much more potent inhibitory effect on the generation of superoxide anions and the release of elastase, with IC_{50} values of 7.18 and 7.83 µM, respectively [85].

2.2.4. Xenicane-Type Diterpene

Xenicane diterpenes are characterized by a nine-membered ring often connected with a six-membered cyclic ether, resulting in a [7.4.0] bicyclic system [86] (Figure 7).

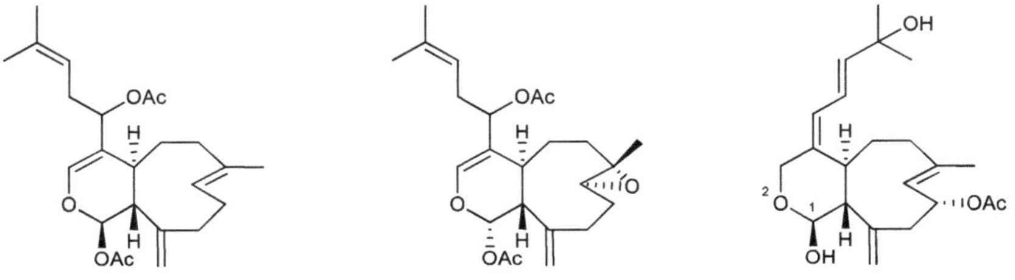

Figure 7. Xenicanes (**27–29**) isolated from soft corals.

Tsitsixenicins A (**27**) and B (**28**), which were isolated from the South African soft coral *Capnella thyrsoidea*, represented the first xenicanes discovered from the family Neptheiidae. Both of these compounds inhibited the production of superoxide anion in human neutrophils, with 68% and 21% inhibitory rates at 1.25 µg/mL [87].

Asterolaurin D (**29**) is a new diterpene isolated from the soft coral *Asterospicularia laurae*, collected from southern Taiwan. The compound possesses a 2-oxabicyclo[7.4.0]tridecane ring system, which is a characteristic feature of xenicane skeletons. Asterolaurin D also contains a hemiacetal moiety at C-1, which might make it much more active than the other analogs in the same series of isolates and even the positive control genistein, with IC_{50} values for the inhibition of superoxide anion generation and elastase release of 23.6 and 18.7 µM, respectively [88].

2.2.5. Miscellaneous Diterpenes

Echinohalimane A (**30**), a new diterpenoid, was isolated from *Echinomuricea* sp. It was the first halimane analog discovered from the phylum Cnidaria. The results of the in vitro experiment revealed that the new halimane-type diterpene exhibited potent anti-inflammatory activity, with an IC_{50} value of 0.38 µg/mL in inhibiting elastase release [89].

Cespitulin G (**31**), a new verticillane-type diterpene, was obtained in a chemical investigation of *Cespitularia taeniata*. It exhibited significant inhibitory activity against elastase release, with an IC_{50} value of 2.7 µg/mL, and against superoxide anion, with an IC_{50} value of 6.2 µg/mL [90].

Tortuosene A (**32**), which was isolated from the Formosan soft coral *Sarcophyton tortuosum*, possesses a new C-2/C-20-cyclized cembranoid skeleton. It showed a potent inhibitory effect against superoxide anion generation by human neutrophils with an IC_{50} value of 7.3 µM [75].

Two new norcembranoids, sinulerectols A (**33**) and B (**34**), were isolated from an extract of the marine soft coral *Sinularia erecta*. Both compounds were found to be potent agents in in vitro anti-inflammatory tests. Compound **33** showed IC_{50} values of 2.3 and

0.9 µM in the inhibition of superoxide generation and elastase release, respectively. In the same assays, the IC$_{50}$ values of compound **34** were 8.5 and 3.8 µM [77].

A new capsosane, 7-epi-pavidolide D (**35**), was isolated from the marine soft coral *Klyxum flaccidum*, collected off the coast of Pratas island. The compound showed good activity against the release of elastase at 10 µM, with an inhibitory rate of 29.96% [78].

A new lobane, lobovarol G (**36**), along with a known analog, loba-8,10,13(15)-trien-14,17,18-triol-14,17-diacetate (**37**), was isolated from the ethyl acetate extract of the soft coral *Lobophytum varium*. Both compounds were found to be effective in the inhibition of elastase release with IC$_{50}$ values of 18.8 and 6.9 µM. Lobovarol I (**38**), a new prenyleudesmane-type diterpene isolated from the same sample of the soft coral, inhibited the release of elastase with an IC$_{50}$ value of 20 µM. The other known eudesmane derivative (**39**) was found to be active with IC$_{50}$ values of 13.7 µM and 4.4 µM in superoxide anion generation and elastase release assays, respectively [91] (Figure 8).

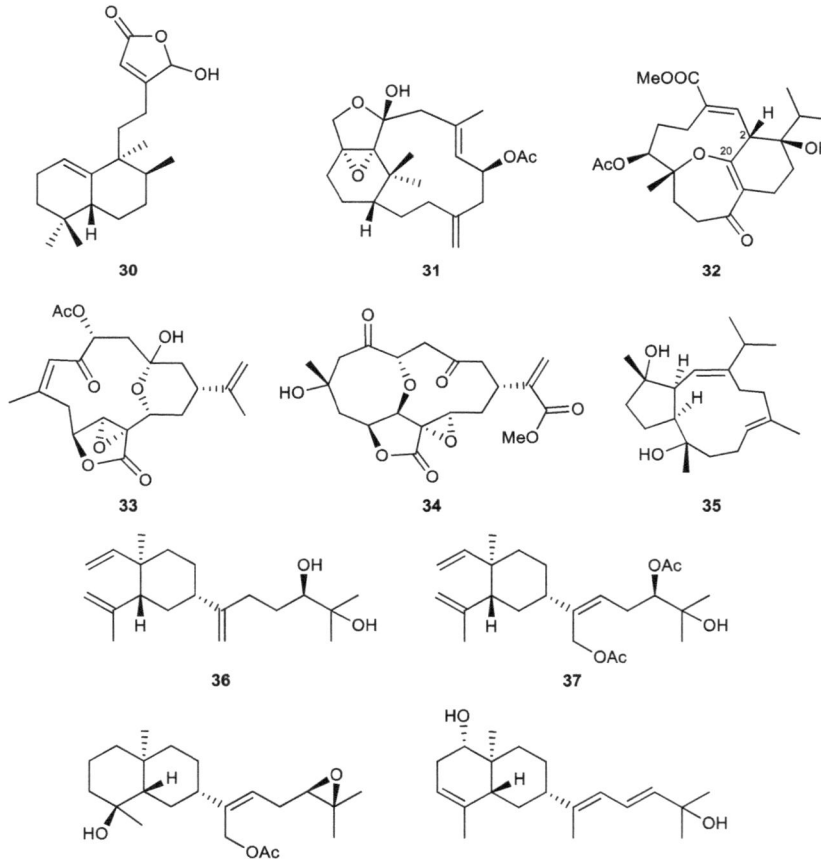

Figure 8. Anti-inflammatory diterpenoids (**30–39**) isolated from different soft corals.

2.3. Biscembranes

Biscembranes are marine natural products that are isolated from the soft coral of the genus *Sarcophyton*. They are characterized by a 14/6/14-membered tricyclic system [79] (Figure 9).

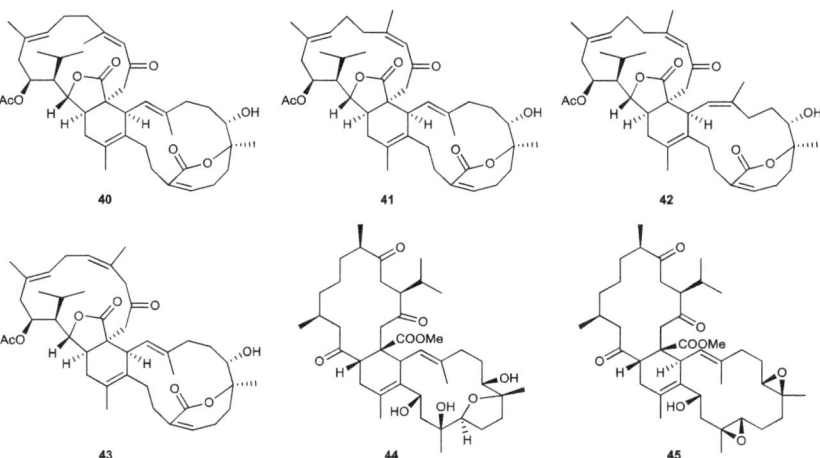

Figure 9. Biscembranes (**40**–**45**) isolated from the genus *Sarcophyton*.

Glaucumolides A (**40**) and B (**41**), novel biscembranes composed of an unprecedented α,β-unsaturated ε-lactone, were isolated from the cultured soft coral *Sarcophyton glaucum*. Both compounds inhibited superoxide anion generation and elastase release with IC_{50} values of 2.79 and 3.97 μM, respectively [76].

Several biscembrane metabolites, which were isolated from the cultured soft coral *Sarcophyton trocheliophorum*, displayed significant anti-inflammatory effects in the in vitro assays. At a concentration of 10 μM, bistrochelides A (**42**) and B (**43**) were found to be good inhibitors of both superoxide anion generation (56.19% and 45.39%, respectively) and elastase release (48.61% and 38.67%, respectively) assays. Meanwhile, methyl tortuoate D (**44**) and ximaolide A (**45**) were less potent than the former two analogs at the same concentration, with 25.67% and 26.64% inhibitory activities against elastase release, respectively [79].

2.4. Steroids

Steroids are tetracyclic compounds that comprise three cyclohexane and cyclopentane rings fused, creating a distinctive perhydro-1,2-cyclopentenophenanthrene core skeleton. The introduction of different side chains and functional moieties, along with some modifications in the core skeleton generated various types of steroids. Methyl groups are normally found at C-10 and C-13, and an alkyl side chain may be also attached to C-17. The integrity of the steroidal scaffold can be disturbed by bond fissions, ring expansions, contractions, or removal of certain functionalities [92].

As per the investigation of related studies, sterols, 9,11-secosterols, gorgostane-type steroids, withanolide-type steroids, steroid glycosides, and several unclassified steroids have been recorded as potential neutrophilic-targeting anti-inflammatory steroids derived from octocorals.

2.4.1. Sterols

Sterols represent a large group of natural steroids that bear a characteristic of a hydroxy group at C-3 in ring A of the steroid skeleton. Oxidation may occur in the side chain or the ring nucleus [55] (Figure 10). New steroids isolated from the Formosan soft coral *Klyxum flaccidum*, klyflaccisteroids J (**46**) and M (**47**), displayed potent anti-inflammatory effects in activated human neutrophils. Klyflaccisteroid J significantly inhibited superoxide anion generation (an IC_{50} value of 5.64 μM) and elastase release (an IC_{50} value of 4.40 μM). Klyflaccisteroid M was inactive against the production of superoxide anions but was a potent inhibitor of elastase release, with an IC_{50} value of 5.84 μM [93,94].

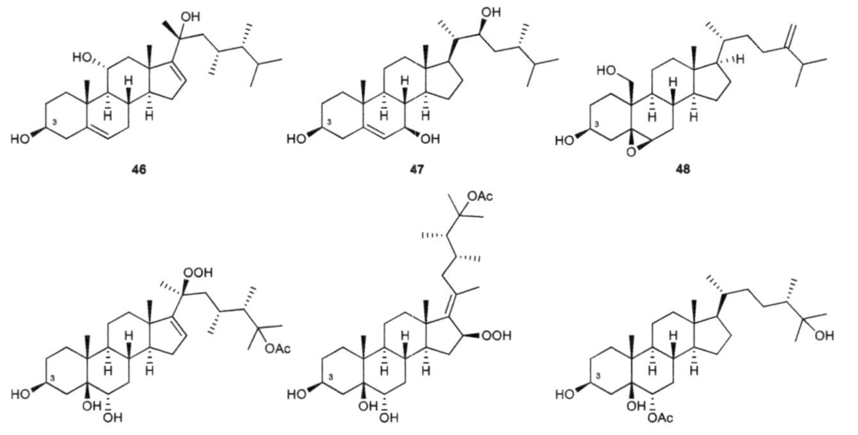

Figure 10. Sterols (**46–51**) isolated from octocorals.

A known steroid, which was identified as 5,6-epoxylitosterol (**48**), was obtained from the octocoral *Litophyton columnaris*. The compound significantly inhibited the generation of superoxide anion generation and the release of elastase, with IC_{50} values of 4.60 μM and 3.90 μM, respectively [95].

Three new polyoxygenated steroids, michosterols A–C (**49–51**), were isolated from the ethyl acetate extract of the soft coral *Lobophytum michaelae*. Michosterol A exhibited IC_{50} values of 7.1 and 4.5 μM against the superoxide anion production and elastase release respectively. Michosterol C was considered a promising inhibitor of elastase release, with an IC_{50} value of only 0.9 μM. Michosterol B (**58**), which possesses a hydroperoxyl group at C-16 and an uncommon double bond between C-17 and C-20, showed the weakest effects in both in vitro assays [96].

2.4.2. 9,11-Secosterols

9,11-secosterols (Figure 11) are a subtype of sterols, which are usually found in marine invertebrates, such as sponges, soft corals, and ascidians. Their structures are featured by the bond cleavage between C-9 and C-11 of ring C. The majority of 9,11-secosterols have a keto group attached to C-9 and a hydroxy group present at C-11 [97].

A known steroid, 5β,6β-epoxy-3β,11-dihydroxy-24-methylene-9,11-secocholestan-9-one (**52**), was obtained from the soft coral *Sinularia nanolobata*. It showed potent activity in in vitro anti-inflammatory assays. The IC_{50} values of the compound were 6.6 μM and 2.9 μM for the inhibition of superoxide anion generation and elastase release, respectively [98].

A series of unprecedented steroid skeletons were discovered from a gorgonian coral *Pinnigorgia* sp., which were assigned as pinnigorgiols A–E (**53–57**). The compounds contained a rare tricyclo[5,2,1,1]decane ring in their structures. Pinnigorgiols D and E were found to be the 11-O-acetyl derivative of pinnigorgiols A and B, respectively. The results of the in vitro experiment demonstrated that all the newly identified metabolites possessed anti-inflammatory potential. The IC_{50} values of pinnigorgiols A–E in the superoxide anion production assay were 4.0, 2.5, 2.7, 3.5, and 3.9 μM, respectively. Their inhibitory effects on the release of elastase were evidenced by IC_{50} values of 5.3, 3.1, 2.7, 2.1, and 1.6 μM [99,100].

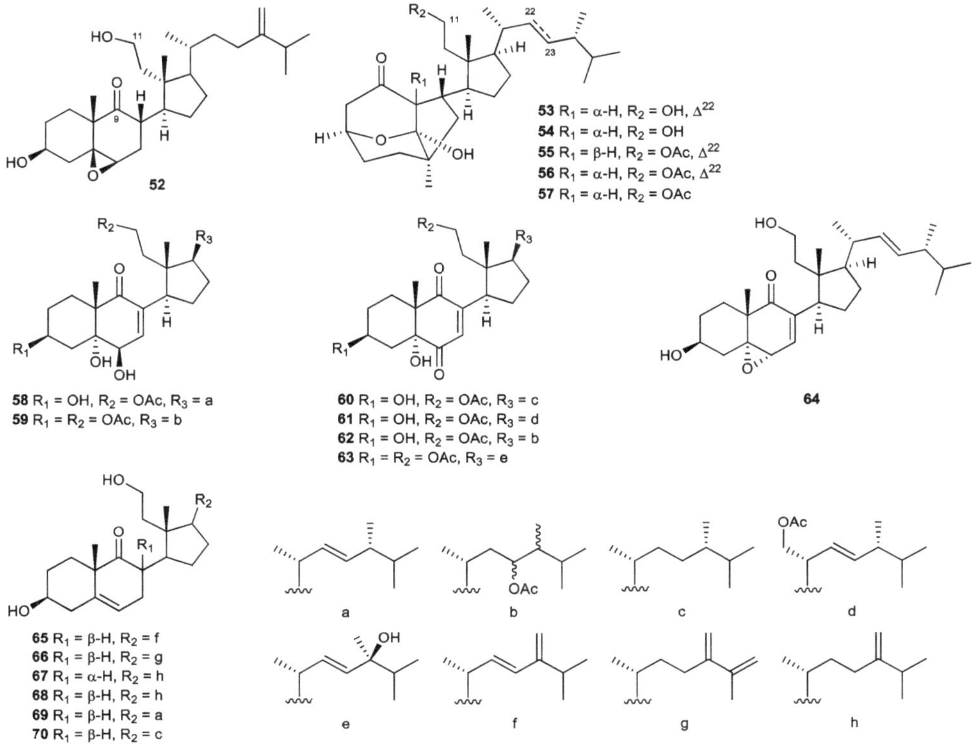

Figure 11. 9,11-secosterols (**52–70**) isolated from the genera *Sinularia* and *Pinnigorgia*.

Ten new 9,11-secosterols were identified in a recent study on the soft coral *Pinnigorgia* sp. More than half of the isolated steroids demonstrated impressive effects on neutrophilic inflammation, including pinnisterols A (**58**), C (**59**), E (**60**), F (**61**), H (**62**), and J (**63**). Except for pinnisterols E and F, which selectively inhibited elastase release and superoxide anion generation, with IC_{50} values of 2.33 and 5.52 µM, respectively, the remaining isolates displayed their effect in both anti-inflammatory assays. For superoxide anion production, their inhibitory effect was demonstrated by low IC_{50} values ranging from 2.33 to 3.89 µM. As inhibitors of elastase release, compounds **58**, **59**, **62**, and **63** exhibited IC_{50} values of 3.32, 2.81, 3.26, and 3.71 µM, respectively [101,102].

A detailed chemical investigation of the gorgonian coral *Pinnigorgia* sp. resulted in the isolation of a new bioactive sterol, 5α,6α-epoxy-(22E,24R)-3β,11-dihydroxy-9,11-secoergosta-7-en-9-one (**64**). This compound displayed inhibitory effects on the generation of superoxide anions and the release of elastase by human neutrophils, with IC_{50} values of 8.65 and 5.86 µM, respectively [103].

The 9,11-secosteroid targeting isolation conducted on the octocoral *Sinularia leptoclados* afforded six bioactive compounds, including two novel steroids, sinleptosterols A (**65**) and B (**66**), along with four known analogs, 8αH-3β,11-dihydroxy-24-methylene-9,11-secocholest-5-en-9-one (**67**), 8βH-3β,11-dihydroxy-24-methylene-9,11-secocholest-5-en-9-one (**68**), leptosterol A (**69**), and (24S)-3β,11-dihydroxy-24-methyl-9,11-secocholest-5-en-9-one (**70**). They exhibited potent anti-inflammatory effects in the in vitro assays. 8αH-3β,11-Dihydroxy-24-methylene-9,11-secocholest-5-en-9-one and 8βH-3β,11-dihydroxy-24-methylene-9,11-secocholest-5-en-9-one were the most potent agents in both superoxide anion production (IC_{50} values of 1.97 and 2.96 µM, respectively) and elastase release (IC_{50} values of 3.12 and 1.63 µM, respectively) assays. For the other four analogs, compound

70 was more active in the inhibition of superoxide anion generation than the others (IC$_{50}$ value of 4.09 μM), but it was the weakest inhibitor of elastase release. Sinleptosterol A was less potent than sinleptosterol B in both assays. Their IC50 values were determined to be 7.07 and 4.68 μM in terms of superoxide anion inhibition, and 7.57 and 4.29 μM for their ability to inhibit elastase release, respectively. The known steroid leptosterol A was also considered a promising anti-inflammatory lead, as it significantly inhibited superoxide anion generation and elastase release, with IC$_{50}$ values of 8.07 and 4.73 μM, respectively [104].

2.4.3. Gorgostane-Type Steroids

Gorgostane steroids (Figure 12) are marine-derived sterols that possess a C30 skeleton with a characteristic three-membered ring present in the side chain attached to C-17 of the cyclopentane ring. In some cases, ring C of the steroidal skeleton loses its integrity due to the oxidative cleavage of the C-9/11 bond, resulting in derivatives named 9,11-secogorgosterols. These metabolites are characterized by the presence of a keto group at C-9 and a carboxyl or a hydroxyl moiety at C-11 [61].

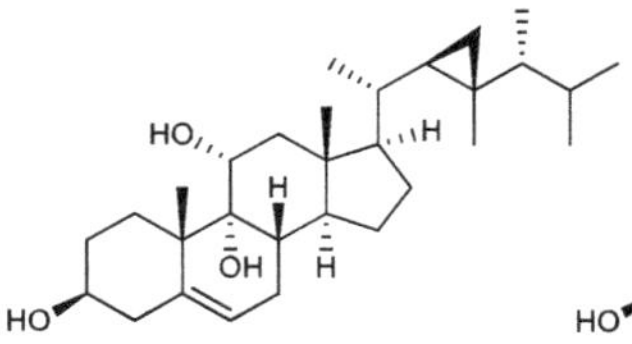

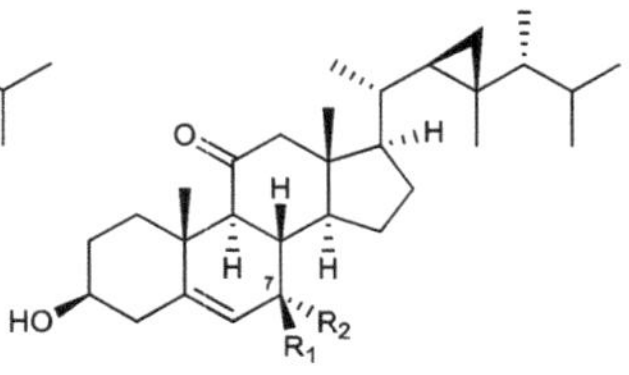

Figure 12. Gorgostane steroids (71–76) isolated from the soft coral *Klyxum flaccidum*.

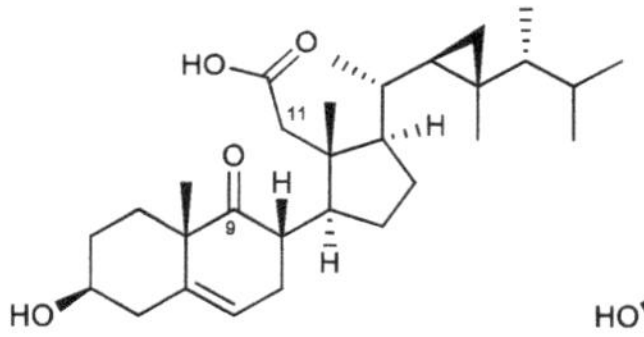

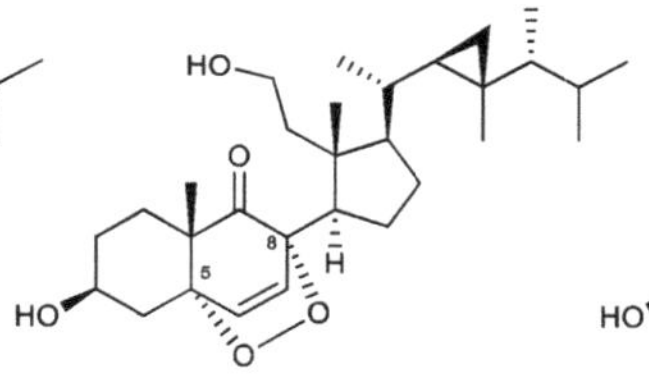

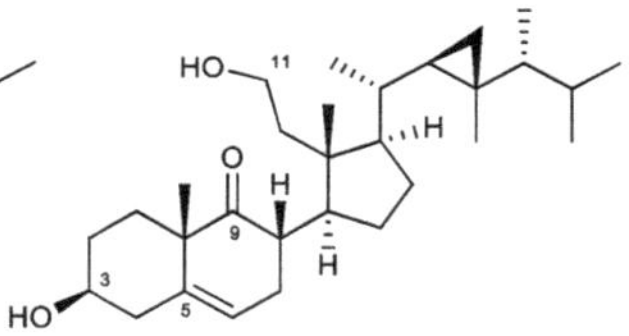

The ethyl acetate extract of the soft coral *Klyxum flaccidum* yielded a series of new and known steroids. Some of these compounds were found to possess anti-inflammatory activity, including gorgost-5-ene-3β,9α,11α-triol (71), klyflaccisteroids C (72), D (73), F (74), K (75), and 3β,11-dihydroxy-9,11-secogorgost-5-en-9-one (76). Gorgost-5-ene-3β,9α,11α-triol was the least active metabolite, with only 27.7% inhibition against elastase release at 10 μM. The new gorgosteroid, klyflaccisteroid C, displayed IC$_{50}$ values of 4.74 μM and 3.97 μM in the inhibition of superoxide anion production and elastase release, respectively. Klyflaccisteroid D, the C-7 oxidized product of klyflaccisteroid C, was less active in both assays when compared to its precursor, with a 30.9% inhibitory rate and an IC$_{50}$ value of 5.37 μM. Klyflaccisteroid F was the first 9,11-secogorgosteroid 11-carboxylic acid isolated from natural sources, which was extremely potent in inhibiting superoxide anion generation (IC$_{50}$ = 0.34 μM) and elastase release (IC$_{50}$ = 0.35 μM). Klyflaccisteroid K, a new steroid possessing a 5,8-epidioxy-9-ene functional group, displayed a similar effect on the suppression of superoxide anion production but was more potent than klyflaccisteroid J in inhibiting elastase release, with IC$_{50}$ values of 5.83 μM and 1.55 μM, respectively. The IC$_{50}$ values of the known secogorgosterol 3β,11-dihydroxy-9,11-secogorgost-5-en-9-one were determined to be 3.84 μM and 2.21 μM in the inhibition of superoxide anion production and elastase release, respectively [94,105].

2.4.4. Withanolide-Type Steroids

Withanolides are a group of C28 polyoxygenated steroidal skeletons that bear a C-22/26 δ-lactone and C-26 or a C-23/26 γ-lactone in the side chain, which is attached to C-17 [106]. A series of withanolide steroids was isolated from the soft coral *Sinularia brassica*, including sinubrasolides A (**77**), H (**78**), J (**79**), K (**80**), and L (**81**) (Figure 13). The known metabolite sinubrasolide A was the most potent agent in the series, with IC$_{50}$ values of 3.5 μM and 1.4 μM for superoxide anion generation and elastase release assays, respectively. Sinubrasolides H and K were found to be novel withanolides with a 16,23-oxo-bridged tetrahydropyran, and sinubrasolide K was the configurational isomer of sinubrasolide H. Regarding biological activity, sinubrasolide H was an effective inhibitor of elastase release (32.4% inhibition), while sinubrasolides J and K were active in the inhibition of superoxide anion generation with inhibitory rates of 32.1% and 34.3% at 10 μM, respectively. The remaining new withanolide, sinubrasolide L, was active in both assays, with inhibitory rates of 26.3% and 25.0% at 10 μM [106].

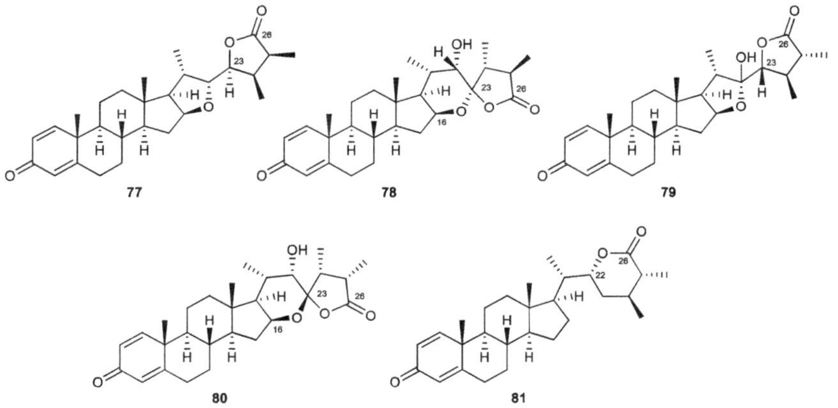

Figure 13. Withanolide steroids (**77**–**81**) isolated from the soft coral *Sinularia brassica*.

2.4.5. Steroid Glycosides

A new bioactive metabolite, carijoside A (**82**), was isolated from an octocoral identified as *Carijoa* sp. The sterol glycoside displayed significant inhibitory effects on superoxide anion generation (IC$_{50}$ = 1.8 μg/mL) and elastase release (IC$_{50}$ = 6.8 μg/mL) by human neutrophils [107].

A new pragnane glycoside, hirsutosteroside A (**83**), was isolated from the soft coral *Cladiella hirsuta*. The compound was evaluated for its anti-inflammatory potential via in vitro tests. It was inactive in the inhibition of superoxide anion production but effectively suppressed the release of elastase with an IC$_{50}$ value of 4.1 μM. At the same time, a known steroid, 24-methylenecholest-5-ene-3β,16β-diol-3-O-α-L-fucoside (**84**), was obtained from another soft coral, *Sinularia nanolobata*. The IC$_{50}$ values of compound **84** were 18.6 μM and 10.1 μM in the inhibition of superoxide anion generation and elastase release assays, respectively [98].

Sinubrasone A (**85**) is a novel steroid collected from the cultured soft coral *Sinularia brassica*. The compound possesses a methyl ester group attached to C-25 and a β-D-xylopyranose connected with C-22 via an O-glycoside bond. Sinubrasone A significantly suppressed superoxide anion generation and elastase release (24.8% and 35.6% inhibition, respectively) at 10 μM [108] (Figure 14).

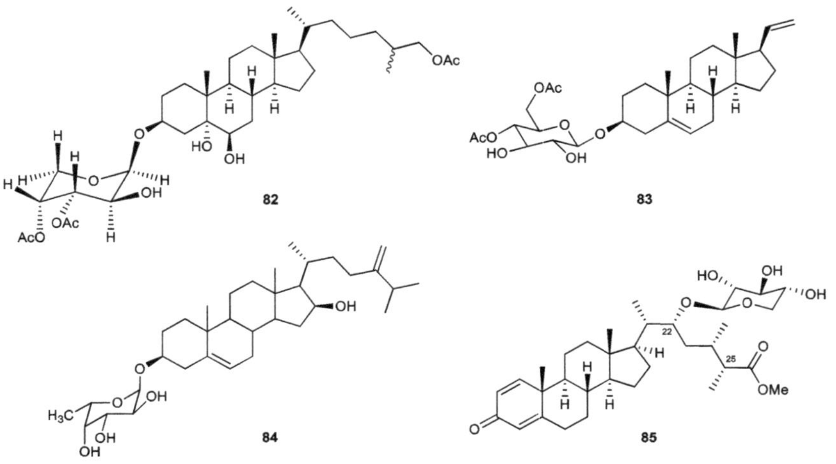

Figure 14. Steroid glycosides (**82–85**) isolated from the soft corals.

2.4.6. Miscellaneous Steroids

6-*epi*-Yonarasterol B (**86**) is a new sterol that was the first steroid isolated from the gorgonian coral of the genus *Echinomuricea*. The compound showed a significant inhibitory effect on the generation of superoxide anions and the release of elastase by human neutrophils, with IC_{50} values of 2.98 and 1.13 µM, respectively [109].

A chemical investigation was conducted on the soft coral *Umbellulifera petasites*, for the first time, resulting in the isolation of three bioactive steroids with potent anti-inflammatory activity. Among these isolates, two new steroids, petasitosterones B (**87**) and C (**88**), demonstrated effective inhibitory activity of superoxide anion generation. The known steroid 5α-pregna-20-en-3-one (**89**) selectively suppressed the release of elastase. Their IC_{50} values were 4.43, 2.76, and 6.8 µM [110].

The Formosan soft coral *Klyxum flaccidum* yielded klyflaccisteroid L (**90**) that displayed notable effects in activated human neutrophils. Klyflaccisteroid L possessed an unusual 11-norsteroid skeleton and was the first representative of an 11-oxasteroid discovered in nature. The compound was inactive against superoxide anion production but demonstrated 25.17% inhibition in elastase release assay at 10 µM [94].

Sinubrasones B–D (**91–93**), which are considered novel steroids with methyl ester groups, were collected from the cultured soft coral *Sinularia brassica*. Sinubrasone B possessing a tetrahydrofuran ring derived from the C-16/22 ether linkage, significantly suppressed superoxide anion generation and elastase release (19.4% and 39.0%, respectively) at 10 µM. Sinubrasones C and D were more effective inhibitors of elastase release with approximately similar IC_{50} values of 6.6 µM and 6.5 µM, respectively. Sinubrasone D also exhibited a potent inhibitory effect against the generation of superoxide anion, with an IC_{50} value of 8.4 µM [108] (Figure 15).

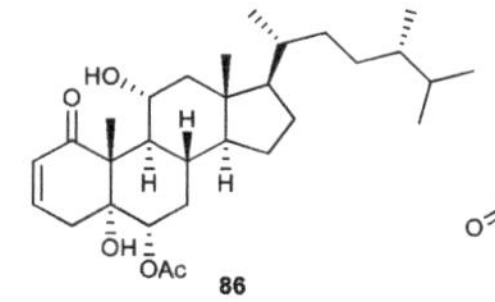

Figure 15. Other steroids (**86–93**) isolated from the octocorals.

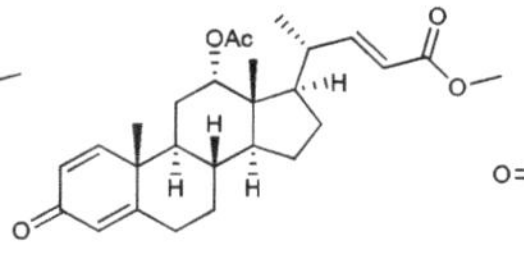

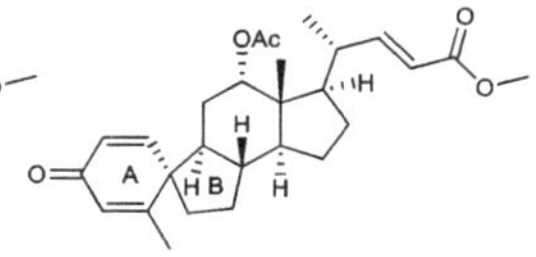

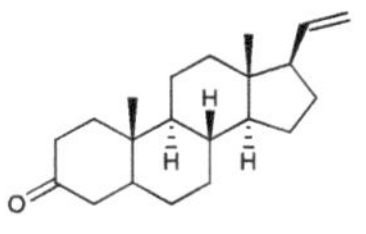

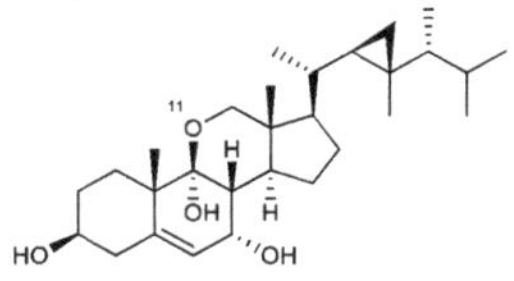

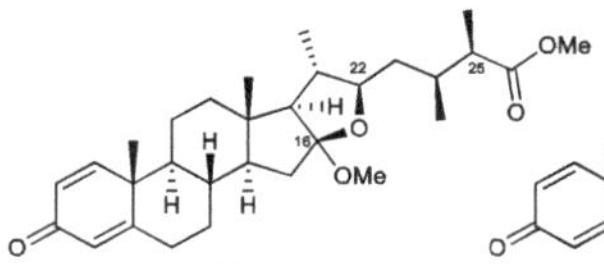

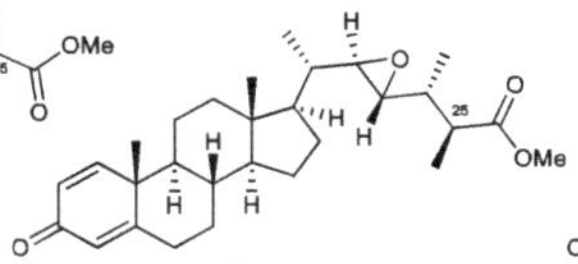

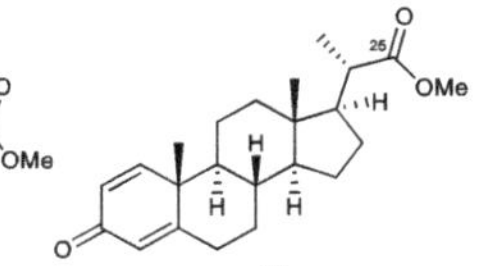

2.5. Miscellaneous

5-(6-Hydroxy-2,5,7,8-tetramethyl-chroman-2-yl)-2-methyl-pentanoic acid methyl ester (**94**), an α-tocopherol derivative, was isolated from the soft coral *Sinularia arborea* for the first time. The bioassay revealed that the metabolite displayed a significant inhibitory effect on the generation of superoxide anion by human neutrophils with an IC$_{50}$ value of 7.42 μM but was inactive toward elastase release [111].

Another new α-tocopherol derivative, hirsutocospiro A (**95**), was discovered in the soft coral *Cladiella hirsuta* with promising anti-inflammatory activity. The compound could be a promising candidate for the development of anti-inflammatory agents, as shown by the IC$_{50}$ values of 4.1 μM and 3.7 μM for the suppression of superoxide anion production and elastase release, respectively [112].

(Z)-N-[2-(4-Hydroxyphenyl)ethyl]-3-methyldodec-2-enamide (**96**), a known nitrogen-containing compound isolated from the soft coral *Sinularia erecta*, was found to be a potent inhibitor of elastase release, with an IC$_{50}$ value of 1.0 μM. The isolate also inhibited superoxide anion generation with an inhibitory rate of 48% at 10 μM [77].

Apo-9′-fucoxanthinone (**97**), isolated from a gorgonian coral *Pinnigorgia* sp., displayed a significant inhibitory effect on the release of elastase by human neutrophils, with an IC$_{50}$ value of 5.75 μM [113] (Figure 16).

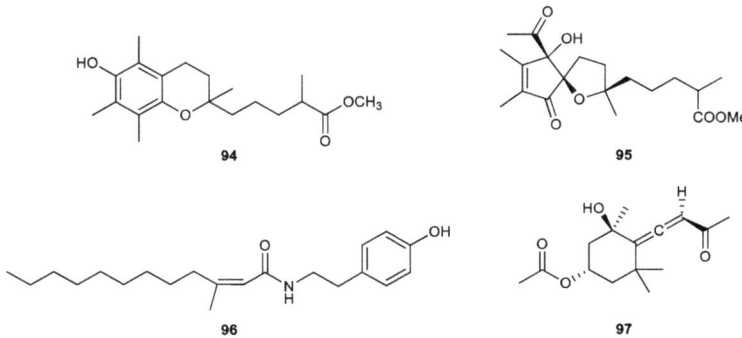

Figure 16. Bioactive metabolites (**94–97**) isolated from octocorals.

3. Preliminary Structure–Activity Relationship of the Octocoral-Derived Secondary Metabolites

As mentioned in the introduction, only 97 of 299 derivatives isolated from octocorals possess significant effects in the in vitro anti-inflammatory tests. The difference regarding their activities may be due to variations in their chemical structures. In this section, some examples regarding the impact of chemical variations on the difference in anti-inflammatory properties of octocoral-origin derivatives are introduced so as to provide the preliminary structure–activity relationship of these marine secondary metabolites.

In a chemical investigation of *Rumphella antipathies*, clovan-2,9-dione (**1**) was found to be the most potent compound among the isolates possessing a similar skeleton. This implies that the presence of the ketone group at C-2 plays a crucial role in the increased effect of sesquiterpenes. In the case of antipacids A and B, the difference is that the side chain at C-8 in the structure of antipacid B (**2**) is shorter than that of antipacid A, which may contribute to the enhanced anti-inflammatory potential of antipacid B in comparison with antipacid A. In addition, antipacid A and clovane-2β,9α-diol were inactive in the in vitro tests, whereas their combination via esterification resulted in rumphellolide L (**3**), which is a potent anti-inflammatory agent [65,66].

Among the polyoxygenated briaranes isolated from the octocoral *Briareum excavatum*, briarenol C was found to be inactive in the anti-inflammatory activity tests. In comparison to briarenols D (**9**) and E, the compound possesses a twisted boat conformation in the methylenencyclohexane ring, indicating that this configuration could significantly affect the anti-inflammatory property of briaranes [71].

Klymollin M (**20**) is one of the new diterpenes obtained from the organic extract of *Klyxum molle*. It was the first eunicelline bearing a phenylacetate group at C-6 and also exhibited the strongest inhibitory activity in the in vitro tests, as compared to other analogs in the study. This indicates that the presence of the substituent at C-6 may enhance the effects of klymollin M [81].

Cladieunicellin X (**26**) isolated from *Cladiella* sp. was found to demonstrate pronounced effects on superoxide anion generation and elastase release in activated neutrophils in comparison with cladieunicellin W. The difference between them is the presence of the methoxy group at C-6 in the structure of cladieunicellin X, implying that the functional group plays a critical role in the activity of these novel 6,7-secoeunicellins [85].

In comparison with the other xenicanes isolated from the same sample of the soft coral *Asterospicularia laurae*, the presence of the hemiacetal group in the chemical structure of asterolaurin D (**29**) was considered to be a critical factor in the enhancement in the inhibitory effects of the compound on elastase release in vitro [88].

Some modifications in the biscembrane skeletons of the derivatives originated from the cultured soft coral *Sarcophyton trocheliophorum* and led to the different extents of their inhibitory effects on superoxide anion generation and elastase release. A 6,7-dihydrooxepin-2(5H)-one moiety and a saturated γ-lactone ring are the common features of the four most potent compounds, glaucumolides A (**40**) and B (**41**) and bistrochelides A (**42**) and B (**43**). In addition to the characteristic functional groups, the bioactivities of the four compounds also varied when compared to each other due to some minor variations in their configurations. Particularly, glaucumolide B exhibits 11Z and 22E double bonds, differing from the E configuration observed at $\Delta^{11(12)}$ and $\Delta^{22(23)}$ in glaucumolide A, as well as the Z configuration at $\Delta^{11(12)}$ and $\Delta^{22(23)}$ in bistrochelide A. Furthermore, a comparison with glaucumolide B reveals that glaucumolide B features a substitution of the 11,12 double bond with a 10,11 double bond. This alteration implies that the slight modification in bistrochelide B, leading to the replacement of the 11,12-double bond, could be accountable for the diminished anti-inflammatory effect observed in it [79].

The two sterols, 5,6-epoxylitosterol (**48**) and litosterol, were obtained from the same sample of *Nephthea columnaris*. However, litosterol was inactive in the anti-inflammatory tests, whereas 5,6-epoxylitosterol showed highly potent effects on superoxide anion generation and elastase release. The difference in their properties implies the crucial role of the 5β,6β-epoxy group in increasing the activity of 5,6-epoxylitosterol [95].

Pinnigorgiols A–E (**53–57**) isolated from *Pinnigorgia* sp. demonstrated promising anti-inflammatory activities. Nonetheless, pinnigorgiol E (**57**) was the most effective inhibitor of elastase release among the isolates, which suggests the important role of an acetoxy substituent at C-11 and the absence of the C-22/23 double bond in the structure of this compound novel compound 9,11-secosterol [99,100].

The gorgonian coral *Pinnigorgia* sp. yielded a potent anti-inflammatory agent and an inactive analog. The difference in their pharmacological properties was believed to be driven by the acetoxy group at C-3 in ring A of pinnisterol C (**59**), as compared to the structure of pinnisterol B [101].

Among the metabolites isolated from the octocoral *Sinularia leptoclados*, 3β,11-dihydroxy-9,11-secogorgost-5-en-9-one presented activity at a concentration greater than 10 μM in both anti-inflammatory in vitro tests. By comparing the chemical structures of these analogs, it was found that 3β,11-dihydroxy-9,11-secogorgost-5-en-9-one possessed a unique gorgosterol side chain, which perhaps accounted for its nullified activities [104].

In a study on the chemical constituents of *Umbellulifera petasites*, petasitosterone C (**88**) was the steroid that possessed a rare A/B spiro[4,5]decane ring system and displayed the strongest activities against superoxide anion generation, as compared to the other steroids isolated from the same sample. This indicates that the unique chemical feature of the compound might be related to its enhanced activity [110].

Table 1. Potent anti-inflammatory compounds derived from octocorals.

Compound Name	Novelty	Chemical Classification	Source	Inhibitory Effects		Ref.
				$O^{\bullet -}$ Generation	Elastase Release	
Clovan-2,9-dione (1)	New	Sesquiterpene	*Rumphella antipathies*	$IC_{50} = 2.72 \pm 0.93$ μg/mL	$IC_{50} = 6.73 \pm 0.85$ μg/mL	[65]
Antipacid B (2)	Novel	Sesquiterpene	*Rumphella antipathies*	$IC_{50} = 11.22$ μM	$IC_{50} = 23.53$ μM	[66]
Rumphellolide L (3)	New	Sesquiterpene	*Rumphella antipathies*	Inh% = 19.57 ± 3.69 (10 μg/mL)	$IC_{50} = 7.63$ μM	[66]
Junceol A (4)	New	Briarane-type diterpene	*Junceella juncea*	Inh% = 45.64 % (10 μg/mL)		[68]
Junceol B (5)	New	Briarane-type diterpene	*Junceella juncea*	Inh% = 159.60 % (10 μg/mL)		[68]
Junceol C (6)	New	Briarane-type diterpene	*Junceella juncea*	Inh% = 124.14 % (10 μg/mL) [68]		[68]
Briarenolide F (7)	New	Briarane-type diterpene	*Briareum* sp.	$IC_{50} = 3.82 \pm 0.45$ μg/mL	Inh% = 27.48 ± 6.60 (10 μg/mL)	[69]
Briarenolide J (8)	Novel	Briarane-type diterpene	*Briareum* sp.	$IC_{50} = 14.98$ μM	$IC_{50} = 9.96$ μM	[70]
Briarenol D (9)	New	Briarane-type diterpene	*Briareum excavatum*		$IC_{50} = 4.65$ μM	[71]
Juncin Z (10)	New	Briarane-type diterpene	*Junceella fragilis*	Inh% = 25.56% (10 μM)		[72]
Lobocrassin B (11)	New	Cembrane-type diterpene	*Lobophytum crassum*	$IC_{50} = 4.8 \pm 0.7$ μg/mL	$IC_{50} = 4.9 \pm 0.4$ μg/mL	[73]
Arbolide C (12)	New	Cembrane-type diterpene	*Sinularia arborea*		$IC_{50} = 5.13$ μg/mL	[74]
Emblide (13)	Known	Cembrane-type diterpene	*Sarcophyton tortuosum*		Inh% = 29.2 ± 6.1 (10 μM)	[75]

Table 1. *Cont.*

Compound Name	Novelty	Chemical Classification	Source	Inhibitory Effects		Ref.
				$O^{\bullet-}$ Generation	Elastase Release	
Isosarcophytonolide D (14)	Known	Cembrane-type diterpene	*Sarcophyton glaucum*	Inh% = 12.40 ± 2.56 (10 μM)	Inh% = 27.12 ± 3.08 (10 μM)	[76]
Sinulerectol C (15)	New	Cembrane-type diterpene	*Sinularia erecta*	Inh% = 24 ± 7 (10 μM)	Inh% = 33 ± 3 (10 μM)	[77]
14-Deoxycrassin (16)	Known	Cembrane-type diterpene	*Sinularia flexibilis*	IC_{50} = 10.8 ± 0.38 μM	IC_{50} = 11.0 ± 1.52 μM	[59]
Flaccidodioxide (17)	New	Cembrane-type diterpene	*Klyxum flaccidum*	Inh% = 8.88 ± 3.33 (10 μM)	Inh% = 27.18 ± 4.05 (10 μM)	[78]
14-O-Acetylsarcophytol B (18)	Known	Cembrane-type diterpene	*Klyxum flaccidum*	Inh% = 11.95 ± 2.53 (10 μM)	IC_{50} = 7.22 ± 0.85 μM	[78]
Cladielloide B (19)	New	Eunicellin-type diterpene	*Cladiella* sp.	IC_{50} = 5.9 ± 0.7 μg/mL	IC_{50} = 6.5 ± 1.9 μg/mL	[80]
Klymollin M (20)	New	Eunicellin-type diterpene	*Klyxum molle*	IC_{50} = 3.13 ± 0.39 μM	IC_{50} = 2.92 ± 0.27 μM	[81]
Krempfielin K (21)	New	Eunicellin-type diterpene	*Cladiella krempfi*		Inh% = 45.51 ± 2.69 (10 μM)	[82]
Krempfielin M (22)	New	Eunicellin-type diterpene	*Cladiella krempfi*		Inh% = 27.30 ± 5.42 (10 μM)	[82]
Krempfielin N (23)	New	Eunicellin-type diterpene	*Cladiella krempfi*		IC_{50} = 4.94 ± 1.68 μM	[83]
Krempfielin P (24)	New	Eunicellin-type diterpene	*Cladiella krempfi*	Inh% = 23.32% ± 5.88 (10 μM)	Inh% = 35.54 ± 3.17 (10 μM)	[83]
Sclerophytin B (25)	Known	Eunicellin-type diterpene	*Cladiella* sp.	Inh% = 28.12 ± 3.61 (10 μM)	Inh% = 16.37 ± 8.14 (10 μM)	[84]
Cladieunicellin X (26)	Novel	Eunicellin-type diterpene	*Cladiella* sp.	IC_{50} = 7.18 ± 1.20 μM	IC_{50} = 7.83 ± 0.83 μM	[85]
Tsitsixenicin A (27)	New	Xenicane-type diterpene	*Capnella thyrsoidea*	Inh% = 68% at 1.25 μg/mL		[87]
Tsitsixenicin B (28)	New	Xenicane-type diterpene	*Capnella thyrsoidea*	Inh% = 21% at 1.25 μg/mL		[87]
Asterolaurin D (29)	New	Xenicane-type diterpene	*Asterospicularia laurae*	IC_{50} = 23.6 μM	IC_{50} = 18.7 μM	[88]
Echinohalimane A (30)	New	Halimane-type diterpene	*Echinomuricea* sp.	Inh% = 20.55 ± 5.18 (10 μg/mL)	IC_{50} = 0.38 ± 0.14 μg/mL	[89]
Cespitulin G (31)	New	Verticillane-type diterpene	*Cespitularia taeniata*	IC_{50} = 6.2 μg/mL	IC_{50} = 2.7 μg/mL	[90]
Tortuosene A (32)	New	Tortuosane-type diterpene	*Sarcophyton tortuosum*	IC_{50} = 7.3 ± 0.8 μM		[75]
Sinulerectol A (33)	New	Norcembrane-type diterpene	*Sinularia erecta*	IC_{50} = 2.3 ± 0.4 μM	IC_{50} = 0.9 ± 0.1 μM	[77]
Sinulerectol B (34)	New	Norcembrane-type diterpene	*Sinularia erecta*	IC_{50} = 8.5 ± 0.3 μM	IC_{50} = 3.8 ± 0.6 μM	[77]
7-Epi-Pavidolide D (35)	New	Capnosane-type diterpene	*Klyxum flaccidum*	Inh% = 24.46 ± 6.99 (10 μM)	Inh% = 29.96 ± 6.14 (10 μM)	[78]
Lobovarol G (36)	New	Lobane-type diterpene	*Lobophytum varium*	Inh% = 18.1 ± 4.0 (10 μg/mL)	IC_{50} = 18.8 ± 1.8 μM	[91]
Loba-8,10,13(15)-trien-14,17,18-triol-14,17-diacetate (37)	Known	Lobane-type diterpene	*Lobophytum varium*	Inh% = 46.5 ± 5.8 (10 μg/mL)	IC_{50} = 6.9 ± 2.7 μM	[91]
Lobovarol I (38)	New	Prenyleudesmane-type diterpene	*Lobophytum varium*	Inh% = 40.2 ± 7.3 (10 μg/mL)	IC_{50} = 20.0 ± 3.0 μM	[91]

Table 1. *Cont.*

Compound Name	Novelty	Chemical Classification	Source	Inhibitory Effects $O^{\bullet-}$ Generation	Inhibitory Effects Elastase Release	Ref.
An eudesmane derivative (39)	Known	Prenyleudesmane-type diterpene	*Lobophytum varium*	$IC_{50} = 13.7 \pm 4.4$ μM	$IC_{50} = 4.4 \pm 0.7$ μM	[91]
Glaucumolide A (40)	Novel	Biscembrane	*Sarcophyton glaucum*	$IC_{50} = 2.79 \pm 0.66$ μM	$IC_{50} = 3.97 \pm 0.10$ μM	[76]
Glaucumolide B (41)	Novel	Biscembrane	*Sarcophyton glaucum*	$IC_{50} = 2.79 \pm 0.32$ μM	$IC_{50} = 3.97 \pm 0.10$ μM	[76]
Bistrochelide A (42)	Known	Biscembrane	*Sarcophyton trocheliophorum*	$IC_{50} = 8.29 \pm 0.48$ μM	Inh% = 48.61 ± 0.96 (10 μM)	[79]
Bistrochelide B (43)	Known	Biscembrane	*Sarcophyton trocheliophorum*	Inh% = 45.39 ± 4.30 (10 μM)	Inh% = 38.67 ± 4.81 (10 μM)	[79]
Methyl tortuoate D (44)	Known	Biscembrane	*Sarcophyton trocheliophorum*	Inh% = 17.61 ± 1.99 (10 μM)	Inh% = 25.67 ± 5.27 (10 μM)	[79]
Ximaolide A (45)	Known	Biscembrane	*Sarcophyton trocheliophorum*	Inh% = 19.69 ± 5.00	Inh% = 26.64 ± 5.02 (10 μM)	[79]
Klyflaccisteroid J (46)	New	Sterol	*Klyxum flaccidum*	$IC_{50} = 5.64 \pm 0.41$ μM	$IC_{50} = 4.40 \pm 0.19$ μM	[93]
Klyflaccisteroid M (47)	New	Sterol	*Klyxum flaccidum*	Inh% = 12.61 ± 1.70 (10 μM)	$IC_{50} = 5.84 \pm 0.33$ 10 μM	[94]
5,6-Epoxylitosterol (48)	Known	Sterol	*Litophyton columnaris*	$IC_{50} = 4.60 \pm 0.85$ μM	$IC_{50} = 3.90 \pm 0.88$ μM	[95]
Michosterol A (49)	New	Sterol	*Lobophytum michaelae*	$IC_{50} = 7.1 \pm 0.3$ μM	$IC_{50} = 4.5 \pm 0.9$ μM	[96]
Michosterol B (50)	New	Sterol	*Lobophytum michaelae*	Inh% = 14.7 ± 5.7 (10 μM)	Inh% = 31.8 ± 5.0 (10 μM)	[96]
Michosterol C (51)	New	Sterol	*Lobophytum michaelae*	Inh% = 17.8 ± 2.8 (10 μM)	$IC_{50} = 0.9 \pm 0.1$ μM	[96]
5β,6β-Epoxy-3β,11-dihydroxy-24-methylene-9,11-secocholestan-9-one (52)	Known	Secosterol	*Sinularia nanolobata*	$IC_{50} = 6.6 \pm 0.6$ μM	$IC_{50} = 2.9 \pm 0.5$ μM	[98]
Pinnigorgiol A (53)	Novel	Secosterol	*Pinnigorgia* sp.	$IC_{50} = 4.0$ μM	$IC_{50} = 5.3$ μM	[99]
Pinnigorgiol B (54)	Novel	Secosterol	*Pinnigorgia* sp.	$IC_{50} = 2.5$ μM	$IC_{50} = 3.1$ μM	[99]
Pinnigorgiol C (55)	Novel	Secosterol	*Pinnigorgia* sp.	$IC_{50} = 2.7$ μM	$IC_{50} = 2.7$ μM	[99]
Pinnigorgiol D (56)	New	Secosterol	*Pinnigorgia* sp.	$IC_{50} = 3.5$ μM	$IC_{50} = 2.1$ μM	[100]
Pinnigorgiol E (57)	New	Secosterol	*Pinnigorgia* sp.	$IC_{50} = 3.9$ μM	$IC_{50} = 1.6$ μM	[100]
Pinnisterol A (58)	New	Secosterol	*Pinnigorgia* sp.	$IC_{50} = 2.33$ μM	$IC_{50} = 3.32$ μM	[101]
Pinnisterol C (59)	New	Secosterol	*Pinnigorgia* sp.	$IC_{50} = 2.50$ μM	$IC_{50} = 2.81$ μM	[101]
Pinnisterol E (60)	New	Secosterol	*Pinnigorgia* sp.		$IC_{50} = 2.33 \pm 0.27$ μM	[102]
Pinnisterol F (61)	New	Secosterol	*Pinnigorgia* sp.	$IC_{50} = 5.52 \pm 1.06$ μM		[102]
Pinnisterol H (62)	New	Secosterol	*Pinnigorgia* sp.	$IC_{50} = 3.26 \pm 0.33$ μM	$IC_{50} = 2.59 \pm 0.29$ μM	[102]
Pinnisterol J (63)	New	Secosterol	*Pinnigorgia* sp.	$IC_{50} = 3.71 \pm 0.51$ μM	$IC_{50} = 3.89 \pm 1.16$ μM	[102]
5α,6α-Epoxy-(22E,24R)-3β,11-dihydroxy-9,11-secoergosta-7-en-9-one (64)	New	Secosterol	*Pinnigorgia* sp.	$IC_{50} = 8.65 \pm 0.19$ μM	$IC_{50} = 5.86 \pm 0.95$ μM	[103]

Table 1. Cont.

Compound Name	Novelty	Chemical Classification	Source	Inhibitory Effects $O^{\bullet-}$ Generation	Elastase Release	Ref.
Sinleptosterol A (65)	Novel	Secosterol	Sinularia leptoclados	$IC_{50} = 7.07 \pm 0.52$ μM	$IC_{50} = 7.57 \pm 0.40$ μM	[104]
Sinleptosterol B (66)	Novel	Secosterol	Sinularia leptoclados	$IC_{50} = 4.68 \pm 0.57$ μM	$IC_{50} = 4.29 \pm 0.25$ μM	[104]
8αH-3β,11-Dihydroxy-24-methylene-9,11-secocholest-5-en-9-one (67)	Known	Secosterol	Sinularia leptoclados	$IC_{50} = 1.97 \pm 0.12$ μM	$IC_{50} = 3.12 \pm 0.07$ μM	[104]
8βH-3β,11-dihydroxy-24-methylene-9,11-secocholest-5-en-9-one (68)	Known	Secosterol	Sinularia leptoclados	$IC_{50} = 2.96 \pm 0.91$ μM	$IC_{50} = 1.63 \pm 0.15$ μM	[104]
Leptosterol A (69)	Known	Secosterol	Sinularia leptoclados	$IC_{50} = 8.07 \pm 0.53$ μM	$IC_{50} = 4.73 \pm 0.57$ μM	[104]
(24S)-3β,11-Dihydroxy-24-methyl-9,11-secocholest-5-en-9-one (70)	Known	Secosterol	Sinularia leptoclados	$IC_{50} = 4.09 \pm 0.50$ μM	Inh% = 25.38 ± 6.68 at 10 μM	[104]
Gorgost-5-ene-3β,9α,11α-triol (71)	Known	Gorgostane-type steroid	Klyxum flaccidum	Inh% = 10.52 ± 2.71 (10 μM)	Inh% = 27.70 ± 5.29 (10 μM)	[105]
Klyflaccisteroid C (72)	New	Gorgostane-type steroid	Klyxum flaccidum	$IC_{50} = 4.78 \pm 0.87$ μM	$IC_{50} = 3.97 \pm 0.10$ μM	[105]
Klyflaccisteroid D (73)	New	Gorgostane-type steroid	Klyxum flaccidum	Inh% = 30.9 ± 4.68 (10 μM)	$IC_{50} = 5.37 \pm 0.20$ μM	[105]
Klyflaccisteroid F (74)	New	Gorgostane-type steroid	Klyxum flaccidum	$IC_{50} = 0.34 \pm 0.01$ μM	$IC_{50} = 0.35 \pm 0.04$ μM	[105]
Klyflaccisteroid K (75)	New	Gorgostane-type steroid	Klyxum flaccidum	$IC_{50} = 5.83 \pm 0.62$ μM	$IC_{50} = 1.55 \pm 0.21$ μM	[94]
3β,11-Dihydroxy-9,11-secogorgost-5-en-9-one (76)	Known	Gorgostane-type steroid	Klyxum flaccidum	$IC_{50} = 3.84 \pm 0.41$ μM	$IC_{50} = 2.21 \pm 0.59$ μM	[105]
Sinubrasolide A (77)	Known	Withanolide-type steroid	Sinularia brassica	$IC_{50} = 3.5 \pm 0.9$ μM	$IC_{50} = 1.4 \pm 0.1$ μM	[106]
Sinubrasolide H (78)	New	Withanolide-type steroid	Sinularia brassica	Inh% = 14.4 ± 3.1 (10 μM)	Inh% = 32.4 ± 5.6 (10 μM)	[106]
Sinubrasolide J (79)	New	Withanolide-type steroid	Sinularia brassica	Inh% = 32.1 ± 5.3 (10 μM)	Inh% = 9.5 ± 5.2 (10 μM)	[106]
Sinubrasolide K (80)	New	Withanolide-type steroid	Sinularia brassica	Inh% = 34.3 ± 6.6 (10 μM)	Inh% = 11.4 ± 3.2 (10 μM)	[106]
Sinubrasolide L (81)	New	Withanolide-type steroid	Sinularia brassica	Inh% = 26.3 ± 0.7 (10 μM)	Inh% = 25.0 ± 1.3 (10 μM)	[106]
Carijoside A (82)	New	Steroid glycoside	Carijoa sp.	$IC_{50} = 1.8$ μg/mL	$IC_{50} = 6.8$ μg/mL	[107]
Hirsutosteroside A (83)	New	Steroid glycoside	Cladiella hirsuta		$IC_{50} = 4.1 \pm 0.1$ μM	[98]
24-Methylenecholest-5-ene-3β,16β-diol-3-O-α-L-fucoside (84)	Known	Steroid glycoside	Sinularia nanolobata	$IC_{50} = 18.6 \pm 1.5$ μM	$IC_{50} = 10.1 \pm 0.8$ μM	[98]

Table 1. Cont.

Compound Name	Novelty	Chemical Classification	Source	Inhibitory Effects $O^{\bullet -}$ Generation	Elastase Release	Ref.
Sinubrasone A (85)	New	Steroid glycoside	*Sinularia brassica*	Inh% = 24.8 ± 6.5 (10 µM)	Inh% = 35.6 ± 1.3 (10 µM)	[108]
6-Epi-yonarasterol B (86)	New	Miscellaneous steroid	*Echinomuricea* sp.	IC_{50} = 2.98 ± 0.29 µg/mL	IC_{50} = 1.13 ± 0.55 µg/mL	[109]
Petasitosterone B (87)	New	Miscellaneous steroid	*Umbellulifera petasites*	IC_{50} = 4.43 ± 0.23 µM		[110]
Petasitosterone C (88)	New	Miscellaneous steroid	*Umbellulifera petasites*	IC_{50} = 2.76 ± 0.92 µM		[110]
5α-Pregna-20-en-3-one (89)	Known	Miscellaneous steroid	*Umbellulifera petasites*		IC_{50} = 6.80 ± 0.18 µM	[110]
Klyflaccisteroid L (90)	New	Miscellaneous steroid	*Klyxum flaccidum*		Inh% = 25.17 ± 6.73 (10 µM)	[94]
Sinubrasone B (91)	New	Miscellaneous steroid	*Sinularia brassica*	Inh% = 19.4 ± 5.0 (10 µM)	Inh% = 39.0 ± 2.3 (10 µM)	[108]
Sinubrasone C (92)	New	Miscellaneous steroid	*Sinularia brassica*	Inh% = 27.7 ± 1.3 (10 µM)	IC50 = 6.6 ± 1.7 µM	[108]
Sinubrasone D (93)	New	Miscellaneous steroid	*Sinularia brassica*	IC_{50} = 8.4 ± 1.1 µM	IC50 = 6.5 ± 1.1 µM	[108]
5-(6-Hydroxy-2,5,7,8-tetramethyl-chroman-2-yl)-2-methyl-pentanoic acid methyl ester (94)	New	α-tocopherol derivative	*Sinularia arborea*	IC_{50} = 7.42 µM		[111]
Hirsutocospiro A (95)	New	α-tocopherol derivative	*Cladiella hirsuta*	IC_{50} = 4.1 ± 1.1 µM	IC50 = 3.7 ± 0.3 µM	[112]
(Z)-N-[2-(4-Hydroxyphenyl)ethyl]-3-methyldodec-2-enamide (96)	Known	Nitrogen-containing compound	*Sinularia erecta*	Inh% = 48 ± 2 (10 µM)	IC50 = 1.0 ± 0.2 µM	[77]
Apo-9'-fucoxanthinone (97)	Known	Allenic norterpenoid ketone	*Pinnigorgia* sp.		IC_{50} = 5.75 µM	[113]

4. Conclusions and Perspectives

The generation of ROS is a crucial component of the antimicrobial effectiveness exhibited by neutrophils. Nevertheless, the excessive production or insufficient removal of ROS can lead to harm to cells and tissues; the oxidation and alteration of DNA, lipids, and proteins; the formation of autoimmune neutrophil extracellular traps (NETs); and the creation of autoantibodies. Indeed, ROS accumulation has been found to be related to psoriasis, a chronic systemic inflammation. The excessive generation of ROS activates dendritic cells so as to display antigens to T cells, leading to an imbalance between T helper (Th)1 and Th2 cells. The equilibrium disruption triggers the growth of keratinocytes and encourages angiogenesis. Subsequently, various inflammatory pathways, such as mitogen-activated protein kinase (MAPK), nuclear factor-kappa B (NF-κB), or those related to Janus kinase-signal transducer and activator of transcription proteins (JAK-STAT), are also activated by ROS [13]. These findings suggest that ROS generation of activated neutrophils could be a potential target for the suppression of inflammation. Therefore, respiratory burst inhibitors have emerged as promising solutions for the treatment of inflammation.

Elastase enzyme is a critical component of extracellular traps which involves in microbicidal activity of neutrophils. Its function links to the digestion of invading microorganisms [114]. However, in case of overproduction, neutrophil elastase can promote prolonged inflammation, which may lead to worsening diseases. Numerous studies have discovered different mechanisms related to chronic lung diseases of extracellular neutrophil elastase, including inducing airway mucus obstruction, modifying cellular differentiation and cellular fate, activating pro-inflammatory signaling, and impairing the innate immune system. The supporting evidence for the crucial role of neutrophil elastase in the pathogenesis of chronic lung diseases related to sustained inflammation, such as bronchopulmonary dysplasia, bronchiectasis, chronic obstructive pulmonary disease, and cystic fibrosis lung disease, has driven more studies regarding antineutrophil elastase agents [115].

Based on a thorough literature investigation, octocorals have proven to be a prolific source of anti-inflammatory natural products that can selectively target neutrophil activities, in particular, superoxide anion generation and elastase release. Up to the present, seven isolates have been discovered to exhibit potent activities in in vitro experiments involving superoxide anion generation and elastase release assays. Half the identified compounds were steroid derivatives, followed by diterpenes, which were the most abundant secondary metabolites isolated from these marine organisms. Several other compounds belonging to sesquiterpenes, biscembrane, and other chemical classes were also demonstrated as potential agents in terms of anti-inflammation. More than 65 out of 97 octocoral derivatives exhibited potent anti-inflammatory properties with IC_{50} values less than 10 μM or equivalent inhibitory rates. More than 50% of the potent compounds were steroids, especially secosterols.

Currently, there has been no in vivo study conducted on marine-derived compounds for the investigation of their mechanisms of action on neutrophils. Nonetheless, the aforementioned potentials of respiratory burst and elastase inhibitors in the resolution of inflammation-related diseases have demonstrated opportunities for the development of these marine natural products as effective therapeutic agents that target neutrophilic inflammation in the future. As a result, detailed studies on the mechanisms of action need to be conducted to support the subsequent development of novel neutrophil-targeting anti-inflammatory agents. The structure–activity relationships also need to be systematically investigated so as to develop the most potent derivatives with the least side effects.

In summary, the discovery and development of lead compounds targeting neutrophilic inflammation is an intriguing aspect of natural product research in recent decades. Octocorals represent a vast reservoir of promising secondary metabolites with interesting biological activity, especially anti-inflammatory effects. More research is needed to fully utilize these new compounds as safe and effective treatments.

Author Contributions: Conceptualization, N.B.A.N., T.-L.H. and K.-H.L.; investigation, N.B.A.N., L.-Y.C., B.-R.P. and P.-J.C.; writing—original draft preparation, N.B.A.N. and K.-H.L.; writing—review and editing, M.E.-S., T.-L.H. and K.-H.L.; supervision, T.-L.H. and K.-H.L.; funding acquisition, T.-L.H. and K.-H.L. All authors have read and agreed to the published version of the manuscript.

Funding: The grants that supported this work were from the Chang Gung Memorial Hospital (CMRPF1M0101~2, CMRPF1M0131~2, CMRPF1N0021, and BMRP450), the Chang Gung University of Science and Technology (ZRRPF3N0101), the Ministry of Education (DP2-111-21121-01-N-01-03), the National Science and Technology Council (NSTC 111-2320-B-255-006-MY3, 111-2321-B-255-001, 112-2321-B-255-001, 112-2321-B-182-003, and 111-2320-B-038-040-MY3), and Taipei Medical University (TMU109-AE1-B15), Taiwan.

Institutional Review Board Statement: Not applicable.

Informed Consent Statement: Not applicable.

Conflicts of Interest: The authors declare no conflict of interest.

References

1. Chen, L.; Deng, H.; Cui, H.; Fang, J.; Zuo, Z.; Deng, J.; Li, Y.; Wang, X.; Zhao, L. Inflammatory responses and inflammation-associated diseases in organs. *Oncotarget* **2018**, *9*, 7204–7218. [CrossRef] [PubMed]
2. Arulselvan, P.; Fard, M.T.; Tan, W.S.; Gothai, S.; Fakurazi, S.; Norhaizan, M.E.; Kumar, S.S. Role of antioxidants and natural products in inflammation. *Oxid. Med. Cell. Longev.* **2016**, *2016*, 5276130. [CrossRef] [PubMed]

3. Serhan, C.N.; Ward, P.A.; Gilroy, D.W. *Fundamentals of Inflammation*; Cambridge University Press: Cambridge, UK, 2010.
4. Germolec, D.R.; Shipkowski, K.A.; Frawley, R.P.; Evans, E. Markers of inflammation. *Methods Mol. Biol.* **2018**, *1803*, 57–79. [PubMed]
5. Medzhitov, R. Origin and physiological roles of inflammation. *Nature* **2008**, *454*, 428–435. [CrossRef] [PubMed]
6. Soehnlein, O.; Steffens, S.; Hidalgo, A.; Weber, C. Neutrophils as protagonists and targets in chronic inflammation. *Nat. Rev. Immunol.* **2017**, *17*, 248–261. [CrossRef]
7. Cruz, N.G.; Sousa, L.P.; Sousa, M.O.; Pietrani, N.T.; Fernandes, A.P.; Gomes, K.B. The linkage between inflammation and type 2 diabetes mellitus. *Diabetes Res. Clin. Pract.* **2013**, *99*, 85–92. [CrossRef]
8. Esteve, E.; Ricart, W.; Fernandez-Real, J.M. Dyslipidemia and inflammation: An evolutionary conserved mechanism. *Clin. Nutr.* **2005**, *24*, 16–31. [CrossRef]
9. Silverstein, D.M. Inflammation in chronic kidney disease: Role in the progression of renal and cardiovascular disease. *Pediatr. Nephrol.* **2009**, *24*, 1445–1452. [CrossRef]
10. Sciarra, A.; Di Silverio, F.; Salciccia, S.; Autran Gomez, A.M.; Gentilucci, A.; Gentile, V. Inflammation and chronic prostatic diseases: Evidence for a link? *Eur. Urol.* **2007**, *52*, 964–972. [CrossRef]
11. Savoia, C.; Schiffrin, E.L. Inflammation in hypertension. *Curr. Opin. Nephrol. Hypertens.* **2006**, *15*, 152–158. [CrossRef]
12. Michels, N.; van Aart, C.; Morisse, J.; Mullee, A.; Huybrechts, I. Chronic inflammation towards cancer incidence: A systematic review and meta-analysis of epidemiological studies. *Crit. Rev. Oncol. Hematol.* **2021**, *157*, 103177. [CrossRef] [PubMed]
13. Chiang, C.C.; Cheng, W.J.; Korinek, M.; Lin, C.Y.; Hwang, T.L. Neutrophils in psoriasis. *Front. Immunol.* **2019**, *10*, 2376. [CrossRef] [PubMed]
14. Bartneck, M.; Wang, J. Therapeutic targeting of neutrophil granulocytes in inflammatory liver disease. *Front. Immunol.* **2019**, *10*, 2257. [CrossRef]
15. Rawat, K.; Shrivastava, A. Neutrophils as emerging protagonists and targets in chronic inflammatory diseases. *Inflamm. Res.* **2022**, *71*, 1477–1488. [CrossRef]
16. Delemarre, T.; Bachert, C. Neutrophilic inflammation in chronic rhinosinusitis. *Curr. Opin. Allergy Clin. Immunol.* **2023**, *23*, 14–21. [CrossRef] [PubMed]
17. Elaine Cruz, R.; Luana Barbosa, C.; Maria das Graças, H. *Neutrophils in Rheumatoid Arthritis: A Target for Discovering New Therapies Based on Natural Products*; IntechOpen: Rijeka, Croatia, 2017; Chapter 5.
18. Margraf, A.; Lowell, C.A.; Zarbock, A. Neutrophils in acute inflammation: Current concepts and translational implications. *Blood* **2022**, *139*, 2130–2144. [CrossRef] [PubMed]
19. Gierlikowska, B.; Stachura, A.; Gierlikowski, W.; Demkow, U. Phagocytosis, degranulation and extracellular traps release by neutrophils-the current knowledge, pharmacological modulation and future prospects. *Front. Pharmacol.* **2021**, *12*, 666732. [CrossRef]
20. Lehman, H.K.; Segal, B.H. The role of neutrophils in host defense and disease. *J. Allergy Clin. Immunol.* **2020**, *145*, 1535–1544. [CrossRef]
21. Naish, E.; Wood, A.J.; Stewart, A.P.; Routledge, M.; Morris, A.C.; Chilvers, E.R.; Lodge, K.M. The formation and function of the neutrophil phagosome. *Immunol. Rev.* **2023**, *314*, 158–180. [CrossRef]
22. Mittal, M.; Siddiqui, M.R.; Tran, K.; Reddy, S.P.; Malik, A.B. Reactive oxygen species in inflammation and tissue injury. *Antioxid. Redox Signal.* **2014**, *20*, 1126–1167. [CrossRef]
23. Zeng, M.Y.; Miralda, I.; Armstrong, C.L.; Uriarte, S.M.; Bagaitkar, J. The roles of NADPH oxidase in modulating neutrophil effector responses. *Mol. Oral Microbiol.* **2019**, *34*, 27–38. [CrossRef] [PubMed]
24. Hwang, T.L.; Su, Y.C.; Chang, H.L.; Leu, Y.L.; Chung, P.J.; Kuo, L.M.; Chang, Y.J. Suppression of superoxide anion and elastase release by C18 unsaturated fatty acids in human neutrophils. *J. Lipid Res.* **2009**, *50*, 1395–1408. [CrossRef]
25. Lucas, S.D.; Costa, E.; Guedes, R.C.; Moreira, R. Targeting COPD: Advances on low-molecular-weight inhibitors of human neutrophil elastase. *Med. Res. Rev.* **2013**, *33*, E73–E101. [CrossRef] [PubMed]
26. Gramegna, A.; Amati, F.; Terranova, L.; Sotgiu, G.; Tarsia, P.; Miglietta, D.; Calderazzo, M.A.; Aliberti, S.; Blasi, F. Neutrophil elastase in bronchiectasis. *Respir. Res.* **2017**, *18*, 1–13. [CrossRef] [PubMed]
27. Ho, A.S.; Chen, C.H.; Cheng, C.C.; Wang, C.C.; Lin, H.C.; Luo, T.Y.; Lien, G.S.; Chang, J. Neutrophil elastase as a diagnostic marker and therapeutic target in colorectal cancers. *Oncotarget* **2014**, *5*, 473–480. [CrossRef]
28. Jiang, K.L.; Ma, P.P.; Yang, X.Q.; Zhong, L.; Wang, H.; Zhu, X.Y.; Liu, B.Z. Neutrophil elastase and its therapeutic effect on leukemia cells. *Mol. Med. Rep.* **2015**, *12*, 4165–4172. [CrossRef]
29. Kelly, E.; Greene, C.M.; McElvaney, N.G. Targeting neutrophil elastase in cystic fibrosis. *Expert Opin. Ther. Targets* **2008**, *12*, 145–157. [CrossRef]
30. Taylor, S.; Dirir, O.; Zamanian, R.T.; Rabinovitch, M.; Thompson, A.A.R. The role of neutrophils and neutrophil elastase in pulmonary arterial hypertension. *Front. Med.* **2018**, *5*, 217. [CrossRef]
31. Chiang, C.C.; Korinek, M.; Cheng, W.J.; Hwang, T.L. Targeting neutrophils to treat acute respiratory distress syndrome in coronavirus disease. *Front. Pharmacol.* **2020**, *11*, 572009. [CrossRef]
32. Mushtaq, S.; Abbasi, B.H.; Uzair, B.; Abbasi, R. Natural products as reservoirs of novel therapeutic agents. *EXCLI J.* **2018**, *17*, 420–451.

33. Newman, D.J.; Cragg, G.M. Natural products as sources of new drugs from 1981 to 2014. *J. Nat. Prod.* **2016**, *79*, 629–661. [CrossRef] [PubMed]
34. Cragg, G.M.; Newman, D.J. Natural products: A continuing source of novel drug leads. *Biochim. Biophys. Acta* **2013**, *1830*, 3670–3695. [CrossRef]
35. Wu, Q.; Sun, J.; Chen, J.; Zhang, H.; Guo, Y.W.; Wang, H. Terpenoids from marine soft coral of the genus *Lemnalia*: Chemistry and biological activities. *Mar. Drugs* **2018**, *16*, 320. [CrossRef]
36. Yan, X.; Liu, J.; Leng, X.; Ouyang, H. Chemical diversity and biological activity of secondary metabolites from soft coral genus *Sinularia* since 2013. *Mar. Drugs* **2021**, *19*, 335. [CrossRef] [PubMed]
37. Elkhawas, Y.A.; Elissawy, A.M.; Elnaggar, M.S.; Mostafa, N.M.; Kamal, E.M.; Bishr, M.M.; Singab, A.N.B.; Salama, O.M. Chemical diversity in species belonging to soft coral genus *Sacrophyton* and its impact on biological activity: A review. *Mar. Drugs* **2020**, *18*, 41. [CrossRef]
38. Nguyen, N.B.A.; Chen, L.Y.; El-Shazly, M.; Peng, B.R.; Su, J.H.; Wu, H.C.; Lee, I.T.; Lai, K.H. Towards sustainable medicinal resources through marine soft coral aquaculture: Insights into the chemical diversity and the biological potential. *Mar. Drugs* **2022**, *20*, 640. [CrossRef] [PubMed]
39. Ermolenko, E.V.; Imbs, A.B.; Gloriozova, T.A.; Poroikov, V.V.; Sikorskaya, T.V.; Dembitsky, V.M. Chemical diversity of soft coral steroids and their pharmacological activities. *Mar. Drugs* **2020**, *18*, 613. [CrossRef]
40. Savic, M.P.; Sakac, M.N.; Kuzminac, I.Z.; Ajdukovic, J.J. Structural diversity of bioactive steroid compounds isolated from soft corals in the period 2015-2020. *J. Steroid Biochem. Mol. Biol.* **2022**, *218*, 106061. [CrossRef]
41. Zhang, Y.; Liu, J.; Shi, D.; Li, Z. Halogenated compounds from corals: Chemical diversity and biological activities. *Mini Rev. Med. Chem.* **2019**, *19*, 1204–1218. [CrossRef]
42. Liang, L.F.; Wang, X.J.; Zhang, H.Y.; Liu, H.L.; Li, J.; Lan, L.F.; Zhang, W.; Guo, Y.W. Bioactive polyhydroxylated steroids from the Hainan soft coral *Sinularia depressa* Tixier-Durivault. *Bioorg. Med. Chem. Lett.* **2013**, *23*, 1334–1337. [CrossRef]
43. Nagappan, T.; Palaniveloo, K. Biological properties and chemical diversity of *Sinularia flexibilis*, an Alcyonacean soft coral. *J. Sustain. Sci. Manag.* **2018**, *13*, 15–34.
44. Liang, L.-F.; Kurtán, T.; Mándi, A.; Yao, L.-G.; Li, J.; Lan, L.-F.; Guo, Y.-W. Structural, stereochemical, and bioactive studies of cembranoids from Chinese soft coral *Sarcophyton trocheliophorum*. *Tetrahedron* **2018**, *74*, 1933–1941. [CrossRef]
45. Ng, S.Y.; Phan, C.S.; Ishii, T.; Kamada, T.; Hamada, T.; Vairappan, C.S. Terpenoids from marine soft coral of the genus *Xenia* in 1977 to 2019. *Molecules* **2020**, *25*, 5386. [CrossRef]
46. Liang, L.F.; Guo, Y.W. Terpenes from the soft corals of the genus *Sarcophyton*: Chemistry and biological activities. *Chem. Biodivers.* **2013**, *10*, 2161–2196. [CrossRef] [PubMed]
47. Nurrachma, M.Y.; Sakaraga, D.; Nugraha, A.Y.; Rahmawati, S.I.; Bayu, A.; Sukmarini, L.; Atikana, A.; Prasetyoputri, A.; Izzati, F.; Warsito, M.F.; et al. Cembranoids of soft corals: Recent updates and their biological activities. *Nat. Prod. Bioprospect.* **2021**, *11*, 243–306. [CrossRef]
48. Putra, M.Y.; Murniasih, T. Marine soft corals as source of lead compounds for anti-inflammatories. *J. Coast. Life Med.* **2016**, *4*, 73–77. [CrossRef]
49. Abdel-Lateff, A.; Alarif, W.M.; Alburae, N.A.; Algandaby, M.M. Alcyonium octocorals: Potential source of diverse bioactive terpenoids. *Molecules* **2019**, *24*, 1370. [CrossRef]
50. Abdelhafez, O.H.; Fahim, J.R.; Desoukey, S.Y.; Kamel, M.S.; Abdelmohsen, U.R. Recent updates on corals from Nephtheidae. *Chem. Biodivers.* **2019**, *16*, e1800692. [CrossRef]
51. Allam, K.M.; Khedr, A.I.; Allam, A.E.; Abdelkader, M.S.A.; Elkhayat, E.S.; Fouad, M.A. Chemical and biological diversity in Nephthea soft corals in the current decade: A review. *J. Adv. Biomed. Pharm. Sci.* **2021**, *4*, 124–133. [CrossRef]
52. Kasimala, M.; Babu, B.H.; Awet, B.; Henok, G.; Haile, A.; Hisham, O. A review on bioactive secondary metabolites of soft corals (Octocorallia) and their distribution in Eritrean coast of Red Sea. *Indian J. Geo-Mar. Sci.* **2020**, *49*, 1793–1800.
53. Available online: https://www.ncbi.nlm.nih.gov/Taxonomy/Browser/wwwtax.cgi?id=6132&lvl=0 (accessed on 29 March 2023)
54. Pérez, C.D.; de Moura Neves, B.; Cordeiro, R.T.; Williams, G.C.; Cairns, S.D. Diversity and distribution of Octocorallia. In *The Cnidaria, Past, Present and Future: The World of Medusa and Her Sisters*; Springer: Berlin/Heidelberg, Germany, 2016; pp. 109–123
55. Sarma, N.S.; Krishna, M.S.; Pasha, S.G.; Rao, T.S.; Venkateswarlu, Y.; Parameswaran, P.S. Marine metabolites: The sterols of soft coral. *Chem. Rev.* **2009**, *109*, 2803–2828. [CrossRef] [PubMed]
56. Coll, J.C. The chemistry and chemical ecology of octocorals (Coelenterata, Anthozoa, Octocorallia). *Chem. Rev.* **1992**, *92*, 613–631. [CrossRef]
57. Han, M.; Wang, Z.; Li, Y.; Song, Y.; Wang, Z. The Application of Coral in Traditional Medicine and Its Chemical Composition Pharmacology, Toxicology, and Clinical Research. *Authorea* **2023**. [CrossRef]
58. Rodrigues, I.G.; Miguel, M.G.; Mnif, W. A brief review on new naturally occurring cembranoid diterpene derivatives from the soft corals of the genera *Sarcophyton, Sinularia,* and *Lobophytum* since 2016. *Molecules* **2019**, *24*, 781. [CrossRef]
59. Wu, C.H.; Chao, C.H.; Huang, T.Z.; Huang, C.Y.; Hwang, T.L.; Dai, C.F.; Sheu, J.H. Cembranoid-related metabolites and biological activities from the soft coral *Sinularia flexibilis*. *Mar. Drugs* **2018**, *16*, 278. [CrossRef]
60. Su, Y.D.; Su, J.H.; Hwang, T.L.; Wen, Z.H.; Sheu, J.H.; Wu, Y.C.; Sung, P.J. Briarane Diterpenoids Isolated from Octocorals between 2014 and 2016. *Mar Drugs* **2017**, *15*, 44. [CrossRef]

61. Abdelkarem, F.M.; Abouelela, M.E.; Kamel, M.R.; Nafady, A.M.; Allam, A.E.; Abdel-Rahman, I.A.M.; Almatroudi, A.; Alrumaihi, F.; Allemailem, K.S.; Assaf, H.K. Chemical review of gorgostane-type steroids isolated from marine organisms and their ^{13}C-NMR spectroscopic data characteristics. *Mar. Drugs* **2022**, *20*, 139. [CrossRef]
62. Chen, L.W.; Chung, H.L.; Wang, C.C.; Su, J.H.; Chen, Y.J.; Lee, C.J. Anti-Acne Effects of Cembrene Diterpenoids from the Cultured Soft Coral Sinularia flexibilis. *Mar Drugs* **2020**, *18*, 487. [CrossRef]
63. Leal, M.C.; Sheridan, C.; Osinga, R.; Dionisio, G.; Rocha, R.J.; Silva, B.; Rosa, R.; Calado, R. Marine microorganism-invertebrate assemblages: Perspectives to solve the "supply problem" in the initial steps of drug discovery. *Mar Drugs* **2014**, *12*, 3929–3952. [CrossRef]
64. Sharma, A.; Bajpai, V.K.; Shukla, S. *Sesquiterpenes and Cytotoxicity*; Springer: Berlin/Heidelberg, Germany, 2013; pp. 3515–3550.
65. Chung, H.-M.; Su, J.-H.; Hwang, T.-L.; Li, J.-J.; Chen, J.-J.; Chen, Y.-H.; Chang, Y.-C.; Su, Y.-D.; Chen, Y.-H.; Fang, L.-S. Rumphellclovanes C–E, new clovane-type sesquiterpenoids from the gorgonian coral *Rumphella antipathies*. *Tetrahedron* **2013**, *69*, 2740–2744. [CrossRef]
66. Chang, Y.C.; Chiang, C.C.; Chang, Y.S.; Chen, J.J.; Wang, W.H.; Fang, L.S.; Chung, H.M.; Hwang, T.L.; Sung, P.J. Novel Caryophyllane-Related Sesquiterpenoids with Anti-Inflammatory Activity from Rumphella antipathes (Linnaeus, 1758). *Mar. Drugs* **2020**, *18*, 554. [CrossRef] [PubMed]
67. Lanzotti, V. *Diterpenes for Therapeutic Use*; Springer: Berlin/Heidelberg, Germany, 2013; pp. 3173–3191.
68. Sung, P.-J.; Pai, C.-H.; Su, Y.-D.; Hwang, T.-L.; Kuo, F.-W.; Fan, T.-Y.; Li, J.-J. New 8-hydroxybriarane diterpenoids from the gorgonians Junceella juncea and Junceella fragilis (Ellisellidae). *Tetrahedron* **2008**, *64*, 4224–4232. [CrossRef]
69. Hong, P.H.; Su, Y.D.; Su, J.H.; Chen, Y.H.; Hwang, T.L.; Weng, C.F.; Lee, C.H.; Wen, Z.H.; Sheu, J.H.; Lin, N.C.; et al. Briarenolides F and G, new briarane diterpenoids from a *Briareum* sp. octocoral. *Mar. Drugs* **2012**, *10*, 1156–1168. [CrossRef] [PubMed]
70. Su, Y.-D.; Cheng, C.-H.; Chen, W.-F.; Chang, Y.-C.; Chen, Y.-H.; Hwang, T.-L.; Wen, Z.-H.; Wang, W.-H.; Fang, L.-S.; Chen, J.-J. Briarenolide J, the first 12-chlorobriarane diterpenoid from an octocoral *Briareum* sp.(Briareidae). *Tetrahedron Lett.* **2014**, *55*, 6065–6067. [CrossRef]
71. Chen, N.F.; Su, Y.D.; Hwang, T.L.; Liao, Z.J.; Tsui, K.H.; Wen, Z.H.; Wu, Y.C.; Sung, P.J. Briarenols C–E, new polyoxygenated briaranes from the octocoral *Briareum excavatum*. *Molecules* **2017**, *22*, 475. [CrossRef] [PubMed]
72. Lin, C.C.; Su, J.H.; Chen, W.F.; Wen, Z.H.; Peng, B.R.; Huang, L.C.; Hwang, T.L.; Sung, P.J. New 11,20-epoxybriaranes from the Gorgonian coral *Junceella fragilis* (Ellisellidae). *Molecules* **2019**, *24*, 2487. [CrossRef] [PubMed]
73. Kao, C.Y.; Su, J.H.; Lu, M.C.; Hwang, T.L.; Wang, W.H.; Chen, J.J.; Sheu, J.H.; Kuo, Y.H.; Weng, C.F.; Fang, L.S.; et al. Lobocrassins A–E: New cembrane-type diterpenoids from the soft coral Lobophytum crassum. *Mar. Drugs* **2011**, *9*, 1319–1331. [CrossRef]
74. Wang, L.H.; Chen, K.H.; Dai, C.F.; Hwang, T.L.; Wang, W.H.; Wu, Y.C.; Sung, P.J. New cembranoids from the soft coral *Sinularia arborea*. *Nat. Prod. Commun.* **2014**, *9*, 361–362. [CrossRef]
75. Lin, K.H.; Tseng, Y.J.; Chen, B.W.; Hwang, T.L.; Chen, H.Y.; Dai, C.F.; Sheu, J.H. Tortuosenes A and B, new diterpenoid metabolites from the Formosan soft coral *Sarcophyton tortuosum*. *Org. Lett.* **2014**, *16*, 1314–1317. [CrossRef]
76. Huang, C.Y.; Sung, P.J.; Uvarani, C.; Su, J.H.; Lu, M.C.; Hwang, T.L.; Dai, C.F.; Wu, S.L.; Sheu, J.H. Glaucumolides A and B, biscembranoids with new structural type from a cultured soft coral *Sarcophyton glaucum*. *Sci. Rep.* **2015**, *5*, 15624. [CrossRef]
77. Huang, C.Y.; Tseng, Y.J.; Chokkalingam, U.; Hwang, T.L.; Hsu, C.H.; Dai, C.F.; Sung, P.J.; Sheu, J.H. Bioactive isoprenoid-derived natural products from a Dongsha atoll soft coral *Sinularia erecta*. *J. Nat. Prod.* **2016**, *79*, 1339–1346. [CrossRef] [PubMed]
78. Tseng, W.R.; Ahmed, A.F.; Huang, C.Y.; Tsai, Y.Y.; Tai, C.J.; Orfali, R.S.; Hwang, T.L.; Wang, Y.H.; Dai, C.F.; Sheu, J.H. Bioactive capnosanes and cembranes from the soft coral *Klyxum flaccidum*. *Mar. Drugs* **2019**, *17*, 461. [CrossRef] [PubMed]
79. Nguyen, N.B.A.; Chen, L.Y.; Chen, P.J.; El-Shazly, M.; Hwang, T.L.; Su, J.H.; Su, C.H.; Yen, P.T.; Peng, B.R.; Lai, K.H. MS/MS molecular networking unveils the chemical diversity of biscembranoid derivatives, neutrophilic inflammatory mediators from the cultured soft coral *Sarcophyton trocheliophorum*. *Int. J. Mol. Sci.* **2022**, *23*, 15464. [CrossRef] [PubMed]
80. Chen, Y.H.; Tai, C.Y.; Hwang, T.L.; Weng, C.F.; Li, J.J.; Fang, L.S.; Wang, W.H.; Wu, Y.C.; Sung, P.J. Cladielloides A and B: New eunicellin-type diterpenoids from an Indonesian octocoral *Cladiella* sp. *Mar. Drugs* **2010**, *8*, 2936–2945. [CrossRef] [PubMed]
81. Lin, M.C.; Chen, B.W.; Huang, C.Y.; Dai, C.F.; Hwang, T.L.; Sheu, J.H. Eunicellin-based diterpenoids from the Formosan soft coral *Klyxum molle* with inhibitory activity on superoxide generation and elastase release by neutrophils. *J. Nat. Prod.* **2013**, *76*, 1661–1667. [CrossRef]
82. Lee, Y.N.; Tai, C.J.; Hwang, T.L.; Sheu, J.H. Krempfielins J-M, new eunicellin-based diterpenoids from the soft coral *Cladiella krempfi*. *Mar. Drugs* **2013**, *11*, 2741–2750. [CrossRef]
83. Lee, Y.N.; Tai, C.J.; Hwang, T.L.; Sheu, J.H. Krempfielins N-P, new anti-inflammatory eunicellins from a Taiwanese soft coral *Cladiella krempfi*. *Mar. Drugs* **2014**, *12*, 1148–1156. [CrossRef]
84. Chen, Y.-F.; Chen, W.-F.; Wen, Z.-H.; Hwang, T.-L.; Zhang, Z.-J.; Sung, P.-J. New bioactive Δ11 (17)-furanoeunicellins from an octocoral *Cladiella* sp. *Phytochem. Lett.* **2019**, *33*, 31–35. [CrossRef]
85. Zhang, Z.-J.; Wang, Y.-H.; Chen, S.-R.; Peng, B.-R.; Yang, S.-N.; Hu, C.-C.; Fang, L.-S.; Hwang, T.-L.; Sung, P.-J. Novel secoeunicellins produced by an octocoral *Cladiella* sp. *Tetrahedron Lett.* **2019**, *60*, 151300. [CrossRef]
86. Betschart, L.; Altmann, K.H. Xenicane natural products: Biological activity and total synthesis. *Curr. Pharm. Des.* **2015**, *21*, 5467–5488. [CrossRef]
87. Hooper, G.J.; Davies-Coleman, M.T. New metabolites from the South African soft coral *Capnella thyrsoidea*. *Tetrahedron* **1995**, *51*, 9973–9984. [CrossRef]

88. Lin, Y.C.; Abd El-Razek, M.H.; Hwang, T.L.; Chiang, M.Y.; Kuo, Y.H.; Dai, C.F.; Shen, Y.C. Asterolaurins A–F, xenicane diterpenoids from the Taiwanese soft coral *Asterospicularia laurae*. *J. Nat. Prod.* **2009**, *72*, 1911–1916. [CrossRef] [PubMed]
89. Chung, H.M.; Hu, L.C.; Yen, W.H.; Su, J.H.; Lu, M.C.; Hwang, T.L.; Wang, W.H.; Sung, P.J. Echinohalimane A, a bioactive halimane-type diterpenoid from a Formosan gorgonian *Echinomuricea* sp. (Plexauridae). *Mar. Drugs* **2012**, *10*, 2246–2253. [CrossRef] [PubMed]
90. Chang, J.Y.; Fazary, A.E.; Lin, Y.C.; Hwang, T.L.; Shen, Y.C. New verticillane diterpenoids from *Cespitularia taeniata*. *Chem. Biodivers.* **2012**, *9*, 654–661. [CrossRef] [PubMed]
91. Chang, C.H.; Ahmed, A.F.; Yang, T.S.; Lin, Y.C.; Huang, C.Y.; Hwang, T.L.; Sheu, J.H. Isolation of lobane and prenyleudesmane diterpenoids from the soft coral *Lobophytum varium*. *Mar. Drugs* **2020**, *18*, 223. [CrossRef] [PubMed]
92. Sultan, A.; Raza, A.R. Steroids: A diverse class of secondary metabolites. *Med. Chem.* **2015**, *5*, 310–317. [CrossRef]
93. Tseng, W.R.; Huang, C.Y.; Tsai, Y.Y.; Lin, Y.S.; Hwang, T.L.; Su, J.H.; Sung, P.J.; Dai, C.F.; Sheu, J.H. New cytotoxic and anti-inflammatory steroids from the soft coral *Klyxum flaccidum*. *Bioorg. Med. Chem. Lett.* **2016**, *26*, 3253–3257. [CrossRef]
94. Tsai, Y.Y.; Huang, C.Y.; Tseng, W.R.; Chiang, P.L.; Hwang, T.L.; Su, J.H.; Sung, P.J.; Dai, C.F.; Sheu, J.H. Klyflaccisteroids K–M, bioactive steroidal derivatives from a soft coral *Klyxum flaccidum*. *Bioorg. Med. Chem. Lett.* **2017**, *27*, 1220–1224. [CrossRef]
95. Whuang, T.Y.; Tsai, H.C.; Su, Y.D.; Hwang, T.L.; Sung, P.J. Sterols from the octocoral *Nephthea columnaris*. *Mar. Drugs* **2017**, *15*, 212. [CrossRef]
96. Huang, C.Y.; Tseng, W.R.; Ahmed, A.F.; Chiang, P.L.; Tai, C.J.; Hwang, T.L.; Dai, C.F.; Sheu, J.H. Anti-inflammatory polyoxygenated steroids from the soft coral *Lobophytum michaelae*. *Mar. Drugs* **2018**, *16*, 93. [CrossRef]
97. Sica, D.; Musumeci, D. Secosteroids of marine origin. *Steroids* **2004**, *69*, 743–756. [CrossRef]
98. Chao, C.-H.; Huang, T.-Z.; Wu, C.-Y.; Chen, B.-W.; Huang, C.-Y.; Hwang, T.-L.; Dai, C.-F.; Sheu, J.-H. Steroidal and α-tocopherylhydroquinone glycosides from two soft corals *Cladiella hirsuta* and *Sinularia nanolobata*. *RSC Adv.* **2015**, *5*, 74256–74262. [CrossRef]
99. Chang, Y.-C.; Kuo, L.-M.; Su, J.-H.; Hwang, T.-L.; Kuo, Y.-H.; Lin, C.-S.; Wu, Y.-C.; Sheu, J.-H.; Sung, P.-J. Pinnigorgiols A–C, 9,11-secosterols with a rare ring arrangement from a gorgonian coral *Pinnigorgia* sp. *Tetrahedron* **2016**, *72*, 999–1004. [CrossRef]
100. Chang, Y.-C.; Hwang, T.-L.; Sheu, J.-H.; Wu, Y.-C.; Sung, P.-J. New anti-inflammatory 9,11-secosterols with a rare tricyclo [5,2,1,1] decane ring from a Formosan gorgonian *Pinnigorgia* sp. *Mar. Drugs* **2016**, *14*, 218. [CrossRef] [PubMed]
101. Chang, Y.C.; Kuo, L.M.; Hwang, T.L.; Yeh, J.; Wen, Z.H.; Fang, L.S.; Wu, Y.C.; Lin, C.S.; Sheu, J.H.; Sung, P.J. Pinnisterols A–C, new 9,11-secosterols from a gorgonian *Pinnigorgia* sp. *Mar. Drugs* **2016**, *14*, 12. [CrossRef]
102. Chang, Y.C.; Hwang, T.L.; Kuo, L.M.; Sung, P.J. Pinnisterols D–J, new 11-acetoxy-9,11-secosterols with a 1,4-quinone moiety from Formosan gorgonian coral *Pinnigorgia* sp. (Gorgoniidae). *Mar. Drugs* **2017**, *15*, 11. [CrossRef] [PubMed]
103. Chang, Y.C.; Hwang, T.L.; Chao, C.H.; Sung, P.J. New marine sterols from a gorgonian *Pinnigorgia* sp. *Molecules* **2017**, *22*, 393. [CrossRef]
104. Chang, Y.C.; Lai, K.H.; Kumar, S.; Chen, P.J.; Wu, Y.H.; Lai, C.L.; Hsieh, H.L.; Sung, P.J.; Hwang, T.L. ^{1}H NMR-based isolation of anti-inflammatory 9,11-secosteroids from the octocoral *Sinularia leptoclados*. *Mar. Drugs* **2020**, *18*, 271. [CrossRef] [PubMed]
105. Tsai, C.-R.; Huang, C.-Y.; Chen, B.-W.; Tsai, Y.-Y.; Shih, S.-P.; Hwang, T.-L.; Dai, C.-F.; Wang, S.-Y.; Sheu, J.-H. New bioactive steroids from the soft coral *Klyxum flaccidum*. *RSC Adv.* **2015**, *5*, 12546–12554. [CrossRef]
106. Huang, C.-H.; Ahmed, A.F.; Su, J.H.; Sung, P.J.; Hwang, T.L.; Chiang, P.L.; Dai, C.F.; Liaw, C.C.; Sheu, J.H. Bioactive new withanolides from the cultured soft coral *Sinularia brassica*. *Bioorg. Med. Chem. Lett.* **2017**, *27*, 3267–3271. [CrossRef]
107. Liu, C.Y.; Hwang, T.L.; Lin, M.R.; Chen, Y.H.; Chang, Y.C.; Fang, L.S.; Wang, W.H.; Wu, Y.C.; Sung, P.J. Carijoside A, a bioactive sterol glycoside from an octocoral *Carijoa* sp. (Clavulariidae). *Mar. Drugs* **2010**, *8*, 2014–2020. [CrossRef]
108. Huang, C.Y.; Su, J.H.; Liaw, C.C.; Sung, P.J.; Chiang, P.L.; Hwang, T.L.; Dai, C.F.; Sheu, J.H. Bioactive steroids with methyl ester group in the side chain from a reef soft coral *Sinularia brassica* cultured in a tank. *Mar. Drugs* **2017**, *15*, 280. [CrossRef]
109. Chung, H.M.; Hong, P.H.; Su, J.H.; Hwang, T.L.; Lu, M.C.; Fang, L.S.; Wu, Y.C.; Li, J.J.; Chen, J.J.; Wang, W.H.; et al. Bioactive compounds from a gorgonian coral *Echinomuricea* sp. (Plexauridae). *Mar. Drugs* **2012**, *10*, 1169–1179. [CrossRef]
110. Huang, C.Y.; Chang, C.W.; Tseng, Y.J.; Lee, J.; Sung, P.J.; Hwang, T.L.; Dai, C.F.; Wang, H.C.; Sheu, J.H. Bioactive steroids from the Formosan Soft coral *Umbellulifera petasites*. *Mar. Drugs* **2016**, *14*, 180. [CrossRef]
111. Chen, K.-H.; Dai, C.-F.; Hwang, T.-L.; Sung, P.-J. 5-(6-Hydroxy-2, 5, 7, 8-tetramethylchroman-2-yl)-2-methyl-pentanoic acid methyl ester. *Molbank* **2014**, *2014*, M822. [CrossRef]
112. Chen, B.W.; Uvarani, C.; Huang, C.Y.; Hwang, T.L.; Dai, C.F.; Sheu, J.H. New anti-inflammatory tocopherol-derived metabolites from the Taiwanese soft coral *Cladiella hirsuta*. *Bioorg. Med. Chem. Lett.* **2015**, *25*, 92–95. [CrossRef]
113. Chang, H.H.; Chang, Y.C.; Chen, W.F.; Hwang, T.L.; Fang, L.S.; Wen, Z.H.; Chen, Y.H.; Wu, Y.C.; Sung, P.J. Pubinernoid A and apo-9′-fucoxanthinone, secondary metabolites from a gorgonian coral *Pinnigorgia* sp. *Nat. Prod. Commun.* **2016**, *11*, 707–708. [CrossRef]

114. Zeng, W.; Song, Y.; Wang, R.; He, R.; Wang, T. Neutrophil elastase: From mechanisms to therapeutic potential. *J. Pharm. Anal.* **2023**, *13*, 355–366. [CrossRef]
115. Voynow, J.A.; Shinbashi, M. Neutrophil Elastase and Chronic Lung Disease. *Biomolecules* **2021**, *11*, 1065. [CrossRef]

Disclaimer/Publisher's Note: The statements, opinions and data contained in all publications are solely those of the individual author(s) and contributor(s) and not of MDPI and/or the editor(s). MDPI and/or the editor(s) disclaim responsibility for any injury to people or property resulting from any ideas, methods, instructions or products referred to in the content.

MDPI AG
Grosspeteranlage 5
4052 Basel
Switzerland
Tel.: +41 61 683 77 34

Marine Drugs Editorial Office
E-mail: marinedrugs@mdpi.com
www.mdpi.com/journal/marinedrugs

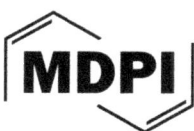

Disclaimer/Publisher's Note: The statements, opinions and data contained in all publications are solely those of the individual author(s) and contributor(s) and not of MDPI and/or the editor(s). MDPI and/or the editor(s) disclaim responsibility for any injury to people or property resulting from any ideas, methods, instructions or products referred to in the content.

www.ingramcontent.com/pod-product-compliance
Lightning Source LLC
LaVergne TN
LVHW070501100526
838202LV00014B/1768